FRCS General Surgery Section 2

Comprehensive vivas

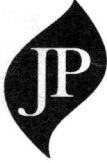

FRCS General Surgery Section 2

Comprehensive vivas

Editors

Sri Ganeshamurthy Thrumurthy MBChB(Hons) MBA LLM FRCS(Gen Surg) FRCP(London) FHEA FAcadMEd
Consultant Surgeon
King's College Hospital and
King Edward VII's Hospital
Honorary Senior Lecturer
King's College London
London, UK

Sacheen Kumar PhD MRSC(Chem) FRCS(Gen Surg)
Consultant Upper GI Surgeon, Royal Marsden Hospital, London
Consultant Upper GI Surgeon
DDSI Institute Cleveland Clinic London Hospital
Upper GI Surgical Oncology Research Group
Institute of Cancer Research, UK

Arnab K Bhowmick MBChB FRCSEd(Gen Surg)
Consultant Colorectal Surgeon, Lancashire
Teaching Hospitals NHS Trust
Preston, UK

Mohamed Baguneid MD MBChB FRCS MBA
Consultant Vascular Surgeon
Sheikh Shakhbout Medical City, Abu Dhabi
Honorary Senior Lecturer
University of Manchester, UK
Adjunct Professor, UAE University
Adjunct Clinical Professor
Khalifa University, UAE

Muntzer Mughal MBChB FRCS ChM
Head of Foregut Surgery and Director of
Clinical Oncology
Cleveland Clinic London Hospital, UK

Muhammad Rafay Sameem Siddiqui
MBChB FRCS PhD DIC PGCert(Clin Ed)
MFSTEd AFFMLM
Consultant General & Colorectal Surgeon South Tyneside & Sunderland NHS Trust
Director of the Clinical Academic Training Office
Honorary Clinical Lecturer
University of Sunderland, UK

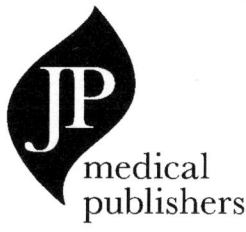

JP medical publishers

London • New Delhi

© 2025 JP Medical Ltd.
Published by JP Medical Ltd, 83 Victoria Street, London, SW1H 0HW, UK
Tel: +44 (0)20 3170 8910   Fax: +44 (0)20 3008 6180
Email: info@jpmedpub.com   Web: www.jpmedpub.com

The rights of Sri Ganeshamurthy Thrumurthy, Sacheen Kumar, Arnab K Bhowmick, Mohamed Baguneid, Muntzer Mughal, and Muhammad Rafay Sameem Siddiqui to be identified as the editors of this work have been asserted by them in accordance with the Copyright, Designs and Patents Act 1988.

All brand names and product names used in this book are trade names, service marks, trademarks or registered trademarks of their respective owners. The publisher is not associated with any product or vendor mentioned in this book.

Medical knowledge and practice change constantly. This book is designed to provide accurate, authoritative information about the subject matter in question. However readers are advised to check the most current information available on procedures included and check information from the manufacturer of each product to be administered, to verify the recommended dose, formula, method and duration of administration, adverse effects and contraindications. It is the responsibility of the practitioner to take all appropriate safety precautions. Neither the publisher nor the editors assume any liability for any injury and/or damage to persons or property arising from or related to use of material in this book.

This book is sold on the understanding that the publisher is not engaged in providing professional medical services. If such advice or services are required, the services of a competent medical professional should be sought. Every effort has been made where necessary to contact holders of copyright to obtain permission to reproduce copyright material. If any have been inadvertently overlooked, the publisher will be pleased to make the necessary arrangements at the first opportunity.

ISBN: 978-1-78779-185-5

British Library Cataloguing in Publication Data
A catalogue record for this book is available from the British Library

Library of Congress Cataloging in Publication Data
A catalog record for this book is available from the Library of Congress

Publishing Manager:	Nikita Chauhan
Editorial Assistant:	Keshav Kumar Baghel
Cover Design:	Seema Dogra

Typeset, printed and bound in India.

Foreword

It is with great pleasure that I introduce this book, written to support surgical trainees in their preparation for the Section 2 of the Intercollegiate Examination in General Surgery. As one of the editors, I have been involved in the evolution and refinement of the content within these pages, drawing from two decades of experience and success of the Alpine FRCS preparation course, which I co-founded with co-editors, Professor Mohamed Baguneid and Mr Arnab K Bhowmick.

This book is the culmination of 20 years of creating scenarios and writing questions for the Alpine course. The scenarios are based on the FRCS curriculum, including Emergency Surgery, General Surgery, Breast, Colorectal, Endocrine, Transplant, Hepatopancreatobiliary (HPB), Oesophagogastric (OG), and Vascular. The scenarios have been rigorously tested and fine-tuned by their use in the Alpine Course. There are also valuable chapters on the structure and marking of the Section 2 examination as well as the Academic Foundation, which can be daunting for those not used to critiquing papers.

The dedication and expertise of the editors and their collaborators have created a resource of such high quality. The success of the Alpine FRCS preparation course can be attributed to the quality and standard of the questions and conduct of the vivas, replicating the Section 2 examination.

This book aims to replicate that experience for those unable to attend a viva course, by asking senior colleagues or peers in a revision group in a viva setting. Excelling in the viva is not simply a matter of having the required knowledge, but the ability to articulate it clearly. By offering clear, structured answers, grounded in knowledge, evidence, and clinical experience, this book will equip trainees to achieve the highest marks possible.

I am delighted to highlight that all profits from the sale of this book are being donated to Cancer Research UK, the world's largest independent cancer research charity, and the single biggest charitable funder of research at The Institute of Cancer Research, UK.

I congratulate all the contributors for producing what I believe is a fantastic resource. I am confident that those preparing for the Section 2 examination will find this book invaluable in preparing for and passing the Section 2 examination in General Surgery.

Professor Muntzer Mughal MBChB FRCS ChM
Head of Foregut Surgery and Director of Clinical Oncology
Cleveland Clinic London Hospital, UK

Preface

In the rapidly evolving field of surgical education, it is crucial that learning resources evolve alongside clinical practice. This book aims to meet that need by offering a comprehensive and practical guide for senior surgical trainees and practising surgeons undertaking Part 2 of the Fellowship of the Royal College of Surgeons (FRCS) General Surgery examination.

The Editors of this book have accrued significant real-world experience in surgical education, from editing mainstream surgical textbooks to delivering acclaimed postgraduate surgical revision courses, such as those for the intercollegiate Membership of the Royal College of Surgeons (MRCS) and FRCS examinations. This collective experience has been incorporated to aid countless cohorts of surgical candidates in passing the examination.

This book stands out for its case-based approach, aligning real-world clinical scenarios with the FRCS General Surgery curriculum. Each chapter is designed not only to provide information, but also to promote critical thinking and effective decision-making. Our goal is to immerse readers in the complexities of patient care, enhancing their ability to apply theoretical knowledge in practical settings within the examination-based environment.

The creation of this textbook was a collaborative effort, with contributions from a diverse group of experts across various surgical and medical specialties. These contributors have brought a wealth of experience and insights, ensuring that the content is both current and relevant to today's medical practice.

Surgical textbooks are typically organised around disease processes and organ systems, often presenting facts in a manner that can be perceived as dry. In contrast, our human minds are hard-wired to respond to stories. This book reorganises the information base for 'General Surgery' around case-based discussions, placing facts within compelling narratives. This approach engages readers, maintaining their interest and encouraging continuous reading.

While the book is targeted at trainees sitting the FRCS General Surgery exit examination in the UK, it will be invaluable for 'General Surgery' trainees in similar training systems globally, including those in Australia and New Zealand. The selected cases comprehensively address clinical scenarios frequently encountered in practice and viva examinations, delivering clinical perspectives and context often hard to glean from conventional textbooks.

On another note, this is not just a book for trainees. Trainers will benefit from the case-based discussions, and established surgeons seeking to refresh their knowledge will find the content equally engaging and practical. The discussions offer opportunities to revisit less frequently encountered areas and provide practical approaches to case management.

The editors emphasise that this book is no substitute for face-to-face viva practice but serves as a key companion throughout the preparation process. It aims to help readers to succeed at the final hurdle before completing their training.

Recognising the rapid advancements in medical science and the growing body of evidence-based practice, we have included the most up-to-date information available. We understand that ongoing learning and adaptation are essential components of any surgeon's career.

We extend our heartfelt thanks to all of our contributors who, despite their busy clinical schedules and family commitments, painstakingly provided the rich background and structure from which these numerous vivas have been derived. Their dedication and expertise have been invaluable. We hope that this book aids in examination preparation towards success in the FRCS General Surgery exit examination and inspires a deeper appreciation for the art and science of surgery. As always, we welcome feedback and suggestions to help to improve future editions.

Yours sincerely,
Sri Ganeshamurthy Thrumurthy
Sacheen Kumar
Arnab K Bhowmick
Mohamed Baguneid
Muntzer Mughal
Muhammad Rafay Sameem Siddiqui

Contents

Foreword	v
Preface	vii
The Editors	xi
Contributors	xv
Acknowledgements	xviii
Abbreviations and acronyms	xx
Introduction	xxix

Chapter 1	**Academic viva**	1
	En Lin Goh, Sri Ganeshamurthy Thrumurthy, Jonathan Moore	
Chapter 2	**Critical care**	23
	Ed Denison-Davies, Irfan Chaudry, Robin Som, Faddy Kamel	
Chapter 3	**Emergency surgery**	129
	Paul Barrow, Ilayaraja Rajendran, Chris Macklin, Finlay Curran, David Monk, Rachael Clifford, Faddy Kamel	
Chapter 4	**General surgery**	243
	Paul Wilson, Robin Som	
Chapter 5	**Breast surgery**	325
	Tracey Irvine, Pooja Padmanabhan, Rachita Mallya, Shramana Banerjee, Carol Norman	
Chapter 6	**Colorectal surgery**	385
	Nick Lees, Adam Rees, Muhammad Rafay Sameem Siddiqui, Faddy Kamel, Tim James Royle, Kapil Sahnan, Rachael Coates	
Chapter 7	**Endocrine surgery**	457
	Helen Elizabeth Doran, Ravi Acharya	
Chapter 8	**Transplant surgery**	493
	David van Dellen, Murali Somasundaram, Manikandan Kathirvel	
Chapter 9	**Hepatopancreatobiliary surgery**	549
	Aali J Sheen, Saurabh Jamdar, Ajith K Siriwardena	

Chapter 10 **Oesophagogastric surgery** 593
Pranav H Patel, Nima Abbassi-Ghadi, Sacheen Kumar

Chapter 11 **Vascular surgery** 657
Abdullah Jibawi, Mohamed Baguneid

Index 681

The Editors

Sri Ganeshamurthy Thrumurthy MBChB(Hons) MBA LLM FRCS(Gen Surg) FRCP(London) FHEA FAcadMEd, is a Consultant Surgeon and Interventional Endoscopist at King's College Hospital and King Edward VII's Hospital, London. Mr Thrumurthy graduated with Honours from the University of Manchester, obtained Membership of the Royal College of Surgeons (MRCS) as a House Officer, and subsequently Membership of the Royal of Physicians (MRCP) as a Senior House Officer. He completed his higher surgical training across South London, and was made a Fellow of the Royal College of Surgeons in England (FRCS). Mr Thrumurthy successfully completed an Advanced Endosurgery Fellowship under Mr Amyn Haji and Professor Bu Hayee at the King's Institute of Therapeutic Endoscopy (King's College Hospital, London), before being appointed as a Consultant Surgeon in the same department. He has a keen interest in medical education and training, and is the editor of a number of medical and surgical textbooks, including the Oxford Handbook of Gastric and Oesophageal Surgery and the upcoming Oxford Handbook of Endoscopy. He is recognised as a Trainer by the British General Medical Council (GMC), as well as an accredited Endoscopy Trainer by the UK Joint Advisory Group (JAG) on gastrointestinal (GI) Endoscopy. He serves as a Course Director for the Basic Surgical Skills Course at the Royal College of Surgeons of England (RCS England). He is an Honorary Senior Lecturer at King's College London (KCL). He is also a Fellow of Higher Education Academy (FHEA) and Fellow of the Academy of Medical Education (FAcadMEd). He has been awarded a Master of Business Administration (MBA) in Healthcare Management under the NHS Leadership Academy, as well as a Master of Laws (LLM) in Medical Law and Ethics. He was appointed as a Fellow of the Royal College of Physicians of London (FRCP) for his contributions to medical education and training. He is a Programme Director for King's Live, one of the world's largest annual international endoscopy symposiums.

Sacheen Kumar PhD MRSC(Chem) FRCS(Gen Surg), is a Consultant Upper Gastrointestinal (GI) Surgeon specialising in the treatment of Oesophago-Gastric Cancer and benign upper GI conditions at The Royal Marsden, Chelsea and Westminster Hospital and Cleveland Clinic London Hospital. He is also an Honorary Clinical Senior Lecturer in the Division of Surgery at Imperial College London and Team Leader of the Upper GI Surgical Oncology Research Group in the Division of Radiotherapy and Imaging at the Institute of Cancer Research (ICR). Mr Kumar qualified in medicine from Imperial College, London, and undertook his General Surgical Training within the London Deanery. His specialist Upper GI Surgical training was undertaken at Royal Free London, Imperial College Healthcare NHS Trust and University College London Hospitals. Upon completion of his training, he spent time at the National Cancer Centre (NCC) in Seoul learning minimally invasive surgical techniques for Upper GI cancer. His postgraduate research was focussed on breath analysis for the early diagnosis of Upper GI cancer. He was awarded his PhD from Imperial College in 2014 and was subsequently appointed to the position of National Institute of Health Research (NIHR) Clinical Lecturer in Surgery. In recognition of his original scientific research, he was elected as a Member of the Royal Society of Chemistry in 2018.

Arnab K Bhowmick MBChB FRCSEd(Gen Surg), graduated from the University of Manchester and then pursued a surgical career in the North West of England, completing basic surgical training.

After being awarded Fellowship of the Royal College of Surgeons of Edinburgh in 1996, he completed Higher Surgical training in the same year and worked in various hospitals in the North West of England, as well as spending 2 years in full time surgical research at Withington Hospital. Mr Bhowmick was awarded the Intercollegiate Fellowship of the Royal College of Surgeons and the Certificate of Completion of Specialist Training in 2005, before embarking on additional training in laparoscopic colorectal surgery. He was then appointed as a Consultant Surgeon in a District General Hospital in North Wales in 2006, and led undergraduate education while developing minimally invasive colorectal surgery. Mr Bhowmick was subsequently appointed as a Consultant Colorectal and General Surgeon at Lancashire Teaching Hospitals NHS Foundation Trust in 2009, and developed advanced laparoscopic colorectal surgery within his Trust. Mr Bhowmick served on the Council of the Association of Coloproctology of Great Britain and Ireland for 6 years, and as Divisional Medical Director for Surgery for 5 years, as well as Deputy Medical Director for Governance and Improvement for 6 years. Mr Bhowmick has been awarded Honorary Senior Lecturer status by three separate Universities for his contributions to surgical education. He has twice been awarded the Bronze National Clinical Excellence Award, and is a current National Clinical Impact Award holder.

Mohamed Baguneid MD MBChB FRCS MBA, is a highly respected Consultant Vascular and Endovascular Surgeon with over 30 years of clinical experience. His expertise includes managing complex aortic and carotid disease, diabetic foot disease and wound healing, with a special focus on peripheral vascular disease. In addition to his clinical expertise, he is a passionate educator and has developed master's programmes in surgical practice and vascular surgery, as well as national and international surgical courses and conferences. Professor Baguneid earned his medical degree from the University of Manchester and holds a global MBA from the Alliance Manchester Business School. He is an active researcher with an MD research thesis from Manchester in tissue engineering. His academic interests include wound healing, diabetic foot disease and soft-tissue infections. He strongly believes in evidence-based clinical practice and has published over 100 articles, including 68 original papers and reviews, in peer-reviewed journals and is the editor of the Oxford Handbook of Key Clinical Evidence and Oxford Handbook of Surgical Guidelines. Throughout his consultant career, Professor Baguneid has held numerous leadership positions, including Medical Director of a strategic partnership of four hospitals in the North West of England, Deputy Medical Director of Strategy in a large teaching hospital in Manchester, and Chair of Surgery in a large hospital in Abu Dhabi. He has been instrumental in developing and implementing clinical strategies to improve patient care and outcomes. He is currently Chair of Vascular Surgery at Sheikh Shakhbout Medical City in Abu Dhabi and building a world class vascular service integrating educational programmes and research into clinical practice.

Muntzer Mughal MBChB FRCS ChM, is a Consultant General and Upper Gastrointestinal Surgeon, Head of the Foregut Surgery Unit and Director of Surgical Oncology at Cleveland Clinic, London. He has been a Consultant General Surgeon for 35 years and has specialist expertise and wide experience in treating upper gastrointestinal (GI) conditions. He is an Honorary Consultant Surgeon at the University College Hospitals, London and Great Ormond Street Hospital for Children and an Honorary Associate Professor at UCL Developmental Biology and Cancer Department. He has been involved in teaching, assessment and designing teaching programmes for 30 years. He has served on the examination panels of the Royal College of Surgeons of England and the Intercollegiate Specialty Board in General Surgery. He has been an external examiner for higher degrees for several universities in the UK and abroad. He developed the format and set up the Alpine FRCS Course with his colleagues, Professor Mohamed Baguneid and Mr Arnab Bhowmick, in 2005, based on his experience as an Examiner for the FRCS Section B examination and running the highly rated North West Higher Surgical Trainee Teaching Programme for General Surgery from 2001 to 2010. He has wide experience in oesophagogastric surgery with particular expertise in oesophageal reconstruction for complex conditions and complications of upper GI surgery. He has regularly assisted thoracic, bariatric, endocrine and paediatric surgeons with complex reconstructions and has developed techniques for rare but serious, life-threatening conditions, such as tracheo-oesophageal fistula, aortoesophageal fistula and chronic oesophageal leaks. He has 25 years of experience in reviewing, designing and reconfiguring clinical services in the National Health Service. He has successfully led major reconfigurations in the North West of England and London. He has a major interest in improving cancer care at a system level and has led the streamlining of cancer multidisciplinary teams for 10 years. He served as a joint Chief Medical Officer of the North Central London Cancer Alliance between 2019 and 2020. He has worked in different capacities with national bodies such as the Royal College of Surgeons of England, the Specialist Advisory Committee for General Surgery, the National Institute for Health and Care Excellence, the Association of Upper GI Surgeons and the National Institute of Health Research. Professor Mughal has published widely, including 'Reconstructive Surgery of the Oesophagus and Stomach', which Springer (International Publisher) will publish in 2024.

Muhammad Rafay Sameem Siddiqui MBChB FRCS PhD DIC PGCert(Clin Ed) MFSTEd AFFMLM, is a Consultant Colorectal and General Surgeon in South Tyneside and Sunderland NHS Trust. He trained in South West London, completed a PhD at Croydon University Hospitals Trust, The Royal Marsden and Imperial College. He then underwent a fellowship in Exeter and completed a PGCert in Clinical Education during his time there. He has extensively published with over 60 peer reviewed publications, over 100 international and national presentations and two books. He has recently been appointed as the Director of the Clinical Academic Training Office at the University of Sunderland overseeing all research activity arising from the department of medicine. He has a keen interest in teaching and most notably is lead for Higher FRCS and Higher VIVA which has helped FRCS candidates to pass the examination, which is complimented by two courses, each runs three times a year. He is a faculty on the Alpine course and the RSM FRCS day.

Contributors

Aali J Sheen MD FRCS(Eng) FEBS(AWS)
Consultant Surgeon
Department of Hepatobiliary Surgery
Manchester University Foundation NHS Trust
Honorary Clinical Professor
The University of Manchester
Manchester, UK

Abdullah Jibawi MBBCh MS AVS FRCS DM
Consultant Vascular, Endovascular and General Surgeon
St George's University Hospitals NHS Foundation Trust
London, UK

Adam Rees MBChB PhD FRCS(Gen Surg)
Consultant Colorectal Surgeon
Manchester Royal Infirmary
Manchester, UK

Ajith K Siriwardena MD FRCS
Consultant Hepatobiliary Surgeon
Manchester Royal Infirmary
Professor of Hepatobiliary Surgery
University of Manchester
Manchester, UK
Past-President, European-African Hepato-Pancreato-Biliary Association (E-AHPBA)

Carol Norman BSc(Hons) MBBS AICSM MS FRCS
Consultant Oncoplastic Breast Surgeon
Croydon University Hospital
London, UK

Chris Macklin BMedSci BMBS FRCS(Gen Surg)
Consultant General and Colorectal Surgeon
Mid Yorkshire Hospitals NHS Trust, Yorkshire
Honorary Senior Lecturer
University of Leeds, UK

David Monk MBChB FRCS(Gen Surg) DipMedEd
Consultant Upper GI and General Surgeon
Cleveland Clinic London, UK

David van Dellen MD FRCS
Consultant Transplant and General Surgeon
Manchester Royal Infirmary, Manchester
Head of School of Surgery NHS England Northwest
Honorary Senior Lecturer
The University of Manchester, UK

Ed Denison-Davies BSc(Hons) MBBS FRCA FFICM DipIMC PGCME
Consultant in Critical Care Medicine and Anaesthesia
Lancashire Teaching Hospitals NHS Foundation Trust, Preston
Major Trauma Network Clinical Director
Lancashire and South Cumbria
HEMS Consultant and Senior Medical Team
North West Air Ambulance, UK

En Lin Goh BSc(Hons) MBBS(Dist) PGCert Med Ed(Dist) MRCS
Academic Clinical Fellow
Oxford Trauma and Emergency Care, NDORMS
Kadoorie Research Centre, University of Oxford
Oxford, UK

Faddy Kamel BM BS PhD FRCS(Gen Surg)
Consultant Colorectal Surgeon
Croydon University Hospital
London, UK

Finlay Curran MBChB FRCS
Consultant General and Colorectal Surgeon
Manchester Royal Infirmary
Manchester, UK

Helen Elizabeth Doran MD FRCS(Gen Surg)
Consultant Endocrine and General Surgeon
Salford Royal Hospital
The Northern Care Alliance NHS Foundation Trust
Salford, UK

Contributors

Hussein Khambalia PhD FRCS
Consultant Transplant Surgeon
Royal Infirmary
Manchester, UK

Ilayaraja Rajendran MBBS FRCS
Consultant General Surgeon
Lancashire Teaching Hospitals NHS Foundation Trust
Preston, UK

Irfan Chaudry MBChB FRCA FFICM FFMLM
Consultant in Critical Care Medicine and Anaesthesia
Lancashire Teaching Hospitals NHS Foundation Trust, Preston
Honorary Senior Lecturer
University of Manchester
Manchester, UK

Jemma Bhoday MBBS BSc FRCS PhD
Post-CCT Advanced Endosurgery Fellow
King's College Hospital
London, UK

Jeremy Ward MBChB MD FRCSEd(Gen Surg)
Consultant Upper GI Surgeon
Lancashire Teaching Hospitals NHS Foundation Trust
Preston, UK

Jonathan Moore FRCS
Specialist Registrar in General Surgery
The Royal Marsden NHS Foundation Trust
School of Cancer and Pharmaceutical Sciences
King's College London
London, UK

Kapil Sahnan MBBS FRCS PhD
Consultant General and Colorectal Surgeon
St Mark's Hospital
London, UK

Manikandan Kathirvel MBBS MS MRCS MCh(GI) FRCS
Consultant General
HPB and Liver Transplant Surgery
Royal Free London and Whittington Health NHS Trust
London, UK

Marc A Gladman MBBS DRCOG DFFP PhD MRCOG FRACS FRCS(Gen Surg)
Consultant Colorectal and Reconstructive Pelvic Floor Surgeon, King's College Hospital
London, UK

Mohamed Baguneid MD MBChB FRCS MBA
Consultant Vascular Surgeon
Sheikh Shakhbout Medical City, Abu Dhabi
Honorary Senior Lecturer, University of Manchester, UK
Adjunct Professor, UAE University
Adjunct Clinical Professor
Khalifa University, UAE

Muhammad Rafay Sameem Siddiqui
MBChB FRCS PhD DIC PGCert(Clin Ed) MFSTEd AFFMLM
Consultant General and Colorectal Surgeon
South Tyneside and Sunderland NHS Trust
Director of the Clinical Academic Training Office
Honorary Clinical Lecturer
University of Sunderland, UK

Murali Somasundaram FRCS DPhil
Senior Clinical Fellow
HPB and Liver Transplant Unit
Royal Free Hospital
London, UK

Nick Lees BA BMBCH MA FRCS DM
Consultant Colorectal Surgeon
Salford Royal Hospital
Salford, UK

Nima Abbassi-Ghadi BMBS BMedSci PhD FRCS
Consultant Upper GI Surgeon
Royal Surrey County Hospital
Guildford, UK

Paul Barrow MBChB(Hons) BSc(Hons) FRCS
Consultant Colorectal Surgeon
Lancashire Teaching Hospitals NHS Foundation Trust
Preston, UK

Paul Wilson FRCSEd FRCS(Gen Surg) MD
Consultant General Surgeon
University Hospitals of Morecambe Bay
Morecambe Bay, UK

Contributors

Pooja Padmanabhan MBBS MRCSEd DNB(Gen Surg) FEBS
Breast Surgeon, Royal Surrey County Hospital
Guildford, UK

Pranav H Patel MBBS PhD FRCS
Consultant Upper GI Surgeon
Royal Marsden Hospital
London, UK

Rachael Clifford MBChB PhD FRCS(Gen Surg)
Specialist Registrar in General Surgery
The Countess of Chester Hospital
Chester, UK

Rachael Coates MBChB BSc FRCS
Consultant General and Colorectal Surgeon
South Tyneside and Sunderland NHS Trust
Sunderland, UK

Rachita Mallya MBChB FRCS
Surgical Registrar and Clinical Research Fellow
Imperial College London, UK

Ravi Acharya MBBS MS(Surg) FRCSEd (Gen Surg)
Senior Fellow in Endocrine Surgery
Salford Royal Hospital
The Northern Care Alliance NHS Foundation Trust, UK

Robin Som MBA FRCS
Post-CCT Fellow in Upper Gastrointestinal Surgery, University Hospital Coventry
Coventry, UK

Sabina Wallace-King BMus BSc MBBS MRCSEd PGCert MedEd
Core Trainee General Surgery
South Tyneside and Sunderland NHS Trust
Sunderland, UK

Sacheen Kumar PhD MRSC(Chem) FRCS(Gen Surg)
Consultant Upper GI Surgeon
Royal Marsden Hospital, London
Consultant Upper GI Surgeon
DDSI Institute Cleveland Clinic London Hospital
Upper GI Surgical Oncology Research Group
Institute of Cancer Research, UK

Saurabh Jamdar BSc(Hons) MBChB MD FRCS(Gen Surg)
Consultant General and Hepatobiliary Surgeon, Manchester Royal Infirmary
Manchester, UK

Schlock Balapuri MBBS FRCS MD
Consultant General and Upper GI Surgeon
Sunderland Royal Hospital
Sunderland, UK

Shramana Banerjee MBBS BSc(Clin Sci) MRCS FEBS PhD(Breast Surg Oncol) Dip Onco-Aesthetics
Breast Surgeon and Breast Fellow
Royal Surrey County Hospital
Guildford, UK

Sri Ganeshamurthy Thrumurthy
MBChB(Hons) MBA LLM FRCS(Gen Surg)
FRCP(London) FHEA FAcadMEd
Consultant Surgeon
King's College Hospital and
King Edward VII's Hospital
Honorary Senior Lecturer
King's College London
London, UK

Thomas Payne MBChB MSc FHEA MRCS
Specialist Registrar in ENT Surgery
St George's University Hospitals NHS Foundation Trust
London, UK

Tim James Royle MBChB FRCS MMedEd
Consultant General and Colorectal Surgeon
South Tyneside and Sunderland NHS Trust
Sunderland, UK

Tracey Irvine MBBS(Hons) MA(Hons) Cantab MSc FRCS(Gen Surg)
Consultant Oncoplastic Breast Surgeon
Royal Surrey County Hospital
Guildford, UK

Acknowledgements

To my family: *Sobanah, Ayishwarriyah, Krishna, Kailash, Sasha, Andy* and *Pedro*.

To *Dr Raj Kumar Menon* for his exemplary mentorship since our days at Raffles.

To *Professor Muntzer Mughal, Professor Mohamed Baguneid, Mr Arnab K Bhowmick, Mr Asif Chaudry, Professor Bu'Hussain Hayee* and *Professor Ameet Patel* for their wisdom, guidance and tutelage.

To *Mr Abdulazeez Bello* and *Mr Ahsan Zaidi* for their paternal support.

To my inspirations: My late father and aviator, *Thrumurthy Krishnamurthy*, who taught me the importance of treating people well; and the unparalleled *Mr Amyn Haji*, who exemplifies this.

Sri Ganeshamurthy Thrumurthy

I would like to thank *all my surgical colleagues* whom I have had the opportunity to work with and learn from over the years, and in particular, my mentor *Professor Muntzer Mughal*, for his unwavering support and guidance.

Sacheen Kumar

I would like to thank *the many excellent colleagues, friends and family* who have supported me with surgical education over the last 20 years culminating in all the efforts to produce this book.

Arnab K Bhowmick

I would like to thank *my family* for their unwavering support and encouragement throughout my career. I am indebted to *my many mentors* whose guidance and wisdom have shaped my knowledge and skills. A heartfelt thanks to *my colleagues* and *all those I have had the privilege to train* over the years.

Mohamed Baguneid

This book is a spin-off from the Alpine FRCS Course, which was created 20 years ago. I would like to express my gratitude to my *co-creators and editors, Professor Baguneid and Mr Bhowmick*, the *core faculty of the course*, and the *nearly 1,000 trainees* who have attended the course. Their participation has kept us on our toes and helped us to create highly discriminative scenarios and questions.

Muntzer Mughal

Acknowledgements

I would like to acknowledge *The One, Habib,* my wife *Bushra Ehsanullah,* my daughters *Aaliyah-Noor* and *Huda-Noor* and *my as of yet unborn child.*

I would also extend my gratitude to my father, *Muhammad Talib Siddiqui,* who gave me the foundations for what I have become today; my mother, *Rana K Siddiqui,* who looked after me; and my sisters, *Rubia Siddiqui* and *Saadia Siddiqui,* for all their help and support, especially during my training years.

Muhammad Rafay Sameem Siddiqui

Abbreviations and acronyms

A&E	Accident and emergency	ANH	Acute normovolaemic haemodilution
AAA	Abdominal aortic aneurysm	AO	Adjuvant! Online
AAC	Acute acalculous cholecystitis	APACHE	Acute Physiology And Chronic Health Evaluation
AAST	American Association of Surgery for Trauma	APC	Adenomatous polyposis coli
ABC	Airway, breathing and circulation	APER	Abdominoperineal excision of rectum
ABG	Arterial blood gas	APTT	Activated partial thromboplastin time
ABPI	Ankle-brachial pressure index	ARDS	Acute respiratory distress syndrome
ABS	Association of breast surgery	ARF	Acute renal failure
ACAS	Asymptomatic carotid artery stenosis	ARR	Absolute risk reduction
ACE	Angiotensin-converting enzyme	ART	Axillary radiotherapy
ACPGBI	Association of Coloproctology for Great Britain and Ireland	ASA	American Society of Anaesthetists
ACS	Abdominal compartment syndrome	ASCO	American Society of Clinical Oncology
ACST	Asymptomatic Carotid Surgery Trial	ASGBI	Association of Surgeons of Great Britain and Ireland
ACTH	Adrenocorticotrophic hormone	AT	Anaerobic threshold
ACTx	Adjuvant chemotherapy	ATA	American Thyroid Association
ADH	Antidiuretic hormone	ATG	Anti-thymocyte globulin
ADQI	Acute dialysis quality initiative	ATLS	Advanced Trauma Life Support
ADRCs	Adipose-derived regenerative stem cells	ATN	Acute tubular necrosis
AF	Atrial fibrillation	ATP	Adenosine triphosphate
AFP	Alpha-fetoprotein	AUC	Area under the curve
AI	Aromatase inhibitor	AV	Arteriovenous
AIDS	Acquired immune deficiency syndrome	AVF	Arteriovenous fistula
AIN	Anal intraepithelial neoplasia	AVG	Arteriovenous grafts
AKIN	Acute kidney injury network	AVM	Arteriovenous malformation
ALI	Acute lung injury	AXR	Abdominal radiograph
AII	Angiotensin II	β-HCG	Beta-human chorionic gonadotrophin
ALP	Alkaline phosphatase	BADS	British Association of Day Surgery
ALT	Alanine transaminase	BAL	Bronchoalveolar lavage
AMPLE	Allergies, medication, past medical history, last meal, events surrounding trauma	BBV	Blood borne viruses
AMR	Antibody-mediated rejection	BCC	Basal cell carcinoma
ANC	Axillary node clearance	BCS	Breast conserving surgery

BCSH	British Committee for Standards in Haematology	CISH	Chromogenic in situ hybridisation
BE	Barrett's oesophagus	CK	Creatine kinase
BE	Base excess	CKD	Chronic kidney disease
BIPAP	Biphasic positive airway pressure	Cl	Chloride
BK	Below knee	CLI	Critical limb ischaemia
BM	Boehringer Mannheim (blood glucose test)	CMF	Cyclophosphamide, methotrexate and fluorouracil
BMI	Body mass index	CMI	Chronic mesenteric ischaemia
BMT	Best medical treatment	CMV	Cytomegalovirus
BP	Blood pressure	CNI	Calcineurin inhibitor
BPD with DS	Biliopancreatic diversion with duodenal switch	CNS	Central nervous system
		CO	Cardiac output
BPH	Benign prostatic hypertrophy	CONSORT	Consolidated Standards for Reporting Trials
bpm	Beats per minute	COPD	Chronic obstructive pulmonary disease
BSA	Body surface area		
BSD	Brainstem dead	COX-2	Cyclo-oxygenase-2
BSG	British Society of Gastroenterology	CP	Chronic pancreatitis
		CPAP	Continuous positive airway pressure
BXO	Balanitis xerotica obliterans		
Ca	Calcium	CPD	Continuing professional development
CABG	Coronary artery bypass graft		
CAD	Coronary artery disease	CPEX	Cardiopulmonary exercise testing
CALI	Chemotherapy assisted liver injury	CPP	Cerebral perfusion pressure
		CPR	Cardiopulmonary resuscitation
cAMP	Cyclic adenosine monophosphate	CPX	Cardiopulmonary exercise test
CAS	Carotid artery stenting	CRM	Circumferential resection margin
CBD	Common bile duct	CRP	C-reactive protein
CCF	Congestive cardiac failure	CRRT	Continuous renal replacement therapy
CCLND	Central compartment lymph node dissection		
		CRT	Capillary refill time
CCrISP	Care of the Critically Ill Surgical Patient	CSF	Cerebrospinal fluid
		CT	Computed tomography
CDI	*Clostridium difficile* infection	CTA	Computed tomography angiogram
CDT	Catheter-directed thrombolysis		
CEA	Carcinoembryonic antigen	CTD	Chronic transplant dysfunction
CETC	Carotid Endarterectomy Trialists Collaboration	CVA	Cerebrovascular accident
		CVC	Central venous catheter
CFA	Common femoral artery	CVI	Chronic venous insufficiency
CgA	Chromogranin A	CVP	Central venous pressure
CHD	Common hepatic duct	CVS	Cardiovascular system
CHOP	Cyclophosphamide, doxorubicin, vincristine and prednisolone	CVVH	Continuous venovenous haemofiltration

Abbreviations and acronyms

CXR	Chest radiograph	ERAS	Enhanced recovery after surgery
D&V	Diarrhoea and vomiting	ERCP	Endoscopic retrograde cholangiopancreatography
DO_2	Oxygen delivery		
D2	Second part of duodenum	ESBL	Extended-spectrum β-lactamases
DBD	Donation after brainstem death	ESD	Endoscopic submucosal dissection
DCD	Donation after cardiac death		
DCIS	Ductal carcinoma in situ	ESR	Erythrocyte sedimentation rate
DCL	Damage control laparotomy	ESRD	End-stage renal disease
DDAVP	Desmopressin (synthetic derivative of antidiuretic hormone l-arginine vasopressin)	ESRF	End-stage renal failure
		ETT	Endotracheal tube
		EUA	Examination under anaesthesia
DEXA	Dual-energy X-ray absorptiometry	EUS	Endoscopic ultrasound
DGH	District General Hospital	EVAR	Endovascular aneurysm repair
DIC	Disseminated intravascular coagulation	FAP	Familial adenomatous polyposis
		FAST	Focussed assessment of sonography in trauma
DIEP	Deep inferior epigastric perforator		
DJ flexure	Duodenojejunal flexure	FBC	Full blood count
DM	Diabetes mellitus	FDG-PET	Fluorodeoxyglucose positron emission tomography
DNA	Deoxyribonucleic acid		
DO	Oxygen delivery	FDP	Fibrin degradation products
DOH	Department of Health	FEA	Flat epithelial atypia
DPG	Diphosphoglycerate	FENa	Fractional excretion of sodium
DRI	Donor risk index	FEV1	Forced expiratory volume in 1 second
DRIL	Distal revascularisation and interval ligation		
		FFP	Fresh frozen plasma
DSA	Digital subtraction angiography	FiO_2	Concentration of inspired oxygen
DU	Duodenal ulcer	FISH	Fluorescent in situ hybridisation
DVLA	Driver and Vehicle Licensing Agency	FLR	Future liver remnant
		FNA	Fine-needle aspiration
DVT	Deep vein thrombosis	FNAB	Fine-needle aspiration biopsy
EBV	Epstein–Barr virus	FNAC	Fine-needle aspiration cytology
ECF	Extracellular fluid	FOB	Faecal occult blood
ECG	Electrocardiogram	FRC	Functional residual capacity
ECMO	Extra-corporeal membrane oxygenation	FRCS	Fellow of the Royal College of Surgeons
ECST	European Carotid Surgery Trials	FRV	Functional residual volume
eGFR	Estimated glomerular filtration rate	FSH	Follicle-stimulating hormone
		FU	Follow-up
EIA	Enzyme immunoassay	FY1	Foundation year 1 doctor
EMR	Endoscopic mucosal resection	FY2	Foundation year 2 doctor
ENT	Ear, nose and throat	G&S	Group and save
ER/OR	Estrogen/Oestrogen receptor	GA	General anaesthesia

GCS	Glasgow Coma Scale	HPS	Hyperplastic pyloric stenosis
G-CSF	Granulocyte colony-stimulating factor	HPV	Human papilloma virus
		HR	Heart rate
GDT	Goal-directed therapy	HRS	Hepatorenal syndrome
GFR	Glomerular filtration rate	HRT	Hormone replacement therapy
GI	Gastrointestinal	HTA	Human Tissue Authority
GIST	Gastrointestinal stromal tumours	HU	Hounsfield units
GIT	Gastrointestinal tract	IAH	Intra-abdominal hypertension
GM	Gynaecomastia	IAP	Intra-abdominal pressure
GN	Glomerulonephropathy	IBD	Inflammatory bowel disease
GOJ	Gastro-oesophageal junction	ICAP	Intercostal artery perforator
GOO	Gastric outlet obstruction	ICD	Implantable cardioverter defibrillator
GORD	Gastro-oesophageal reflux disease	ICF	Intracellular fluid
GP	General practitioner	ICP	Intracranial pressure
GSV	Great saphenous vein	ICS	Intraoperative cell salvage
GTN	Glyceryl trinitrate	ICU	Intensive care unit
GU	Genitourinary	IFTA	Interstitial fibrosis and tubular atrophy
Gy	Gray		
HAI	Hospital-acquired infection	IgG	Immunoglobulin G
HAP	Healthcare-associated pneumonia	IH	Intermittent haemodialysis
		IHD	Ischaemic heart disease
HAT	Hepatic arterial thrombosis	IJV	Internal jugular vein
Hb	Haemoglobin	IMA	Inferior mesenteric artery
HBV	Hepatitis B virus	IMCA	Independent mental capacity advocate
HCO_3	Bicarbonate		
HCC	Hepatocellular carcinoma	INR	International normalised ratio
HCG	Human chorionic gonadotrophin	IOC	Intraoperative cholangiography
HCV	Hepatitis C virus	IPF	Initial poor function
HDU	High dependency unit	IPMN	Intraductal papillary mucinous neoplasm
HER2	Human epidermal growth factor receptor 2	IPPV	Intermittent positive pressure ventilation
HGD	High-grade dysplasia	ISCP	Intercollegiate Surgical Curriculum Programme
HIAA	Hydroxyindoleacetic acid		
HIT	Heparin-induced thrombocytopaenia	ISE	Intercollegiate Speciality Examination
HIV	Human immunodeficiency virus	ITC	Isolated tumour cells
HLA	Human leukocyte antigen	ITGCN	Intratesticular germ cell neoplasia
HNA	Human neutrophil antigen	ITP	Idiopathic thrombocytopaenic purpura
HNPCC	Hereditary nonpolyposis colorectal cancer		
		ITU/ICU	Intensive treatment/care unit
HPB	Hepatopancreaticobiliary	IV	Intravenous

IVC	Inferior vena cava	MAP	Mean arterial pressure
IVF	In vitro fertilisation	MBL	Massive blood loss
JSCFE	Joint Surgical Colleges Fellowship Examination	MC&S	Microscopy, culture and sensitivity
K	Potassium	MCN	Mucinous cystic neoplasm
KCl	Potassium chloride	MDM	Multidisciplinary team meeting
kHz	Kilohertz	MDRD	Modification of diet in renal disease
LA	Local anaesthetic		
LAGB	Laparoscopic adjustable gastric band	MDT	Multidisciplinary team/meeting
		MELD	Model for end-stage liver disease
LBO	Large bowel obstruction	MEN	Multiple endocrine neoplasia
LC	Laparoscopic cholecystectomy	Met-Hb	Methaemoglobin
LC-CRT	Long course chemoradiotherapy	Mg	Magnesium
LCIS	Lobular carcinoma in situ	mHz	Megahertz
LDH	Lactate dehydrogenase	MI	Myocardial infarction
LFT	Liver function test	MIBG	Meta-iodobenzylguanidine
LGD	Low-grade dysplasia	MIP	Minimally invasive parathyroidectomy
LGIB	Lower gastrointestinal bleed		
LH	Luteinising hormone	MMF	Mycofenolate mofetil
LHM	Laparoscopic Heller's myotomy	MNG	Multinodular goitre
LHRH	Luteinising hormone receptor hormone	MODS	Multi-organ dysfunction syndrome
LIF	Left iliac fossa	MOOSE	Meta-analyses of Observational Studies in Epidemiology
LIFT	Ligation of the intersphincteric fistula tract		
		MRA	Magnetic resonance angiogram
LLQ	Left lower quadrant	MRC	Medical Research Council
LMA	Laryngeal mask airway	MRCP	Magnetic resonance cholangiopancreatography
LMWH	Low molecular weight heparin		
LOS	Lower oesophageal sphincter	MRE	Magnetic resonance enterogram
LRINEC	Laboratory risk indicator for necrotising fasciitis	MRI	Magnetic resonance imaging
		MRSA	Methicillin-resistant *Staphylococcus aureus*
LRTI	Lower respiratory tract infection		
LRYGB	Laparoscopic Roux-en-Y gastric bypass	MS	Multiple sclerosis
		MSSA	Methicillin sensitive *Staphylococcus aureus*
LSG	Laparoscopic sleeve gastrectomy		
LSV	Long saphenous vein	MSU	Midstream urine
LVEDP	Left ventricular end-diastolic pressure	MTC	Medullary thyroid carcinoma
		MTOR	Mammalian target of rapamycin
LVEF	Left ventricular ejection fraction	MUGA	Multigated acquisition
LVI	Lymphovascular invasion	Na	Sodium
MA	Microwave ablation	NAC	Nipple areolar complex
MALT	Mucosa-associated lymphoid tissue	NaCl	Sodium chloride
		NAI	Non-accidental injury

Abbreviations and acronyms

NASCET	North American Symptomatic Carotid Endarterectomy Trial	PCA	Patient controlled analgesia
NASH	Nonalcoholic steatohepatitis	PCC	Prothrombin complex concentrate
NBM	Nil by mouth	PCR	Pathological complete response
NBO	Nil by oral route	PCT	Percutaneous tracheostomy
NCTx	Neoadjuvant chemotherapy	PD	Peritoneal dialysis
NET	Neuroendocrine tumour	PDS	Polydiaxonone
NEX	Neoadjuvant endocrine treatment	PE	Pulmonary embolism
NF	Neurofibromatosis	PEC	Percutaneous endoscopic colostomy
NFATc	Nuclear factor of activated T cells	PEEP	Positive end-expiratory pressure
NG	Nasogastric	PEG	Percutaneous endoscopic gastrostomy
NGT	Nasogastric tube	PEI	Percutaneous ethanol injection
NHS	National Health Service	PEP	Post-exposure prophylaxis
NHSBSP	NHS Breast Screening Programme	PET	Positron emission tomography
NICE	National Institute for Clinical Excellence	PFA	Profunda femoris artery
NIDDM	Non-insulin-dependent diabetes mellitus	PFC	Peripancreatic fluid collection
NIV	Non-invasive ventilation	PH	Primary hyperhidrosis
NJ	Nasojejunal	PHPT	Primary hyperparathyroidism
NNT	Number needed to treat	PICC	Peripheral indwelling central catheter
NODAT	New-onset diabetes after transplantation	PMHx	Past medical history
NOGCA	National Oesophagogastric Cancer Audit	PN	Parenteral nutrition
NOMI	Non-occlusive mesenteric ischaemia	PNF	Primary nonfunction
NSAID	Non-steroidal anti-inflammatory drug	PNS	Parasympathetic nervous system
NSGCT	Non-seminomatous germ cell tumours	PO	Per oral
OCP	Oral contraceptive pill	POCT	Point-of-care testing
OGD	Oesophagogastroduodenoscopy	POEM	Per oral endoscopic myotomy
OPSI	Overwhelming postsplenectomy infection	PONV	Postoperative nausea and vomiting
OR	Odds ratio	POSSUM	Physiological and Operative Severity Score for the enUmeration of Mortality and morbidity
OSNA	One-step nucleic acid amplification	PPH	Procedure for prolapsed haemorrhoids
PA	Pulmonary artery	PPI	Proton pump inhibitor
PAD	Pre-deposit autologous blood donation	PPPD	Pylorus preserving pancreatico-duodenectomy
PAWP	Pulmonary artery wedge pressure	PPV	Patent processus vaginalis
PBC	Primary biliary cirrhosis	PR	Per rectum
		PRBC	Packed red blood cells

PRISMA	Preferred Reporting Items for Systematic Reviews and Meta-Analyses	RUQ	Right upper quadrant
		S/C	Subcutaneous
		SAFARI	Subintimal arterial flossing with antegrade-retrograde intervention
PSA	Prostate specific antigen		
PT	Prothrombin time		
PTC	Percutaneous transhepatic cholangiogram	SCA	Sickle cell anaemia
		SCC	Squamous cell carcinoma
PTFE	Polytetrafluoroethylene	SCF	Supraclavicular fossa
PTH	Parathyroid hormone	SCIWORA	Spinal cord injury without radiological abnormality
PTLD	Post-transplant lymphoproliferative disorder		
		SCM	Sternocleidomastoid
PTS	Post-thrombotic syndrome	SCPRT	Short course preoperative radiotherapy
PTT	Prothrombin time		
PTU	Propylthiouracil	SFA	Superficial femoral artery
PVS	Persistent vegetative state	SGAP	Superior gluteal artery perforator
PYE	Portal vein embolisation	SHA	Strategic Health Authority
QA	Quality assurance	SIADH	Syndrome of inappropriate antidiuretic hormone
QALY	Quality-adjusted life year		
QARC	Quality Assurance Reference Centre	SIRI	Serious incident requiring investigation
QoL	Quality of life	SIRS	Systemic inflammatory response syndrome
QPTH	Quick parathyroid hormone assay		
RAAS	Renin angiotensin aldosterone system	SIRT	Selective internal radiotherapy
		SISH	Silver in situ hybridisation
RAI	Radioiodine ablation	SLE	Systemic lupus erythematosus
RBC	Red blood cells	SLN(B)	Sentinel lymph node (biopsy)
RCC	Renal cell carcinoma	SMA	Superior mesenteric artery
RCT	Randomised controlled trial	SMG	Submandibular gland
RFA	Radiofrequency ablation	SNS	Sacral nerve stimulation
Rh	Rhesus	SOB	Short of breath
RIF	Right iliac fossa	SPECT	Single-photon emission computed tomography
RIG	Radiologically inserted gastrostomy		
		SRH	Stigmata of recent haemorrhage
RLN	Recurrent laryngeal nerve	SSI	Surgical site infection
RLQ	Right lower quadrant	SSV	Short saphenous vein
RNA	Ribonucleic acid	ST (years 1–8)	Speciality trainee doctor (years 1–8)
ROC	Receiver operating characteristic		
RR	Respiratory rate	STARR	Stapled transanal rectal resection
RRR	Relative risk reduction	STC	Slow transit constipation
RRT	Renal replacement therapy	STROBE	STrengthening the Reporting of OBservational studies Epidemiology
RT	Radiotherapy		
RUDI	Revision using distal inflow	SVC	Superior vena cava

SVR	Systemic vascular resistance	TTG	Tissue transglutaminase antibody
TACE	Transarterial chemotherapy	TTS	Through the scope
TAMIS	Transanal minimally invasive surgery	TUG	Transverse upper gracilis
		U&E	Urea and electrolytes
TAPP	Transabdominal preperitoneal repair	UC	Ulcerative colitis
		UDT	Undescended testicle
TB	Tuberculosis	UGFS	Ultrasound-guided foam sclerotherapy
TBSA	Total body surface area		
Tc	Technetium	UGI	Upper gastrointestinal
TEDs	Thromboembolism deterrant stockings	UIQ	Upper inner quadrant
		US(S)	Ultrasound scan
TEG	Thromboelastogram	UTI	Urinary tract infection
TEMS	Transanal endoscopic microsurgery	VAB	Vacuum-assisted biopsy
		VAC	Vacuum-assisted closure
TEO	Transanal endoscopic operation	VACB	Vacuum-assisted core biopsy
TEP	Totally extraperitoneal repair	VAP	Ventilator-associated pneumonia
TFT	Thyroid function tests	VARD	Video-assisted retroperitoneal dissection
Tg	Thyroglobulin		
TIA	Transient ischaemic attack	VEGF-A	Vascular endothelial growth factor A
TIC	Touch imprint cytology		
TIPS	Transjugular intrahepatic portosystemic shunt	VMA	Vanillylmandelic acid
		VOC	Vaso-occlusive crisis
TM	Therapeutic mammoplasty	VRD	von Recklinghausen's disease
TME	Total mesorectal excision	VRE	Vancomycin-resistant enterococci
TNF	Tumour necrosis factor	VTE	Venous thromboembolism
TOS	Thoracic outlet syndrome	vWF	von Willebrand factor
TPMT	Transpurine methyltransferase	WBI	Whole breast irradiation
TPN	Total parenteral nutrition	WCC	White cell count
TRALI	Transfusion-related acute lung injury	WHO	World Health Organisation
		WLE	Wide local excision
TRAM	Transverse rectus abdominis myocutaneous (flap)	WOPN	Walled off pancreatic necrosis
		ZES	Zollinger–Ellison syndrome
TSH	Thyroid stimulating hormone		
TT	Thrombin time		

Introduction

The Intercollegiate specialty fellowship examination in general surgery

The Intercollegiate Specialty Fellowship Examination in General Surgery comprises two sections. This book is dedicated to preparing for and passing Section 2. Section 1 is a written test composed of two papers, each containing Single Best Answer (SBA) questions. Paper 1 consists of 120 SBAs and lasts 2 hours and 15 minutes, while Paper 2 also consists of 120 SBAs and lasts 2 hours and 15 minutes. Section 1 examinations are delivered via computer-based testing at accredited test centres worldwide. Candidates must meet the required standard in Section 1 to proceed to Section 2.

Section 2 comprises the clinical component of the examination, consisting of a series of meticulously designed and structured scenario-based interviews. These examinations will be conducted at preselected host centres worldwide. It is worth noting that the format of Section 2 has changed significantly since the coronavirus disease 2019 (COVID-19) pandemic. There is now less reliance on patient contact (i.e. patients will only be used in the long cases, and candidates will not be required to examine patients). It is likely that FRCS General Surgery curriculum and format will continue to undergo periodic updates, so candidates are advised to refer to contemporary published guidance at all times.

The format includes both clinical and oral examinations covering all aspects of General Surgery, incorporating relevant anatomy, physiology, pathology, research methodology, levels of evidence, and statistical analysis. The syllabus is available on the Joint Committee on Intercollegiate Examinations (JCIE) website (www.jcie.org.uk). Depending on where the examination is attempted, candidates may be required to follow specific guidance from the Joint Surgical Colleges Fellowship Examination (JSCFE) website (www.jscfe.co.uk).

Candidates must choose their special interest from Breast, Colorectal, Oesophago-gastric (OG), Hepatopancreaticobiliary (HPB), Endocrine, Trauma, Transplant, and 'GI Surgery and Surgery of Childhood'. *It is important to note that the OG and HPB candidates are now assessed separately, and no longer under a common 'upper GI' theme.*

Clinical examinations

There will be two clinical examinations:
1. General surgery:
   - 2 x 10 minutes short cases
   - 1 x 20 minutes long case
2. Specialist interest:
   - 2 x 10 minutes short cases
   - 1 x 20 minutes long case

Patients may only be used for the long case, and will not be examined (i.e. they will only be used for history taking and communication skills). For the short cases, no patients will be present, instead, clinical scenarios will be used for each short case. These examinations will assess history taking, examination, and planning of surgical care, including relevant pathology, investigations, and operative surgery.

Oral (viva) examinations

There will be four oral (viva) examinations:
1. Emergency surgery/Trauma/Critical care—clinical topics with discussion of published evidence supporting practice.
2. General surgery principles and clinical practice—including applied anatomy, physiology and pathology.
3. Specialist interest surgery—clinical practice—clinical topics with discussion of published evidence supporting practice
4. Specialist interest surgery:
   - Basic principles—applied anatomy, physiology and pathology (15 minutes)
   - Academic foundation (15 minutes). Candidates will be given 30 minutes to read one general paper.

The aim of the oral (viva) examination is to sample three areas of the curriculum in 15 minutes (two emergency surgery, two trauma surgery and two critical care in 30 minutes).

Marking of section 2 of the examination

The viva/oral examination begins with the academic viva, with topics decided at the examiners' meeting prior to the examination. Examiners start with easier questions to help candidates to settle in, then progress to more challenging ones. Each examiner independently awards marks (8—outstanding, 7—good, 6—pass, 5—fail, 4—poor) without prior discussion. The final mark is the mean of all individual marks in each section. A strong performance in one section can compensate for a weaker performance in another, as the overall score is an aggregate.
The marking allocation for each station is as follows:

Section	Pass mark	Highest mark	Weighting (%)
General surgery: Clinical	120	160	23
Special interest: Clinical	120	160	23
Special interest surgery: Clinical practice oral	72	96	14
Special interest surgery: Basic principles and academic	60	80	12
Emergency surgery/Trauma/Critical care oral	72	96	14
General surgery/Principles and clinical practice oral	72	96	14

When to take the examination? There is no perfect time to take the examination, but candidates are generally ready from ST6 onwards (or equivalent). Procrastination may only delay the inevitable. Commitment to the application process and a structured approach to preparation are essential. The examination tests clinical decision-making, prioritisation, and thought process rather than rote knowledge. Candidates must be prepared to discuss cases as if referred by a consultant colleague.

Preparation for section 2: Thorough preparation is crucial, with a focus on technique and presentation. The examination tests clinical decision-making skills and judgement. Key preparation strategies include:
- Group revision for collaborative learning and practice
- Viva practice with consultants to cover a wide range of topics
- Practicing under realistic conditions to handle examination pressure
- Comprehensive coverage of the syllabus to avoid surprises

- Attending relevant multidisciplinary teams (MDTs) for subspecialty knowledge
- Maintaining health and well-being to enhance performance
- Leveraging past examination success strategies
- Attending relevant courses for consolidation and mock examination experience

Viva technique

Mastering your viva technique is the most critical and decisive step towards passing the examination. Success hinges not only on the depth of your knowledge but also on your ability to deliver answers with clarity and structure. Developing these delivery skills is essential, enabling you to communicate in an organised, clear and structured manner. Confidence will come with practice. For instance, try reading a topic from a book, then close the book and recite what you have just studied—you may be surprised at the difficulty. Integrating viva practice into your revision, especially focussing on weaker areas, is crucial. Given the practical nature of surgery, emphasise viva practice over rote reading of textbooks.

Expect a degree of nervousness

It is natural to feel nervous, and it may take time to settle into the examination. Ignore other candidates and focus on your performance, as the outcome is determined by you and the examiners. Hearing others give polished answers which can be distracting, but you do not know how they performed in other parts of the examination. Examiners expect nerves and are more interested in how you manage under pressure.

Systematic thinking and answering

Organise your answers to demonstrate a clear, systematic thought process, which is key to producing succinct responses. Before delving into details, consider what the examiner is asking. Opening phrases are crucial; start with statements like, 'Patient safety is paramount here...' or 'I would first establish haemorrhage control before considering definitive intervention...' Compartmentalise and categorise your answer to show that you practice surgery in a systematic and safe manner.

Speak from experience

In the examination, speak as if you are the consultant, not a trainee. Constantly calling for help or senior's advice can irritate examiners and indicate a lack of confidence. Most scenarios will be within your scope of practice and experience. For example, when asked, 'How would you achieve temporary abdominal closure in this patient while awaiting relook laparotomy?' a suitable response could be, 'In my experience, I have most often used the ABThera NPT System for temporary bridging of abdominal wall openings, especially where primary closure is not indicated or impossible.' Avoid responses that defer decisions to a consultant.

Avoid 'reading the examiner'

Do not read into the examiner's body language. Even the most enthusiastic examiner can become monotonous after repeatedly asking the same questions. Most examiners take pleasure in good performance and aim to pass candidates wherever possible. Ignore any poker-faced or negative reactions, and stay focussed.

Avoid distractions

One examiner will mark while the other asks questions. Do not attempt to see the marking examiner's scores, as this is distracting and can be irritating. Never argue with the examiner, regardless of your conviction. Be diplomatic, state your beliefs based on your experience, and acknowledge that there may be other valid approaches.

Structured vivas

The structured format of the examination ensures fairness, preventing examiners from focussing unfairly on their areas of expertise. Remember, an examiner may ask questions outside their specialty, to which you might have more experience. Draw confidence from this while respecting the examiner's experience.

Maximising the use of this book

This book is intended as a revision companion and guide, not a comprehensive textbook of surgery or its subspecialties. We encourage using this book with a partner or in a small group, emphasising interactive revision. Take turns asking each other questions and reflect on your answers to make them clearer and more concise. Although this book primarily targets the viva section, much of the clinical examination involves similar questions. We have covered as many topics as possible, though some may not be included, as evident in the Intercollegiate Surgical Curriculum Programme (ISCP) syllabus. We welcome feedback and suggestions for future improvements to benefit upcoming candidates.

Chapter 1

Academic viva

En Lin Goh, Sri Ganeshamurthy Thrumurthy, Jonathan Moore

Critical appraisal

Analysis

A structured approach is essential in appraising a manuscript. In general, the analysis should focus on the internal and external validities of the study. The internal validity refers to the conduct of the study and is generally centred on potential bias and confounding factors. The external validity describes the interpretation of the study, which relates to the generalizability and applicability of the results. The methods and results sections will typically provide information regarding internal validity while the discussion and conclusion sections will provide information regarding external validity. The following describes key questions to consider when appraising each section of a manuscript.

Abstract
- Is the abstract clear and easy to understand?
- Does the abstract reflect the content of the full manuscript?

Introduction
- What is the justification for the study?
- Does clinical equipoise exist between the diagnostic or therapeutic modalities being compared? (i.e. does the study have real-world purpose?)
- How does the study fit in with currently accepted practices, perspectives or standards?
- Is the aim of the study clearly stated?
- Is the aim of the study appropriate in answering the research question?

Methods
- What is the study design?
- How were participants identified and allocated to their respective groups?
- Was the study open-label, single-blind or double-blind?
- Were there any *a priori* hypotheses or assumptions used to calculate a sample size?
- What are the pre-specified outcomes?

Results
- Are all prespecified outcomes reported?
- Are individual or composite outcomes reported?
- Are clinically relevant outcomes reported?
- How do the relative and AR compare?
- What is the attrition rate?
- How was missing data handled?

Discussion
- Are the results (including expected and unexpected findings) adequately explained?
- How do the results fit in with currently accepted practices, perspectives or standards?
- Are the findings appropriately stated in terms of significance and importance?

Conclusion
- Are the conclusions justified based on the results?
- Do the conclusions address the aim of the study?
- What is the generalizability and applicability of the results?

Presentation
A succinct summary of the study is an important component of the academic viva. This can be given at the beginning or the end depending on the examining style. It is essential to develop an approach that one is comfortable with. The following is a proposed structure to provide a summary with detailed examples to follow later on in this chapter.
- Aims and study design
- Sample size and selection
- Intervention
- Analysis and results

To conclude the summary, you should provide your overall impression of the study and how relevant this will be to current clinical practice.

Key definitions

Basic definitions
- *Accuracy of a test:* The proportion of subjects given the correct result
- *Bias:* The introduction of a systematic error into sampling or testing by selecting one outcome over others
- *Confounder:* An unaccounted variable that influences both the dependent variable and independent variable, causing a spurious association
- *Effectiveness*: Describes whether interventions have the intended or expected effect under ordinary (clinical) circumstances
- *Efficacy*: Describes the impact of interventions under optimal (trial) conditions

- *Incidence*: The number of new cases divided by the number of people at risk during a specified time period
- *Null hypothesis*: The assumption that any difference observed in the results of two or more groups is due to chance (nonsignificant)
- *Type 1 error:* A false positive result – wrongful rejection of null hypothesis
- *Type 2 error:* A false negative result – wrongful acceptance of null hypothesis
- *Power:* The probability that a type 2 error will not be made in the study – finding a true difference when present. It is generally accepted that power should be 0.8 or greater (i.e. you should have an 80% or greater chance of finding a statistically significant difference when one exists)
- *Prevalence*: The number of existing cases divided by the total number of people in a population
- *Reliability*: How consistent a test is on repeated measurements
- *Sensitivity*: The proportion of subjects with the disorder who have a positive result (i.e. the proportion of true positives)
- *Specificity*: The proportion of subjects who do not have the disorder and who have a negative test (i.e. the proportion of true negatives)
- *Validity*: The extent to which a test measures what it is supposed to measure

Statistical definitions
- *Absolute risk (AR)*: The incidence rate of the outcome
- *Absolute risk reduction (ARR)*: Difference in AR between the control group and experimental group
- *Alpha level*: Threshold to decide whether to accept or reject the null hypothesis (typically set at 0.05)
- *Confidence interval (CI)*: A range of certainty within which the true population result lies (typically set as 95%)
- *Hazard rate*: Probability of an endpoint event in a time interval divided by the duration of the time interval
- *Hazard ratio*: Hazard rate in the experimental arm divided by the hazard rate in the control arm – compares experimental and control groups throughout the study duration unlike the relative risk (RR) and odds ratio (OR)
- *Likelihood ratio for a negative test result*: How much more likely is a negative test to be found in a person with as opposed to without the condition?
- *Likelihood ratio for a positive test result*: How much more likely is a positive test to be found in a person with as opposed to without the condition?
- *Mean*: Sum of all values divided by the sample size
- *Median*: Middle value when data from a sample is sorted into ascending order
- *Mode*: Most frequent value in a sample
- *Negative predictive value (NPV)*: The proportion of subjects with a negative test result who do not have the disorder
- *Number needed to harm (NNH)*: Number of subjects treated for one extra subject to have the adverse outcome compared with the control intervention
- *Number needed to treat (NNT)*: Number of subjects who must be treated with the intervention compared with the control for one additional subject to experience the beneficial outcome

- *Odds*: Expression of chance – the ratio of the number of times an event is likely to occur divided by the number of times it is likely not to occur
- *Odds ratio*: Ratio of the odds of having the outcome in the experimental group relative to the odds of having the outcome in the control group (log OR of 0 reflect the same outcome rates)
- *P-value*: The probability of getting the observed results by chance
- *Positive predictive value (PPV)*: The proportion of subjects with a positive test result who do have the disorder
- *Relative risk (RR)*: Ratio of the probability of the outcome in the experimental group to the probability of the outcome in the control group
- *Relative risk reduction (RRR)*: Difference in the risk of the outcome in the experimental group, expressed as a proportion of the risk in the control group
- *Risk*: Probability of something happening – number of times an event is likely to occur divided by the total number of events possible
- *Risk/benefit ratio*: Number needed to harm to number needed to treat ratio
- *Standard deviation (SD)*: Square root of the variance – measures the spread of data relative to the mean
- *Variance:* Average of squared differences around the mean – indicates the amount of variation in the data

Bias

Background

Bias refers to the introduction of a systematic error into sampling or testing by selecting one outcome over others. This can occur at any stage in the design, running, analysis and reporting of a study, and has the potential to influence results. Numerous forms of bias exist, which can be broadly classified into selection, observation and reporting bias (see **Table 1**).

Table 1 Types of bias		
Type of bias		**Definition**
Selection bias	Berkson bias	Arises when the sample population is taken from a hospital setting but the hospital cases do not reflect the rate or severity of the condition in the community population
	Diagnostic purity bias	Arises when co-morbidity is excluded in the sample population, such that the sample population does not reflect the true complexity of cases in the population
	Neyman bias	Occurs when the prevalence of a condition does not reflect in its incidence – usually due to a time gap between the onset of a condition and the actual selection of the study population (e.g. rapidly progressive conditions such as pancreatic cancer)

Continues opposite

Table 1 *Continued*		
Type of bias		**Definition**
Observation bias	Interviewer bias	Arises when the researcher is not blinded to the subject's group allocation in the study, and this alters the researchers' approach to the subject and the recording of results
	Response bias	Arises in any study in which the subjects answer questions in the way they believe the researcher wants them to answer, rather than according to their true beliefs
	Hawthorne effect	Arises when subjects alter their behaviour, usually positively because they are aware they are being observed in a study
	Recall bias	Arises when subjects selectively remember details from the past – can be particularly problematic in case-control studies and in cross-sectional surveys
	Attrition bias	Arises due to drop out of subjects such that the final study population is no longer representative of the true population
	Lead-time bias	Arises when a disease is detected by a screening or surveillance test earlier than it would have been if it had been diagnosed by its clinical appearance. This time lag or 'lead time' during which the disease is asymptomatic is not taken into account during the survival analysis
Reporting bias	Publication bias	Arises from the failure to publish the results of a study on the basis of the direction or strength of the study findings
	All's well bias	Arises when a dominant theory precludes the publication of opposing theories

Types of studies

Background

Clinical research can be categorised into observational studies, experimental studies or evidence summaries. Observational studies include case reports, case series, case-control studies, cohort studies and cross-sectional studies. Experimental studies include randomised controlled trials (RCTs) and crossover trials. Evidence summaries comprise narrative reviews, systematic reviews and meta-analyses (see **Table 2**).

Principles of study design

Table 2 Types of studies			
Types of study		**Description**	**Advantages and disadvantages**
Observational (descriptive)	Case report	Description of a single case, which is typically rare, has unique characteristics, poses a diagnostic or management challenge	*Advantages*: Useful for identifying new or rare diseases and for generating a hypothesis
			Disadvantages: Anecdotal, cannot be repeated, prone to chance association and bias

Continues overleaf

Table 2 Continued			
Types of study		Description	Advantages and disadvantages
	Case series	Description of a series of cases, which is typically rare, has unique characteristics, poses a diagnostic or management challenge	*Advantages:* Useful for studying rare diseases and treatment approaches *Disadvantages:* Anecdotal, prone to chance association and bias
Observational (analytical)	Case-control study	Subjects who have the outcome (cases) are matched with subjects who do not have the outcome (controls) and assessed whether they have been exposed to one or more risk factors in the past *Aim:* To evaluate if odds of prior exposure or risk factor differs by disease state	*Advantages:* Quick, cheap, few subjects required, useful for demonstrating rare associations *Disadvantages:* Recall bias, confounding factors
	Cohort study	A group of subjects exposed to a risk factor are matched to a group of subjects not exposed to a risk factor, at the beginning of the study no subject has the outcome *Aim:* To evaluate if exposure or risk factor is associated with later development of disease	*Advantages:* Direct estimation of disease incidence rates, assess temporal relationships and multiple outcomes *Disadvantages:* Expensive to set up and maintain, bias if subjects drop out, confounding factors
	Cross-sectional study	Prevalence of the exposure and the outcome in a population at one point in time is determined *Aim:* To establish disease prevalence	*Advantages:* Useful to establish association, cheap *Disadvantages:* No information on temporal sequence of events, cannot determine any cause-and-effect relationship between the exposure and outcome
Experimental	RCT	Subjects in the study are randomly allocated to a treatment and control group, for comparison and differences are measured *Aim:* To investigate therapeutic efficacy of an intervention	*Advantages:* Gold standard, reliable measure of efficacy *Disadvantages:* Time-consuming, expensive, affected by noncompliance and missing outcomes

Continues opposite

Table 2 *Continued*			
Types of study		**Description**	**Advantages and disadvantages**
	Crossover trial	All subjects receive one treatment and then switch to the other treatment halfway through the study *Aim*: To investigate therapeutic efficacy of an intervention	*Advantages*: Useful for studying rare disease (lack of subjects would make conventional trial underpowered), subjects act as own controls *Disadvantages*: Results affected if dissimilar conditions exist at the two time points
Evidence summary	Narrative review	A review summarising the evidence of specific topic from one or more perspectives *Aim:* To provide an up-to-date summary of current available evidence	*Advantages*: Provides useful summary of current available evidence *Disadvantages*: Influenced by authors' perspective and potential sources of reporting bias
	Systematic review	A review of a clearly formulated question that uses systematic and explicit methods to identify, select, and critically appraise relevant research, and to collect and analyse data from the studies that are included in the review *Aim*: To provide an unbiased summary of current available evidence	*Advantages*: Provides useful, unbiased summary of current available evidence *Disadvantages*: Limited by the quality of included studies
	Meta-analysis	A quantitative systematic review *Aim*: To provide an unbiased summary of current available evidence	*Advantages*: Provides useful, unbiased summary of current available evidence *Disadvantages*: Limited by the quality of included studies

Levels of evidence

Evidence-based medicine relies on the use of current best evidence in making decisions about patient care. The quality of evidence is graded using a hierarchical system, and one such example is the Oxford Centre for Evidence-Based Medicine (CEBM) levels of evidence (see **Table 3**). Additionally, the Grading of Recommendations Assessment, Development and Evaluation (GRADE) working group has developed an approach to grading of quality of evidence and strength of recommendations. With this approach, the overall quality of evidence is categorised as high, moderate, low or very low.

Table 3 Oxford CEBM levels of evidence

Level	Description
1a	Evidence from a systematic review or meta-analysis of RCTs
1b	Evidence from an individual RCT
1c	Evidence from all or none RCT
2a	Evidence from a systematic review or meta-analysis of cohort studies
2b	Evidence from an individual cohort study or low quality RCT
2c	Evidence from 'outcomes' research or ecological studies
3a	Evidence from a systematic review or meta-analysis of case-control studies
3b	Evidence from an individual case-control study
4	Evidence from case series or low-quality cohort and case-control studies
5	Expert opinion without explicit critical appraisal, or based on physiology, bench research or 'first principles'

Graphical representation of data

Data from systematic reviews and meta-analyses

Forest plots
- A forest plot is a graphical summary of results from clinical or scientific studies addressing a specific outcome (see **Table 4** below)

Table 4 Example forest plot displaying results of a fictitious meta-analysis

Study IDs	Intervention group n/N[1]	Control group n/N	Relative risk (fixed) 95% CI[2]	Weight[3] (%)	Relative risk (fixed) 95% CI[2]
Rowling JK 2000	1/131	2/133		17.8	0.50 (0.05–5.49)
Albus D 2003	7/279	9/290		77.7	0.84 (0.36–1.93)
Hermione G 2005	3/102	1/101		4.5	3.00 (0.12–72.77)
Total	512	542	Left Right	100.0	0.87 (0.41–1.87)[4]
			0.01 0.1 1 10	100	

Continues opposite

Table 4 *Continued*
Test for heterogeneity Chi-square = 0.79, df = 2, ρ = 0.67, I^2 = 0.0%[5]
Test for overall effect ζ = 0.35, ρ = 0.7[6]
1. N = total number in group, n = number in group with the outcome
2. Outcome of interest in picture and in number. Fixed effect model used for meta-analysis
3. Influence of studies on overall meta-analysis. Overall effect
5. Heterogeneity (I^2) – 0%. So, we use fixed effect model
6. p value indicating level of statistical significance
Source: Figure reused with permission from 'Forest plot at a glance', by Tran Quang Hong originally posted on Students 4 Best Evidence, 1st July 2016.

- The result from each individual study is presented as a weighted estimate with confidence intervals, which are pooled together to provide a summary estimate and confidence interval

See sample Forest plot above:

- The fourth column: Relative risk (fixed) 95% CI – visually represents the outcomes. The boxes show effect estimates from single studies, while the diamond shows the pooled result. The horizontal lines through the boxes illustrate the length of the CI (i.e. the longer the horizontal line, the wider the CI, and the less reliable the study results). The width of the diamond similarly represents the CI. The vertical line is the 'line of no effect', at which point there is no clear difference between the intervention and control groups. For adverse outcomes (e.g. mortality), those results left of the line of no effect favour the intervention over the control (i.e. RR ratio less than 1). Similarly, for desirable outcomes (e.g. disease-free survival), those results right of the line favour the intervention over the control (i.e. RR ratio more than 1). Finally, if the diamond touches the vertical line, the overall (combined) result is not statistically significant (i.e. the outcome rates are similar between the intervention and control groups)
- The fifth column: Weight (%) – numerically estimates the effect that an individual study has on the pooled result. For example, the bigger the sample size and the narrower the CI, the greater the percentage weight, the bigger the box, and the greater the overall effect that the study has on the pooled outcome
- The sixth column: Relative risk (fixed) 95% CI – numerically represents the data in column four. When the 95% CI does not include 1, the result is considered statistically significant
- Further information in the lower left corner of the plot:
  - *p*-value indicates the level of statistical significance. It can be said that the difference between the groups is statistically significant ($p < 0.05$) if the diamond shape does not touch the 'line of no effect'.
  - I^2 indicates the level of heterogeneity (0–100%). Studies are considered homogenous if $I^2 \leq 50\%$, indicating that a fixed-effect model meta-analysis can be used. $I^2 > 50\%$ indicates high heterogeneity, in which case a random effects model for meta-analysis should be used.

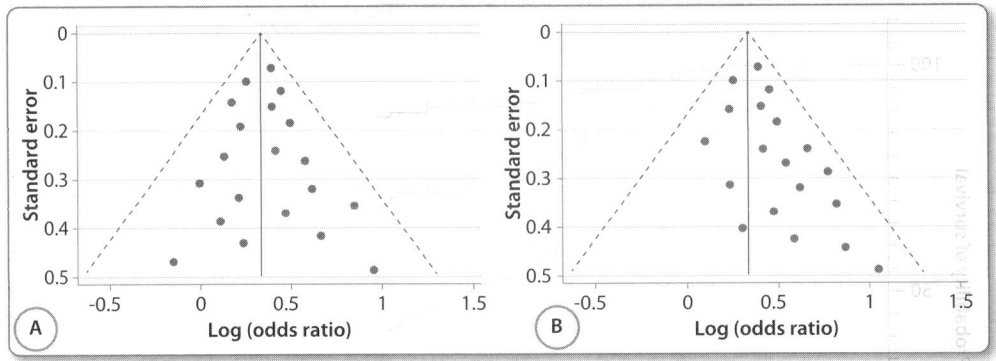

Figure 1 Example of funnel plots from two hypothetical meta-analyses A and B. The grey dots represent individual studies included in the meta-analyses, the dotted lines indicate the 95% confidence interval, and the central vertical line indicates the overall effect. Example A demonstrates plot symmetry indicating a low risk of publication bias, whereas example B demonstrates plot asymmetry indicating a high risk of publication bias.

Funnel plots
- A funnel plot evaluates the presence of publication bias and is typically used in systematic reviews and meta-analysis (**Figure 1**)
- In the absence of publication bias, results from high-quality studies should be plotted near the average, while results from low-quality studies will be spread evenly on both sides of the average, creating a funnel-shaped appearance.
- The presence of asymmetry in the funnel plot is suggestive of publication bias.
- Egger's test is a commonly used statistical test to assess potential publication bias via funnel plot asymmetry. As a general rule, this test is unreliable if the meta-analysis contains fewer than 10 studies. A p-value of < 0.05 using Egger's test indicates a high risk of publication bias

Data for survival and regression analysis
Kaplan–Meier curves
- A Kaplan–Meier curve is a form of survival analysis (**Figure 2**)
- Looks at event rates over the study period, rather than at a specific time point
- Commonly used for survival analyses (death) but may be used for any dichotomous outcome with an associated time quantifier (i.e. time to event)
- Determines survival probabilities and proportions of individuals surviving, providing estimation of a cumulative survival probability
- Should be accompanied by a 'number at risk' table. The number at risk at any specific time point will be equal to the total number of patients remaining in the study (i.e. those that have not experienced the event of interest or have been censored at this time point)

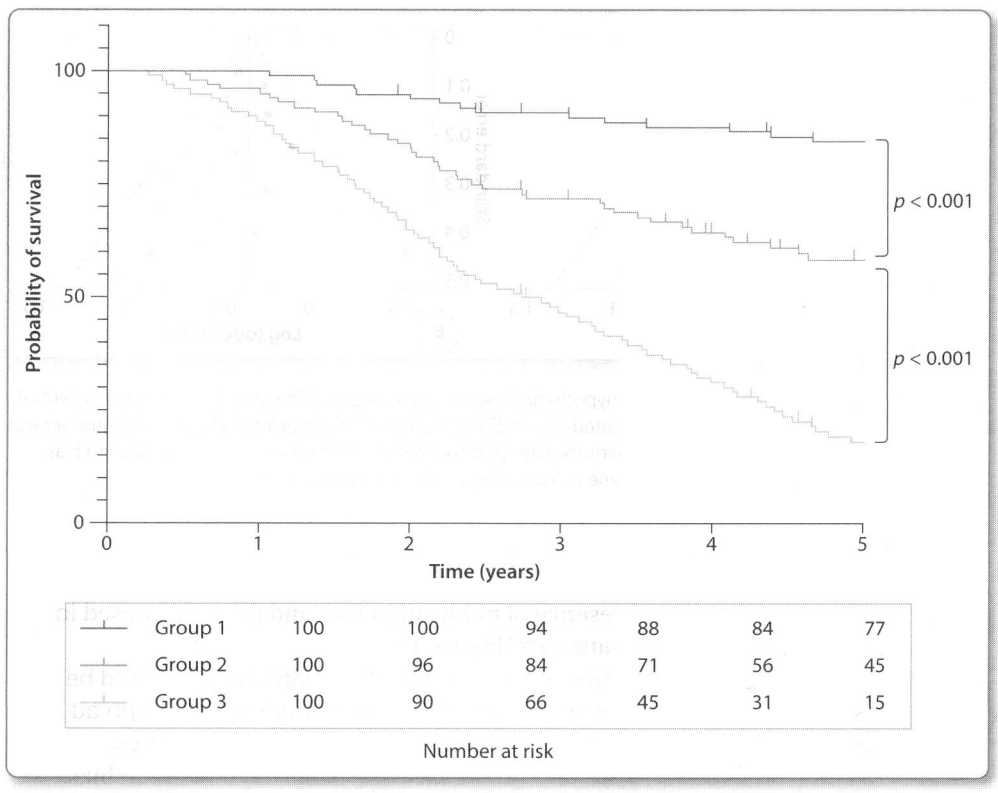

Figure 2: Kaplan–Meier survival curves comparing three hypothetical groups. The significance of the difference between groups has been compared using the Log-Rank test. A p-value of < 0.05 indicates a significant difference in survival between groups.

Regression analysis
- Regression expresses the relationship between two or more variables in the form of an equation
- Regression equation has predictive value but does not prove causality
- Linear regression is performed if the dependent variable is continuous, and logistic regression performed for a dichotomous dependent variable
- There are two types of regression:
  i. *Simple (univariate regression)*: Describes the relationship between a dependent variable and single explanatory variable
  ii. *Multiple (multi-variable) regression:* Describes the relationship between a dependent variable and two or more independent variables, which can be continuous or categorical

Data for diagnostic tests
Receiver operating characteristic (ROC) curves:
- A ROC curve is a graphical description of a test's performance in relation to a dichotomous outcome (**Figure 3**)

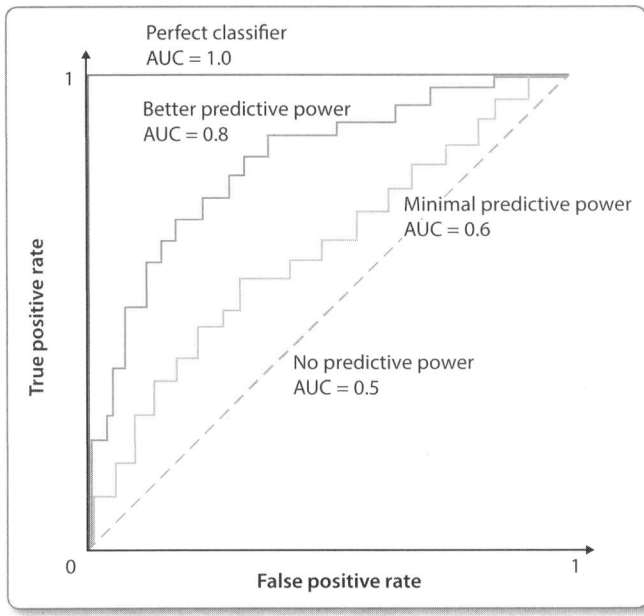

Figure 3 ROC curve demonstrating different AUC values.

- This is quantified by the area under the curve (AUC), which is generated by plotting the true positive rate (sensitivity) against the false positive rate (1 minus specificity) at various thresholds
- An AUC value of 0.5 means the test performs no better than chance, and an AUC of 1.0 indicates perfect performance/predictive ability of the test, i.e. the closer the AUC value is to 1.0, the better the test. See example of ROC curve below

Categories of data and statistical tests

Background
Data can be categorical, ordinal or continuous. Examples are as follows:
- Categorical data – gender
- Ordinal data – Likert scales
- Continuous data – height

Both ordinal and continuous data may demonstrate either a parametric (Gaussian) or non-parametric (non-Gaussian) distribution. Data with a non-parametric distribution can be either positively or negatively skewed. One method to determine the distribution is by comparing the mean, median and mode as demonstrated below:
- Parametric distribution – mean = median = mode
- Positive skew – mean > median > mode
- Negative skew – mode > median > mean

Statistical tests
Parametric tests are statistical tests that are based on the assumption that the data follows a Gaussian distribution. In contrast, non-parametric tests are statistical

tests that do not rely on assumptions of the data following a Gaussian distribution. Differences between parametric and non-parametric statistical tests are summarised in **Tables 5** and **6**.

Table 5 Comparison of parametric and non-parametric statistical tests

Parametric statistical tests	Non-parametric statistical tests
More assumptions	Fewer assumptions
More statistically powerful	Less statistically powerful
Uses actual values in the dataset for analysis	Uses ranking of values in the dataset for analysis
Results are easier to interpret	Results are more difficult to interpret

Table 6 Statistical tests used to analyse a given dataset

Sample type		Parametric data	Non-parametric data	Categorical data
Single sample		One-sample *t* test	Wilcoxon's signed rank test	Chi-squared test Fisher's exact test (small sample)
Two groups	Paired	*t* test	Wilcoxon's matched pairs test	McNemar's test
	Unpaired	*t* test	Mann–Whitney U test	Chi-squared test Fisher's exact test (small sample)
More than two groups	Paired	Repeated-measures ANOVA	Friedman's test	McNemar's test
	Unpaired	One-way ANOVA	Kruskal–Wallis	Chi-squared test

Screening tests

Background

Screening is a population-based strategy that aims to detect the presence of a disease before symptoms and/or signs are present so that treatment can be implemented at a stage where it is more effective – ultimately, reducing disease-related mortality (**Table 7**). The criteria required to justify the benefits of screening for a disease are as follows:
- The condition should be an important health problem
- There should be a recognisable latent or early symptomatic stage
- The natural history of the condition, including development from latent to declared disease, should be adequately understood
- There should be an accepted treatment for patients with recognised disease
- There should be a suitable test or examination that has a high level of accuracy
- The test should be acceptable to the population
- There should be an agreed policy on whom to treat as patients
- Facilities for diagnosis and treatment should be available

Table 7 Advantages and disadvantages of screening	
Advantages of screening	Disadvantages of screening
• Early detection and treatment of disease • Reduction in disease-related morbidity and mortality • Potential for improved cost-effectiveness	• Risk of false positives – leads to unnecessary intervention, anxiety • Risk of false negatives – leads to false reassurance, delay in treatment • Overdiagnosis may result in unnecessary treatment • Lead time bias • Low absolute risk reduction

- The cost of screening (including diagnosis and treatment of patients diagnosed) should be economically balanced in relation to possible expenditure on medical care as a whole
- Screening should be a continuing process and not a 'once and for all' project

There are two main screening strategies:
1. Universal screening – this strategy aims to screen an entire population defined by a certain characteristic
2. Selective screening – this strategy aims to screen selected members of a population with certain risk factors

For successful screening, the screening test in question should be sufficiently accurate to detect the disease earlier than in the absence of screening. The sensitivity and the specificity of the screening test are important considerations when evaluating accuracy and are discussed below.

Sensitivity and specificity

Sensitivity

- Refers to the true positive rate – the proportion of all people with the disease who test positive
- A test with a sensitivity of 100% will have 0 false negatives
- A test with a high sensitivity is used to rule out disease – this is useful for screening diseases with low prevalence

Specificity

- Refers to the true negative rate – the proportion of all people without the disease who test negative
- A test with a specificity of 100% will have 0 false positives
- A test with a high specificity is used to rule in disease – this is useful for confirming a disease after initial screening

Positive and negative predictive values

Positive predictive value

- Refers to the probability that a person with a positive test result has the disease

- This varies directly with pre-test probability (disease prevalence) – the higher the pre-test probability, the higher the PPV

Negative predictive value
- Refers to the probability that a person with a negative test result does not have the disease
- This varies inversely with pre-test probability – the lower the pre-test probability, the higher the NPV

Types of statistical error

Type 1 and 2 errors
Statistical testing is based on null hypothesis, which the test aims to accept or reject. Type 1 and 2 errors occur when the null hypothesis is incorrectly accepted or rejected.

Type 1 error
- Arises when the null hypothesis is incorrectly rejected (false positive) – a difference is identified when none exists
- Alpha (α), which is the threshold for significance (typically 0.05) refers to the probability of a type 1 error occurring – at an α of 0.05, a type 1 error would occur in 1 out of 20 tests
- The probability of a type 1 error can be reduced by lowering the α level (e.g. 0.05 → 0.01) – there is an increase in probability of a type 2 error with this

Type 2 error
- Arises when the null hypothesis is incorrectly accepted (false negative) – no difference is identified when one exists
- Beta (β) (typically set at 0.2) refers to the probability of a type 2 error occurring – at a β of 0.2, a type 2 error would occur in 1 out of 5 tests
- The probability of a type 2 error can be reduced by increasing the sample size

Power
Power refers to the probability that a type 2 error will not be made in the study (defined as 1 – beta). A power cut-off of 0.8 is typically used. Several measures can be made to increase power including:
- Increasing sample size
- Increasing expected effect size
- Increasing precision of measurement

Sub-group analysis

Background
Sub-group analysis involves analysis of data from study subjects split into sub-groups defined by a specific set of variables. The aim of this form of analysis is to

determine if the treatment effect observed differs in magnitude across selected subsets of interest. Sub-group analysis can be used to investigate heterogeneous results, or to answer specific questions about particular patient groups, types of intervention or types of study. Analysis of effect size estimates can be within (sub-group analysis) or between (interaction analysis) sub-groups.

Limitations
Nonetheless, there are important limitations to be aware of when interpreting this form of analysis. Firstly, sub-group analyses are inherently observational and are not based on randomised comparisons. Secondly, the sample size of sub-groups tends to be smaller, which increases the probability of a type 2 error. Thirdly, the probability of false positive and false negative significance tests increases as more sub-group analyses are performed. This raises the concern of data dredging, which refers to the collection of excessive amounts of data on the groups in the study with multiple comparisons of the groups looking for any differences in outcomes.

Miscellaneous key concepts

Impact factor
Impact factor is a measure of the frequency with which an average article in a journal has been cited in a particular year or period and is commonly used as a surrogate measure of the importance of a journal. Impact factors are calculated by dividing the number of current year citations by the source items published in that journal during the previous 2 years. These are published annually in the Journal of Citation Reports and may vary from year to year.

It is important to understand that impact factors are subject to manipulation as journals may choose to publish highly citable papers early in the year (i.e. to maximise time to accrue citations). Editors may also encourage authors to preferentially reference from their own journal to increase subsequent impact factors.
The following are the impact factors for key surgical journals from 2018.
- JAMA Surgery – 10.668
- Annals of Surgery – 9.476
- British Journal of Surgery – 5.572

Reporting checklists

CONSORT statement
- Evidence-based minimum set of recommendations for reporting RCTs
- Provides a standard approach for authors to prepare reports of trial findings
- Comprises a 25-item checklist and flow diagram

PRISMA
- Evidence-based minimum set of recommendations for reporting in systematic reviews and meta-analyses

- Provides a standard approach for authors to prepare reports of systematic reviews and meta-analyses
- Comprises a 27-item checklist and flow diagram

Quality assessment

Jadad scale (Oxford quality scoring system)
- Procedure to independently assess the methodological quality of a clinical trial
- A three-point questionnaire forms the basis of the scale:
    i. Was this a randomised study? (Maximum score of 2)
    ii. Was the study double blind? (Maximum score of 2)
    iii. Was there a description of dropouts and withdrawals? (Maximum score of 1)
- A score out of a maximum of five is allocated, with a score of 0 indicating poor methodological quality and a score of 5 indicating rigorous methodological quality

Modified Cochrane Collaboration's tool for assessing risk of bias:
- Tool to assess the risk of bias in RCTs
- Covers six domains of bias including selection bias, performance bias, detection bias, attrition bias, reporting bias and other bias
- A judgement of high, low or unclear risk of material bias is allocated for each item

Sample academic viva

The following two papers have been selected to illustrate core statistical concepts and provide examples of the type of viva questions that are frequently asked during the FRCS academic station. They have not been chosen based on their individual merits or limitations and will be appraised in a constructive fashion. The full journal articles can be viewed open access via the respective journal websites.

Sample 1

Title: Use of Prophylactic Mesh when Creating a Colostomy does not Prevent Parastomal Hernia: A Randomised Controlled Trial - STOMAMESH
Authors: Odensten et al.
Published: Annals of Surgery
Date: March 2019
DOI: 10.1097/SLA.0000000000002542
PMID: 29064900

Q. 1.1 How would you summarise this paper?

This paper was authored by a Swedish group and reports the outcomes of a double-blinded multi-centre randomised controlled trial (STOMAMESH). It was published in Annals of Surgery in 2019. The research question was whether the use of prophylactic mesh when creating a permanent end colostomy during open colorectal surgery prevents parastomal hernia formation. Patients in the intervention group had a lightweight polypropylene mesh inserted in the sublay position at the site of colostomy formation and patients in the control group had no mesh inserted. The primary outcome measure was parastomal hernia rate. The secondary outcome was peri-operative complication rates. This is a clinically relevant research question since parastomal hernia is a common complication after colorectal surgery with significant associated morbidity. This study randomised 232 patients, with 211 included in the final analysis. The rate of both clinically and radiologically detected parastomal hernia at 1-year follow-up was approximately 30%, with no significant difference between the mesh and non-mesh groups. There was no significant difference in peri-operative complications between treatment groups. The authors conclude that the use of prophylactic reinforcing mesh does not alter the rate of parastomal hernia.

Q. 1.2 What is the study hypothesis and null hypothesis?

The study hypothesis was that polypropylene mesh placed in the sublay position around a colostomy decreases the risk of parastomal hernia. The null hypothesis is that prophylactic mesh does not decreases the risk of parastomal hernia.

Q. 1.3 What is a CONSORT diagram and why is this important?

The CONSORT (Consolidated Standards of Reporting Trials) statement consists of a checklist and flow diagram to improve the quality of reporting of RCTs. A CONSORT diagram is a flow diagram which provides information about how a trial was conducted, reporting enrolment, allocation, follow-up and analysis of patients involved in the RCT. It is important to analyse the presence and quality of any CONSORT diagram in an RCT, since it provides a broad view of how the trial was conducted, in addition to concisely reporting the employed methodology. In this study, the CONSORT diagram clearly illustrates how many patients were randomised into the mesh ($n = 114$) and non-mesh groups ($n = 118$), how many patients were lost to follow-up (mesh; $n = 10$, non-mesh; $n = 11$) and how many were included in the final analysis in each treatment arm. An attrition rate of <10–20% is generally considered acceptable in RCTs for minimising the chance of attrition bias, therefore the 9% loss to follow-up rate observed in this study is reasonable, however.

Q. 1.4 What is a power calculation and has it been performed appropriately?

Power calculations are used to determine the minimum study sample size required to answer a research question (or null hypothesis) avoiding a type 2 error (i.e. accept a false null hypothesis). There are three main components of a power calculation: (1) The statistical power – usually set at 80%. (2) The significance level – usually set at 95%. (3) The expected effect size – the magnitude of the expected study result, usually based on similar studies or a pilot study. In this study, the authors have performed a power calculation which is appropriately described in the methods section to calculate the required sample size for this RCT. The factors considered in this calculation were a parastomal hernia incidence rate of 20% without and 5% with mesh, a 5-year survival rate of just over 50% (based on the fact the majority of patients were operated on for colorectal cancer) and an accepted significance level of 95%. To achieve a power of 80% the authors have calculated that 220 patients were required, subsequently randomising 232 for the study.

Q. 1.5 What is the difference between intention-to-treat and per-protocol analysis?

Intention-to-treat (ITT) analysis includes all patients in the groups to which they were randomised, regardless of their adherence to the entry criteria, treatment received or any deviation from the study protocol. ITT analysis ensures comparability between groups as obtained through randomisation, maintains sample size, and eliminates bias. This is the recommended method of analysis in RCTs aiming to detect superiority. Per-protocol analysis is a comparison of treatment groups that includes only those patients who completed the treatment originally allocated and strictly adhered to protocol. If done alone, this analysis may lead to bias. In non-inferiority trials per-protocol analysis is important but should be reported alongside ITT analysis. Data from this study was analysed on an ITT basis.

Q. 1.6 Are there any potential limitations of this study?

Design: This was a well-designed RCT with well explained and suitable methodology for randomisation, data collection and analysis. However, the endpoint of parastomal hernia recurrence at 1 year is a potential limitation of this study since, as stated in the opening sentence, 'parastomal hernias mostly develop within 2 years of surgery but can occur up to 30 years later', and longer-term results would be of clinical interest. This is true for both parastomal hernia rate and detection of mesh-related complications which may feasibly present after 1 year follow-up. However, as is the case with many RCTs, longer-term follow-up results may well be reported in a future publication.

Generalisability of results: This study included only patients undergoing open colorectal surgery and the chosen technique of mesh insertion required a midline incision. Since a large proportion of elective colorectal surgery is now performed laparoscopically these results may not be generalisable to current practice. Furthermore, as illustrated in Tables titled as 'Types of studies' and 'Oxford CEBM levels of evidence', a large number of eligible patients from participating hospitals were not included in the trial with some notable differences in patient characteristics including ASA grade, age and surgical timing (elective vs. emergency) which may have introduced selection bias into the study.

Q. 1.7 Would this paper change your practice?

This was a well-designed RCT investigating a clinically relevant research question. The study population appears homogenous between treatment groups and there is a relatively low attrition rate. Parastomal hernia remains a significant problem in clinical practice, particularly in patients with end colostomies, and it is of interest to evaluate techniques for reducing its incidence. Based on the results of this study I would not routinely utilise light-weight polypropylene mesh inserted in the sublay position at the site of colostomy formation during open colorectal surgery. However, I would want to assess the long-term results of the present study and evaluate the literature regarding the efficacy of other surgical approaches before definitively deciding whether to use prophylactic mesh during colostomy formation.

Sample 2

Title: C-reactive protein level as a predictor of difficult emergency laparoscopic cholecystectomy
Authors: Ng et al.
Published: BJS open
Date: July 2019
DOI: 10.1002/bjs5.50189
PMID: 31592082

Q. 2.1 How would you summarise this paper?

This paper was authored by a group from Scotland and published in BJS open in 2019. The research question was whether pre-operative CRP levels are able to predict the degree of operative difficulty in emergency laparoscopic cholecystectomy. The study included patients undergoing emergency laparoscopic cholecystectomy and intra-operative cholangiography by a single surgeon in a single centre between September 2012 and December 2017 for any biliary pathology who had a pre-operative documented CRP value. The exposure was pre-operative peak CRP level, and the primary outcome measure was surgical difficulty based on a pre-determined (Nassar) scale. This is a relevant research question since NICE guidelines currently recommend consideration of emergency laparoscopic cholecystectomy for patients with acute cholecystitis up to 7 days following onset of symptoms; however, some surgeons may be put off in patients with high CRP values owing to the perceived operative difficulty and associated morbidity. This was a retrospective, cohort study which included 804 patients in the final analysis. The key findings were that a CRP value of >90 predicted higher operative difficulty with 71.5% sensitivity and 70.5% specificity, and that pre-operative peak CRP level was predictive of higher operative difficulty when adjusting for confounding variables using multi-variable logistic regression analysis. The authors conclude that raised pre-operative CRP levels were associated with greater operative difficulty and could be of use in planning surgical management in patients with acute biliary admissions.

Q. 2.2 What is receiver operating characteristic analysis and what is the significance of these results?

Receiver operating characteristic (ROC) analysis is a graphical approach for analysing the performance of a classifier (in this case CRP) to predict a binary outcome (in this case operative difficulty grade 1–3 vs. grade 4–5). The continuous variable CRP can be plotted graphically, with false positive rate on the X-axis and true positive rate on the Y-axis, to compare the relative performance of different CRP levels in predicting the outcome variable. In this study, the optimum CRP value for predicting operative difficulty in this patient cohort was unknown so ROC analysis was used to determine a threshold which maximised sensitivity and specificity of this classifier to predict the outcome. Results demonstrated this threshold to be a CRP level of 90 mg/L which predicted operative difficulty with 71.5% sensitivity and 70.5% specificity. The area under the curve (AUC) for peak pre-operative CRP level to predict operative difficulty was 0.78 indicating acceptable prediction value.

Q. 2.3 What is the difference between sensitivity and specificity?

Sensitivity refers to the true positive rate of a test. In this context, for patients with grade 4–5 operative difficulty a CRP threshold value of >90 mg/L predicted this 71.5% of the time. Specificity refers to the true negative rate of a test. In this context, for patients with grade 1–3 operative difficulty a CRP threshold value of <90 mg/L predicted this 70.5% of the time.

Q. 2.4 What is an odds ratio and what does this result signify? Why has the author used odds ratios rather than relative risk?

An OR is the ratio of the odds of having a particular outcome in one group relative to the odds of having the outcome in another (control) group. In this study, the odds of a patient with a peak CRP value of >90 mg/L having a higher operative difficulty was 5.9 times greater compared to the control group of patients with a peak CRP < 90 mg/L, giving an OR of 5.90. This result is statistically significant (with a p-value set at <0.05) since the 95% CI does not cross 1.0, in this case 2.80 to 12.50. The author has used multi-variable logistic regression analysis; therefore, the output will always be reported as an OR rather than RR. The other variables apart from CRP which were included in the multi-variable analysis were number of days from admission to surgery, age and sex.

Q. 2.5 In Table titled as 'Statistical tests used to analyse a given dataset' the author has reported both mean and median CRP values. What is the difference between mean and median and when should they be used?

The mean is the sum of all values divided by the sample size. The median is the middle value when data from a sample is sorted into ascending order. Both mean and median values can be calculated for any continuous data set. As a general rule, mean (and standard deviation) are reported for parametric (normally distributed) data and median (and interquartile range) are reported for non-parametric data. It is unusual to report both median and mean values for the same variable. If it is unknown whether a data set is normally distributed, then statistical tests may be used to test for normality (e.g. the *Kolmogorov–Smirnov test*). Since this has not been reported in this study it is difficult to determine (without evaluating the original dataset) whether CRP level was normally distributed and hence reporting mean or median more appropriate.

However, the fact that the mean and median values are noticeably different would suggest that the data is unlikely to be normally distributed. The author has performed a student's t-test to test for significance of the differences between CRP group means, this test should only be used for parametric data. The non-parametric equivalent is the *Mann–Whitney U* test.

Q. 2.6 Are there any potential limitations of this study?

Design: This study allowed for the evaluation of a large cohort of patients undergoing emergency cholecystectomy. Although data were collected prospectively, the retrospective, observational study design remained susceptible to bias and impossible to rule out confounding despite adjustments for several prognostic factors. The prognostic/confounding factors included in the multi-variable logistic regression model seem reasonable; however, the authors have not detailed the rationale as to why they were chosen and there might be an argument for including the indication for surgery (e.g. biliary colic, cholecystitis, and pancreatitis) since this is likely to be a confounder affecting both the exposure (CRP) and outcome (operative difficulty). The inclusion of all biliary pathologies in the analysis may also have introduced heterogeneity in relation to both operative difficulty and CRP levels. It would also have been of interest to evaluate whether CRP levels and operative difficulty were associated with operative morbidity (e.g. bile leak) in this cohort, since this is arguably a more clinically relevant outcome. This may be due to the low rate of complications observed in the study cohort (3.9%); however, the authors do not provide further information regarding the severity or nature of these complications.

Generalisability of results: As a single-centre study, one potential advantage was that all procedures were performed by the same surgeon, in the same institution, thereby reducing heterogeneity surrounding peri-operative patient management. However, this also reduced the generalisability of the findings compared with a multi-centre, population-based approach. Furthermore, the author's routine use of intra-operative cholangiography and laparoscopic bile duct exploration instead of MRCP/ERCP is commendable, however, this may not reflect current practice in many hospitals. As stated by the authors, one potential limitation of this approach to managing patients with biliary disease relates to logistical difficulties and lack of early access to emergency theatre or a dedicated biliary surgical team which may further affect generalisability of these results.

Q. 2.7 Would this paper change your practice?

This is an interesting paper evaluating a clinically relevant research question. The primary outcome that a CRP value of >90 mg/L predicts operative difficulty with approximately 70% sensitivity and specificity is a useful clinical metric. The authors have provided a useful threshold level beyond which emergency laparoscopic cholecystectomy is more likely to be challenging which I will consider in my clinical practice. However, since this threshold will fail to predict a difficult laparoscopic cholecystectomy in almost 1 in 3 patients, I will also consider other patient and surgical factors when planning surgical management of acute biliary disease.

Chapter 2

Critical care

Ed Denison-Davies, Irfan Chaudry, Robin Som, Faddy Kamel

Scenario 1

Respiratory failure

A 62-year-old gentleman is on the ward 2 days after an elective right hemicolectomy. He has no other comorbidities. He has developed an oxygen requirement overnight, with saturations of 85% on 15 L/min oxygen.

Q. 1.1 How would you assess this patient on the ward round?

This patient should be managed with the initial approach used for all acutely unwell patients – the ABCDE approach:

Assessment, investigations, and interventions should ideally occur simultaneously:

Airway: Ensure the patient has a patent airway.
Place the patient on oxygen, ensuring he has intermittent saturation monitoring aiming for an oxygen saturation of 94–98%, unless he has a history of chronic obstructive pulmonary disease (COPD) when the target should be reduced to 88–92%.

Breathing: Look at the respiratory pattern. Is he using accessory muscles to help with breathing (e.g. sat bolt upright; nasal flaring)?
Are both sides of the chest moving equally?
Count the respiratory rate.
Percussion and auscultation of the chest
Is a chest X-ray (CXR) indicated?
Confirm saturations; does the patient need an arterial blood gas (ABG)?

Circulation: Does the patient feel warm or cool peripherally?
Peripheral versus central capillary refill time
Is there a good radial pulse; what is the pulse rate; is it regular?
Examine the abdomen.
What is the blood pressure (BP) and urine output?
Perform and interpret an electrocardiogram (ECG).
Is other imaging required?

Disability: Perform a Glasgow Coma Scale (GCS) on the patient using eyes, voice, and motor response:

E1 = no eye opening
E2 = eye opening to pain
E3 = eye opening to voice
E4 = eye opening spontaneously

V1 = no verbal response
V2 = incomprehensible sounds
V3 = inappropriate words
V4 = confused
V5 = orientated

M1 = no motor response
M2 = extension to pain
M3 = flexion to pain
M4 = withdrawal from pain
M5 = localising pain
M6 = obeys commands

Exposure: Perform a temperature.
Expose the patient to ensure no clinical clues are missed.

Your assessment reveals that this gentleman's saturations are 85% on 60% humidified oxygen. His postoperative CXR shows consolidation at the right base, and you diagnose a pneumonia; his ABG demonstrates – pH 7.38; pO_2 7 kPa; pCO_2 5 kPa; HCO_3^- 24; BE −1.

Q. 1.2 Explain the different types of respiratory failure and how these are treated.

Type 1 respiratory failure (RF1) is defined as:
Hypoxaemia (PaO_2 < 8 kPa) with a normal carbon dioxide (CO_2) level ($PaCO_2$ < 6.7 kPa)

Causes of RF1 include:
- Acute respiratory distress syndrome (ARDS)
- Pulmonary embolism (PE)
- Pneumonia

Treatment of RF1 involves:
- Increasing the fractional inspired oxygen concentration (FIO_2) that your patient is receiving targeting an oxygen saturation of 94–98%. If the patient has COPD, an oxygen saturation of 88–92% is acceptable if indicated (check patient's observations to determine what their normal oxygen saturation is)
- As the patient's oxygen requirements increase ensure a medical registrar and a critical care outreach/registrar review takes place
- Ensure you treat the underlying cause of the RF1 – e.g. if caused by a pneumonia then start antibiotics

Type 2 respiratory failure (RF2) is defined as:
Hypoxaemia (PaO_2 < 8 kPa) with a raised CO_2 level ($PaCO_2$ ≥ 6.7 kPa)

Causes of RF2 include:
- Chronic obstructive pulmonary disease
- Alcohol
- Flail chest
- Guillain-Barré syndrome (autoimmune condition which can be triggered by surgery leading to muscle weakness)
- Life-threatening/near fatal asthma

Treatment of RF2 involves:
- Increasing the FiO_2 that your patient is receiving targeting an oxygen saturation of 94–98%. If the patient has COPD, an oxygen saturation of 88–92% is acceptable if indicated (check patient's observations to determine what their normal oxygen saturation is; patients at risk of RF2 have moderate to severe COPD and may be on long-term oxygen therapy). Hypoxia kills before hypercarbia so ensure a patient receives adequate oxygen therapy
- As the patient's oxygen requirements increase ensure a medical registrar and a critical care outreach/registrar review takes place
- Ensure you treat the underlying cause of the RF2

You increase this gentleman's inspired oxygen by applying a 15 L Hudson mask with reservoir bag (non-rebreather) targeting an oxygen saturation of 94–98%.

Q. 1.3 What oxygen masks do you know; what oxygen flow rates are required and what FiO_2 do they deliver?

Oxygen delivery devices are divided into fixed and variable performance oxygen masks.

Fixed performance masks, also known as 'Venturi' masks, use the Bernoulli's principle. This principle states that if oxygen (a 'fluid') travels through a narrow opening it speeds up while the surrounding air pressure drops. This pressure drop to below atmospheric means that air can be entrained see diagram below for schematic representation of Bernoulli's principle.

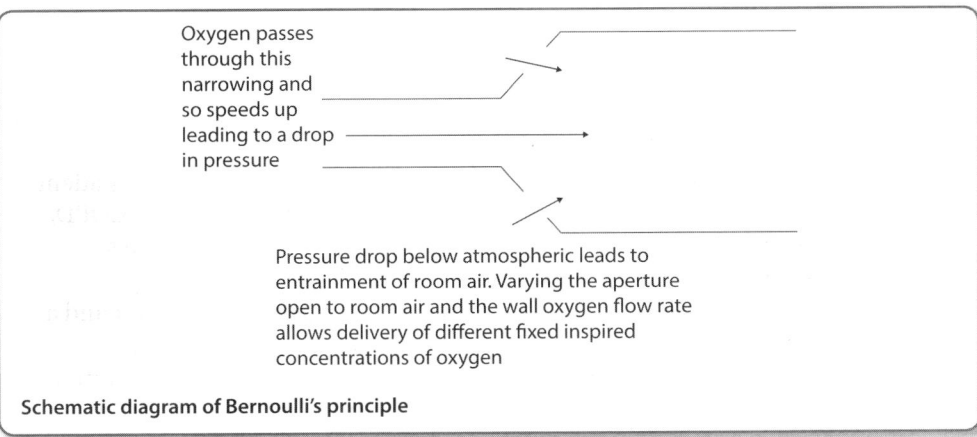

Schematic diagram of Bernoulli's principle

Colour	Oxygen flow	Fraction of inspired oxygen (FiO_2)
Blue	2 L/min	24%
White	4 L/min	28%
Orange	6 L/min	31%
Yellow	8 L/min	35%
Red	10 L/min	40%
Green	15 L/min	60%

Variable performance mask FIO_2 is much more susceptible to patient factors such as peak inspiratory flow rate and the presence of a respiratory pause than the fixed performance masks. For all types of masks, tightness of fit will also affect FIO_2. Below is a table of estimated FIO_2 for variable performance masks:

Oxygen delivery device	Oxygen flow	Fraction of inspired oxygen (FIO_2)
Nasal cannulae – also dependent on how much a patient mouth breathes	2 L/min	28%
	4 L/min	36%
	6 L/min	44%
Hudson mask	5–6 L/min	40%
	9–10 L/min	60%
Non-rebreather mask – may require higher flow rates and flow should be adjusted so that the reservoir bag does not deflate more one-third third during inspiration	10–12 L/min	80–100%

The critical care team review this gentleman at your request and decide to admit him to the intensive care unit for further management.

Q. 1.4 What additional respiratory support can critical care offer for types 1 and 2 respiratory failure?

Advanced respiratory support can be divided into:
- Continuous positive airway pressure (CPAP)
- Non-invasive ventilation (NIV) – also known as BiPAP
- Invasive ventilation
- CPAP – generally used in RF1 as it improves oxygenation
  Continuous positive airway pressure provides positive airway pressure throughout all phases of spontaneous ventilation. It increases the functional residual capacity (FRC) of the lung (the amount of gas in the lung at end exhalation) and opens collapsed alveoli. By splinting alveoli open more oxygen is able to get into the bloodstream – therefore leading to improved oxygenation. CPAP also reduces left ventricular transmural pressure and therefore increases cardiac output – hence it is a very effective for treatment of pulmonary oedema. Normal starting pressures are 5 cm H_2O and can be increased to up to 15 cm H_2O [though at this level patients do swallow a lot of air and the stomach may need to be decompressed with a nasogastric (NG) tube].
  - NIV – generally used in RF2 – improves oxygenation and ventilation (CO_2 clearance)
  Non-invasive ventilation provides positive airway pressure at two different levels throughout all phases of spontaneous ventilation. As with CPAP, it increases the FRC and will lead to an improvement in oxygenation. However, its main use is to increase a patient's minute volume by increasing the volume of each breath (tidal volume) and so lower the patient's CO_2 levels. Hence why this is favoured for RF2

or in patients who purely have a raised pCO_2 (where additional oxygen may not need to be administered). Starting pressures are usually 5 cm H_2O for the lower level and 10–15 cm H_2O for the higher level
- Invasive ventilation – used in all types of respiratory failure
This involves performing an emergency anaesthetic and placing an endotracheal tube (ETT) to assist with oxygenation/ventilation. Three basic modes are:
1. *Continuous mandatory ventilation (CMV):* In this mode, the ventilator is set at a specific tidal volume and a set number of breaths per minute. The machine does all the work of breathing
2. *Synchronised intermittent mandatory ventilation (SIMV):* In this mode, the ventilator is set to deliver a set number of breaths per minute. However, the patient can spontaneously breath with the machine. If the patient breaths then the ventilator helps support that breath with 5–10 cm H_2O positive pressure (this is because there is a lot of resistance in an ETT, and the patient will also be weaker than normal as they are so unwell). When the patient breaths the ventilator then registers that breath as one of the set numbers required per minute
3. *Pressure support ventilation:* This mode is usually used when weaning a patient off a ventilator. The patient initiates all breaths, and the machine then supports each breath with 5–10 cm H_2O. As weaning progresses, the amount of support delivered by the ventilator is reduced until the patient is ready for a trial of extubation. The ventilator does have a backup breathing rate if the patient does not take a breath after a certain amount of time (usually 15 seconds)

Further reading

O'Driscoll BR, Howard LS, Earis J, et al. British Thoracic Society Guideline for oxygen use in adults in healthcare and emergency settings. BMJ Open Respir Res 2017; 4:e000170.

Scenario 2

Neurotrauma

A 26-year-old gentleman is brought in by the ambulance service. He fell from a ladder while clearing leaves from a gutter. The crew estimate that this was from a height of 6–8 m. The patient landed on the left side of his head on concrete and his most recent GCS was 8 (E1, V2, M5).

Q. 2.1 How would you assess this patient?

This patient should be managed using Advanced Trauma Life Support (ATLS) or the European Trauma Course (ETC) principles. This initially involves performing a primary survey to identify any life-threatening injuries prior to imaging being performed.

A. i. Catastrophic Haemorrhage – obvious visible catastrophic haemorrhage from arterial bleeds (usually from the extremities) will lead to exsanguination within a few minutes.

Manage aggressively using combat action tourniquets (CATs) as well as haemostatic dressings (e.g. Celox). This should have been performed prehospital by ambulance crews; however, dressings and tourniquets can become dislodged in transit and must be checked.

If tourniquets have been applied, they should have the time of application written on them.

ii. Airway – maintenance of a patent airway is essential. In patients with a reduced GCS, airway manoeuvres may need to be performed – ideally a jaw thrust; however, if this is unsuccessful then neck extension may be needed to ensure oxygenation.

Airway adjuncts include an oropharyngeal airway (Guedel) or bilateral nasopharyngeal airways – even in patients with suspected head injury, including base of skull fractures (otorrhoea/rhinorrhoea, Panda eyes, Battle's sign).

Oxygenation is the priority – patients are much more likely to develop brain injury from prolonged hypoxia than from the theoretical risk of penetration of a correctly inserted nasopharyngeal airway through a disrupted cribriform plate.

iii. Ensure the C-spine is immobilised. Historically patients had triple immobilisation with blocks, collar, and tape. However, current practice is moving away from collars as they are often ill fitting and lead to pressure injuries. Blocks and immobilisation with tape is often seen as sufficient now.

Airway (i.e. adequate oxygenation) *always* takes priority over the cervical spine, and as such the head should be extended if adequate oxygenation is not achievable with other manoeuvres and adjuncts.

B. Breathing – look for evidence of bruising or swelling over the chest and neck.
What is the respiratory rate?
Assess bilateral chest expansion (ideally from the feet looking up at the chest).
Feel the chest and ribs. Start with clavicles and then individually palpate the ribs. Is there crepitus, pain, subcutaneous emphysema or soft tissue swelling?
Tracheal deviation is a very late sign of tension pneumothorax and will likely mean the patient is close to respiratory arrest – consequently it is rarely clinically useful.
Listen – over the anterior chest wall and in the axillae. Wheeze in the context of trauma is a potential sign of pneumothorax, especially if the patient has no history of asthma.

C. Circulation – is there a radial pulse; what is the BP and heart rate?
Are the peripheries cold or warm (is it cold outside to explain cold peripheries)?
What is the capillary refill time – peripheral versus central.
Palpate the abdomen – is it tender, is the abdomen expanding?
Does the pelvis look intact, is there any bruising around it, is there blood at the urethral meatus? Has a pelvic binder been applied prehospital and is it in the correct position (at the level of the greater trochanters). *Do not spring the pelvis.*
Assess the legs – are there femoral fractures; are the legs neurovascularly intact?

D. Is there evidence of a head injury?
Is the patient complaining of back pain?
Does the patient move all limbs or is there weakness, a sensory level or lateralising signs?
Calculate the GCS.
Assess the pupils – what size are they and are they reactive to light?
Is the patient's physiology suggestive of neurogenic shock – this is spinal cord injury leading to loss of sympathetic tone presenting as bradycardia as well as vasodilatation resulting in hypotension, warm peripheries, and priapism?

E Ensure the patient is fully exposed.
What is the temperature and blood sugar?
Is there suspicion of a medical cause for the trauma [e.g. low speed road traffic collision (RTC) with minimal damage to the vehicle reported where the patient actually had a myocardial infarction (MI) at the wheel of the car]?
Take an AMPLE history (Allergies, Medications, Past medical history, Last meal or other intake, Events leading to the presentation).

Your primary survey reveals that this gentleman has a GCS of 8 (E1, V2, M5) with an obvious boggy swelling to the left side of the head and blood and cerebrospinal fluid (CSF) coming out of his left ear. His left pupil is 6 mm, dilated and unresponsive to light, his right pupil is 3 mm and sluggishly reactive. He also has lateralising signs as he is not moving the right side of his body.

Q. 2.2 What is the next intervention that the trauma team should perform?

The airway needs to be secured, and all major trauma teams will have a doctor who can perform advanced airway interventions on them (usually an anaesthetist or intensivist).
Intubating the airway has two goals in this scenario:
1. To protect the airway from blood/aspiration of vomit
2. To aid in the management of this patient's obvious severe head injury. Severe head injury is defined as any patient with GCS < 9 secondary to traumatic brain injury. Taking control of the airway allows optimisation of parameters such as oxygenation and ventilation (CO_2 clearance) to minimise the rise in intracranial pressure (ICP)

Your patient is now intubated.

Q. 2.3 What is the next step in the management of this patient?

If a major trauma patient is stable enough, then they should have a computed tomography (CT) scan. A typical major trauma CT involves a non-contrast CT head and then a contrast chest, abdomen, and pelvis. The point of a major trauma CT scan is to:
1. Rapidly identify life-threatening injuries including bleeding sites
2. Identify head or spinal injury
3. Triage of patients to the operating theatre for surgery on the correct body compartment (chest or abdomen/pelvis) or the angiography suit for interventional radiology; or potentially to a hybrid theatre for simultaneous surgical and interventional radiology (IR) control of injuries

If a patient is too unstable for a major trauma CT scan (rare nowadays) then the use of a focused assessment with sonography for trauma (FAST) is indicated. This allows assessment of which body compartment potentially needs to be opened first in theatres while undergoing damage control surgery.

Your patient has a major trauma CT scan and the report states that this gentleman has a large left extradural haematoma (EDH) (see figure below).

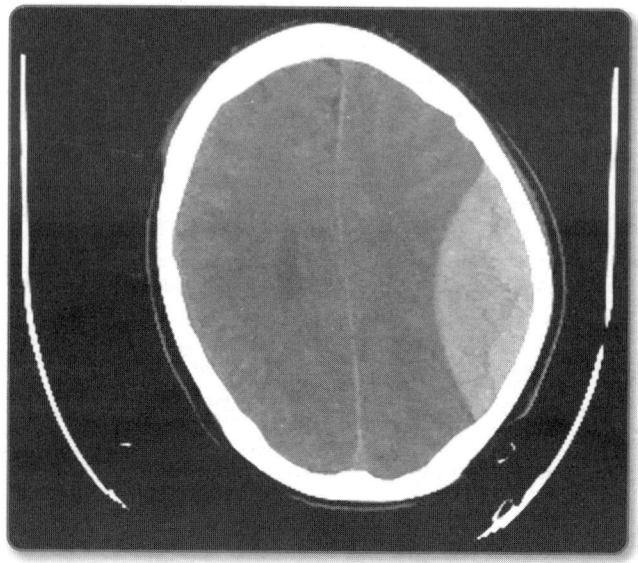

Q. 2.4 What is an EDH?

The brain has three layers of membrane (meninges) around the outside of it – the pia mater (adherent to the brain), the arachnoid mater (CSF lives between the pia and arachnoid maters), and the dura mater. An EDH forms outside the dura mater and is often due to a tear in an artery (often the middle meningeal), although it can be from skull base fractures or venous injury if it is adjacent to major dural venous sinuses. It is often associated with a temporal skull fracture. The blood from this artery expands into the potential space between the skull and the dura mater until it reaches one of the cranial sutures. The dura mater is adherent to the sutures and so the ongoing bleeding leads to a lens (or lemon!) shaped haematoma pushing against the brain. There is no damage to the brain initially, however the pressure effects of this haematoma can lead to brain injury. EDHs are relatively uncommon but can be rapidly fatal. The classical history is of a 'lucid interval' followed by coma, though this may be absent. Prognosis is excellent if surgical evacuation is timely before the pressure effects cause brain injury.

Q. 2.5 What measures can be used in the acute situation to reduce ICP?

As mentioned previously intubation in itself is a means of controlling ICP by three main mechanisms (the three **Ps**):

1. **Positioning:** It allows the patient to be sat 30 degrees head up (reverse Trendelenburg if spine not cleared) with the neck central without worrying about managing the airway – so improving venous drainage from the head and reducing ICP
2. **Physiology:** It allows the patient's oxygenation and CO_2 to be normalised minimising the cerebral vasodilatation seen with hypoxaemia or hypercapnia, so reducing ICP
3. **Pharmacology:** It allows the patient to be heavily sedated and muscle relaxed, thereby decreasing the brain's metabolic rate and so reducing ICP in this manner

Osmotherapy is the next step which consists of either using a bolus of hypertonic saline or mannitol to help lower ICP.

Further reading

Chakraverty S, Zealley I, Kessel D. Damage control radiology in the severely injured patient: what the anaesthetist needs to know. Br J Anaesth 2014; 113:250–257.

Scenario 3

Perioperative analgesia

A 45-year-old lady has undergone an open right hemicolectomy electively. The procedure was planned as laparoscopic but was converted to open intra-operatively. The patient underwent spinal anaesthesia, and had postoperative analgesia prescribed.

Q. 3.1 Where is the spinal space and what drugs do anaesthetists place in this space?

Anaesthetists usually place a spinal anaesthetic by inserting a needle into the patient's back between the third and fourth lumbar vertebrae (based on a landmark technique). Patients are usually sat up, but this procedure can also be performed on the side. The needle advances through the various tissue layers and comes to rest in the subarachnoid space in between the arachnoid mater and pia mater. This space contains the CSF.

Once CSF is seen to come out of the spinal needle drugs can be injected. This usually consists of local anaesthetic ('heavy' 0.5% bupivacaine) and an opioid (e.g. diamorphine). Other drugs can also be injected. Dependent on how the patient is positioned after the spinal is performed determines the height and density of the block. The analgesic effects of a spinal can last up to 24 hours (especially if diamorphine is placed); though the effects will usually start to wear off after a few hours.

Q. 3.2 What is the difference between an epidural and spinal regional anaesthetic technique?

An epidural technique deposits drugs into the epidural space – the potential space outside the dura mater – the outermost layer of meninges of the central nervous system. This is the same potential space where an EDH forms in the brain. A spinal technique deposits drugs in the subarachnoid space, where CSF is. Spinal anaesthetics are delivered with very thin needles – 24 or 25 gauge (thickness of a hair). The volumes used are also small – total of 2–3 ml. For an epidural technique the needle used is much larger (16 gauge) and once a catheter is placed in the epidural space larger volumes of local anaesthetic are placed (up to 20–30 mL) as the drug has to diffuse through two layers of membrane to reach the subarachnoid space where the nerves that are being targeted are.

You review this patient on the ward round the following morning and she complains that she is in significant pain.

Q. 3.3 What analgesia can you offer her?

The World Health Organization (WHO) uses the analgesic ladder which consists of:

Step 1 = mild pain – non-opioid [non-steroidal anti-inflammatory drugs (NSAIDs)/paracetamol] ± adjuvant

Step 2 = moderate to strong pain – opioid for mild to moderate pain ± non-opioid ± adjuvant

Step 3 = strong to severe pain – opioid for severe pain ± non-opioid ± adjuvant

Adjuvants:
- Antidepressants – e.g. amitriptyline for neuropathic pain
- Anticonvulsants – e.g. gabapentin for neuropathic pain
- Corticosteroids – e.g. dexamethasone
- Anxiolytics – e.g. diazepam

Neuropathic pain is chronic pain resulting from injury to the nervous system. The injury can be to either the central nervous system or the peripheral nervous system. Neuropathic pain can occur after trauma and many diseases such as multiple sclerosis and stroke.

This WHO three-step approach is effective in 80–90% of patients with cancer pain when optimally used.

For postoperative pain, additional analgesia is often required in the form of patient-controlled analgesia (PCA).

Q. 3.4 How does each of the above drugs work?

Paracetamol: The exact mechanism of action remains to be determined. However, a variant of the cyclooxygenase (COX-1) enzyme (COX-3) has been described in the brain and spinal cord and is proposed to be the site of action for the antipyretic and analgesic effects.

Other theories include:
- Inhibition of prostaglandin synthesis
- Modulation of pain via stimulation of descending pain pathways

Non-steroidal anti-inflammatory drugs – e.g. ibuprofen, naproxen, diclofenac:
These drugs block the synthesis of prostaglandins by inhibition of the enzyme COX. Prostaglandins are important mediators of inflammation sensitising nerve endings to the chemical mediators that cause pain. NSAIDs reduce pain by both peripheral and central mechanisms.

Inhibition of prostaglandins also causes the side effects associated with NSAIDs such as reduced platelet aggregation, damage to the stomach lining, reduced blood flow to the kidneys and bronchospasm.

Codeine phosphate: It is a prodrug and 10% is converted to morphine and the analgesic and constipating effects are due to this morphine metabolite. It is used as an opioid for mild to moderate pain.

Tramadol: It is a non-selective agonist at mu-, kappa-, and delta-opioid receptors. It also inhibits neuronal uptake of noradrenaline and enhances serotonin release. It too is used for mild to moderate pain.

Morphine: It is an agonist at mu- and kappa-opioid receptors. Opioids work by increasing intracellular calcium which ultimately reduces membrane excitability and decreased pain fibre firing. It is used for severe pain.

Fentanyl (a synthetic opioid): It is occasionally used in PCAs instead of morphine and may be started by your pain team. It is a highly selective mu agonist – the mu-opioid receptor is specifically involved in the mediation of analgesia. Fentanyl is used for severe pain.

Further reading

Venermo MA, Farber A, Schanzer A, et al. Reduction of major amputations after surgery versus endovascular intervention: The BEST-CLI randomized trial. Eur J Vasc Endovasc Surg. 2024:S1078-5884(24)00492-1.

Scenario 4

Surgery in the context of altered mental capacity

A 62-year-old man has been conservatively managed for small bowel obstruction for the last 3 days. He has a background of severe COPD and is housebound. Your junior colleague rings to tell you that he has deteriorated and needs senior review.

On examination:
A – maintain own
B – respiratory rate 45 breaths/min, sat upright using all accessory muscles; oxygen saturations of 95% on 15 L/min oxygen with a reservoir bag in place
C – BP 90/40 mmHg, pulse rate 125 bpm
D – GCS 14 – confused
E – temperature 37.9°C abdomen peritonitis

Your junior colleague has performed an ABG showing pH 7.25; pO_2 20 kPa; pCO_2 4 kPa; HCO_3^- 16 mmoL; BE 8 mmol/L

Q. 4.1 What is your plan?

This gentleman's condition has now progressed to a life-threatening condition. He is septic and acidotic from his perforated abdomen. He is attempting to compensate for this acidaemia by blowing off CO_2. Unfortunately, due to his underlying respiratory condition, this compensatory effort is not particularly effective.

Without an operation this gentleman will die.

Q. 4.2 What scoring systems do you know that will help in your decision making regarding his likely outcome?

Historically the P-POSSUM (Portsmouth Physiological and Operative Severity Score for the enUmeration of Mortality and morbidity) score has been used for the prediction of mortality and morbidity in patients due for emergency or elective surgery. This was first reported in the British Journal of Surgery in 1998. Since then, the National Emergency Laparotomy Audit (NELA) has emerged, led by the National Institute of Academic Anaesthesia's Health Services Research Centre. It has developed a separate NELA risk calculator which provides an estimate of the risk of death within 30 days of emergency abdominal surgery. The initial data used to validate this risk tool was from NELA patients recorded between 2014–2016. The audit is ongoing and presumably the NELA model will be further refined based on this data.

Of note P-POSSUM and NELA often give significantly different risk numbers. There are a number of contributors to this difference, the main one being the move away from categorisation of data (in P-POSSUM) towards continuous variables (in NELA). Therefore, a small difference in numbers will be reflected in NELA, whereas P-POSSUM variables need to cross a threshold to change the outcome mortality. These scoring systems are clearly only a guide and are only one element used to determine what a patient's likely outcome will be.

Your NELA risk calculator gives you a NELA mortality of 55.2% and a P-POSSUM mortality of 99.9%.

Q. 4.3 What other information can be used to inform your decision making?

Obviously given the history and mortality scoring this gentleman is at very high risk if he is operated upon. Speaking to the patient's family to gain a corroborating history and further elucidate what his functional history was like prior to this hospital admission will be very useful. Furthermore, an understanding of any previously expressed wishes will help in your decision making.

When this patient's wife is spoken with, she tells you that he has severe COPD and is on home nebulisers. He has also been on long-term oxygen therapy (LTOT) for 14 hours per day for the last 2 years. Prior to this hospital admission he has not left the house for the last 6 months and she has to perform his activities of daily living (ADLs) for him. On further questioning, she goes on to say that he has been very unhappy these last few months and would not want any further deterioration in his quality of life.

Based on all the information you have gathered you feel that operating on this gentleman would not be in his best interests or consistent with his wishes. You decide that palliation is the correct decision for this gentleman.

Q. 4.4 If you were uncertain as to whether or not to operate, whom else could you speak to help with decision making?

As surgeons you do not work in isolation, so discussion with a consultant colleague would be an appropriate first step. Other colleagues that you could speak to would be the consultant anaesthetist covering the emergency list or the duty critical care consultant. Both these doctors will have experience of managing critically unwell patients and a good understanding of what their likely outcomes will be.

When you initially assessed this patient, you had assessed his capacity and had determined that he lacked capacity; you had therefore acted in the patient's best interests at all times, with input from the family as to what his wishes would have been.

Q. 4.5 What is the Mental Capacity Act and how do you assess capacity?

The Mental Capacity Act (MCA) is designed to protect and empower people who may lack the mental capacity to make their own decisions about their care and treatment. It applies to people aged 16 and over.

The principles of this act are:
1. A person must be assumed to have capacity unless it is established that he or she lacks capacity
2. A person is not to be treated as unable to make a decision unless all practicable steps to help to do so have been taken without success
3. A person is not to be treated as unable to make a decision merely because he they make an unwise decision
4. An act done, or decision made, under this act for or on behalf of a person who lacks capacity must be done, or made, in their best interests
5. Before the act is done, or the decision is made, regard must be had to whether the purpose for which it is needed can be as effectively achieved in a way that is less restrictive of the person's rights and freedom of action

All patients are assumed to have capacity unless proven not to. For a patient to be assessed as having capacity, the following four criteria must be met.
1. The patient must understand the information relevant to the decision
2. Be able to retain that information
3. Use or weigh up that information as part of making the decision
4. Be able to communicate this decision back to the clinician

These criteria also mean that patients may have capacity for simpler decisions, but lack the ability to make more complex decisions as they are unable to either understand the relevant information or weigh up the relevant information as part of making a decision.

Q. 4.6 How would your decision making have been affected if this patient's wife had been a lasting power of attorney for health and welfare?

In England, patients can appoint a lasting power of attorney (LPAs) for health – their legal proxy. The LPAs can consent to treatment deemed necessary by doctors and can refuse life-sustaining treatment if specifically authorised to do so by the patient.

Further reading

Menon D, Chatfield D. Mental Capacity Act 2005 Guidance for Critical Care. Intensive Care Society 2011. [online] Available from http://icmwk.com/wp-content/uploads/2014/02/mental_capacity_act.pdf [Last accessed February, 2022].

Scenario 5

Postoperative myocardial infarction

A 72-year-old woman underwent an open appendicectomy yesterday. The procedure was uncomplicated and she went back to the ward. She has a background of obesity, hypertension, hypercholesterolaemia, diabetes and smokes 40 a day.

As you review her on your ward round, she says that she has been complaining of central chest pain for the last hour, and the nursing staff placed her on a Hudson mask due to low oxygen saturations.

Q. 5.1 What is the differential diagnosis for this lady?

When answering viva questions, you need to have a structure; one such structure is to divide your differential diagnosis into surgical and medical causes to ensure you reliably capture them all.

Looking at the medical causes of chest pain, the three most common to think of are chest infection, myocardial infarction (MI), and pulmonary embolus (PE). There are also rarer causes such as spontaneous pneumothorax which this author has seen twice!

In the postoperative patient, it is unusual for a chest infection to develop on day 1 postoperatively unless either

1. The patient was clearly developing a chest infection prior to theatre, but the emergent nature of the surgery required meant the operation had to go ahead – your patient will therefore be more likely to go to a critical care unit (CCU) postoperatively
2. The patient obviously aspirated perioperatively – though your anaesthetist should communicate this to you

Investigations include performing a CXR, starting appropriate antibiotics, increasing observation frequency for this patient and potentially discussing with the medical or critical care team dependent on severity of symptoms.

It is unusual for a patient to develop a PE immediately postoperatively; classically PE develops at round about 1 week postoperatively. Symptoms include severe hypoxaemia, often requiring a sudden increase in oxygen requirements associated with chest pain and sometimes haemoptysis. Patients develop RF1 and the CXR is usually clear. CT pulmonary angiogram (CTPA) is the investigation of choice and should be performed urgently. Treatment is with treatment dose anticoagulation [usually low-molecular-weight heparin (LMWH)], and this should be started even before CTPA is obtained if there is strong clinical suspicion (even if the patient has had recent surgery – dependent on severity of symptoms and the weighing up of risks vs. benefits). For life-threatening PE (unable to oxygenate/haemodynamic instability), thrombolysis should be considered.

You feel, given her cardiac risk factors, that this lady may well be having an MI.

Q. 5.2 What other symptoms might she have and how are you going to diagnose that she is having an MI?

In addition to the classical reporting of 'crushing' central chest pain like 'somebody is sitting on my chest', patients also report radiation of pain down the left arm (sometimes the right!) and into the left jaw. They may also experience shortness of breath and hypoxaemia secondary to heart failure, palpitations and nausea.

The umbrella term acute coronary syndrome is used to group together the three conditions of unstable angina, non-ST elevation MI (NSTEMI), and ST elevation MI (STEMI). To differentiate between these three conditions, two investigations must be performed – a 12-lead ECG and cardiac troponins.

Unstable angina = no ST elevation on ECG and no troponin rise (no cardiac muscle death)
NSTEMI = no ST elevation and a significant troponin rise (dependent on troponin measured, timing of blood samples and sensitivity of assays)
STEMI = ST elevation and a significant troponin rise

You have the nursing staff perform an ECG on the ward. This clearly demonstrates a STEMI.

Q. 5.3 Which leads on the ECG look at which walls of the heart?

Septal wall = V1 and V2
Anterior wall = V3 and V4
Lateral wall = V5, V6, I, and aVL
Inferior wall = II, III, and aVF

Having an emergency echocardiogram performed by an appropriately trained individual will also identify if there is any regional wall motion abnormality (RWMA) in the corresponding area of the heart.

Q. 5.4 What are your treatment options for this lady?

Treatment of a STEMI includes morphine, oxygen, up to two puffs of GTN spray (the patient may have her own) and 300 mg aspirin as a loading dose. If the patient is already on 75 mg aspirin/day and has taken her daily dose, then this can be supplemented with 225 mg aspirin. Consider loading with clopidogrel 300 mg (or your local hospital equivalent – e.g. ticagrelor). Ultimately this lady needs to be discussed with a cardiologist to determine the risk/benefit of her having primary percutaneous coronary intervention (PPCI) in the face of an open appendicectomy within the last 24 hours. Further anticoagulation is required for PPCI.

Further reading

Verbree-Willemsen L, Grobben RB, van Waes JA, et al. Causes and prevention of postoperative myocardial injury. Eur J Prev Cardiol 2019; 26:59–67.

Scenario 6

Burns

A 25-year-old gentleman is brought in by the ambulance service. He had been out drinking and left his oven on when he returned home last night, leading to a fire. After he was extricated by the fire crew he was brought to A&E. It was unclear how many hours he was in the burning house for before he was removed.

Q. 6.1 What elements will you be particularly looking for in your primary survey that relate to burn injury?

A   Airway – maintenance of a patent airway is essential. Warning signs in patients with burn injury include voice changes (secondary to burning of the vocal cords), singeing of facial hair; burns of the mouth and tongue and coughing up of carbonaceous sputum. There should be a low threshold to intubate these patients early as swelling of facial structures can develop rapidly, especially in the face of fluid resuscitation for extensive burns

B   Breathing – inhalational injury of superheated air and other products of combustion can lead to significant lung injury. Early intubation will also help to manage this; oxygenation can deteriorate to such an extent that patients develop ARDS, especially in the face of significant fluid resuscitation. In rare cases, patients may need to be placed on extracorporeal membrane oxygenation (ECMO).

Carbon monoxide (CO) poisoning should be considered, especially if there has been prolonged exposure to smoke in a confined space. CO displaces oxygen from the haemoglobin molecule. Saturation probes falsely interpret carboxyhaemoglobin (COHb) as oxygenated haemoglobin such that a patient's saturation may read 100% with significant COHb on board. Symptoms of COHb poisoning vary from mild confusion through to seizures and coma. ST segment changes may also be present on the ECG. Coma and/or COHb levels >40% always indicate serious poisoning (smokers may have up to 10% COHb). COHb levels can be measured at the bedside on an ABG machine. Treatment is 100% oxygen until levels are <2%.

Rarely patients may have circumferential burns of the torso. This leads to significant problems oxygenating and ventilating patients. In these cases, escharotomy should be performed. Wounds can bleed excessively and therefore ensure patients are cross-matched

C   All patients with significant burn injury should have a high index of suspicion for trauma. The default position for these patients should be triage to a Major Trauma Centre (MTC) unless there is good reason not to go there. Any patient that has sustained recent burn injury and is hypotensive should be assumed to have traumatic injury causing this hypotension (e.g. bleeding/spinal injury) until proven otherwise.

The Parkland formula is frequently used as a guide for fluid resuscitation in burn injury patients. This is calculated as:

% body surface area of burn × weight in kg × 2–4 mL/kg

This calculates the total volume of fluid to be infused over 24 hours from time of injury, not hospital admission. Half of this should be given over the first 8 hours and the other half over the following 16 hours. To be clear, this is only a guide for fluid infusion rate at the start of resuscitation – i.e. the initial few hours. It should then be tailored on an individual patient basis using urine output, other vital signs and investigations. In adults, a urine output of 0.5 mL/kg/h would be a reasonable initial target.

When placing IV cannulae, try not to go through burnt skin if possible; however sometimes there may be no choice.

D Again, think about whether the patient has suffered traumatic injury prior/during the burn episode – e.g. explosion/collapsing building
E Assessment of extent and depth of burn injury occurs at this point; not before

Q. 6.2 How are you going to assess the extent of burn injury for this patient?

There are a number of commercial charts that can be used for this – e.g. Lund and Browder.

The 'rule of nines' is also useful in adults:

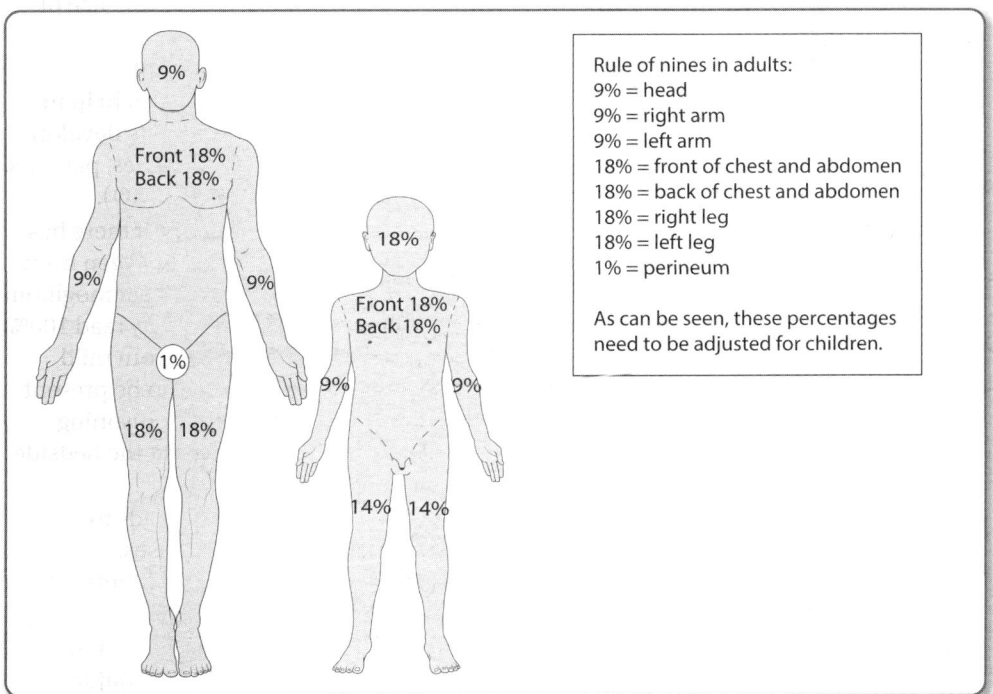

There are also various apps that are now available for assessing extent of burn injury.

Q. 6.3 How will you assess the depth of burn injury?

Depth of burn injury is classified by which structures are involved:

Depth	Structures damaged	Clinical	Course
Superficial	Epidermis	Painful and red	Pain for 48 hours Desquamation in 3–7 days
Partial thickness	Epidermis and dermis	Painful, wet with blisters and oedema	Heals over 14–28 days
Full thickness	Down to subcutaneous tissue and muscle	Dry surface, little or no pain	Removal of burn eschar and skin grafting

Only partial and full thickness burn injuries are used in the calculation of percentage burn. In addition, partial and full thickness areas often overlap, rather than being discrete entities.

Causes of burns other than flame injury include scalding liquids, steam, acid, alkali and electrical injury including lightning. With an electrical injury, there may only be small entry and exit points; however, all the tissue plains between these points may have been disrupted and injured. Furthermore, if the path of current passes through the chest, there is a risk of cardiac injury and cardiac arrest.

Further reading

https://www.britishburnassociation.org/national-burn-care-referral-guidance/ [Accessed 1st April 2023]

https://www.britishburnassociation.org/first-aid-guidelines/[Accessed 1st April 2023]

Scenario 7

Levels of care

You are booking a patient for an emergency Hartmann's procedure for perforated diverticular disease. The CEPOD anaesthetist asks you to speak to ITU as the patient will require a level 3 bed postoperatively.

Q. 7.1 What are the different levels of care within the hospital environment and what are the differences between each of them?

There are four levels of care within a hospital:

Level 0:
- Standard ward
- Maximum frequency of observations is 4-hourly
- 1:8 nursing to patient ratio

Level 1:
- Standard ward
- Observations more frequent than 4-hourly
- Can include:
  - Oxygen therapy
  - IV infusions
  - Patient-controlled analgesia
- 1:8 nursing to patient ratio

Level 2:
- Traditionally high-dependency unit (HDU)/CCU
- Up to single organ support (excluding mechanical ventilation)
- Step down from level 3
- Extended monitoring (can be invasive, e.g. arterial line)
- 1:2 nursing to patient ratio

Level 3:
- Traditionally ITU
- Patients requiring mechanical ventilation
- Multi-organ support
- 1:1 nursing to patient ratio

Further reading

Inspection framework: NHS acute hospitals. Core service: critical care. [online] Available from https://www.cqc.org.uk/sites/default/files/20160713_NHS_core_service_inspection_framework_critical_care.pdf [Last accessed February, 2022].

Scenario 8

Pulse oximetry

You are called to see a 45-year-old patient on the surgical ward on day 2 after an emergency laparotomy. The nurse is concerned about the patient's respiratory rate of 21/min and SpO_2 of 88% on pulse oximetry. The patient appears comfortable at rest, and there are no significant findings on chest or abdominal examination.

Q. 8.1 What are the principles behind pulse oximetry?

- Blood reflects light, with oxygenated and deoxygenated haemoglobin reflecting different wavelengths
- The oximeter contains two light-emitting diodes:
  i. 600 nm (red) that measures total amount of haemoglobin
  ii. 940 nm (infrared) measures the amount of oxygenated haemoglobin
- The oximeter compares the two measurements to give a percentage saturation of oxygen (SO_2)
- This is the reading shown on the monitor

Q. 8.2 What sources of error are there for pulse oximetry?

- Cool peripheries
- Nail varnish use
- Nicotine-stained fingers
- Jaundice
- Carboxyhaemoglobin (gives falsely high reading)

Q. 8.3 How reliable is pulse oximetry?

- It is a good bedside test
- It lacks enough information to give true assessment of a patient's oxygenation
- SO_2 can be high but Pao_2 can still be low (the relationship is not linear)
- Does not give any information on $Paco_2$ (especially important in RF2)

Further reading

Chan ED, Chan MM, Chan MM. Pulse oximetry: understanding its basic principles facilitates appreciation of its limitations. Respir Med 2013; 107:789–799.
Jubran A. Pulse oximetry. Crit Care 2015; 19:272.

Scenario 9

Oxygen delivery

A 65-year-old patient undergoes an emergency laparotomy and Hartmann's procedure for perforated sigmoid diverticulitis. On postoperative day 2, he remains intubated on the intensive care unit, and on low-dose inotropic support. Abdominal examination reveals a marginally dusky stoma, prompting the surgeon to consider the patient's oxygenation-perfusion status.

Q. 9.1 How is oxygen carried in the blood?

- Oxygen is mainly bound to haemoglobin
- A negligible amount (<1%) is dissolved in blood

Q. 9.2 What factors determine oxygen delivery to tissues?

- The concentration of haemoglobin
- Cardiac output
- Oxygen saturations
- $DO_2 = (O_2 \text{ in Hb}) + (O_2 \text{ dissolved in blood}) \times CO$

Cardiac output:
- $CO = HR \times SV$
- Controlled by heart rate and stroke volume

Oxygen saturation:
- Can be increased by using supplemental oxygen

Haemoglobin concentration:
- This should be optimised where possible to ensure adequate oxygenation

Q. 9.3 What is the oxygen dissociation curve?

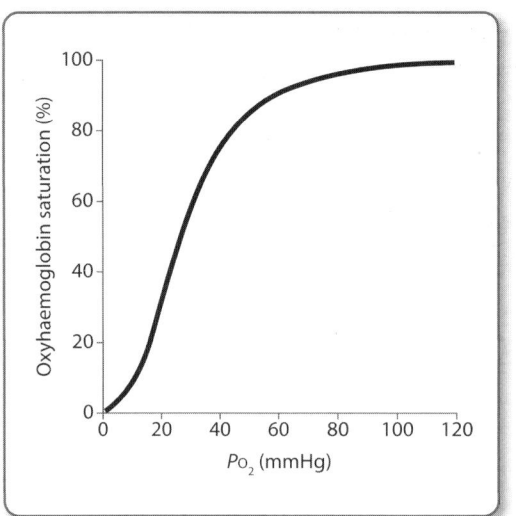

Source: Poli G. (2017). Oxyhaemoglobin dissociation curve, pt 3: what the curve means. [online] Available from https://www.vettimes.co.uk/oxyhaemoglobin-dissociation-curve-pt-3-what-the-curve-means/ [Last accessed February, 2022].

Q. 9.4 What shifts the curve to the right?

CADET face right

C – increase in $Paco_2$
A – acidosis
D – increase in 2,3-diphosphoglycerate (DPG)
E – exercise
T – increase in temperature

Q. 9.5 What shifts the curve to the left?

- Alkalosis
- Decrease in 2,3 DPG
- Hypothermia
- Decreased $Paco_2$
- Foetal Hb

Q. 9.6 What is the significance of oxygen saturation of 90% with relation to the oxygen dissociation curve?

When saturations fall below 90%, this is where the sigma curve is much steeper on the graph. Therefore, any further drop in oxygen saturation leads to an exponential drop in Pao_2.

Q. 9.7 What is the Bohr effect?

This is a description of a shift in the curve in direct response to a change in pH. Most commonly this is due to a right shift from acidosis.

Q. 9.8 What is 2–3 DPG?

- It is a by-product of the glycolytic pathway
- It binds to the beta chain of haemoglobin
- The effect is to reduce the affinity of Hb to oxygen (thus allowing Hb to release oxygen more freely)

Q. 9.9 What do you know of the oxygen cascade?

This is a description of the transfer of oxygen from the air we breathe down to the mitochondria in the cells.

Within each section of the cascade, the Pao_2 drops.

It requires the passive transfer of gas down partial pressure gradients.

The steps are:
- Atmospheric air
- Humidified tracheal gas
- Alveolar gas
- Arterial blood
- Mitochondria
- Venous blood

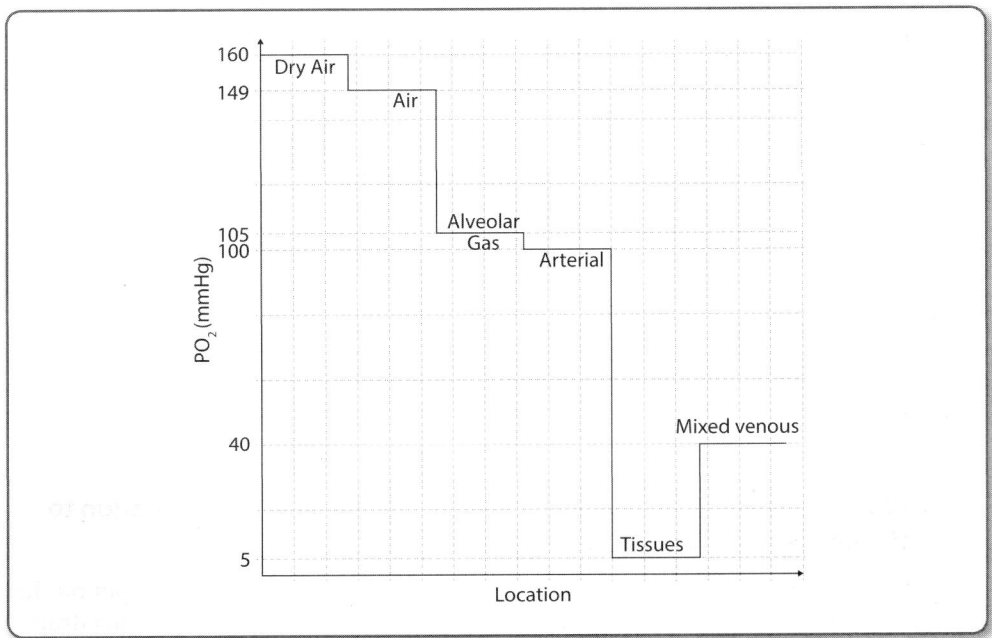

Source: Nickson C. (2020). Tissue oxygenation assessment. [online] Available from https://litfl.com/tissue-oxygenation-assessment/ [Last accessed February, 2022].

Further reading

Hamilton C, Steinlechner B, Gruber E, Simon P, Wollenek G. The oxygen dissociation curve: quantifying the shift. Perfusion 2004; 19:141–144.

Shepherd JR, Dominelli PB, Roy TK, et al. Modelling the relationships between haemoglobin oxygen affinity and the oxygen cascade in humans. J Physiol 2019; 597:4193–4202.

Scenario 10

Cardiovascular monitoring

You have performed an emergency laparotomy on an 80-year-old female patient for ischaemic bowel. She will be admitted to ITU postoperatively for close monitoring.

Q. 10.1 What types of cardiovascular monitoring are you are of?

- Central venous pressure (CVP) monitoring
- Pulmonary artery catheter (rare in current practice)
- Peripheral arterial line

Q. 10.2 How is CVP monitoring carried out?

- This requires a central line to be inserted
- The most common sites are:
  - Internal jugular vein
  - Subclavian vein
  - Femoral vein

Q. 10.3 What is CVP?

- This is a measure of the hydrostatic pressure within the great vessels.
- Reference range of 0–8 mmHg

Q. 10.4 What does CVP measure?

- It is an estimate of right atrial pressure
- Can be used to assess cardiac preload
- Can be used to assess a patient's volume status

Q. 10.5 Can you draw a CVP trace and explain the different components?

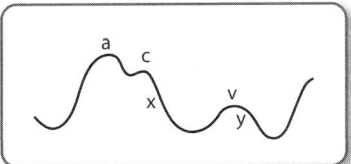

Waveform	Phase of cardiac cycle	Mechanical event
A wave	End diastole	Atrial contraction
C wave	Early systole	Tricuspid bulging
V wave	Late systole	Systolic filling of atrium
X descent	Mid systole	Atrial relaxation
Y descent	Early diastole	Early ventricular filling

Q. 10.6 How is the CVP indicative of a patient's fluid status?

- It does not accurately measure the volume status of a patient
- The exact value is not in itself the important factor
- It is the change in value secondary to fluid bolus challenges that aids clinicians in assessing whether a patient is fluid depleted

Q. 10.7 What are the indications for CVP line insertion?

- Cardiovascular monitoring
- Infusion of specific drugs
    - Inotropes
    - Vasopressors
    - Total parenteral nutrition (TPN)
- Access for patients with difficult peripheral access

Q. 10.8 What are the complications of CVP line insertion?

Early:
- Incorrect placement
    - Includes tip of the line
    - Includes accidental placement into artery
- Bleeding
- Pneumothorax/haemothorax
- Arrhythmias
- Air embolism

Late:
- Infection [lines should not be left for longer than 10 days (5–7 in groin)]
    - Includes systemic sepsis
- Occlusion
- Thrombosis of the vessel

Q. 10.9 What is a peripheral arterial catheter?

- This is a line inserted into a peripheral artery most commonly the radial artery
- It is used for invasive BP monitoring

Q. 10.10 Can you draw an arterial line waveform?

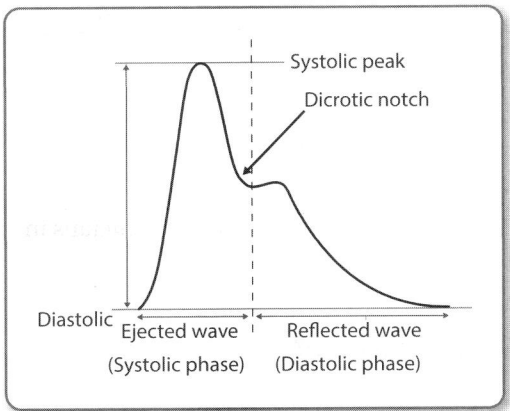

Source: https://dokumen.tips/documents/hemodynamicsfinalpptx.html?page=25 [Accessed 1st April 2023]

The dicrotic notch is representative of when the aortic valve closes.

Further reading

Stewart RM, Park PK, Hunt JP, et al. Less is more: improved outcomes in surgical patients with conservative fluid administration and central venous catheter monitoring. J Am Coll Surg 2009; 208:725–735; discussion 735–737.

Scenario 11

Perioperative risk stratification

You have admitted an 81-year-old patient with an acute abdomen, and a CT-confirmed diagnosis of small bowel perforation. The patient has been consented and booked for an emergency laparotomy. However, the patient's family wishes to discuss the appropriateness of surgery given the patient's functional status and perioperative risk.

Q. 11.1 What methods of risk stratifying patients preoperatively are you aware of?

- American Society of Anesthesiologists (ASA) grade
- P-POSSUM score
- APACHE and APACHE II (mostly used in ITU setting)

Q. 11.2 What are the different ASA grades?

ASA I:
- Fit and well patient
- No comorbidities

ASA II:
- Mild systemic disease
- Not affecting quality of life

ASA III:
- Severe systemic disease
- Directly affects quality of life
    - E.g. COPD with reduced exercise tolerance

ASA IV:
- Severe systemic disease that is a constant threat to life
- This includes an acute surgical condition

ASA V:
- Moribund patient
- Not expected to survive without surgery
    - Abdominal aortic aneurysm (AAA) rupture
    - Massive trauma

ASA VI:
Patient with confirmed brainstem death.

Q. 11.3 What is the significance of ASA grading?

- A higher grade is associated with a higher risk of morbidity and mortality to the patient
- It is, however, a crude assessment but the most commonly used

Q. 11.4 What is the P-POSSUM score?

- Portsmouth – Physiological and Operative Severity Score for the enumeration of mortality and morbidity
- Versions exist for:
  - Colorectal surgery
  - Oesophagogastric (OG) surgery
  - Vascular surgery
  - However, these are not widely used and can be inaccurate
- Commonly used for emergency surgery
- It is part of the NELA protocol
- Online tools are used to calculate
- Current guidelines state the morbidity and mortality risk must be:
  - Discussed with the patient ± relatives
  - Clearly documented in the notes
  - Clearly documented in the consent form
- Can both over and underestimate risk

Q. 11.5 How can risk be formally assessed in elective patients?

- Assess cardiac function
  - ECG
  - ECHO
  - Stress ECHO
- Assess lung function
  - Spirometry
  - Lung function tests
- Cardiopulmonary exercise testing (CPET)
  - Measures the bodies physiological response to stress
  - Looks at:
    - Anaerobic threshold
    - Peak oxygen intake
    - Ventilatory efficiency
  - This is used routinely in OG surgery

Q. 11.6 What methods of optimising patients are you aware of?

The main principle of optimisation is to ensure that the physiological parameters are as close to normal as possible:

Elective:
- Haemoglobin is within range
- Diabetes is under good control
- Hypertension is under good control
- Use of high calorie drinks in the immediate preoperative period

Emergency:
- Adequate fluid resuscitation
- Adequate BP
  - Includes use of inotropes/vasopressors
- Correct electrolyte disturbances

Patients who need emergency surgery and are haemodynamically unstable may benefit from optimisation in the ITU setting prior to surgery.

However, it is a delicate balance between optimisation and timing of surgery, as delay in surgery may itself lead to poor outcomes in the patient.

Further reading

Helkin A, Jain SV, Gruessner A, et al. Impact of ASA score misclassification on NSQIP predicted mortality: a retrospective analysis. Perioper Med (Lond) 2017; 6:23.

Mahler DA, Franco MJ. Clinical applications of cardiopulmonary exercise testing. J Cardiopulm Rehabil 1996; 16:357–365.

NELA RISK calculator. [online] Available from https://data.nela.org.uk/riskcalculator/ [Last accessed February, 2022].

Scenario 12

Sedation

You are about to perform a colonoscopy on a 50-year-old male patient for change in bowel habit (CIBH). You are consenting the patient, and he asks you if he will be put to sleep. You explain that he will be given sedation.

Q. 12.1 What do you understand by the term conscious sedation?

This is when medication is used to make a patient feel relaxed coupled with analgesia without affecting levels of consciousness or awareness of surroundings.

Q. 12.2 What common sedative medications that are used in endoscopy are you aware of?

Midazolam:
- Benzodiazepine that binds to GABA receptors
- Short half-life
- Caution in renal and hepatic failure

Fentanyl:
- An opioid drug with greater potency than morphine
- Rapid onset and short half-life
- Has potential for respiratory depression

Pethidine:
- Another opioid drug
- More potent than morphine
- Can cause myocardial depression alongside respiratory depression

Q. 12.3 What precautions should be taken before administering conscious sedation?

- Monitoring of oxygen saturations and BP before, throughout and after administration of the sedative drug
- Oxygen should be administered throughout
- Titrate doses accordingly starting with small doses

Q. 12.4 Which patients are high risk for sedation?

- Elderly patients
- Any patient with a known chronic respiratory illness
  - Asthma
  - COPD
- Patients with comorbidities
- Patients already taking benzodiazepines

Q. 12.5 What must you monitor for in patients having conscious sedation and how would you deal with it?

- Respiratory depression is the most dangerous acute complication of sedatives
- If there are any signs of this the patient must be monitored closely and naloxone given if indicated
- Airway protection should be considered if severe respiratory depression ensues

Q. 12.6 What must you check before giving a patient conscious sedation?

- They have someone to take them home after the procedure
- There is a responsible adult at home with them for a 24-hour period following sedation
  - If not, the patient must stay in hospital for 24 hours post-sedation or the procedure be rebooked
- Inform the patient they should not drink any alcohol or take any other drugs that can cause sedation (including recreational drugs) for 24 hours postsedation as a minimum

Further reading

Cosmo GD, Congedo E. Is sedation for endoscopy as safe as you think? Minerva Anestesiol 2017; 83:1118–1120.

Shehabi Z, Flood C, Matthew L. 2018. Midazolam use for dental conscious sedation: how safe are we? Br Dent J 2018; 224:98–104.

Scenario 13

Principles of general anaesthesia

You are consenting a patient for a laparoscopic cholecystectomy, and the patient asks if they will be asleep for the procedure. You inform the patient that the procedure will be performed under general anaesthesia.

Q. 13.1 What are the principles of a general anaesthetic?

A general anaesthetic requires the following:
- Unconsciousness (hypnosis)
- Analgesia
- Muscle relaxation (dependant on the procedure)

General anaesthesia has two phases:
- Induction
- Maintenance

Q. 13.2 What can be used to induce and maintain hypnosis?

It can be either IV or gaseous.

Intravenous:
- Propofol
  - Rapid onset
  - Rapidly metabolised with little accumulation of metabolites
  - Good antiemetic properties
  - Can cause myocardial depression
  - Can be used for maintenance of sedation on ITU, total IV anaesthesia and for day-case surgery
- Ketamine
  - Can also be used for induction of anaesthesia
  - Has good analgesic properties
  - Little myocardial depression – suitable for haemodynamically unstable patients
  - Can cause nightmares
- Etomidate
  - Negligible myocardial depression – suitable for haemodynamically unstable patients
  - Unsuitable for maintaining sedation
  - Can cause adrenal suppression with prolonged use

- Thiopentone
  - Very rapid onset of action – used for rapid sequence induction
  - Can cause severe myocardial depression
  - Metabolites build up quickly
  - Unsuitable for maintenance infusion

Gaseous (more commonly used for maintenance):
- Halothane
- Sevoflurane
- Isoflurane

Q. 13.3 What analgesia is used during anaesthesia?

Opioids are the choice of analgesia used in anaesthesia.
- Morphine
- Fentanyl
- Remifentanil

Q. 13.4 What muscle relaxants are used in general anaesthesia?

These are either depolarising or non-depolarising.

Depolarising:
- Suxamethonium
- Rapid onset and short half-life
- Mechanism via non-competitive blockade of neuromuscular junction
- Broken down by plasma cholinesterase

Non-depolarising:
- Rocuronium
- Atracurium
- Long onset of action
- Mechanism via competitive blockade of the neuromuscular junction
- Reversed with acetylcholinesterase

Further reading

Bigatello L, Pesenti A. Respiratory physiology for the anesthesiologist. Anesthesiology 2019; 130:1064–1077.

Scenario 14

Thermoregulation

You are in theatre about to start an emergency laparotomy for small bowel obstruction. After the WHO checklist, one of the medical students approaches you asking why there is a need to use a Bair Hugger for the patient.

Q. 14.1 What are the normal parameters for body temperature?
Normal parameters for body temperature: 36.5–37.5°C.

Q. 14.2 Why is it important to ensure body temperature is maintained?
This is to ensure that enzymatic function remains optimally functioning. Enzymes which are proteins will denature at a temperature of 32°C.

Q. 14.3 Why is temperature regulation important in an operating theatre?
The temperature in an operating theatre is often cooler, at around 21°C. This coupled with the stress response of surgery can lead to heat loss. Thus, patients are at risk of becoming hypothermic, which is a preventable complication and is associated with adverse outcomes for patients.

Q. 14.4 What are the different mechanisms of heat loss that you are aware of?

Radiation:
- This is the process where heat is transferred from a warmer object to a cooler one
- An example of this would be a cold operating table
- 40% of heat loss

Convection:
- This is where convection currents remove the layer of warm air around the skin
- 30% of heat loss

Evaporation:
- This is where moisture evaporates
- Important in open surgery
- 25% of heat loss

Conduction:
- Occurs with cold fluid washout for example
- Rare

Respiration:
- Loss of heat by inspiring cold air
- 10% of heat loss

Q. 14.5 What are the physiological responses to hypothermia?

- Overall increase in oxygen demand, from two- to five-fold
- Reduction in cardiac output
- Vasoconstriction
- Increased chance of developing cardiac arrhythmias
- Metabolic acidosis
- Renal and liver function suppression
- Increased rate of wound infection
- Behaviour changes
- Shivering
- Hairs on body becoming erect

Q. 14.6 What measures can be put into place to prevent hypothermia in theatres?

Respiratory:
- Warmed inspired air for any GA procedure lasting longer than 30 minutes
- Ensure patient has a temperature of at least 36°C prior to induction of anaesthesia

Fluids:
- Fluids including blood should be warmed to 37°C before infusion where possible
- This includes fluid for wash

Warming:
- For any procedure over 30 minutes, a warming device should be used for the patient such as a 'Bair Hugger'

Further reading

Ruetzler K, Kurz A. Consequences of perioperative hypothermia. Handb Clin Neurol 2018; 157:687–697.

Scenario 15

Stress response to surgery

You are assessing a 67-year-old male patient who is 24 hours post laparoscopic right hemicolectomy. He is catheterised and has had a low urine output over the last 4 hours.

Q. 15.1 What is the cause of this patient's reduced urine output?

The main cause in this patient is the activation of the renin–angiotensin–aldosterone system which occurs as a direct response of the body to surgery. This is couples with release of ADH. Both are stimulated to conserve fluid.

It may continue for 3–5 days postsurgery. Dehydration postoperatively and potential ileus with fluid extravasation into the gut lumen can further exacerbate the oliguria.

Q. 15.2 Describe the renin–angiotensin–aldosterone system.

- Renin is secreted by the juxtaglomerular cells in the kidney – this is activated by the sympathetic nervous system
- Renin converts angiotensinogen (produced by the liver) to angiotensin I
- Angiotensin I is converted to angiotensin II by angiotensin-converting enzyme (ACE) (present in the lung capillaries)
- Angiotensin II is a potent vasoconstrictor
- It also activates the adrenal cortex (glomerulosa) to produce aldosterone
- Aldosterone leads to sodium and water retention from the distal convoluted tubule at the expense of potassium
- Both angiotensin II and aldosterone lead to an increase in BP

Q. 15.3 What is the metabolic response to surgery or trauma?

There are two phases:
- Ebb phase (<24 hours)
- Flow phase (after 24 hours)
  - Catabolic phase (3–10 days)
  - Anabolic phase (10–60 days)

Ebb phase:
- This occurs within the first few hours of surgery
- The goal of this phase is to protect. It conserves circulatory volume and minimises demands on the body
- It is modulated by catecholamines, cortisol, and aldosterone
- The effects include reduction in:
  - Oxygen consumption
  - Enzyme activity
  - Cardiac output
  - Basal metabolic rate
  - Body temperature
- There is an increase in production of acute phase proteins

Flow phase:
- This occurs after 24 hours, with a dramatic increase in the metabolic rate
- There is an increase in the following:
  - Oxygen consumption
  - Glucose production (glucose is incredibly important in the response to trauma and the metabolic response is geared to providing as much as possible)
  - Cardiac output
  - Metabolic rate
  - Body temperature
  - Weight loss
- This is divided into a catabolic phase initially followed by an anabolic phase

Q. 15.4 What do you understand by the catabolic phase, and can you describe the effects this has on the body?

The catabolic phase is where the body breaks down molecules such as glucose into ATP to release energy.

Glucose:
- Insulin levels decrease and glucagon levels increase
- Cortisol also results in insulin resistance
- This all leads to glycolysis and release of glucose from the liver
- State of glucose intolerance with high serum glucose
- Body glycogen stores last for about 24 hours after which blood glucose is maintained by other methods (i.e. gluconeogenesis from breakdown products of lipids or proteins)

Fat:
- Lipolysis is stimulated by the sympathetic nervous system, ACTH, cortisol, glucagon, and decreased insulin
- Triglycerides broken down to glycerol and fatty acids
- Glycerol is used for gluconeogenesis, and fatty acids are oxidised for energy

Protein:
- Suppressed insulin levels encourage the release of amino acids from the skeletal muscle
- A three- to four-fold increase in serum amino acids is usually required after major trauma
- This requirement reaches its peak about a week after injury
- These amino acids are used for gluconeogenesis and for synthesis of acute phase proteins
- There is a negative nitrogen balance

Q. 15.5 What do you understand by the anabolic phase, and can you describe the effects this has on the body?

The anabolic phase is where the process of cell differentiation and growth, which is controlled by growth hormones and androgens.
During this phase, the following occurs:
- Repair of tissues
- Replenishing glycogen reserves
- Replenishing of fat and protein stores
- Weight gain

The overall duration and increase in metabolic rate in the flow phase depends on the type of stimulus, increasing from elective surgery to trauma.

Q. 15.6 How may the systemic response to surgery be minimised?

Preoperatively:
- High protein loading preoperative
- Control of preoperative sepsis where possible

Intraoperatively:
- Good tissue handling
- Minimally invasive surgery
- Shorter surgery time

Postoperatively:
- Correct hypovolaemia including replacement of fluids and electrolytes
- Transfuse as required
- Correct metabolic abnormalities
- Control of postoperative sepsis
- Enteral feeding
- Ensure adequate analgesia
- Correct hypoxia

Further reading

Desborough JP. The stress response to trauma and surgery. Br J Anaesth 2000; 85:109–117.
Hoo B, Boshier PR, Freethy A, et al. Redefining the stress cortisol response to surgery. Clin Endocrinol (Oxf) 2017; 87:451–458.

Scenario 16

Inotropes and circulatory support

You have admitted a 67-year-old gentleman with ascending cholangitis. He has undergone an endoscopic retrograde cholangiopancreatography (ERCP) with partial stone extraction and stent insertion. He is on ITU and remains septic with a consistently low systolic BP < 90 mmHg despite adequate fluid replacement and a raised heart rate of 120 bpm.

Q. 16.1 Can you define shock?

Shock is defined as reduced end-organ perfusion leading to end-organ dysfunction with an associated mortality.

Q. 16.2 What drugs can be used to provide circulatory support?

These can either be:
- Inotropes
  - Increase myocardial contractility
- Vasopressors
  - Cause vasoconstriction

Q. 16.3 What is cardiac output?

Cardiac output = Stroke volume × heart rate

Q. 16.4 What is Starling's law of the heart?

The force of contraction of the left ventricle is proportional to the stretch on the myocardial fibres.

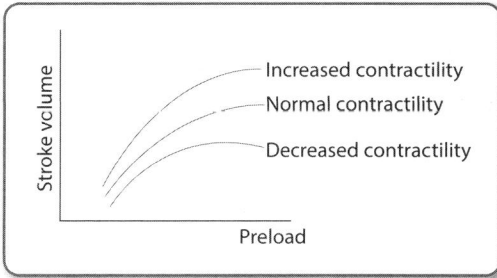

Source: The Frank-Starling mechanism. [online] Available from https://derangedphysiology.com/main/cicm-primary-exam/required-reading/cardiovascular-system/Chapter%20027/frank-starling-mechanism [Last accessed February, 2022].

X-axis can be stroke volume or cardiac output.
Preload is equal to the end diastolic volume.
Inotropes push the curve upwards and increase cardiac output.

Q. 16.5 What is blood pressure?

- Blood pressure is the product of cardiac output and SVR
- Therefore, to increase BP you can either:
  - Increase CO
  - Increase SVR

Q. 16.6 What examples of inotropes do you know?

Inotropes work by increasing the available amount of calcium within the cardiac myocytes through activation of adenylyl cyclase, leading to increased production of cAMP which in turn leads to activation of protein kinase A. This results in an increased influx of calcium, and this increases myocardial contractility.

	Type of drug	Mode of action	Notes
Dobutamine	Synthetic catecholamine	Beta-1	Nil
Milrinone/ Enoximone	Synthetic	Phosphodiesterase II inhibitors	Also causes vasodilation
Dopexamine	Synthetic analogue of dopamine		Also causes vasodilation (specifically splanchnic vasodilation)

Q. 16.7 What examples of vasopressors do you know?

	Type of drug	Mode of action	Notes
Adrenaline	Endogenous catecholamine	Alpha-1 agonist (mainly) Beta-1 agonist (in lower doses)	In low doses – has inotropic effects via beta-1 receptors
Noradrenaline	Endogenous catecholamine	Alpha-1 agonist	
Vasopressin (ADH)	Endogenous hormone	Acts on collecting ducts to increase water resorption	
Dopamine	Endogenous precursor of noradrenaline	Dopamine receptor (D1 and D2) agonist	Has inotropic properties depending on dose

Q. 16.8 What is the drug of choice for circulatory support in sepsis?

The drug of choice is noradrenaline in septic shock.

Further reading

Annane D, Ouanes-Besbes L, De Backer D, et al. A global perspective on vasoactive agents in shock. Intensive Care Med 2018; 44:833–846.

Kislitsina ON, Rich JD, Wilcox JE, et al. Shock – classification and pathophysiological principles of therapeutics. Curr Cardiol Rev 2019; 15:102–113.

Scenario 17

Rhabdomyolysis

A 34-year-old man was admitted 24 hours ago following a road traffic collision, where he was trapped in the vehicle for over 6 hours before being retrieved. He suffered multiple traumatic injuries including an open pelvic fracture and intra-abdominal haemorrhage. He underwent an ex-fix for his pelvis fracture, a laparotomy and packing with a defunctioning sigmoid colostomy (secondary to the pelvic fracture) with a laparostomy. While reviewing him on the ward round and you notice he is now developing acute renal failure with dark urine.

Q. 17.1 What are you concerned about with regards to his renal function?

His renal failure can be attributed to two causes:
1. Pre-renal failure due to hypovolaemia and hypoperfusion to the kidneys due to the SIRS response from trauma
2. Rhabdomyolysis secondary to crush injury

Q. 17.2 What is rhabdomyolysis?

This is a severe condition secondary to the breakdown of skeletal muscle and subsequent release of intracellular toxins that has a mortality of up to 60%.

Q. 17.3 Are there any investigations that will guide you towards a diagnosis of rhabdomyolysis?

- Creatine kinase
- Imaging to rule out obstructive cause
  - Retroperitoneal haematoma for example in this case
- Urine dip to check for myoglobinuria

Q. 17.4 What is the pathophysiology of the disease?

- There is a breakdown of muscle tissue
  - Commonly back/thigh/calf
- This leads to a release of the following due to tissue breakdown
  - Potassium (hyperkalaemia)
  - Phosphate (hyperphosphataemia)
  - Creatine kinase
  - Lactate dehydrogenase (LDH)

- Myoglobin is released as a direct consequence of muscle breakdown
- This binds to the Tamm-Horsfall protein in the thick ascending loop of Henle
- This leads to the formation of a precipitate which causes obstruction within the tubules thus leading to renal failure

Q. 17.5 What is the treatment?

- Aggressive fluid resuscitation to try and 'flush' out the precipitates formed in the tubules is the only known agreed treatment
- Other controversial treatments include:
    - Mannitol
    - Alkalinisation of urine

Further reading

Zimmerman JL, Shen MC. Rhabdomyolysis. Chest 2013; 144:1058–1065.
Bosch X, Poch E, Grau JM. Rhabdomyolysis and acute kidney injury. N Engl J Med 2009; 361:62–72.

Scenario 18

Hepatorenal syndrome

You are doing a ward round and have been asked to review a patient on ITU with abdominal pain on a background of alcoholic liver disease. The team are concerned that there has been a sharp decline in renal function over the last 48 hours.

Q. 18.1 What condition are you worried about?

Hepatorenal syndrome

Q. 18.2 What is hepatorenal syndrome?

It is the development of renal failure on a background of:
- Advanced chronic liver disease
- Portal hypertension
- Ascites

Q. 18.3 What is the pathophysiology of the disease?

- Due to reduced renal perfusion
- Portal hypertension leads to splanchnic vasodilation
- Leads to reduced renal perfusion
  - Activation of renin-angiotensin system
  - Renal vasoconstriction
- The renal vasoconstriction is insufficient to compensate the effects of the splanchnic vasodilation
- This all leads to persistent decreased renal perfusion and worsening renal vasoconstriction
- The result is renal failure

The process is precipitated by an acute event:
- GI bleeding
- Acute alcoholic hepatitis
- Infection/Sepsis
- Diuretic overuse

Q. 18.4 What are the types of HRS that you are aware of?

There are two types:

Type 1:
- This is a rapid progressive worsening in renal function
- Commonly precipitated by spontaneous bacterial peritonitis (SBP)
- Average survival is <2 weeks
- Overall survival is 10 weeks at most

Type 2:
- Chronic stable worsening in renal function
- Commonly caused by ascites that is refractory to diuretic treatment
- Average survival 3–6 months

Q. 18.5 What is the treatment?

The only curative treatment is a liver transplant. Without this, it is a fatal disease.
   Other treatments are designed to keep patient alive long enough to find a donor if they are suitable for a transplant.

Medical:
- Splanchnic vasopressors
- Somatostatin analogues
- Noradrenaline

Surgical treatment:
- Transjugular intrahepatic portosystemic shunt (TIPS)

Further reading

Amin AA, Alabsawy EI, Jalan R, Davenport A. Epidemiology, pathophysiology, and management of hepatorenal syndrome. Semin Nephrol 2019; 39:17–30.

Francoz C, Durand F, Kahn JA, Genyk YS, Nadim MK. Hepatorenal syndrome. Clin J Am Soc Nephrol 2019; 14:774–781.

Scenario 19

Postoperative respiratory complications

You are leading a ward round and come across a 72-year-old male patient who has had a laparotomy and patch repair of a perforated duodenal ulcer. It is now the 3rd postoperative day, and she has developed increasing oxygen requirements.

Q. 19.1 What are your differential diagnoses?

- Basal atelectasis
- Pneumonia
- PE

Q. 19.2 What is the pathophysiology of atelectasis?

- Most commonly occurs in the first 3 days postoperatively
- Secondary to a ventilation/perfusion mismatch in the dependent areas of the lungs
  - The bases are mostly affected
- Can be due to hypoventilation of these areas secondary to poor pain control postoperatively and therefore patients do not take deep breaths
- Atelectasis itself also causes a ventilation/perfusion mismatch
  - Leads to shunt
  - Leads to increased work of breathing

Q. 19.3 What is the management of basal atelectasis?

- Oxygen therapy to ensure saturations are at appropriate level for the patient
  - Beware the patient with COPD
- Nurse the patient upright where possible
- Ensure adequate analgesia
- Chest physiotherapy
- Mobilisation

Q. 19.4 How can the risk of basal atelectasis be reduced?

- Ensure adequate postoperative analgesia
  - Patient-controlled analgesia
  - Epidural

- Encourage early mobilisation (ERAS where possible)
- Early chest physiotherapy in high-risk patients
- Nurse upright

Q. 19.5 When does a diagnosis of pneumonia commonly occur?

- This usually occurs 3–5 days postoperatively
- Is nosocomial in origin
    - Antibiotics should be tailored as per hospital guidelines
- Can be due to aspiration especially in patients who are elderly or are in ileus

Q. 19.6 When does a pulmonary embolism classically occur?

- 5 days postoperatively is the most common time
- Usually presents with pleuritic chest pain and an associated tachycardia with hypoxia

Q. 19.7 How would you assess the likelihood of PE being the diagnosis?

- Assess the patient's symptoms
- Look for ECG changes of S1Q3T3
    - Large S wave in lead I
    - Q wave in lead III
    - Inverted T wave in lead III
- Calculate the Well's score
    - Used to calculate the probability of a PE

Well's criteria:

Criteria	Points
Clinical signs and symptoms of DVT	3
PE is most likely diagnosis or equally likely	3
Heart rate >100	1.5
Reduced mobility for 3 days or surgery in previous 4 weeks	1.5
Previous confirmed diagnosis of DVT or PE	1.5
Haemoptysis	1
Malignancy within last 6 months	1

Score	Management
<4	D-dimer
	If negative no further investigations
4–6	D-dimer
	Consider imaging (CTPA or $\dot{V}/\dot{Q}$ scan)
>6	Straight to urgent imaging (CTPA or $\dot{V}/\dot{Q}$ scan)

Q. 19.8 What is a D-dimer?

- Measures levels of fibrin-degradation products
- Very high sensitivity of >95%
- Poor specificity as raised by multiple inflammatory conditions
  - Infection
  - Surgery

Q. 19.9 How can you classify a PE?

- Stable PE:
  - Haemodynamically stable
  - No right ventricular dysfunction
- Submassive PE:
  - Haemodynamically stable
  - Evidence of right ventricular dysfunction
- Massive PE:
  - Haemodynamic instability
  - Right ventricular dysfunction

Q. 19.10 What treatment options are available?

- The most common treatment for stable and sub-massive PEs is anticoagulation
  - Warfarin
  - Direct oral anticoagulant (DOAC)
- For some sub-massive PEs and massive PEs
  - Thrombolysis
  - Thrombectomy

Q. 19.11 What is the best way to prevent a PE?

- Ensure appropriate deep vein thrombosis (DVT) prophylaxis is prescribed
  - Ted stockings
  - Low-molecular-weight heparin
- Patients undergoing surgery for colorectal cancer should receive 28 days of DVT prophylaxis postoperatively as per NICE guidelines.

Further reading

Beckerman Z, Bolotin G. Surgical treatment of acute massive pulmonary embolism. Adv Exp Med Biol 2017; 906:75–88.

Howard L. Acute pulmonary embolism. Clin Med (Lond) 2019; 19:243–247.

Jolly M, Phillips J. Pulmonary embolism: current role of catheter treatment options and operative thrombectomy. Surg Clin North Am 2018; 98:279–292.

Scenario 20

Ventilator-associated pneumonia

An intubated and ventilated 80-year-old male patient is under your care after a laparotomy and Hartmann's procedure for perforated diverticular disease. He has a history of lung fibrosis, and he is becoming difficult to ventilate on day 5 postoperatively. He has raised inflammatory markers, and a CT of the abdomen and pelvis shows no collections.

Q. 20.1 What do you understand by the term ventilator-associated pneumonia (VAP)?

This is a nosocomial pneumonia [hospital-acquired pneumonia (HAP)] that occurs 48 hours or more after intubation. There should be infiltrates present on CXR plus at least two of the following:
- Temperature > 38.3°C
- White cell count (WCC) < 4 or > 12
- Purulent tracheal secretions

Q. 20.2 What is the pathophysiology of VAP?

- It is associated with prolonged mechanical ventilation
- The most common cause is aspiration
  - This may be due to ileus/delayed gastric emptying
  - Can also be secondary to sedation
- There is colonisation of bacteria on the inner lining of the ET tube
- Initially, this causes ventilator-associated tracheobronchitis, which is the precursor to VAP
- Onset > 4 days has poorer prognosis as it is more likely to be drug resistant

Q. 20.3 What specific measures can be taken to reduce the incidence of VAP?

- Ensure the patient is nursed upright (around 45°)
- Ensure optimal sedation of the patient, i.e. as light as the patient tolerates
- Good oral hygiene
- Regular suction
- Ensure adequate ET tube cuff pressure is maintained to help prevent leakage of bacteria
- Ensure stress ulcer prophylaxis (ranitidine)

Q. 20.4 What are the most common causative organisms?
- *Pseudomonas aeruginosa*
- *Staphylococcus aureus*
- *Klebsiella*
- *Haemophilus*

Q. 20.5 What is the treatment?
- Requires early recognition and clinical suspicion
- Broad-spectrum antibiotics
- Multidisciplinary team (MDT) approach with microbiology team

Further reading

Metersky ML, Kalil AC. Management of ventilator-associated pneumonia: guidelines. Clin Chest Med 2018; 39:797–808.

Oliveira J, Zagalo C, Cavaco-Silva P. Prevention of ventilator-associated pneumonia. Rev Port Pneumol 2014; 20:152–161.

Spalding MC, Cripps MW, Minshall CT. Ventilator-associated pneumonia: new definitions. Crit Care Clin 2017; 33:277–292.

Scenario 21

Tracheostomy

You have a patient in ITU who has suffered polytrauma secondary to multiple stabbings. It is decided that he will require a prolonged period of ventilation before weaning can be achieved.

Q. 21.1 What are the types of surgical airway that you are aware of?

- Needle cricothyroidotomy (usually in emergencies)
- Cricothyroidotomy
- Tracheostomy

Q. 21.2 What indications for a tracheostomy are you aware of?

- Long-term management of ventilated patient
- Failed extubation in ITU
- Airway obstruction (trauma in surrounding area including larynx)
- Failed intubation
- Acute epiglottitis
- Chronic respiratory insufficiency

Q. 21.3 What are the benefits of using a tracheostomy?

- Shortens weaning time form ventilation
- Reduces need for sedative drug use
- Improved patient comfort
- Reduced incidence of nosocomial respiratory infections
- Reduced overall hospital stay

Q. 21.4 Describe how you would insert a tracheostomy.

- This is performed under GA with the patient supine
- Make transverse incision between cricoid cartilage and sternal notch
- Then use blunt dissection to identify the trachea
- Identify 1st tracheal ring, then make a small window between the 2nd and 3rd tracheal rings by removing a small piece of cartilage
- Then ask the anaesthetist to withdraw the ET tube in place, and then immediately insert the tracheostomy tube under direct vision

- Ensure there is adequate ventilation and equal bilateral chest expansion
- Secure tube and close layers

Q. 21.5 What are the complications of tracheostomy insertion?

Immediate:
- Bleeding
- Asphyxia
- Oesophageal injury

Early:
- Aspiration
- Blockage
- Mucus plugging
- Infection

Late:
- Tracheal stenosis
- Subglottic stenosis
- Difficult decannulation
- Delayed bleeding

Q. 21.6 What is the immediate postoperative management of a patient with a tracheostomy?

- Nurse the patient upright
- Check for equal bilateral breath sounds and chest expansion
- CXR
- Suction PRN
- Humidified oxygen

Q. 21.7 What are the advantages and disadvantages of using a double cannula tracheostomy tube?

Advantages:
- Lower incidence of obstruction
- Easier to clean by allowing removal of inner tube
- Allows for vocalisation

Disadvantage:
- Increased resistance to breathing

Further reading

Arora A, Hettige R, Ifeacho S, Narula A. Driving standards in tracheostomy care: a preliminary communication of the St Mary's ENT-led multi-disciplinary team approach. Clin Otolaryngol 2008; 33:596–599.

Scenario 22

Bleeding disorders

You are in clinic and have booked a patient for a laparoscopic right hemicolectomy. The patient has a background of haemophilia.

Q. 22.1 Can you describe the clotting cascade?

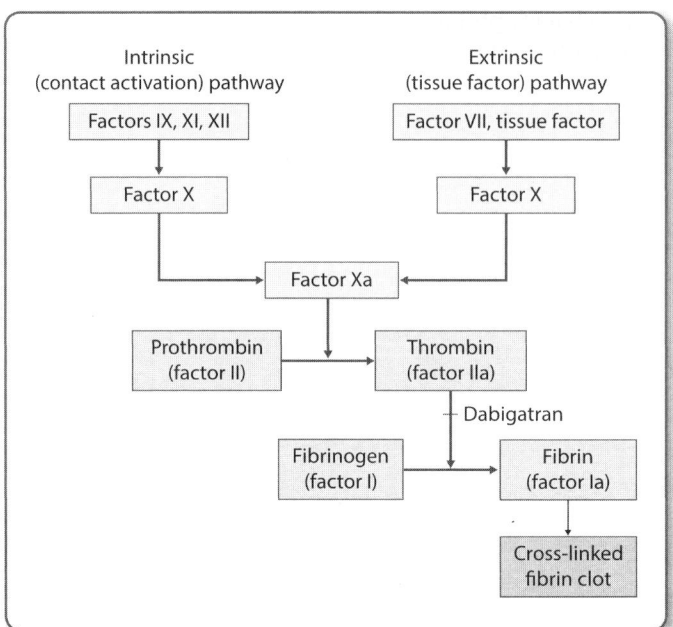

Source: Simplified diagram of the coagulation cascade demonstrating pharmacology of dabigatran. [online] Available from https://www.researchgate.net/figure/Simplified-diagram-of-the-coagulation-cascade-demonstrating-pharmacology-of-dabigatran_fig1_51615136 [Last accessed February, 2022].

Q. 22.2 What do you understand by the term bleeding disorder?

A disorder that may be acquired or congenital that predisposes a patient to bleeding.

Q. 22.3 What congenital bleeding disorders are you aware of?

Haemophilia A:
- X-linked recessive
- Affects factor VIII
- Presents with spontaneous bleeding:
  - Brain
  - Joints/Muscles
  - Brain
  - GI tract
- Preoperatively can be treated with desmopressin or factor VIII transfusion

Haemophilia B:
- X-linked recessive disorder
- Affects factor XI
- Presents in identical fashion to haemophilia A
- Preoperatively can be treated with prothrombin complex or factor XI

von Willebrand disease:
- Both autosomal dominant and recessive
- Affects von Willebrand factor
  - Plasma carrier of factor VIII
  - Aids in platelet adhesion at sites of vascular injury
- Presents with bleeding:
  - Epistaxis
  - Mucosal
  - Petechiae
- Preoperatively can be treated with cryoprecipitate, factor VIII or desmopressin

Q. 22.4 What acquired bleeding disorders are you aware of?

Platelet dysfunction:
- Drug induced:
  - Non-steroidal anti-inflammatory drugs
  - Antiplatelet medications, e.g. aspirin/clopidogrel
  - Heparin
- Alcohol

Thrombocytopaenia:
- Increased platelet consumption
  - Sepsis
    Disseminated intravascular coagulation (DIC)
- Decreased platelet production
  - Bone marrow failure
  - Increased chronic alcohol intake
- Decreased platelet longevity
  - Idiopathic thrombocytopenic purpura (ITP)

Vitamin K deficiency:
- Reduced bile salts
- Malabsorption
- Poor diet

Liver failure:
- Affects vitamin K-dependent clotting factors
- Decreased synthesis of clotting factors
- Decreased synthesis of clotting inhibitors
  - Protein C
  - Protein S
  - Antithrombin III

Q. 22.5 What are the vitamin K-dependent clotting factors?

Mnemonic 1972:
Factors:
- X
- IX
- VII
- II

Q. 22.6 What common anticoagulant medications are you aware of?

Warfarin:
- Affects vitamin K-dependent clotting factors
- Reversed using vitamin K

Direct oral anticoagulant:
- Rivaroxaban/Edoxaban
- Inhibitor of activated factor X (Xa)
- Most commonly use Beriplex across trusts, however, not 100% effective
- Andexanet alfa has been provisionally approved in UK (not widely available)

Dabigatran:
- Non-peptide direct thrombin inhibitor
- Reversed with idarucizumab

Heparin:
- Antithrombin II activator
- Reversed with protamine

Further reading

Mensah PK, Gooding R. Surgery in patients with inherited bleeding disorders. Anaesthesia 2015; 70:112–120, e39–40.

Scenario 23

Diagnosis of death using neurological criteria (brainstem testing) and organ donation

You are asked to review a 46-year-old man on the HDU who was admitted overnight with an extensive traumatic brain injury. He was intubated at scene with a GCS of 3 and remained on the ICU, his CT scan showed an extensive traumatic subarachnoid haemorrhage which the neurosurgical team has deemed inoperable. You are asked to review the patient as he is to be considered for organ donation.

Q. 23.1 What types of organ donation are you aware of?

Broadly speaking types of organ donation can fall into several categories:
- Live organ donation
- Donation after circulatory death
- Donation after brain death
- Tissue donation

(Organ donation and specific classification will be covered in more detail in the Transplant Chapters)

Q. 23.2 The nurse at the bedside report that his infusion of propofol and alfentanil have been stopped for 24 hours. The patient continues to have an output and is maintaining a MAP without requiring vasopressors, he has not 'triggered' the ventilator in that time. What are your thoughts on how next to proceed?

The patient is most likely brainstem dead however, he will need to undergo formal diagnosis of death by neurological criteria – brainstem testing.

Q. 23.3 What are the criteria for brainstem testing? What are the physiological principles behind the tests? How will you do the tests?

Criteria for brainstem testing:
Preconditions:
- The patient should be unconscious, apnoeic, and mechanically ventilated
- The cause of the irreversible coma should be from brain damage of known aetiology, e.g. spontaneous intracranial haemorrhage, hypoxic brain injury, ischaemic stroke, and trauma

- If the primary diagnosis of coma is unclear, a prolonged period of clinical observation may be required before understanding any underlying pathology

Caution must be used if 'Red Flag signs' are present:
1. Testing < 6 hours since the loss of the last brainstem reflex
2. Patients with any neuromuscular disorders
3. Prolonged fentanyl infusions
4. Testing < 24 hours since the loss of the last brainstem reflex, where aetiology primarily anoxic damage
5. Steroids given in space-occupying lesions such as abscesses
6. Aetiology primarily located to the brainstem or posterior fossa
7. Hypothermia (24-hour observation period following re-warming to normothermia recommended)

Exclusion criteria:
The apnoeic coma must not be due to reversible causes:

Body temperature at time of testing	If core temperature is ≤34°C, testing cannot be carried out
Serum sodium (Na⁺) at time of testing	Serum sodium should be between 115 and 160 mmol/L. Rapid rises or falls in Na⁺ should be avoided
Serum potassium (K⁺) at time of testing	Serum potassium should be >2 mmol/L
Serum phosphate (PO_4^{3-}) at time of testing	Serum phosphate should not be profoundly elevated (>3.0 mmol/L) or lowered (<0.5 mmol/L) from normal
Serum magnesium (Mg^{2+}) at time of testing	Serum magnesium should not be profoundly elevated (>3.0 mmol/L) or lowered (<0.5 mmol/L) from normal
Blood glucose at time of testing	Blood glucose should be between 3.0 and 20.0 mmol/L and should be tested prior to each test
If there is any clinical reason to expect endocrine disturbances?	Hormonal assays should be undertaken as appropriate
Is the apnoea due to neuromuscular blocking agents, other drugs or a non-brainstem cause (e.g. cervical injury, any neuromuscular weakness)?	The answer should be NO before proceeding to tests

Physiological principles:
- Aiming to test brainstem function by assessing the function of the cranial nerves (which arise from the brainstem)
- Apnoea test is testing the central respiratory drive to hypercapnia. During the period of apnoea, CO_2 within the blood will increase due to the lack of excretion from the lungs. As the $PaCO_2$ rises, this diffuses across the blood brain barrier and as per the Henderson–Hasselbalch equation (below) the concentration of H^+ will

increase. This is detected by central chemoreceptors and is a strong central drive to increase ventilation.

$$CO_2 + H_2O \leftrightharpoons H_2CO_3 \leftrightharpoons H^+ + HCO_3^-$$

Performing the tests:
- Ensure all preconditions are met and decide on appropriate personnel to perform the test
- Inform the family as they may wish to be present for the first set of tests
- Equipment required: Pen torch, cotton swab, auriscope (to check for ear wax), bladder syringe, ice cold water, tongue depressor (or laryngoscope blade), Yankauer sucker, bag valve circuit (to provide oxygenation during apnoea and to observe any respiratory effort), capnography – this will be already attached as the patient is intubated and ventilated
- Ensure the patient is ventilated on 100% O_2, allow the $ETCO_2$ to rise to 6.0 kPa.
- Ensure the tympanic membranes can be seen in both ears
- Take the first set of ABGs
- Perform cranial nerve examination:
  - Pupillary reaction to light: Cranial nerves II, III
  - Corneal reflex (use light touch with sterile gauze): Cranial nerves V, VII
  - Vestibulo-ocular reflex: flex head to 30°, slowly inject 50–60 mL ice cold water in each ear observing for any eye movement: Cranial nerves III, VI, VIII
  - Gag reflex: spatula or Yankauer sucker or laryngoscope to stimulate the posterior pharynx: Cranial nerves IX, X
  - Cough reflex: pass a suction catheter down the ETT to the carina: Cranial nerves IX, X
  - Supraorbital pressure: any motor response observed either central or peripheral: Cranial nerves V, VII. Reflex limb and trunk movements (spinal reflexes) can be present
  - Take second set of ABGs, there must have been a minimum rise > 0.5 kPa from the first set of results and no respiratory effort observed for a minimum of 5 minutes
  - Once all the above have been observed and if the criteria are fulfilled then the time of brainstem death can be recorded. Then a second set of tests must also take place

Further reading

Diagnosing death using neurological criteria. [online] Available from https://www.odt.nhs.uk/deceased-donation/best-practice-guidance/donation-after-brainstem-death/diagnosing-death-using-neurological-criteria/ [Last accessed February, 2022].
Form for the diagnosis of death using neurological criteria {short version}. [online] Available from https://www.ficm.ac.uk/sites/ficm/files/documents/2021-10/Form_for_the_Diagnosis_of_Death_using_Neurological_Criteria-short%20version.pdf [Accessed 1st April 2023]
Oram J, Murphy P. Diagnosis of death. Contin Educ Anaesth Crit Care Pain. 2011; 11:77–81.

Scenario 24

Local anaesthetics

You have been asked to review a 24-year-old female for removal of four lipomas situated on her back and shoulders. She would like to have them removed under local anaesthetic in the outpatient clinic.

Q. 24.1 What types of local anaesthetic agents do you know?

Broadly speaking there are two main types of anaesthetic agents commonly used. These are Amide and Ester local anaesthetics; this refers to the compound linking the lipophilic amide ring to the hydrophilic portion.

Common amide local anaesthetics include bupivacaine, lidocaine, prilocaine and ropivacaine. Isomeric forms of bupivacaine are also used as they have an improved cardiotoxic profile, these include L-bupivacaine.

Common ester local anaesthetics used include cocaine, procaine, amethocaine and chloroprocaine. Ester local anaesthetics have a higher incidence of allergic reactions and anaphylaxis compared to the amides.

Q. 24.2 What local anaesthetic agent would you use and why? What is the toxic dose?

Factors governing choice of local anaesthetic:
- Safety profile
- Speed of onset
- Density and duration of block provided
- Toxic dose/volume to be injected
- Any additives
    - Safety profile: For the reasons listed above, the most commonly used local anaesthetic agents for this procedure would be from the amide group
    - Speed of onset: Local anaesthetic agents work by first crossing the cell membrane of the neurone

Membrane permeability is related to ionisation, and many drug molecules exist as weak acids or bases and therefore, in an ionised and un-ionised form. The ratio of the two forms varies with the surrounding pH.

$$BH^+ \text{ (ionised)} \rightleftharpoons B + H^+ \text{ (un-ionised)}$$

In an acid environment, the above equation will shift towards the left, i.e. the ionised form.

In an alkaline environment, the above equation will tend towards the right, i.e. un-ionised form.

Local anaesthetics block action potential generated by blocking Na^+ channels within the neurone. The majority of local anaesthetic agents are mainly but not completely ionised at physiological pH.

The un-charged species (B) penetrates the nerve sheath of the neurone and then is converted to the BH^+ active form, which blocks the Na^+ channels and transmission of the action potential.

Increasing the acidity of the external solution would favour ionisation and render local anaesthetics ineffective. Local anaesthetics are therefore, ineffective in infected/inflamed tissue (acidic).

The speed of onset of a local anaesthetic, therefore, depends on the amount of un-ionised drug present when injected and how close to the nerve fibre it is injected.

Drugs such as lidocaine exist in a greater un-ionised portion at physiological pH compared to the commonly used bupivacaine and so have a quicker onset of action when injected subcutaneously.

The toxic doses of commonly used local anaesthetic drugs are in the table here:

Local anaesthetic	Plain		With ephedrine	
	Maximum dose (mg/kg)	Maximum dose (mg)	Maximum dose (mg/kg)	Maximum dose (mg)
Bupivacaine	2	175	3	225
L-bupivacaine	2	200	3	225
Lidocaine	5	350	7	500
Mepivacaine	5	350	7	500
Ropivacaine	3	200	3	250
Prilocaine	6	400	8	600

- Density and duration of block provided:
  - The duration of the block provided is determined by the percentage of protein binding of drug within the plasma. Commonly used agents such as lidocaine have a lower percentage of protein-bound drug (76%) versus bupivacaine (96%) and hence a shorter duration of action (4–6 hours) versus (8–12 hours)
  - The density of the block can be affected by several factors:
    - Patient variables, e.g. age, obesity
    - Concentration and the dose used
    - Site of injection, e.g. spinal anaesthesia versus subcutaneous injection
    - Additives, e.g. epinephrine (localised vasoconstriction to reduce recirculation of drug), hyaluronidase, opiates

Q. 24.3 You are carrying out the procedure in the outpatient setting how will you ensure a safe environment?

- Ensure adequate IV access
- Ensure full resuscitation facilities available
- Ensure full monitoring of patient
- Ensure skilled assistance/help available
- Calculate safe maximum dose for patient prior to injection

Q. 24.4 While you are injecting bupivacaine, the patient starts to complain of feeling strange, having a metallic taste and tingling around her mouth. What are your next steps? What is the most probable explanation?

The patient is having an adverse reaction to toxic levels of local anaesthetic agent, or she may have suffered from an intravenous injection. The course of action now would be to stop administering the bupivacaine and continue to monitor the patient for any further signs of toxicity.

Q. 24.5 What are the signs and symptoms of local anaesthetic toxicity? What is the treatment required?

The toxicity of local anaesthetics is mainly secondary to their membrane stabilising effects on cells, especially within the heart and CNS. Features include:
- Periorbital tingling
- Metallic taste
- Light headedness, agitation, and tremor
- Cardiac arrhythmias particularly resistant ventricular arrhythmias
- Loss of consciousness and/or convulsions

The treatment for local anaesthetic toxicity is as per the Association of Anaesthetists of Great Britain and Ireland guidelines listed here.
1. Stop injecting the local anaesthetic (remember infusion pumps)
2. Call for help and inform immediate clinical team of problem
3. Call for cardiac arrest trolley and lipid rescue pack
4. Give 100% oxygen and ensure adequate breathing:
   - Maintain the airway and if necessary secure it with a tracheal tube (if anaesthetic help is available)
   - Hyperventilation may help reduce acidosis
5. Confirm or establish intravenous access
6. If circulatory arrest:
   - Start continuous CPR using standard protocols
   - Give intravenous lipid emulsion
   - Recovery may take > 1 hour
   - Consider the use of cardiopulmonary bypass if available

If no circulatory arrest:
- Conventional therapies to treat hypotension, brady-, and tachyarrhythmia
- Consider intravenous lipid emulsion
7. Control seizures with small incremental doses of benzodiazepine, thiopental or propofol

Intralipid is a 20% lipid emulsion for IV use (propofol is not an alternative). The mechanism of action is that it will bind any unbound local anaesthetic within plasma.

If the patient suffers a cardiac arrest, the period of resuscitation will be prolonged due to the resistant nature of any underlying arrythmias.

Further reading

The Association of Anaesthetists of Great Britain and Ireland 2018. [online] Available from www.aagbi.org/qrh [Last accessed February, 2022].

Scenario 25

Acute kidney injury

You are asked to review a 54-year-old male patient on the surgical HDU. He underwent a right hemicolectomy just over 24 hours ago and the sister in charge is concerned as he has not passed much urine (100 mL over 24 hours).

Q. 25.1 What is your initial approach?

You would approach the patient and take a careful history and assessment based on ABC/CCrISP principles.

On assessment you find that the patient has a history of chronic kidney disease (CKD 3) and hypertension. ABC assessment reveals a respiratory rate of 24, SaO_2 94% on nasal cannulae, HR 90 bpm, BP 115/65 mmHg, his urine output is as above, and he is apyrexial. His pain is well controlled with a working epidural.

Q. 25.2 What are you most concerned about? What is your differential diagnosis?

You are most concerned about the development of an acute kidney injury (AKI). In the above case, the patient has a predisposition to developing an AKI due to his background CKD.

Acute kidney injury covers a wide range of insults to the kidney, the differential diagnoses can be categorised as:

Pre-renal (~30–60% of AKI):
- True volume depletion, e.g. diarrhoea
- Reduction in effective circulating volume, e.g. oedema, postsurgery
- Reduced cardiac output
- Renovascular disease, e.g. stenosis or embolus

Renal (~20–40%):
- Glomerular disease, e.g. primary glomerulonephritis (anti-GBM, ANCA), secondary, e.g. due to infection or vasculitis
- Nephrotic syndrome
- Vascular, e.g. embolic disease, haemolytic uraemic syndrome
- Drug induced, e.g. NSAIDs, cyclosporine

Post-renal (~1–10%):
- Obstructive uropathy: Blocked urinary catheter, surgical damage to ureters, bladder, urethra

Q. 25.3 Can you describe how AKI is staged?

There are two main validated scoring systems used for classification of AKI.

In 2004, the RIFLE score was introduced Risk, Injury, Failure, Loss, End stage. RIFLE enables monitoring of the progression of AKI severity during hospitalisation and RIFLE classes are strongly associated with increased lengths of stay, renal replacement therapy (RRT) requirement, renal function recovery, and discharge from hospital.

Class	Creatinine/GFR	Urine output mL/kg/h
Risk	↑ Cr × 1.5 or ↓ GFR > 25%	<0.5 × 6 h
Injury	↑ Cr × 2 or ↓ GFR > 50%	<0.5 × 12 h
Failure	↑ Cr × 3 or ↓ GFR > 75% Or if baseline Cr ≥ 353.6 µmol/L (≥4 mg/dL) ↑ Cr > 44.2 µmol/L (>0.5 mg/dL)	<0.3 × 24 h or anuria × 12 h
Loss	Complete loss of kidney function > 4 weeks	
End stage	Complete loss of kidney function > 3 months	

Limitations of RIFLE:
- Requires baseline creatinine (not always available)
- Endogenous secretion of creatinine is variable, (e.g. according to age, muscle mass); additionally, tubular secretion of creatinine can be affected by drugs (e.g. trimethoprim)
- Does not define aetiology of AKI
- The requirements for RRT not included

The AKIN (Acute Kidney Injury Network) scoring system (2007) was defined:

Score	Creatinine requirements	Urine output mL/kg/h
AKIN 1	↑ Cr ≥ 26.5 µmol/L (≥0.3 mg/dL) or Cr 1.0–2 times baseline	<0.5 (>6 h)
AKIN 2	↑ Cr > 200 or > 2–3 times baseline	<0.5 (>12 h)
AKIN 3	↑ Cr > 3 times baseline or if baseline Cr ≥ 353.6 µmol/L (≥4 mg/dL) Or requirement for RRT	<0.3 (24 h) Or anuria (12 h)

The AKIN score is used once a patient is fully hydrated. It relies on serum creatinine only and baseline creatinine is not required. Serum creatinine has to be measured at least twice within a 48-hour period. The AKIN score also includes the requirement for RRT.

Disadvantages:
- Does not account for any rise in creatinine outside of 48 hours
- Does not account for wide variability in indications for the use of RRT

Q. 25.4 What indications are you aware of for the use of RRT in AKI?

- Refer adults, children, and young people immediately for RRT if any of the following are not responding to medical management:
    - Hyperkalaemia
    - Metabolic acidosis
    - Symptoms or complications of uraemia (e.g. pericarditis or encephalopathy)
    - Fluid overload
    - Pulmonary oedema
- Base the decision to start RRT on the condition of the adult, child, or young person as a whole and not on an isolated urea, creatinine, or potassium value
- All of the above would be in discussion with critical care or nephrology teams

Despite adequate hydration, the patient has deteriorated with signs of persistent metabolic acidosis, and he is now struggling to breathe. You have called the critical care team and on assessment the team has decided that the patient requires RRT.

Q. 25.5 What methods of RRT are you are aware of?

- Peritoneal dialysis (more for chronic renal failure)
- Continuous veno-venous haemofiltration (CVVH)
- Haemodialysis

NB: There are different modes and types of CVVH and haemodialysis, but these are not required for the examination.

Q. 25.6 Can you briefly explain the mechanism of action and the differences between CVVH and haemodialysis?

Continuous veno-venous haemofiltration:
- Requires large vein cannulation with a dual bore catheter (usually a femoral line, e.g. Vascath)
- Pressure gradient is created by the use of a pump
- Convection – pressure gradient pushes water across the membrane and carries solutes with it (solvent drag)
- This *ultrafiltrate* is then replaced with specialised, sterile replacement fluid
- Anticoagulation is required, e.g. heparin or citrate

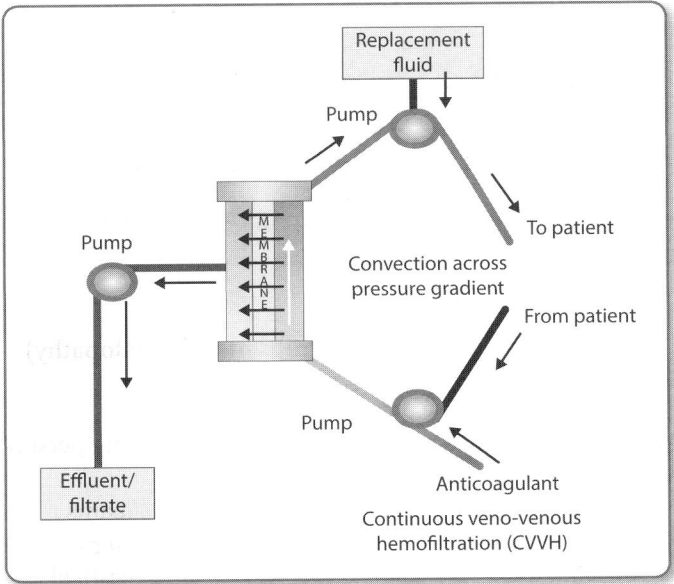

Haemodialysis:
- Requires large vein cannulation with a dual bore catheter (usually a femoral line, e.g. Vascath)
- Pressure gradient is created by the use of a pump
- Semipermeable membrane; counter current flow
- Diffusion across concentration gradient (osmosis)
- Electrolyte manipulation (especially K^+)
- Larger fluid shifts than CVVH
- Anticoagulation is required, e.g. heparin or citrate

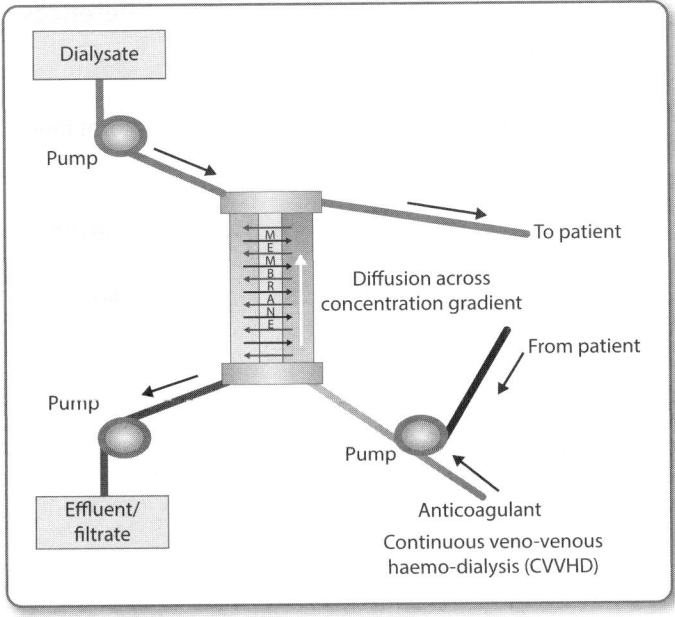

Further reading

Lopes JA, Jorge S. The RIFLE and AKIN classifications for acute kidney injury: a critical and comprehensive review. Clin Kidney J 2013; 6:8–14.

NICE. (2019). Acute kidney injury: prevention, detection and management. [online] Available from www.nice.org.uk/guidance/ng148 [Last accessed February, 2022].

Scenario 26

Sepsis

You have been asked to review a 52-year-old female patient who underwent a laparoscopic cholecystectomy for acute cholecystitis 3 days ago. She has been complaining of increased shortness of breath and the nurse looking after her is worried.

Q. 26.1 Describe how you would approach the patient and what your initial thoughts regarding differential diagnoses would be.

Initial approach would be a history and examination, and an assessment according to ABC/CCrISP principles.

Possible causes for increased shortness of breath in the postoperative patient can be classified as: (Although not mutually exclusive categorisation in this way will give the answer structure and also help order your thoughts.)

Medical causes:
- *Respiratory:* Chest infection
- *Cardiovascular:* Acute coronary syndrome, PE
- *Metabolic:* Respiratory compensation for metabolic acidosis
- *Pain:* Increased pain causing increased work of breathing

Surgical causes:
- Biliary leak, sepsis
- Retained stone – causing pain
- Pancreatitis

Q. 26.2 On ABCDE assessment, the following parameters are noted:

A – maintaining own, Sao_2 88% on nasal cannulae oxygen
B – RR 24 breath/min using accessory muscles
C – HR 120 bpm, BP 84/58 mmHg
D – GCS 15/15
E – mild abdominal tenderness on palpation, soft, temperature 38.8°C

MEWS score: 12
The team have ordered baseline blood investigations, ABGs, ECG, and a CXR.

The ECG is here:

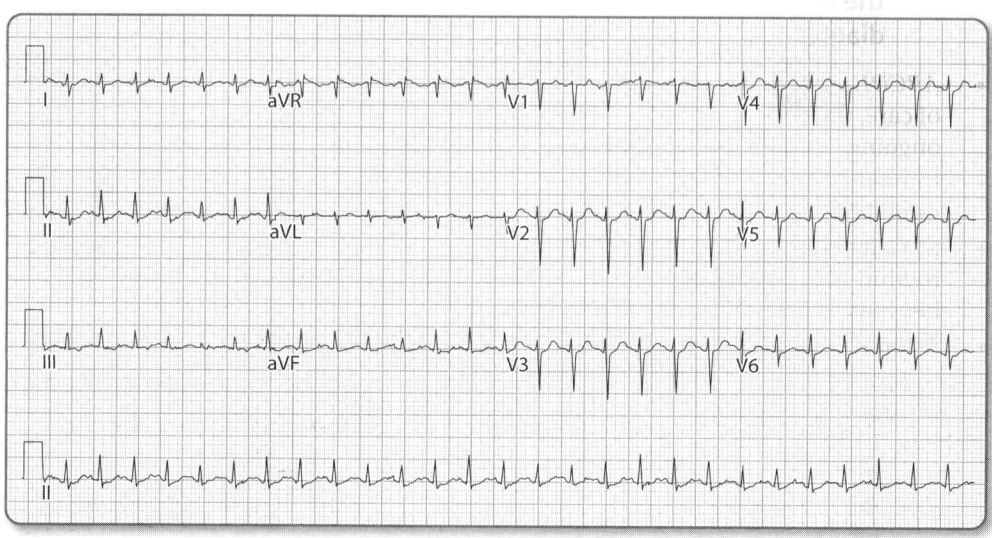

Arterial blood gas results:
On 2 L O_2 via nasal cannulae:

PaO_2	9.6 kPa
$PaCO_2$	3.6 kPa
pH	7.1
HCO_3^-	18
BE	−6.2
Lactate	4.1

The CXR is here:

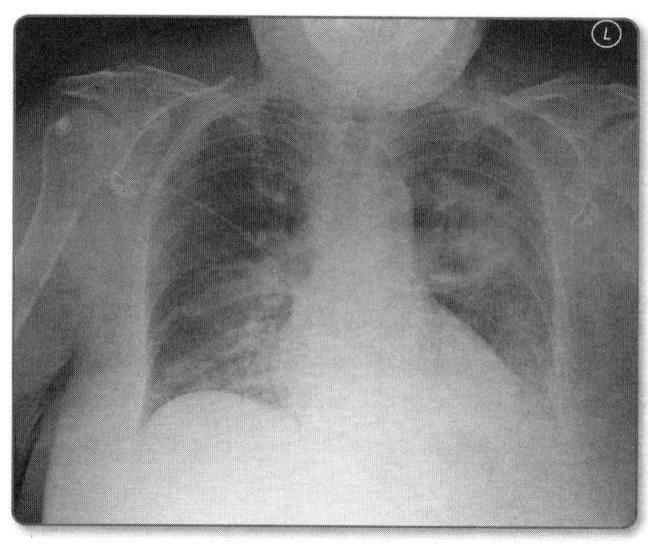

Scenario 26 **Sepsis**

Q. 26.3 Can you summarise the results of the investigations above, explain the metabolic picture shown by the ABG and give your differential diagnosis?

- *ABCDE assessment:* This patient is clearly unwell and will need an increased level of care, the critical care team would need to be contacted. The patient will require ongoing resuscitation, treatment, and assessment
- Immediate resuscitation would include 15 L O_2 via a non-rebreather mask, establishment of IV access if not already and initial fluid bolus
- *ECG:* It shows sinus tachycardia (P waves present, regular rhythm as per lead II – rhythm strip), HR approximately 150 bpm (300 divided by number of large squares between QRS complexes)
- Arterial blood gas:
  - *Look at Pao_2:* Hypoxia – need to increase the FIO_2
  - *Look at pH:* Acidosis, what is the cause?
    - Lactate is increased – either due to increased production (from anaerobic respiration) or reduced excretion (from the liver)
    - Base excess is more negative – metabolic acidosis (BE is increased, i.e. more positive in metabolic alkalosis)
    - $Paco_2$ is decreased, secondary to respiratory compensation for metabolic acidosis – clinically seen as increased work of breathing
- *Metabolic picture:* Metabolic acidosis most likely driven by increased lactate production with respiratory compensation
- *Chest X-ray:* Bilateral haziness greater in the lower and midzones
- *Differential diagnosis:* Sepsis secondary to a chest infection

Q. 26.4 Can you define SEPSIS? What is the underlying pathological response? What are the treatment priorities?

New 'Sepsis' guidelines were published in 2021 and updated in 2023.

New terms and definitions:
- Sepsis is defined as life-threatening organ dysfunction caused by a dysregulated host response to infection
- Organ dysfunction can be identified as an acute change in total SOFA score ≥ 2 points consequent to the infection. (SOFA = Sequential Organ Failure Assessment)

The SOFA score is a mortality prediction score based on the degree of organ dysfunction (6 organ systems used). The score is calculated on admission and every 24 hours until discharge using the worst parameters measured during the prior 24 hours.
- The baseline SOFA score can be assumed to be zero in patients not known to have pre-existing organ dysfunction
- A SOFA score ≥ 2 reflects an overall mortality risk of approximately 10% in a general hospital population with suspected infection. Even patients presenting with modest dysfunction can deteriorate further, emphasising the seriousness of this condition and the need for prompt and appropriate intervention, if not already being instituted

- Septic shock is a subset of sepsis in which underlying circulatory and cellular/metabolic abnormalities are profound enough to substantially increase mortality
- Patients with septic shock can be identified with a clinical construct of sepsis with persisting hypotension requiring vasopressors to maintain MAP > 65 mmHg and having a serum lactate level > 2 mmol/L (18 mg/dL) despite adequate volume resuscitation. With these criteria, hospital mortality is in excess of 40%

Pathophysiology of sepsis:
- Pathogen stimulates host defence cells, resulting in systemic inflammation and activation of proinflammatory mediators, ultimately leading to tissue damage
    - Primary source of infection most commonly lung, abdomen, or urinary tract
    - Exact pathogenesis unknown; factors involved may include:
        - Surge of proinflammatory cytokines
        - Delayed apoptosis of neutrophils
        - Decline in lymphocytes due to apoptosis
        - Dysfunction of coagulation and inappropriate deposition of intravascular fibrin
- Proinflammatory mediators reported to be involved in sepsis include:
    - Tumour necrosis factor-alpha
    - Interleukins
    - Macrophage migration inhibitory factor (MIF)
    - Soluble triggering receptor expressed on myeloid cell-1 (sTREM-1)
    - High mobility group box protein (HMGB-1)
    - Platelet-activating factor (PAF)
    - Prostaglandins
    - Leukotrienes
    - Thromboxane
    - Tissue factor
- Organ and tissue involvement:
    - Local infection progresses to mild systemic inflammation and possibly septic shock with major changes in cardiovascular system
    - Endothelial changes such as increased leukocyte adhesion, procoagulant state, vasodilation, and loss of barrier function can result in generalised tissue oedema
    - Microcirculatory changes may include impaired response to local stimulation and obstruction of microvessel lumens by microthrombi and plugs of white and red blood cells
    - Widespread tissue factor expression, fibrin deposition, and impaired anticoagulation can contribute to development of DIC and subsequent organ dysfunction, bleeding (via consuming platelets and clotting factors), and mortality
    - Sepsis as a disease occurs across a wide spectrum and is a heterogeneous disease state
    - It is a disease of the micro- and macrovascular systems
    - At the cellular level, there is mitochondrial dysoxia which leads to a failure of aerobic metabolism and a reduction in the production of ATP

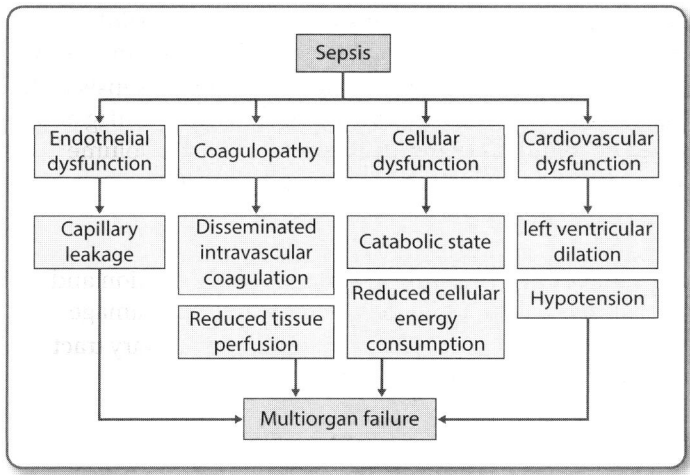

Treatment of sepsis:
- Rapid diagnosis of sepsis and early resuscitative treatment as required ('the golden hour'). The use of a care 'bundle' approach to early resuscitation – the sepsis 6:
  1. Administer oxygen. Aim to keep saturations > 94% (88–92% if at risk of CO_2 retention, e.g. COPD)
  2. Take blood cultures. At least a peripheral set. Consider source of sepsis, e.g. CSF, urine, sputum
  3. Give IV antibiotics: Broad spectrum (can be guided once microbiology results are available) – within 1 hour in sepsis with shock or high likelihood of sepsis. Unconfirmed/suspected sesspsis – investigate rapidly – antibiotics within 3 hours.
  4. Give IV fluids – balanced crystalloids. If hypotensive/lactate > 2 mmol/L, 500 mL stat. May be repeated if clinically indicated – do not exceed 30 mL/kg
  5. Check serial lactates: Used to guide effectiveness of resuscitation and severity of sepsis
  6. Measure urine output: Strict fluid balance may need catheterisation
- Assessment of severity of the septic response, e.g. the use of MEWS, the presence of 'Red Flag' signs (as per UK sepsis trust)
- Decide on early escalation of appropriate care, e.g. early involvement of critical care team. Involvement with relevant advanced diagnostic teams, e.g. CT abdomen
- Continual reassessment of treatment, consider primary source control and when appropriate, e.g. laparotomy

Further reading

Lever A, Mackenzie I. Sepsis: definition, epidemiology, and diagnosis. BMJ 2007; 335:879–883.
Sepsis Six and Red Flag Sepsis are copyright to and intellectual property of the UK Sepsis Trust, registered charity no. 1158843. sepsistrust.org.
Singer M, Deutschman CS, Seymour CW, et al. The Third International Consensus Definitions for Sepsis and Septic Shock (Sepsis-3). JAMA 2016; 315:801–810.
Stearns-Kurosawa DJ, Osuchowski MF, Valentine C, Kurosawa S, Remick DG. The pathogenesis of sepsis. Annu Rev Pathol 2011; 6:19–48.

Scenario 27

Pulmonary embolism

You are asked to assess a 54-year-old obese female patient who underwent a laparoscopic low anterior resection yesterday. She has become suddenly breathless and is tachycardic.

Q. 27.1 Describe how you would approach the patient, in terms of assessment and differential diagnoses.

- Initial approach would be a history and examination with an ABCDE/CCrISP assessment of severity
- Differential diagnoses; sudden onset of breathlessness in the postoperative patient
- Medical causes:
  - Atelectasis, acute collapse
  - Pulmonary embolism
  - Acute coronary syndrome
  - Exacerbation of underlying respiratory disease, e.g. asthma, COPD
  - Chest infection
- Surgical causes:
  - Pneumothorax
  - Peritonitis – acute rupture of viscus
  - Haemorrhage
  - Hypovolaemia

On arrival she is being administered 15 L O_2 via a non-rebreather mask, her ABCDE observations are:
- A – own
- B – RR 24 breath/min, SaO_2 86%
- C – BP 110/60 mmHg, HR 120 bpm – ECG sinus tachycardia
- D – GCS 15
- E – temperature 37.7°C, abdomen soft non-tender, chest pain on inspiration

Routine blood investigations have been ordered. A CXR showed no gross abnormality. ABGs show RF1.

Q. 27.2 What will you instruct the team to do next?

- The initial assessment shows that the patient is critically unwell and will require higher levels of care. You would contact the critical care team for further discussion

- Looking at the list of differential diagnoses you would order a CTPA and cardiac enzymes
- A CTPA with contrast has been done

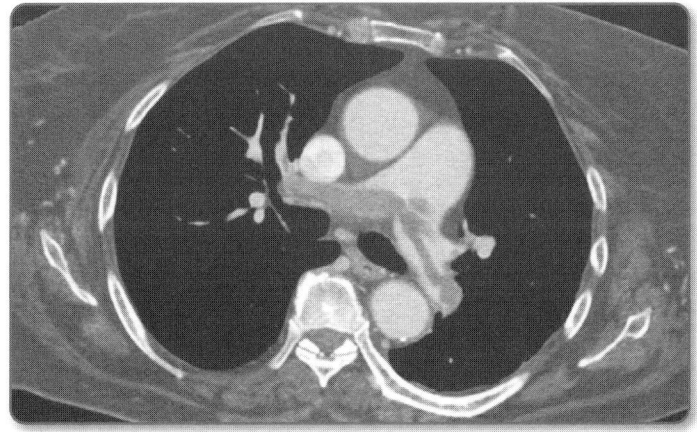

Q. 27.3 What is your diagnosis? What are the principles of management?

- A large perfusion defect is seen in the pulmonary trunk due to a saddle PE
- The principles of treatment are related to minimising the effects of a large $\dot{V}/\dot{Q}$ shunt, prevention of further clot propagation and clot lysis if relevant
- Need to classify the type of PE to guide further treatment:

American Heart Association classification of PE:
- Massive PE – acute PE with any of the following:
  - Sustained hypotension
    - Systolic BP < 90 mmHg for ≥15 minutes or requiring inotropic support
    - Not due to a cause other than PE, such as arrhythmia, hypovolaemia, sepsis, or left ventricular (LV) dysfunction
  - Persistent profound bradycardia (heart rate < 40 bpm with signs or symptoms of shock)
  - Pulselessness
- Sub-massive PE – acute PE without systemic hypotension (systolic BP ≥ 90 mmHg) but with either right ventricular (RV) dysfunction or myocardial necrosis
- Low-risk PE – acute PE without clinical markers of adverse prognosis that define massive or sub-massive PE

A bedside echocardiogram shows that the right ventricle is dilated, and she is becoming hypotensive (BP 85/53 mmHg) despite fluid resuscitation.

Q. 27.4 What are your treatment options?

As outlined above this is a massive PE, with significant haemodynamic compromise. The clot will require removal, options available are:

Systemic thrombolysis:
- Use of pharmacological agents, e.g. tenecteplase, risk of haemorrhage balanced against life-threatening PE
- Preferred over catheter-directed thrombolysis

Catheter-directed thrombolysis:
- Use in patients with acute hypotensive PE in case of high bleeding risk, failed systemic thrombolysis, and/or shock likely to result in death before systemic thrombolysis takes effect
- Use as an alternative to surgical treatment if systemic thrombolysis is contraindicated or has failed

Surgical pulmonary embolectomy:
- Use if shock or hypotension is present and there is a contraindication to or failed thrombolysis
- Consider if: Sub-massive acute PE with clinical evidence of poor prognosis
- Intermediate-high risk PE if anticipated bleeding risk with thrombolysis is high
- Will need to start continuous prophylaxis with either LMWH or unfractionated heparin or insertion of an IVC filter on discussion with radiology colleagues
- Continue with supportive therapy on a critical care unit

Q. 27.5 What do you understand by a physiological shunt?

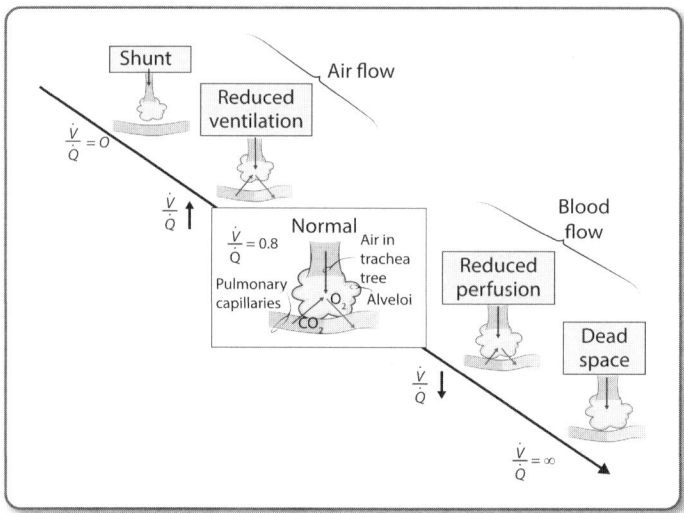

- In the above figure, we can see the relationship between the alveolus and the pulmonary capillary. Air flow into and out of the alveolus is ($\dot{V}$) and blood flow in the pulmonary capillary is ($\dot{Q}$)
- $\dot{V}/\dot{Q}$ is critical to oxygen delivery and the excretion of CO_2. In the normal lung, there is a small $\dot{V}/\dot{Q}$ mismatch due to a physiological shunt. (Anatomical dead space within the trachea and large bronchial tree where no gas exchange occurs and also mixing of venous and arterial blood in the bronchial and Thebesian veins)

- You can now use the above shunt figure to explain the pathophysiology of a PE. The blood flow has been occluded via a large clot causing a massive increase in alveolar dead space. There will be a large number of alveoli where although ventilated there is no capillary flow to allow gas exchange. This also explains the fact that while increasing the $F\text{IO}_2$ administered to the patient there is minimal or no increase in the observed $S\text{aO}_2$
- The figure can also be used to explain the pathophysiology of virtually all respiratory conditions that will arise in the critical care vivas by explaining the presence of $\dot{V}/\dot{Q}$ mismatch and shunt

Further reading

Jaff MR, McMurtry MS, Archer SL, et al. Management of massive and submassive pulmonary embolism, iliofemoral deep vein thrombosis, and chronic thromboembolic pulmonary hypertension: a scientific statement from the American Heart Association. Circulation 2011; 123:1788–1830.

NICE. (2020). Pulmonary embolism [online] Available from https://cks.nice.org.uk/pulmonary-embolism [Last accessed February, 2022].

Scenario 28

Acute respiratory distress syndrome

You are reviewing a previously fit 42-year-old man with acute pancreatitis, who underwent NG tube insertion yesterday for frequent vomiting. The ward staff are concerned as his NEWS score is 9 and he has become very short of breath.

Q. 28.1 What do you think the likely differential diagnoses are?

You can classify them into medical and surgical causes:
- *Medical:* Aspiration pneumonia, ARDS, PE
- *Surgical:* An acute abdomen – perforation of viscus, complicated peritonitis, pancreatitis

ABCDE assessment reveals the following:
- A – maintaining, 15 L O_2 via non-rebreather mask
- B – SaO_2 87%, RR 25 breath/min, using accessory muscles
- C – BP 178/98 mmHg, capillary refill 3 seconds
- D – Alert
- E – Temperature 38.2°C, abdomen soft, mild epigastric tenderness

Q. 28.2 What are you going to do?

As with previous questions you will now understand that the first thing to get across to the examiner is the appreciation of the severity of the acute presentation. The immediate priority will be ongoing resuscitation, appropriate investigations and escalation of care to an appropriate setting, e.g. critical care and involvement of appropriate teams.

You will need to order some basic investigations including routine blood tests, ABGs, and a CXR as a minimum.

The results of investigations are as follows:
Arterial blood gas results:
pH   7.34
PaO_2 7.8 kPa
$PaCO_2$ 5.8 kPa
BE   −2.4
Lactate   1.0

Scenario 28 Acute respiratory distress syndrome

The CXR is here:

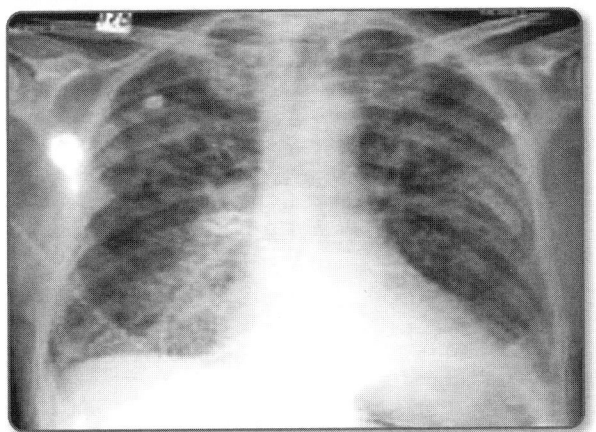

Q. 28.3 What is your likely diagnosis? What is your management plan?

- The ABG reveals a RF1
- The CXR reveals bilateral extensive pulmonary shadowing
- The most likely diagnosis in this scenario is developing ARDS secondary to aspiration of gastric contents
- The priorities for management are to improve the primary hypoxia which is not achievable in a ward setting. The patient will need improved oxygen delivery either by high-flow nasal cannulae or a trial of CPAP on the ICU

Q. 28.4 What are the diagnostic criteria for ARDS?

- Acute respiratory distress syndrome is a clinical syndrome of diffuse lung injury characterised by acute onset with hypoxemia and bilateral radiographic infiltrates and without left atrial hypertension
- The 2012 Berlin definition (which replaced the 1994 American-European Consensus Conference definition) of ARDS consists of:
  - Onset within 1 week of a known clinical insult or new or worsening respiratory symptoms
  - Bilateral opacities not fully explained by effusions, lobar/lung collapse, or nodules on CXR or CT
  - Respiratory failure not fully explained by a cardiac failure or fluid overload (in the absence of risk factors for ARDS, an objective assessment such as echocardiography is required to exclude these causes of hydrostatic oedema)
  - The severity of ARDS is measured by calculating the ration of the Pao_2/Fio_2. Which essentially shows how effective the lungs are at processing the amount of oxygen administered to the oxygen seen in the pulmonary artery
  - **Mild** ARDS: Pao_2/Fio_2 > 200 mmHg but ≤ 300 mmHg with positive end-expiratory pressure (PEEP) or CPAP ≥ 5 cm H_2O

- **Moderate** ARDS: $Pao_2/Fio_2 > 100$ mmHg but ≤ 200 mmHg with PEEP ≥ 5 cm H_2O
  - **Severe** ARDS: $Pao_2/Fio_2 \leq 100$ mmHg with PEEP ≥ 5 cm H_2O
- Mortality of ARDS varies with its severity:
  - Mild is associated with 27% mortality
  - Moderate is associated with 32% mortality
  - Severe is associated with 45% mortality
- ARDS can be caused by direct lung injury or indirectly by inflammatory processes focused on other organs:
  - The most common causes of direct lung injury leading to ARDS are pneumonia and aspiration of gastric contents
  - The most common causes of indirect lung injury leading to ARDS are non-pulmonary sepsis, severe trauma, and large amounts of blood transfused over a short period of time [> 8 units/24 hours, termed transfusion-related acute lung injury (TRALI)]

Management:
- The priority is to treat any underlying causes, e.g. antibiotics for pneumonia and to provide organ support as necessary
- On the ICU, the mainstay of treatment is with ventilation either non-invasive as tolerated or invasive ventilation as required
- PEEP is used to improve alveolar recruitment, and ventilation strategies are centred on the use of low tidal volume usually 6 mL/kg. Neuromuscular paralysis may be required to achieve volume control in patients who are invasively ventilated

Q. 28.5 Can you explain the underlying pathophysiology of ARDS?
- There are three pathological stages to ARDS, the important thing to be aware of is that ARDS is a heterogeneous disease in that different parts of the lungs are affected differently and can present in any of the varying disease states. This makes the treatment of ARDS complex
  1. **Exudative phase:** First 2-4 days onset after lung injury. Loss of alveolar surfactant leads to alveolar exudate from inflammatory mediator release - alveoli filled with fluid and some units collapse
  2. **Fibroproliferative phase:** Proliferation of connective tissue and structural lung proteins causing extensive lung damage and air leakage into surrounding tissue, secondary infection is common
  3. **Resolution and recovery:** Reorganising of underlying lung tissue formation of scar tissue and traction bronchiectasis, lung improvement may continue for 6-12 months

Further reading
ARDS Definition Task Force; Ranieri VM, Rubenfeld GD, et al. Acute respiratory distress syndrome: the Berlin definition. JAMA 2012; 307:2526–2533.
Leaver SK, Evans TW. Acute respiratory distress syndrome. BMJ 2007; 335:389–394.

Scenario 29

Pneumothorax

You attend a major trauma call. The patient is a 27-year-old male who has been stabbed in the left chest. During the primary survey the following observations are recorded: saturations = 89% on 15 L of O_2; pulse = 130 bpm; BP = 85/60 mmHg. Your colleague who is performing the primary survey reports distended neck veins.

Q. 29.1 What is the most likely cause for this? What are the other possibilities, and how can one differentiate between them?

The history, the presence of shock and the distended neck veins strongly suggest either a tension pneumothorax or cardiac tamponade. Another important cause to consider is haemorrhagic shock, though one would not expect the neck veins to be distended in this case.

The distinction should be made clinically in the trauma setting, rather than radiologically. The displacement of the trachea away from the affected side, and hyper-resonant percussion notes and diminished air entry on the affected sided would indicate a tension pneumothorax.

Muffled heart sounds suggest cardiac tamponade. A dull percussion note would be heard in the presence of a massive haemothorax.

It is of course possible for the patient to have all three of these, and the team need to treat in the order of 'ABCDE', as per ATLS.

Q. 29.2 Describe how to adequately assess for shift of the trachea.

First, look. Then, feel, using your second, third and fourth fingers – place the second and third finger on each sternoclavicular joint, then run the middle finger down the trachea. It should end in between your second and third finger.

Q. 29.3 The patient does indeed have tracheal deviation to the right, hyper-resonant percussion notes and absent breath sounds on the left. However, the heart sounds are also muffled. What should you and the trauma team do next? Outline how you would do this.

Although this patient appears to have both tension pneumothorax and cardiac tamponade, ATLS guidelines dictate that injuries compromising breathing will kill before those affecting circulation – therefore, the tension pneumothorax – which can kill quickly – needs to be decompressed first. This is done by inserting a large bore cannula into the pleural space on the affected side. The site of choice used to be the 2nd intercostal space in the midclavicular line, but the most recent ATLS guidelines are to place it at the 5th intercostal space anterior to the midaxillary line (for paediatric patients, the 2nd intercostal space, midclavicular line is still appropriate). Of course, do not forget to quickly clean the site, and remove the needle. A hiss of air will be heard.

Q. 29.4 What is the next step? Outline how would do this.

Needle decompression converts a tension pneumothorax to a simple pneumothorax, and this needs treating with a surgical chest drain.

First, check you have all the necessary equipment:
- Sterile gloves, gown, and drapes
- Cleaning antiseptic
- Local anaesthetic
- Scalpel
- Blunt instrument, e.g. Roberts clip, or medium haemostat
- 28–32 F chest tube
- Chest drain bottle with underwater seal
- Silk sutures
- Dressing and tape

Then, position the patient – extend their arm over their head and flexed at the elbow. This may be limited by concomitant injury, and you may need an assistant to hold the arm.

Widely prep and drape the chest wall. Identify the 'triangle of safety'. The borders of this are: the lateral border of pectoralis major, the lateral border of latissimus dorsi; the base of the axilla and the 5th intercostal space. The site of insertion should be the 4th or 5th intercostal space, anterior to the midaxillary line.

Infiltrate the site with local anaesthetic, and infiltrate the layers all the way down to the pleura.

Make 2–3 cm transverse incision at the site. Bluntly dissect down to the pleura. Gently push the blunt instrument through the pleura, staying on top of the rib to avoid the intercostal neurovascular bundle. Hold the instrument close to its tip so that it is advanced under control. Use the instrument to spread the tissues and widen the opening. Perform a finger thoracostomy – use your finger to sweep away any clot or adherent tissue. Advance the fenestrated end of the tube into the space, and place the other end underwater in the chest tube bottle. Secure it with a silk suture; if time permits, place a purse string which can be used to close the thoracostomy when the drain is eventually removed. Apply a sterile dressing. Perform a CXR, which would also be an adjunct to the primary survey in this case.

Further reading

MacDuff A, Arnold A, Harvey J; BTS Pleural Disease Guideline Group. Management of spontaneous pneumothorax: British Thoracic Society Pleural Disease Guideline 2010. Thorax 2010; 65:ii18–31.

Hallifax RJ, Roberts M, Russell N, et al. Pneumothorax management: current state of practice in the UK. Respir Res 23 (2022). https://doi.org/10.1186/s12931-022-01943-9

Scenario 30

Abdominal compartment syndrome

You are reviewing an 86-year-old gentleman on ICU. He underwent an emergency EVAR for a ruptured AAA in the morning. The ICU staff tell you that they have found ventilation increasingly difficult for the past few hours; he is anuric, having maintained a good urine output throughout his procedure; and his intra-abdominal pressure (IAP) is 23 mmHg.

Q. 30.1 What is the likely diagnosis? What risk factors for this does the patient have?

There is evidence of abdominal compartment syndrome (ACS). In this case, the risk factors are:
- Intra-abdominal: in his case, retroperitoneal haematoma from the ruptured AAA
- Intra-luminal: it is possible that he has developed ileus or pseudo-obstruction as a result of the physiological insult of the rupture and the surgery
- Extra-abdominal: acidosis, fluid overload due to heart failure and worsened by transfusion and fluid resuscitation, in combination with the physiological 'hit' result in leaky capillaries that put pressure on the abdominal compartment

A further risk factor decreased abdominal wall compliance. This can occur in patients with major burns.

Another way to think of risk factors is:
- Primary: insults/injuries to the abdominal organs themselves, e.g. perforation
- Secondary: extra-abdominal causes, e.g. sepsis, burns
- Chronic, e.g. ascites

Q. 30.2 What things in particular concern you?

He is developing new organ failure – he is now anuric – with an IAP over 20, which is the definition of ACS. This, in combination with an IAP over 20, and the difficulty ventilating tell you that he is at risk of mortality.

Q. 30.3 What is intra-abdominal hypertension and how would you grade it?

Intra-abdominal hypertension (IAH) is intra-abdominal pressure > 12 mmHg. It is graded I–IV:
- I = 12–15 mmHg
- II = 16–20 mmHg

- III = 21–25 mmHg
- IV = Over 25 mmHg

Q. 30.4 How do you measure IAP?

Intra-abdominal pressure can be measured directly or indirectly. Direct measurement involves placing a needle or catheter into the abdominal space, and so there is risk of bowel perforation or other injury with this. Indirect measurement is done by measuring the pressure in the bladder.

The equipment needed for this indirect measurement includes (on the assumption that the patient already has a urinary catheter):
- Three-way tap × 2
- Pressure transducer and tubing
- Luer lock connector
- 30 and 50 mL Luer lock syringe
- Clamp
- Normal saline

Steps:
1. Use aseptic technique
2. Prime transducer and monitoring lines with normal saline
3. Attach end of urinary catheter to one of the three-way taps (tap 1); using the Luer lock connector, attach to the other three-way tap (tap 2), and then connect this to the urinary drainage bag
4. Connect the pressure transducer to tap 1
5. Place the patient in the supine position as much possible. If the patient is prone or lying at an angle, IAP will be higher
6. Have the transducers arranged so that tap 2 is levelled at the point where the mid-axillary line meets the iliac crest
7. Ensure lines are not kinked
8. Clamp the urinary drainage bag
9. Infiltrate the bladder with 1 mL/kg of normal saline
10. Wait 60 seconds for equilibrium
11. Take the pressures that occur at end expiration

Q. 30.5 How would you manage this patient?

The management depends on the degree of organ failure, the likely causes and the persistence of IAH.

In this case, he seems to have just started to show signs of ACS. It would be worth trying conservative measures first, and these relate to the risk factors discussed earlier. So, intra-luminal decompression can be achieved with an NG tube. Acidosis can be corrected. If there is heart failure, off-loading of fluid can help. Sedation, neuromuscular blockade and placing the patient at 30° can improve muscle wall compliance.

Serial measurements are important. If IAP and/or organ failure persists, decompressive laparostomy will be needed. As this patient is already anuric, there should be a low threshold for doing this.

Q. 30.6 What different ways of temporary abdominal closure do you know of?

- Bogota bag
- Vacuum-assisted closure (VAC)

Further reading

Sartelli M, Viale P, Catena F, et al. 2013 WSES guidelines for management of intra-abdominal infections. World J Emerg Surg 2013:3.

De Laet IE, Malbrain MLNG, De Waele JJ. A Clinician's Guide to Management of Intra-abdominal Hypertension and Abdominal Compartment Syndrome in Critically Ill Patients. Crit Care 2020; 24:97.

Scenario 31

Nutrition

During the ward round, you see a patient who underwent an oesophagectomy by a colleague of yours. Unfortunately, there has been a large anastomotic leak detected on a postoperative water-soluble swallow. The patient has not tolerated the insertion of NG tubes, and no feeding jejunostomy was performed during the operation. You decide to keep the patient nil by mouth and commence TPN.

Q. 31.1 The patient has heard TPN is risky. Explain to him why he needs it and the risks.

The candidate should explain to the patient that in order to be supplied with their daily calories, salts and electrolytes, nutrition will be provided through a line in the vein. The candidate should reference that ideally, nutrition should go straight to the gut, either through the mouth, or via tubes straight to the intestine – as this is not an option in his case, TPN is necessary. The benefits are to provide their daily requirements so that they do not lose weight and strength, and to aid recovery from the operation.

The risks of TPN can be divided into risks associated with the line, and metabolic risks. Risks associated with the line are:
- Pneumothorax during or just after line insertion
- Bleeding during or just after line insertion
- Infection
- Clotting off of the line

Metabolic risks are:
- Disturbance of blood salts and electrolytes, e.g. high or low potassium
- Immunosuppression
- Deranged liver function tests

Q. 31.2 What are the indications for TPN?

Broadly speaking, TPN is indicated in any patient whose gastrointestinal (GI) tract is not functioning adequately in order that nutrients, electrolytes and calories can be absorbed from it. These include:
- Short bowel syndrome
- Prolonged ileus
- Severe diarrhoea
- Severe vomiting

- Bowel obstruction
- Enterocutaneous fistula
- Persistent, non-enterotomies
- Inability to access the enteral tract
- Following surgery where it is not expected that enteral feed can resumed for at least 5 days

Q. 31.3 Through what routes can TPN be delivered?

Total parenteral nutrition must be delivered via an appropriate line/catheter into a central vein. The high osmolality of TPN can lead to thrombophlebitis if delivered via simple cannula into a peripheral vein. The types of line are:
- Peripherally inserted central catheter (PICC)
- Hickman line
- Groshong catheter
- Central venous pressure line
- Femoral line

Q. 31.4 Through what routes can enteral nutrition be delivered?

- Per oral
- Nasogastric tube
- Nasojejunal tube
- Feeding gastrostomy
- Feeding jejunostomy

Q. 31.5 You review the blood for another patient on the round. She has not received any form of nutrition for 6 days. What are they at risk of developing?

Potassium = 2.4, magnesium = 0.58, phosphate = 0.47

This patient has hypokalaemia, hypomagnesaemia, and hypophosphataemia. When associated with prolonged starvation, these results would suggest that this patient is at risk of refeeding syndrome. This would manifest itself clinically as any one of the sequelae of these electrolyte disturbances, e.g. neurological symptoms of confusion, seizure, cardiac symptoms such as arrhythmias, cardiac failure.

Further reading

https://www.bapen.org.uk/resources-and-education/education-and-guidance/guidelines

Scenario 32

Acute kidney injury and renal replacement therapy

You are asked to review a patient under the medics. The patient is 73-year-old and has been admitted with lethargy and deranged electrolytes. The patient's serum creatinine was 273. You have been asked to see her as she underwent an anterior resection with loop ileostomy 4 weeks ago.

Q. 32.1 What is the definition of acute kidney injury?

Acute kidney injury can be defined clinically or biochemically. Clinically, it is a urine output of <0.5 mL/kg/h for 6 hours.

Biochemically, it is an increase in serum creatinine 1.5–2 times the baseline (stage 1); 2–3 times the baseline (stage 2); or >3 times the baseline (stage 3).

Q. 32.2 What do you suspect is the cause in this case? How do you classify the causes?

It is possible she has a high output ileostomy which has caused pre-renal AKI. Other causes of AKI are renal and postrenal.

Q. 32.3 What are the principles of management in AKI?

- Consider which is the most likely cause – pre-renal, renal or postrenal
- Obtain up to date electrolytes and ABG
- Administer IV fluids and titrate against fluid status and urine output
- Correct cause of pre-renal causes – in this case, treat the high output ileostomy with dietary measures, restricting oral intake, codeine, loperamide, and ruling out an intra-abdominal cause for it
- Review drug chart and stop nephrotoxic medications
- Perform urine dip
- If there is a catheter, check it is not obstructed
- Renal ultrasound to exclude postrenal cause
- Contact HDU to assess for need for RRT

Q. 32.4 What are the life-threatening complications of AKI?

- Hyperkalaemia
- Pulmonary oedema

Q. 32.5 What are the indications for acute RRT?

- Hyperkalaemia (K > 7)
- Pulmonary oedema
- Severe acidosis (pH < 7.1)
- Anuria
- Uraemic encephalopathy
- Toxin overdose

Q. 32.6 What are the types of RRT?

- Dialysis
- Haemofiltration
- Renal transplant

Q. 32.7 What is the difference between haemofiltration and haemodialysis?

- Both haemofiltration and haemodialysis are used to treat renal failure. Both rely on blood being pumped through an extracorporeal circuit, and solutes moving across a semi-permeable membrane
- The key difference between haemofiltration and haemodialysis is the method in which solute removal takes place. Haemofiltration relies on convection; haemodialysis utilises diffusion
- In haemofiltration, the patient's blood creates a positive hydrostatic pressure that drives water and molecules that are small enough to pass through the membrane into filtrate; the filtrate is then discarded. The patient is given fluid to correct any fluid loss
- In haemodialysis, a crystalloid solution known as dialysate is separated from the patient's blood by the semi-permeable membrane. Here, molecules move across their concentration gradient by diffusion. Thus, potassium and urea move from the blood to the dialysate; bicarbonate moves the other way. Dialysate moves counter-current to the blood to maintain this concentration gradient

Q. 32.8 List the different types of dialysis.

- Peritoneal dialysis
- Haemodialysis via central venous catheter
- Haemodialysis via arteriovenous fistula

Further reading

Vadakedath S, Kandi V. Dialysis: A Review of the Mechanisms Underlying Complications in the Management of Chronic Renal Failure. Cureus 2017; 9:e1603.

Scenario 33

Shock

You attend a trauma call. The patient is an 83-year-old female who tripped and fell down a flight of 5 stairs. The primary survey is as follows:
- Airway – intact
- Breathing – RR = 24 breath/min, saturations are 93% on 15 L, no external chest injuries, both sides of chest moving symmetrically, auscultation and percussion notes normal throughout and on both sides
- Circulation – BP = 105/75 mmHg, pulse = 90 bpm, capillary refill is 3 seconds; abdomen is soft and non-tender; no evidence of pelvic or long bone injury
- Disability – GCS 15; scalp laceration present

Q. 33.1 What is the most common type of shock that occurs in trauma? What are the other types that can occur in trauma?

The most common type of shock is haemorrhagic shock. Patients can also suffer obstructive shock in the form of tension pneumothorax and cardiac tamponade. Patients can also suffer neurogenic and spinal shock.

Q. 33.2 What features in this scenario suggest haemorrhagic shock?

She is tachypnoeic, diastolic pressure is raised, and capillary refill is 3 seconds.

Q. 33.3 What stage of shock do you think she is in?

She is in at least class II shock, because of the aforementioned clinical features, and could very well be in class III.

Q. 33.4 Complete this blank table:

	Class I	Class II	Class III	Class IV
Blood loss (mL)				
Blood loss (% volume)				
Heart rate				
Systolic BP				
Diastolic BP				
Respiratory rate				
Urine output				
Extremities				
Mental state				

	Class I	Class II	Class III	Class IV
Blood loss (mL)	750	750–1,500	1,500–2,000	>2,000
Blood loss (% volume)	0–15	15–30	30–40	>40
Heart rate	<100	>100	>120	>140
Systolic BP	No change	No change	Reduced	Significantly reduced
Diastolic BP	No change	Raised	Reduced	Significantly reduced/ unrecordable
Respiratory rate	<20	>20	>30	>40
Urine output	>30	20–30	10–20	<10
Capillary refill	Normal	Slow	Slow	Very slow
Mental state	Normal	Anxious	Anxious/ Aggressive/ Drowsy	Drowsy/ Unconscious

Q. 33.5 What in particular about her raises your suspicion that she is more seriously injured than the observations and signs indicate?

She is 83, and there is a chance that polypharmacy may falsely reassure, or put her at risk of haemorrhage – e.g. she may be on a beta-blocker that is preventing her from mounting a tachycardia; or she may also be on anticoagulants or antiplatelets.

Q. 33.6 A fluids bolus of 1 L of crystalloid is administered. Her BP goes up to 130 systolic, but then soon comes back down to 100 systolic. Classify her response, and state what you would do next.

She is a transient responder. In the trauma setting, transient responders are likely to be actively bleeding. She should therefore be transfused blood.

Responders to fluids have an increase, and a sustained increase in BP and are unlikely to be bleeding, and so are unlikely to need transfusion.

The vital signs of non-responders do not change with fluids, and this should alert the team to life-threatening causes of shock – either severe haemorrhagic (class IV), or obstructive causes (tension pneumothorax or cardiac tamponade).

Further reading

https://www.emergencymedicinekenya.org/wp-content/uploads/2021/09/ATLS-10th-Edition.pdf
 [Accessed 1st April 2023]

Scenario 34

Atrial fibrillation

You are in clinic junior member of your team calls you to say a patient under your care is in fast atrial fibrillation (AF). The patient is day 3 post oesophagectomy.

Q. 34.1 What is your immediate concern?

Your immediate concern is that this patient's life is at risk. Fast AF with haemodynamic compromise is an emergency. Though it may indicate an anastomotic leak, the priority to assess using the advanced life support protocol.

Q. 34.2 What are the principles of management of AF?

First, assess for chest pain and haemodynamic instability. If these are present, a peri-arrest/medical emergency call should be put out.

If these are not present, clarify if the patient has long-standing AF. Patients who are postsurgery may miss their usual medications if they have been kept nil by mouth. Seek to correct electrolyte disturbances, i.e. potassium and magnesium, ensure the patient is well hydrated, assess for sepsis. Seek urgent advice from a cardiologist or the medical team about controlling rate, rhythm and prevention of cerebrovascular events.

Q. 34.3 Name the most common agents used in treating AF.

- Digoxin
- Beta-blockers
- Amiodarone

If beta-blockers are being given intravenously, patients should be monitored preferably in an HDU setting. Amiodarone, in the acute setting, is given through a central line, and patients will certainly need HDU level of care.

Q. 34.4 Do you know of any scores that can be used to assess a patient's risk of developing cerebrovascular events?

The CHA_2DS_2-VASc score is the most recent method:

Age	65–74: +1	>75: +2
Sex	Female: +1	Male: 0
Congestive heart failure	No: 0	Yes: +1
Hypertension	No: 0	Yes: +1
History of stroke/TIA/thromboembolism	No: 0	Yes: +2
History of cardiac or peripheral vascular disease	No: 0	Yes: +1
Diabetes mellitus	No: 0	Yes: +1

Further reading

https://www.england.nhs.uk/south/wp-content/uploads/sites/6/2018/10/AF-GUIDANCE.pdf [Accessed 1st April 2023]

Scenario 35

Disseminated intravascular coagulation

You are part of the trauma surgery team. On a ward round, you are about to see a patient who was admitted 2 days ago after a severe road traffic accident. He sustained multiple long bone fractures requiring surgery. He has been unwell overnight. You and the team are looking at the patient's latest blood results; the normal range is in brackets:
- Haemoglobin = 9.1 (120–180 g/L)
- Platelet count = 15 (150–140 × 10^9/L)
- International normalised ratio (INR) = 4.79 (0.8–1.2)
- Activated partial thromboplastin time (APTT) = >200 (23–30 seconds)
- D-dimer = >4,000 (0.1–0.45 mg/L)
- Fibrinogen = 1.49 (1.5–4.5 g/L)

Q. 35.1 What do the blood tests indicate?

These suggest the patient has DIC – there is evidence of concurrent activation of coagulation and fibrinolytic pathways, e.g. the platelet count has fallen, while the D-dimer (a fibrin degradation product) is elevated.

Q. 35.2 What clinical features would you expect?

- Haematological – evidence of thrombosis, followed by bleeding
- Systemic – evidence of shock and end-organ failure

Q. 35.3 What conditions pre-dispose patients to DIC?

- Sepsis
- Surgery
- Shock, including trauma and/or burns
- Malignancy, e.g. promyelocytic leukaemia
- Pregnancy, e.g. eclampsia
- Autoimmune conditions, e.g. systemic lupus erythematosus (SLE)

Disseminated intravascular coagulation can be thought of as the haematological component of systemic inflammatory response syndrome (SIRS). The patient in this scenario has multiple risk factors for DIC.

Q. 35.4 What is the treatment?

Treat the underlying cause – in this case, assess for sepsis, underlying undiagnosed trauma, malignancy or autoimmune conditions.

Treat bleeding – if the patient is bleeding, give platelets; cryoprecipitate may be required in those with low fibrinogen.

Treatment of thrombosis – with care, low-dose heparin.

Further reading

M Levi, CH Toh, J Thachil, H G Watson. Guidelines for the diagnosis and management of disseminated intravascular coagulation. Br J Haematol 2009; 145:24–33.

Wada H, Thachil J, Di Nisio M, et al. Guidance for diagnosis and treatment of disseminated intravascular coagulation from harmonization of the recommendations from three guidelines. J Thromb Haemost 2013; 11: 761–767.

Scenario 36

Hyponatraemia

An 89-year-old lady was admitted with collapse, abdominal pain, and vomiting. She has an incarcerated femoral hernia. You notice that her serum sodium = 125 mmol/L.

Q. 36.1 What is the normal plasma concentration of sodium?
135–145 mmol/L

Q. 36.2 What is the daily sodium requirement?
1 mmol/kg/day

Q. 36.3 What is the most likely cause of her low sodium?
Vomiting as a result of her obstructed, incarcerated hernia.

Q. 36.4 What are the causes of hyponatraemia?
The causes of low sodium can be thought of as either fluid loss or fluid excess.
Fluid loss:
- Renal losses, e.g. diuretics
- GI losses, e.g. high stoma output, vomiting

Fluid excess:
- Excessive intake, e.g. over-administration of IV fluids, polydipsia
- Retention of fluid, e.g. cardiac failure, liver failure, syndrome of inappropriate antidiuretic hormone secretion (SIADH)

Q. 36.5 What are the symptoms of hyponatraemia?
The symptoms are largely neurological, and include headaches, confusion, irritability, muscle cramps, and spasm. Seizures may occur at levels < 115 mmol/L.

Q. 36.6 What are the principles of management of hyponatraemia?

Treatment should be initiated when sodium is <130 mmol/L. Patients with severe neurological symptoms such as seizures require joint management with intensive care and the medical team. The cause must be identified – is it due to fluid loss, or fluid excess – and then treated accordingly.

In the case of fluid loss, the losses need to be replaced, usually with 0.9% saline.

In the case of fluid excess, fluid restriction is required.

Where the cause is not clear, a urinary sodium should be sent off and compared with the plasma sodium.

Further reading

https://cks.nice.org.uk/topics/hyponatraemia/ [Accessed 1st April 2023]

Scenario 37

Heparin-induced thrombocytopenia

A 71-year-old lady who underwent an emergency Hartman's for perforated sigmoid diverticulitis is readmitted 5 days after discharge. Platelet count on admission is $172 \times 10^9/L$. She is found to have a swollen right leg that is tender on palpation. A venous duplex confirms a DVT, and a heparin infusion is commenced as per the local guidelines.

Five days later, her leg swelling persists, and a repeat duplex shows a thrombosis of the right common and superficial femoral vein, as well as the popliteal, tibial, and saphenous systems. Her platelet count is now 80. Assay tests confirm heparin-induced thrombocytopenia (HIT).

Q. 37.1 What is HIT? What are the types of HIT, and which type does this lady have?

Heparin-induced thrombocytopenia is thrombocytopenia caused by heparin therapy. There are two types – type I and type II. Type I is non-immune mediated. The fall in platelet count moderate and transient, and patients do not develop complications. Type II is immune mediated. Antibodies against heparin-platelet factor 4 complexes, and is of clinical significance, thus this lady has type II.

Q. 37.2 How is the diagnosis made?

Clinically, as assays can take a long time to come back. The criteria are as follows:
1. Normal platelet count prior to heparin therapy
2. Fall in platelet count of 50% from patient's baseline that starts 5–10 days after heparin is started.
3. Acute arterial or venous thrombosis
4. Thrombocytopenia resolves once heparin is stopped.

Q. 37.3 What is the management?

- Stop heparin immediately.
- Start a non-heparin anticoagulant, e.g. direct thrombin inhibitors such as argatroban.

Further reading

Watson H, Davidson S, Keeling D. Guidelines on the diagnosis and management of heparin-induced thrombocytopenia: second edition. Br J Haematol 2012, 159:528–540.

Scenario 38

Massive blood loss

You have been asked by your department to represent surgery on a local transfusion committee. The committee is updating the protocol on massive blood loss and wants to produce a guideline that will be available for staff to review in the form of a poster.

Q. 38.1 List some features that need to be on this poster.

Familiarise yourself with your own local massive blood loss protocol. They generally contain most of the following:
- Definition of what massive blood loss is
- Contact number to activate protocol: usually an emergency number through switch
- Other contact numbers, e.g. intensive care, haematology, theatres, interventional radiology, obstetricians, endoscopy
- Immediate management: this usually needs outlining the ABC approach to resuscitation, calling for help, placing large bore cannulae, which blood tests to order and giving fluids
- Components of massive blood loss packs, and how to administer, e.g. instructions on when to give group O blood, platelets, cryoprecipitate

Q. 38.2 What is your definition of massive blood loss?

There are many definitions, each usually contains a *volume* of blood loss within a *time period*:
- Entire blood volume in 24 hours
- Half of entire volume in 3 hours
- 150 mL/min

Q. 38.3 When should platelets be given in massive blood loss?

Platelets should be given when the platelet count is $<100 \times 10^9/L$.

Q. 38.4 When should cryoprecipitate be given in massive blood loss?

This should be considered when the fibrinogen is <1.5 g/L. Fibrinogen falls in DIC.

Q. 38.5 What are the deleterious effects of massive blood transfusion?

Haematological:
- Coagulopathy
- Thrombocytopenia

Biochemical:
- Hyperkalaemia
- Hypocalcaemia
- Metabolic acidosis

Infectious:
- Hepatitis B and C
- HIV
- CMV
- Prions

Respiratory:
- Transfusion-related lung injury
- Pulmonary oedema

Systemic:
- Hypothermia

Further reading

Stanworth SJ, Dowling K, Curry N, et al. A guideline for the haematological management of major haemorrhage: A British Society for Haematology Guideline. Br J Haematol 2022; 198:654– 667.

Scenario 39

Intravenous fluids and electrolytes

You are seeing a 37-year-old man in the emergency department who appears to have perforated appendicitis. You are going to take him to theatre as soon as possible. His pulse is 115 bpm, BP 90/70 mmHg, temperature 38.3°C. He will be going to HDU in the meantime.

Q. 39.1 What do you need to consider when prescribing intravenous fluids for this patient?

This patient has evidence of septic shock. Therefore, the fluids need to be started immediately, and protocolised to meet targets. These targets are:
- Maintaining a mean arterial pressure of at least 65 mmHg
- Achieving a urine output of at least 0.5 mL/kg/h
- A central venous pressure of at least 8 mmHg
- Central venous saturations of at least 70%

Q. 39.2 What fluid will you give this patient and why?

This patient requires resuscitation, and should therefore have fluid has a relatively smaller volume of distribution, as this improves vascular expansion. Fluids containing sodium are best for this. Too much 0.9% saline can lead to hyperchloraemic acidosis though, so Hartmann's – which has less chloride – may be preferential.

Colloids have been shown to have some harmful side effects – they can also cause hyperchloraemic acidosis – and are no longer in favour.

Q. 39.3 What causes of hyperchloraemic acidosis do you know of?

Causes are usually either GI, renal or exogenous. In GI causes, the underlying pathophysiology is loss of bicarbonate from the GI tract. This leads to unopposed hydrogen ions in the body's bicarbonate-CO_2 pH buffer system. GI causes include:
- Diarrhoea
- Vomiting
- Excessive nasogastric/nasojejunal losses
- Pancreatic fistula

Renal causes are proximal or distal renal tubular acidosis. In proximal renal tubular acidosis, bicarbonate is not absorbed, and is excreted in the urine. In distal acidosis, the distal nephron does not secrete hydrogen into the urine. Therefore, in both types, there is acidosis of the blood, with alkaline urine.

Exogenous causes include resuscitation with too much 0.9% saline, and ingestion of substances such as hydrochloric acid and ammonium chloride.

Q. 39.4 What ions are lost in large volumes from biliary and pancreatic fistulas?

Bicarbonate and sodium

Q. 39.5 What ions are lost from nasogastric suctioning?

Potassium and chloride

Further reading

Barlow A, Barlow B, Tang N, et al. Intravenous Fluid Management in Critically Ill Adults: A Review. Crit Care Nurse 2020; 40:e17–e27.

Chapter 3

Emergency surgery

*Paul Barrow, Ilayaraja Rajendran, Chris Macklin, Finlay Curran,
David Monk, Rachael Clifford, Faddy Kamel*

Scenario 1

Damage control laparotomy

Q. 1.1 Can you describe what is meant by the term damage control laparotomy?

- Damage control surgery is a concept of abbreviated laparotomy, designed to prioritise short-term physiological recovery over anatomical reconstruction in the seriously injured and compromised patient

> A 30-year-old man is admitted to the emergency department with a history of a heavy weight falling on his abdomen 2 hours previously. He is hypothermic with a temperature of 34.5°C. His blood pressure is 80/60 mmHg and pulse is 120/min with cool peripheries. He has high-flow oxygen via a rebreathe mask and two large-bore cannulae with blood transfusion in progress. He is maintaining this blood pressure but it is not rising. A CT scan shows pancreatic oedema and evidence of haemorrhage between the pancreatic parenchyma and the splenic vein.

Q. 1.2

A. What criteria would you consider preoperatively to guide you into performing a damage control laparotomy?

B. What intraoperative findings would make you decide against a definitive procedure?

A.
- Temperature <34°C
- Arterial pH <7.2
- Laboratory-confirmed (international normalised ratio/prothrombin time and/or partial thromboplastin time >1.5 times normal) or clinically observed coagulopathy in the pre- or intraoperative setting
- Administration of >10 units of packed red blood cells
- Requirement for a resuscitative thoracotomy in the emergency department
- Limited surgical expertise
- Time pressures due to multiple casualties
- Lack of necessary blood products
- Priority for immediate surgery on other body system
- Embolisation needed for extra-abdominal injury (e.g. pelvic fracture)
- Abdominal wall closure not possible due to oedema
- Relook needed (e.g. bowel viability)

B.
- Inaccessible venous injury, e.g. identification of a juxta-hepatic venous injury
- Devascularised or destroyed pancreas, duodenum, or pancreaticoduodenal complex injury discovered during operation

Q. 1.3
A. What are the benefits of damage control laparotomy?
B. What are the disadvantages of damage control surgery?

A.
- Physiological optimisation
- Opportunity for transfusion, chance to optimise circulating volume, improve body temperature, and correction of clotting deficiencies
- Avoid further injury and restore physiological disturbance
- Achieve haemostasis without a prolonged physiological insult
- Avoid the lethal triad of hypothermia, acidosis, and coagulopathy
- Direct compression on the aorta at the level of the diaphragm to allow resuscitation catch up
- Leave the abdomen open for return for definitive procedure
- Staple off multiple bowel injuries quickly to prevent contamination and sepsis
- Limit contamination
- Protect abdominal contents and minimise protein loss

B.
- Increase in hospital mortality
- Increase in ileus
- Increase in anastomotic leakage
- Increase in wound dehiscence
- Increase in superficial surgical site infection

As a consequence of the disadvantages of damage control laparotomy, there is a move towards careful decision-making regarding damage control laparotomy and achievement of definitive management if possible.

Further reading

Harvin JA, Kao LS, Liang MK, et al. Decreasing the use of damage control laparotomy in trauma: a quality improvement project. J Am Coll Surg 2017; 225:200–209.

Harvin JA, Wray CJ, Steward J, et al. Control the damage: morbidity and mortality after emergent trauma laparotomy. Am J Surg 2016; 212:34–39.

Moore EE, Thomas G. Orr memorial lecture. Staged laparotomy for the hypothermia, acidosis, and coagulopathy syndrome. Am J Surg 1996; 172:405–410.

Rotondo MF, Schwab CW, McGonigal MD, et al. "Damage control": An approach for improved survival in exsanguinating penetrating abdominal injury. J Trauma 1993; 35:375–383.

Voiglio EJ, Dubuisson V, Massalou D, et al. Abbreviated laparotomy or damage control laparotomy: Why, when and how to do it? J Visc Surg 2016; 153:13–24.

Weale RD, Kong V, Buitendag J, et al. Damage control or definitive repair? A retrospective review of abdominal trauma at a major trauma centre in South Africa. Trauma Surg Acute Care Open 2019; 4:e000235.

Scenario 2

Laparoscopic injuries

Q. 2.1 Which are the significant generic complications of laparoscopic surgery? How would you recognize them clinically?

- The most common injuries occur during access to the abdominal cavity with trocar injuries causing mainly visceral and vascular injuries, and Verres needles causing vascular injuries and the potential for carbon dioxide embolus. Secondly, thermal injuries can occur by direct contact, heat conduction or arcing from the use of energy devices including unipolar or bipolar diathermy as well as the harmonic scalpel. The limited field of view means that operators also have to be wary of off camera and traction injuries when instruments may typically injure the intestine
- The gastrointestinal tracts, particularly the small intestine, are most affected by access trauma or energy devices. The vascular system is also affected by access injuries, particularly with trocar insertion. The most susceptible patients are thin females with minimal intra-abdominal fat. The risk of small bowel injury varies from 0.08 to 0.3% in minor to more major laparoscopic procedures. Although vascular injuries will have little delay to presentation, the average time for presentation of symptoms for small intestinal injury is 2–3 days for cannula and needle injuries, and 10–12 days for energy device-induced injury. Low abdominal or suprapubic trocar insertion can injure the bladder, and risk can be minimised by encouraging patients to empty their bladder prior to surgery or catheterisation if the bladder is full and therefore at risk
- Vascular injuries will demonstrate themselves quickly, with fresh blood within the abdominal cavity or an expanding retroperitoneal haematoma. The patient may become hypotensive and tachycardic, with a developing requirement for inotropes. Intestinal injury may present with abdominal pain requiring opioid analgesia, abdominal distention, ileus, peritonism, pyrexia, tachycardia, reduced urine output, increased respiratory rate, cardiac arrhythmia, and rising inflammatory markers. Bladder injury may present in a similar way, with both types of injury affecting the colour of drain contents. It is important to note, however, that symptoms can be subtle and non-specific. In 2011, the NPSA published the results of a review of patients who had suffered complications after laparoscopic surgery. Due to the less invasive nature of the surgery, it should be emphasised that subtle symptoms could include anorexia, nausea, or vomiting and reluctance to drink or mobilise

An 82-year-old man is 2 days post laparoscopic right hemicolectomy with primary anastomosis. He is found to have abdominal distention, left-sided abdominal pain, and pyrexia.

Scenario 2 Laparoscopic injuries

Q. 2.2 How would you assess and manage this patient?
- The main concern for this patient is of a postoperative complication. Although an anastomotic leak is possible at this stage, an iatrogenic injury should also be considered for this clinical presentation
- Management should follow Care of the Critically Ill Surgical Patient (CCrISP) principles of A to E with an assessment of whether the patient is stable or unstable. After the initiation of high-flow oxygen, intravenous fluids, and appropriate monitoring, the patient should have blood tests including a serum lactate and blood cultures. Broad-spectrum intravenous antibiotics should be administered as soon as possible. An urgent contrast-enhanced CT scan of the abdomen will be required unless the patient is unstable or has signs of peritonitis in which case resuscitation and immediate transfer to the operating theatre is the appropriate management

Q. 2.3 A CT scan shows free fluid within the abdomen and the patient has generalised abdominal tenderness with guarding.

How would you manage this scenario?
- A decision needs to be made to proceed to surgery. Firstly, the patient needs to be adequately fluid resuscitated and broad-spectrum antibiotics should be given. There should be a discussion with an intensivist regarding transfer to a postoperative critical care bed
- An estimate of the operative mortality should be undertaken and a consultant surgeon and anaesthetist should be present as mortality is likely to be >5% (NELA)
- It needs to be decided whether the approach will be by laparoscopy or laparotomy. While laparoscopy offers continued minimally invasive therapy for the patient, there are the issues of distended bowel hampering a thorough examination and increasing risk of access injury as well as potential for missing bowel injury due to visualisation difficulties. If laparoscopy is chosen then the decision to convert will need to be made on the basis of whether it is possible to make a full examination of the gastrointestinal tract, including the anastomosis. If there is free intestinal content and no cause seen, a conversion to laparotomy will be required. It is good practice is to examine structures multiple times to reduce the chance of missing an abnormality

Q. 2.4 You find an intact anastomosis but an isolated defect in a mid-small bowel loop with leaking of enteric content. What are going to do?
- At 2 days after the original operation if the patient is haemodynamically stable with no inotrope requirement and a serum albumin of over 25 g/L with minimal intra-abdominal oedema, a primary repair of the defect may be performed. This is best performed with a single seromuscular layer of 3/0 absorbable sutures
- Care needs to be taken to ensure that there is no other local or more distant injury
- A thorough washout should be carried out and non-suction drains inserted
- Intravenous broad-spectrum antibiotics should be given and a low threshold for reoperation in 48–72 hours if there is failure to progress

- Clear, open, and honest communication with the relatives is necessary (Duty of Candour) regarding a likely iatrogenic injury during the first operation

Further reading

Jacobson M, Osias J, Bizhang R, et al. The direct trocar technique: an alternative approach to abdominal entry for laparoscopy. JSLS 2002; 6:169–174.

Lamont T, Watts F, Panesar S, Macfie J, Matthew D. Safety alerts early detection of complications after laparoscopic surgery: summary of a safety report from the National Patient Safety Agency. BMJ (Clinical Research Ed) 2011; 342:c7221.

National Emergency Laparotomy Audit (NELA) Standards. https://www.nela.org.uk/downloads/NELA%20Standards_Mar%202023_approved_V2.pdf

Scenario 3

Bile leak following laparoscopic cholecystectomy

A 34-year-old female presents 2 days after being discharged following a laparoscopic cholecystectomy performed within 2 weeks of an episode of moderate gallstone pancreatitis on APACHE II scoring. She is complaining of right-sided abdominal pain, and has raised inflammatory markers, and pyrexia.

Q. 3.1 A CT scan shows right upper quadrant (RUQ) and right iliac fossa (RIF) free fluid and a small amount of air within the abdominal cavity, with improved peripancreatic changes. What would be the differential diagnoses and possible causes?

- This is likely to be due to a bile leak following a complex operation (post-pancreatitis): In this situation, the surgeon may have performed a subtotal cholecystectomy with a sutured endo-loop or stapler closure of the Hartmann's pouch stump. The importance of review of the operation note should be stated to try and ascertain the possible aetiology
- It is possible that there may be a bile leak due to a bile duct injury. Factors leading to this include severe inflammation that can distort the anatomy, aberrant ductal anatomy, or diathermy injury to the ductal system
- The possibility of iatrogenic bowel injury also needs to be considered
- A haematoma is also possible although the fluid density should enable it to be distinguished on CT scanning

Q. 3.2 How would you manage this patient?

- The first priority is a full assessment to establish evidence of signs of sepsis. The hydration state of the patient needs to be assessed and a decision made regarding fluid replacement requirements. If there are signs of sepsis then consideration needs to be given for initiating the sepsis 6 protocol (IV fluid challenge, broad-spectrum antibiotics, high-flow oxygen, serum lactate measurement, blood for culture, and urine output measurement)
- Blood tests to be requested included a full blood count, group and save, urea and electrolytes, and bilirubin and liver enzymes
- A contrast-enhanced CT scan of the abdomen and pelvis should be performed
- The notes should be looked including the operation note for any indication of intraoperative difficulty. The extent of cholecystectomy whether total or subtotal and the technique for remnant closure should be noted as this may be a potential site of bile leakage

- If the patient has any signs of peritonism, they will require a diagnostic laparoscopy and washout

Q. 3.3 At laparoscopy, there is free bilious fluid within the abdominal cavity, how would you proceed?

- The patient requires a careful laparoscopy and thorough washout. Care exploration of the gallbladder fossa should be undertaken if the amount of inflammation in and around the gallbladder fossa permits. Occasionally, a biliary radicle arising from the liver and can be identified with careful lavage, and facilitated by reduced insufflation pressure
- A non-suction drain should be placed in the right subhepatic space
- Broad-spectrum intravenous antibiotics should be continued as secondary infection of bile is a potential risk causing peritonitis

Q. 3.4 A postoperative magnetic resonance cholangiopancreatography (MRCP) reveals a bile duct injury. What are the principles for description of a bile duct injury?

There are several classifications:
- Strasberg classification (Type A–E)
- Bismuth classification (Type 1–5)
- Hannover classification (Types A–E with further subdivision): Uniquely, this includes a description of associated vascular injury in types C and D
- Stewart–Way classification (Class I–IV)
- The principle is to define the site of the injury. The involvement of the common bile or common hepatic duct versus a segmental or sectoral duct. The proximity to the liver hilum and whether complete or not are key features in these classifications. The classifications correlate with more significant injuries with more serious prognostic consequences for the patient

Q. 3.5 What are the principles of managing an iatrogenic bile leak?

- The immediate priority is to deal with the inflammatory impact on the peritoneal cavity and drainage to prevent sepsis. This should be done by an urgent laparoscopy after resuscitation with a thorough washout and the placement of drains. The patient should be given broad-spectrum antibiotics to prevent secondary infection of the bile within the peritoneal cavity. Careful attention should be made to analgesia, fluid balance, and prevention of respiratory complications
- Imaging of the biliary tract needs to be performed to look at the source of the bile leak. This can be by endoscopic retrograde cholangiopancreatography (ERCP) or noninvasively by MRCP. However, the former does give the option for stenting to reduce the pressure on the biliary system that in some cases may be the only intervention required

- If a more serious injury (one in three of bile leaks after cholecystectomy) is identified, urgent discussion with a hepatobiliary specialist should be undertaken to formulate a strategy for further surgical intervention. It some cases, this may need to be immediately or it may be delayed for 6 weeks. At all stages, the patient and their family to be kept informed of the current condition and future plans
- At the tertiary centre, once the sepsis is controlled, injuries without total common bile duct (CBD) occlusion or transection can be managed with endoscopic techniques. These are percutaneous transhepatic cholangiography or ERCP with sphincterotomy to reduce pressure on the biliary system with a stent to cover the opening into the ductal system
- In the case of complete transection or total occlusion, operative management is required. The options are direct end-to-end suturing if tension free over a T tube (Kehr T tube or internal Y-drainage tube) or Roux-en-Y hepaticojejunostomy
- There are reports of endoscopic biliary stenting and pedicled omental patch repair as a bridge to definitive Roux-en-Y if friable inflamed tissues are present. It should be noted that direct anastomosis does have a risk of stricturing. Stricture development, recurrent biliary sepsis, and cirrhosis are factors which lead to a lower life expectancy for patients who suffer iatrogenic bile duct injury

Further reading

Ahmad F, Saunders RN, Lloyd GM, Lloyd DM, Robertson GS. (2007). An algorithm for the management of bile leak following laparoscopic cholecystectomy. Ann R Coll Surg Engl 2007; 89:51–56.

Bismuth H. Postoperative strictures of the bile ducts. In: Blumgart LH (Ed). The Biliary Tract V. NY: Churchill-Livingstone; 1982. pp. 209–218.

Strasberg SM, Hertl M, Soper NJ. An analysis of the problem of biliary injury during laparoscopic cholecystectomy. J Am Coll Surg 1995; 180:101–125.

Scenario 4

Blunt chest trauma

A 78-year-old female presents following a fall down an entire flight of stairs and is complaining of shortness of breath and right-sided chest pain. Her oxygen saturations are 94% on room air, with a respiratory rate of 29 breaths per minute.

Q. 4.1 How would you assess and manage this patient?

- The Advanced Trauma Life Support (ATLS) protocol, spinal immobilisation until clearance from trauma CT that includes a full spinal view
- *AMPLE* (*A*llergies, *M*edications, *P*ast medical *history*, *L*ast meal or other intake, and *E*vents leading to presentation) to ensure medical background known. In the elderly, the events leading to the presentation need special consideration
- Oxygen, IV access with two large-bore cannulas, IV tranexamic acid 1 g, consider activation of major haemorrhage protocol (RBCs, FFP, and platelets), and analgesia
- Have in mind the immediate life-threatening injuries from blunt trauma including tension pneumothorax, aortic injury, haemothorax with severe active bleeding, pericardial tamponade from myocardial injury, or tracheobronchial disruption
- On assessment of the chest exclude tension pneumothorax with midline shift (shifted trachea, absent sounds single side of chest, unequal chest expansion) – if so, consider needle decompression (give landmarks – triangle of safety) and formal surgical chest drain with under water seal (give landmarks – 5th ICS, AAL)
- Consider FAST scanning in the ED to look for pericardial effusion, haemothorax, or free intra-peritoneal fluid. A Trauma CT scan should be performed as soon as possible once the patient is stable. As well as free fluid, air, and solid organ assessment remember careful assessment of thoracic aorta for signs of intimal dissection
- Complete assessment with secondary survey and full history to exclude any symptoms prior to fall which may need investigating

She has a trauma CT scan which reveals a large right-sided haemopneumothorax and multiple displaced posterior rib fractures. There are no intra-cranial or abdominal injuries. You successfully insert a surgical chest drain.

Q. 4.2 What would be the factors to consider with regards to the next steps of management for this patient?

- The main concern to be monitored is the volume coming out of the chest drain. Indications for thoracotomy include 1,500 mL (20 mL/kg) evacuated within the

first hour or >200 mL/h for the first 2–4 hours. The other consideration is the volume of ongoing transfusion requirements to maintain haemodynamic stability assuming there is no other source of blood loss
- There may be a need for involvement of the tertiary cardiothoracic centre
- It is important to review the CT scan to identify rib fractures. The questions to be answered are how many ribs are fractured, is there any displacement, and is there a flail segment. A flail segment is defined as when there are three or more ribs fractured in two or more places – leading to a flail chest. The segment of chest wall does not have bony continuity with the rest of the thoracic cage leading to a paradoxical movement, i.e. outward on inspiration and inward on expiration. Rib fixation may be indicated with certain injuries. Generally, a thoracic surgical opinion should be sought if there are more than three ribs fractured or if there is a flail segment. Otherwise, the management is nonoperative
- The nonoperative management includes analgesia, chest physiotherapy, oxygen, and nebulisers. Consideration may need to be given to antibiotic therapy if secondary infection is developing. The full range of oral analgesia with the addition of regional anaesthesia should be discussed
- Chest drains should be removed when there is no air leak and fluid drainage is only serous. It is not necessary to wait until serous fluid drainage stops as the drain creates some irritation by its presence

Q. 4.3 **3 days later post-removal of chest drain, a repeat chest X-ray (CXR) reveals a persistent pneumothorax and worsening surgical emphysema in the soft tissues of the chest and neck. How would you manage the patient?**

- A thorough clinical assessment should be made to include assessment of airway maintenance, chest sounds and expansion, oxygen saturations, and respiratory rate
- Developing emphysema in the soft tissues around the neck raises concerns over airway integrity and early involvement of the anaesthetic team should be considered
- A radiological assessment of the pneumothorax should be made to assess size and comparison to initial imaging
- Reinsertion of a surgical chest drain to drain pneumothorax using full aseptic technique in the triangle of safety and connected to an under-water seal. A CXR post-insertion should then be performed to ensure correct positioning
- Possibilities of the failure of re-expansion include blockage of the initial drain due to clot to prevent adequate drainage or persistent leak due to fistula (often indicated if the patient has extensive surgical emphysema)

The patient should be monitored for their respiratory rate and oxygen saturations with early discussion with a tertiary cardiothoracic centre to discuss possible need for transfer for VATS and injection of sealant into fistula.

Further reading

National Institute for Health and Clinical Excellence. Insertion of metal rib reinforcements to stabilise a flail chest wall [Interventional procedure guidance 36]. London: National Institute for Health and Clinical Excellence; 2010.

Pieracci FM, Majercik S, Ali-Osman F, et al. Consensus statement: Surgical stabilisation of rib fractures rib fracture colloquium clinical practice guidelines injury. Int J Care Injured 2017; 48:307–321.

Scenario 5

Urinary retention

A 77-year-old male complains of the inability to pass urine following a planned day case open inguinal hernia repair under general anaesthesia (GA).

Q. 5.1 What are the causes of urinary retention?

- Inefficient detrusor muscle
- Outflow obstruction
- Prostatic hyperplasia (BPH)
- Constipation
- Prostate or bladder cancer
- Urethral stricture
- Urolithiasis
- Phimosis
- Paraphimosis
- Medications
- Infection
- Trauma
- Neurologic impairment
- Spinal cord injuries from trauma, infarct, or demyelination
- Epidural abscess and epidural metastasis
- Guillain–Barré syndrome, diabetic neuropathy, and stroke
- Anatomic distortion – pelvic organ prolapse, pelvic masses, or urethral diverticulum
- Postoperative
- Postpartum

Q. 5.2 How would you manage this patient?

- If the patient is in pain and unable to void, it is entirely reasonable to proceed to urethral catheterisation. If there is no urgency for catheterisation, a bladder ultrasound may be performed. If <400 mL residual urine, a fluid challenge should be given with encouragement to mobilise and observation undertaken for successful voiding. If >400 mL urine then a urinary catheter should be inserted using standard two-way catheter under full asepsis and the patient should be kept overnight for removal of the catheter the following morning

- A full history and examination should be carried out. This should include review of fluid charts to assess perioperative and postoperative fluid balance. Previous urinary problems and current medications should be identified
- If the patient has recently undergone prostatic or urethral surgery then consideration of discussion with the urology team prior to catheterisation should be considered
- It should be remembered that in men there is a 50% recurrence of acute urinary retention in 1 week and 66% in 1 year. This can be mitigated by the prescription of an α1 adrenergic blocker at time of initial catheterisation in acute urinary retention secondary to benign prostatic hypertrophy. 5α reductase inhibitors are also used. Generally, with the institution of medical therapy, two trials without a catheter (at 1–2 weeks and 2 weeks after that) before embarking on prostate surgery. Urodynamics are done prior to surgery to establish if retention is due to outlet obstruction or detrusor insufficiency. If the latter then relief of any obstruction will be ineffective

Q. 5.3 You find that you are unable to pass a standard two-way catheter. How would you proceed?

- Alternative anatomy should be considered such as an enlarged prostate, strictures, or previous creation of false passages
- A larger diameter foley catheter should initially be considered, followed by a coudé tip or three-way catheter
- If there is still no success, a urologist should be consulted who may consider a flexible cystoscope-guided catheterisation or a supra-pubic catheter

Q. 5.4 The patient reports that for some time they have been struggling with nocturia up to five times per night and hesitancy. When you inserted a larger size catheter, there is an 1,800 mL residual despite the patient not complaining of any pain. How would you proceed?

- This is indicative of chronic urinary retention, likely due to an enlarged prostate. Consideration needs to be given that this may be malignant. Clinical examination should include a digital rectal examination. Routine bloods including urea and electrolytes, bone profile and prostate-specific antigen should be taken
- The volume of IV fluids administered and fluid balance should be taken into account and the possibility of post-catheterisation diuresis should be considered. A renal ultrasound scan needs to be performed to assess for hydronephrosis. The patient needs to be informed that a catheter may be required until a diagnosis is made

Further reading

Desgrandchamps F, De La Taille A, Doublet JD, Reten France Study Group. The management of acute urinary retention in France: a cross-sectional survey in 2618 men with benign prostatic hyperplasia. BJU Int 2006; 97:727–733.

Fisher E, Subramonian K, Omar MI. The role of alpha blockers prior to removal of urethral catheter for acute urinary retention in men. Cochrane Database Syst Rev 2014; CD006744.

Fitzpatrick JM, Kirby RS. Management of acute urinary retention. BJU Int 2006; 97:16.

Marshall JR, Haber J, Josephson EB. An evidence-based approach to emergency department management of acute urinary retention. Emerg Med Pract 2014; 16:1.

Wasson JH, Reda DJ, Bruskewitz RC, et al. A comparison of transurethral surgery with watchful waiting for moderate symptoms of benign prostatic hyperplasia. The Veterans Affairs Cooperative Study Group on Transurethral Resection of the Prostate. N Engl J Med 1995; 332:75.

Scenario 6

Testicular pain

A 35-year-old male presents to accident and emergency (A & E) with a short history of severe left-sided testicular pain.

Q. 6.1 How would you clinically evaluate this patient?

- A full history and examination should be conducted including pain history (site, duration, sudden or gradual onset, previous episodes, radiation into groin or back), associated swelling, change in positioning of testicle, urinary or bowel symptoms, personal medical and family history, and sexual activity history
- On examination, one should look for localised or general tenderness and swelling of the testicle and scrotum. The position of the testicle is checked to see if it is high lying or a clapper-bell type testis with the long pole lying horizontally. Examination to see if the tenderness was detectable in the spermatic cord and whether the cord could be felt to be twisted. A cremasteric reflex should be tested for by lightly stroking the superior and medial part of the thigh to see if the cremaster muscle contracts and pulls up the ipsilateral testis. The absence of a cremasteric reflex is associated with testicular torsion. However, cremasteric reflex is a less reliable sign after the age of 12. One should also look for a blue dot sign and localisation of testicular pain when the cause may be a torted appendix testis (hydatid of Morgagni). A positive Prehn sign is when manual elevation of the scrotum relieves pain and is more suggestive of epididymitis than testicular torsion

Q. 6.2 What are the differential diagnoses?

- The most likely diagnoses to consider are epididymo-orchitis or testicular torsion. Testicular torsion is more common in neonates and post-pubertal boys but 40% of cases are in men over 21. Between 1/2 and 1/4 men over 21 hospitalised with testicular pain will have torsion of the testis
- A scrotal abscess or Fournier's gangrene is less common but the most serious condition that has to be considered particularly if the patient is unwell, febrile, or has signs of haemodynamic instability
- Other causes include inguinoscrotal hernia, testicular cancer, renal colic, post-traumatic pain, post-vasectomy pain, Henoch–Schönlein purpura, mumps orchitis, and referred pain

Q. 6.3 The patient has an acutely swollen tender left testicle. How would you manage the patient?

- Initial management should include analgesia, keep nil by mouth, and arrange for standard or high-resolution ultrasound with Doppler flow study to the testicle. The lack of a colour Doppler signal to the testis is a highly sensitive indicator of testicular torsion
- Epididymo-orchitis is the most common cause of testicular pain often due to the organisms *N. gonorrhoea* and *C. trachomatis* in younger men and *E. coli* and *Pseudomonas* in older men. There is an increased risk among active homosexual men. A positive Prehn's sign (manual elevation of the scrotum relieves pain) is more often seen with epididymitis than testicular torsion. The cremasteric reflex is usually positive
- In males of <35 years old, there is a higher risk of sexually transmitted diseases. The antibiotics of choice are ceftriaxone (250 mg intramuscular injection in one dose) plus doxycycline (100 mg orally twice a day for 10 days). For the over 35 age group where coliforms and pseudomonas are more likely than levofloxacin 500 mg orally once daily for 10 days. 48–72 hours should be allowed to assess the effect of treatment then if there is no improvement, an alternative cause should be considered. If *N. gonorrhoeae* or *C. trachomatis* are the cause then contact tracing of sexual partners is required to allow them to be referred for assessment
- Torsion is due to inadequate fixation of the lower pole of the testis to the tunica vaginalis. It may be precipitated by trauma or vigorous physical activity. 8 hours of ischaemia will result in reduction in fertility even with normal contralateral testis. This is probably due to reduction in volume of germ cell-generating tissue. Consider in differential diagnosis when there is acute presentation with abdominal pain, nausea, and vomiting. The clinical findings may be of bell clapper deformity with high-riding testis and transverse lie. There will probably be a negative cremasteric reflex although this is an unreliable sign
- If there is any problem in obtaining an ultrasound and the probability of testicular torsion is high then surgical exploration should be performed. If there is any delay in access to the operating theatre, it is stated that a manual detorsion can be attempted but pain and tenderness may prevent this. The operation of choice is three-point fixation of both testes as the contralateral testis is also at risk of torsion

Further reading

Cummings JM, Boullier JA, Sekhon D, Bose K. Adult testicular torsion. J Urol 2002; 167:2109.

Scenario 7

Postoperative ileus

You are called by the F1 doctor for advice regarding a patient who underwent an anterior resection for a rectal adenocarcinoma 5 days ago. They have a distended abdomen and you discern they have not opened their bowels or passed flatus since the operation. They have vomited twice.

Q. 7.1 How would you assess this patient?

- Take a full history and examine the patient, in particular wishing to exclude the presence of abdominal wall or acute incisional hernias
- The patient should be managed according to CCrISP guidelines, and obtain good IV access for fluid resuscitation, monitoring of urine output/catheterisation and critical care input for organ support if required
- A nasogastric tube (NGT) should be used to decompress the stomach and reduce the risk of further vomiting and aspiration

Q. 7.2 What is your differential diagnosis?

- Given the presence of abdominal distension and the history of not opening bowels since the operation, it is necessary to determine if there is evidence of mechanical bowel obstruction or a paralytic/postoperative ileus
- Given the recent history of surgery, conditions such as anastomotic leak will need to be excluded as a cause of these symptoms

Q. 7.3 How would you investigate this patient?

- Parameters of systemic infection should be measured including white cell count and C-reactive protein (CRP). Urea and electrolytes should be tested – hypokalaemia may be a cause of functional ileus and would exclude the development of acute kidney injury from fluid third space losses
- Amylase/lipase should be checked as pancreatitis is a potential cause of functional ileus
- A plain abdominal radiograph may be obtained although this is not sensitive or specific to differentiate between mechanical or paralytic ileus. A CT scan has >90% sensitivity and specificity for diagnosis of mechanical obstruction; and will exclude anastomotic leak. CT should therefore be utilised to investigate this patient

Q. 7.4 What are the radiological features of ileus?

The CT would demonstrate dilatation of both large and small bowel without any evidence of transition or hold up from dilated bowel to non-dilated bowel, and no associated fluid collection, abscess or pneumoperitoneum that would suggest infection or anastomotic leak.

Q. 7.5 This patient's CT is reported as ileus. What are the potential causes of postoperative ileus?

This is an acquired abnormality of motility of the bowel following surgery manifested by the inability to pass flatus or stool and/or tolerate oral diet, although there is no consensus of a strict definition of postoperative ileus.

In the postoperative patient, the causes of ileus could be due to the following:
- Paralytic – a neurogenic condition mediated by adrenergic and non-adrenergic inhibitory reflexes
- Intra-abdominal or retroperitoneal lesions, e.g. haemorrhage and infection
- Drug-induced – due to use of opioids, neuroleptic drugs, etc.
- Metabolic – e.g. hypokalaemia or diabetes mellitus
- Vascular – hypoperfusion of the bowel due to inadequate blood supply

Q. 7.6 What options are available to reduce the risk of postoperative ileus?

There have been two main strategies employed:
1. Establishment of early oral intake
2. Reduction of opioid use via multimodal analgesic techniques or surgical techniques that are known to reduce postoperative pain.
   - Perioperative chewing of gum may reduce the development of ileus, but the evidence is weak (often only reported as a matter of hours benefit to return of bowel function). In a similar vein, early enteric feeding does not conclusively prevent ileus
   - Reports of the various strategies to avoid opioids such as perioperative epidural anaesthesia and lidocaine infusions have not demonstrated any reduction on postoperative ileus, nor have using prokinetic agents such as gastrografin, $5HT_4$ receptor agonists (such as prucalopride), magnesium oxide, choline citrate, metoclopramide, or bisacodyl. The μ receptor agonist, alvimopan, may reduce length of stay and time to return of bowel function in patients having major urological surgery, but yet to be investigated for colorectal or general surgery patients
   - Laparoscopic surgery may improve the time to bowel function, due to reduced analgesic requirements so should be used when possible. However, there are limited quality publications on the benefits in terms of ileus prevention

Q. 7.7 It is now postoperative day 8 and the patient's bowels have not opened, suggestive of prolonged ileus. What nutrition options are available for the patient?

- Within 7 days of surgery, it is unlikely such a patient would need nutritional support unless they were at high risk of intestinal failure or were assessed as being malnourished preoperatively. Oral/enteral nutritional support should be utilised first, as remaining nil by mouth may prolong the ileus
- Use of parenteral nutrition (PN) should only be considered when there are no features of bowel function returning and the patient is at risk of nutritional failure, as PN requires central venous access which has risks of infection. They can be referred to the nutrition team for assessment of the pros and cons for assessment for PN

Further reading

Chapman SJ, Pericleous A, Downey C, Jayne DG. Postoperative ileus following major colorectal surgery. Br J Surg 2018; 105:797–810.

Lim P, Morris OJ, Nolan G, et al. Sham feeding with chewing gum after elective colorectal resectional surgery: A randomized clinical trial. Ann Surg 2013; 257:1016–1024.

Paulson EK, Thompson WM. Review of small-bowel obstruction: The diagnosis and when to worry. Radiology 2015; 275:332–342.

Taylor BE, McClave SA, Martindale RG, et al. Guidelines for the provision and assessment of nutrition support therapy in the adult critically ill patient: Society of Critical Care Medicine (SCCM) and American Society for Parenteral and Enteral Nutrition (A.S.P.E.N.). Crit Care Med 2016; 44:390–438.

Vather R, Trivedi S, Bissett I. Defining postoperative ileus: results of a systematic review and global survey. J Gastrointest Surg 2013; 17:962–972.

Vilz TO, Stoffels B, Strassburg C, Schild HH, Kalff JC. Ileus in Adults. Dtsch Arztebl Int 2017; 114:508–518.

Scenario 8

Intussusception

A 61-year-old female is admitted via her GP to the surgical assessment unit with a short history of RIF pain, vomiting, and bloating. She is otherwise fit and well. Your registrar informs you that abdominal examination reveals mild distension with tenderness and localised guarding in the RIF. Her haemoglobin (Hb) is 102 g/L, white blood cell (WBC) is 15, and C-reactive protein (CRP) is 45.

Q. 8.1 How would you proceed?

- A full history and examination of the patient. History will be focused on onset, course, and duration of symptoms. Important aspects of her history would include migratory pain? Any change in bowel habit? Any weight loss? Last time bowels opened/passed wind? Any family history of colorectal cancer (CRC) or any recent colonic investigations? Any gynae/urinary symptoms? Examine the patient ensuring a rectal examination is performed
- Initial investigations would include routine blood work up including a group and save, urine dip stick (including pregnancy test in a younger patient). Ensure the patient remains NBM with adequate IVI access/IV fluids/IV antibiotics analgesia with a tentative initial diagnosis of acute appendicitis
- Due to her age, anaemia, and the wide differential diagnosis of RIF pain, request an urgent portovenous phase CT scan of the abdomen and pelvis ensuring renal function is adequate for intravenous contrast. Other differentials would include colonic neoplasm, right ovarian/tubal pathology, diverticulitis (caecal or sigmoid lying in the right iliac fossa), epiploic appendagitis, or ureteric coli

Q. 8.2 The CT is performed that evening and is reported as ileo-colic intussusception. What do you know about this condition, in relation to adults?

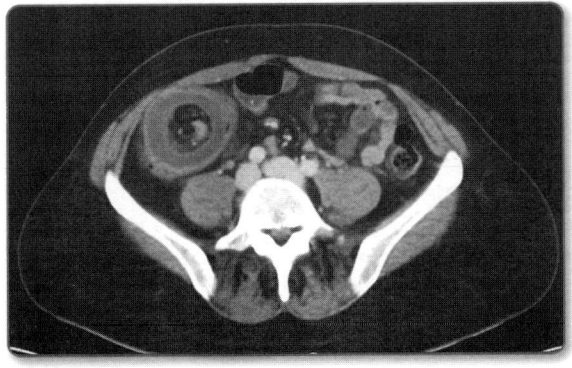

- Adult intussusception is extremely rare, occurring two to three times per 1,000,000 adult population per year. It accounts for <5% of all intestinal obstructions. The classical triad of vomiting, rectal bleeding (redcurrant jelly), and abdominal pain in paediatric intussusception is rarely seen in adults and where paediatric intussusception can be commonly treated non-operatively with pressure techniques such as barium hydrostatic reduction, surgery is almost always required in the adult population. Symptoms can be vague and long-standing or acute and obstructive and may mimic other intra-abdominal conditions. The predominant symptoms are of colicky abdominal pain and vomiting with the next being rectal bleeding
- *The four main types of intussusception are enteroenteric (small bowel only), colocolic (large bowel only), ileocolic* (terminal ileum prolapses within the ascending colon), *ileocecal (ileocecal valve is the lead point)*
- Approximately, 50% are found to be either enteroenteric or ileocolic. In adults 90% of cases a lead point will be identified, with 10% idiopathic, possible lead points include carcinoma, Meckel's diverticulum, colonic diverticulum, lymphoma, lipoma, strictures, metastatic lesions, polyps, or inflammatory lesions. 50% of small bowel and large bowel intussusception are due to malignant tumours

Q. 8.3 How would you proceed in this particular case?

- This patient has signs of localised peritonism and a radiological diagnosis of ileo-colic intussusception. Her WBC is raised indicating a systemic inflammatory response. If left untreated, this would lead to progressive bowel distension, ischaemia, intestinal perforation, and subsequent peritonitis
- Ensure the patient is prepped for theatre and inform the anaesthetic team that she requires surgery overnight. Request a nasogastric (NG) tube and ensure antibiotics have been administered. If possible, a preoperative discussion with the radiologist would be helpful to try and identify the lead-point or possibility of malignancy
- Patient would be consented for a laparoscopic/open right hemicolectomy ± stoma. Predictive morbidity and mortality would be calculated with the National Emergency Laparotomy Audit (NELA) risk prediction calculator and documented on the consent form, if the risk of mortality is >10%, a Critical Care unit bed should be made available

Q. 8.4 What operative factors should be considered when dealing with intussusception in adults and this case in particular?

In this case, the patient has minimal abdominal distension and a 'virgin abdomen', and a laparoscopic approach could be feasible depending on facilities and availability. However, in patients with significant abdominal distension due to dilated small or large bowel or with multiple previous abdominal operations, an open approach might be more appropriate. Careful consideration should be made in regard to attempted intraoperative manual/laparoscopic reduction of the intussusception. The risk in attempted reduction is perforation and risk of malignant cells disseminating in the abdominal cavity. The advantage of reduction, especially in small bowel is to preserve bowel length, to prevent possible short bowel syndrome in particular in patients with Crohn's disease. There are arguments that resection without reduction should be the treatment of choice in all inflamed, ischaemic, or friable segments and certainly colocolic intussusception as the high incidence of malignancy in this location

Q. 8.5 At operation you find an ileocolic intussusception, what operation do you perform?

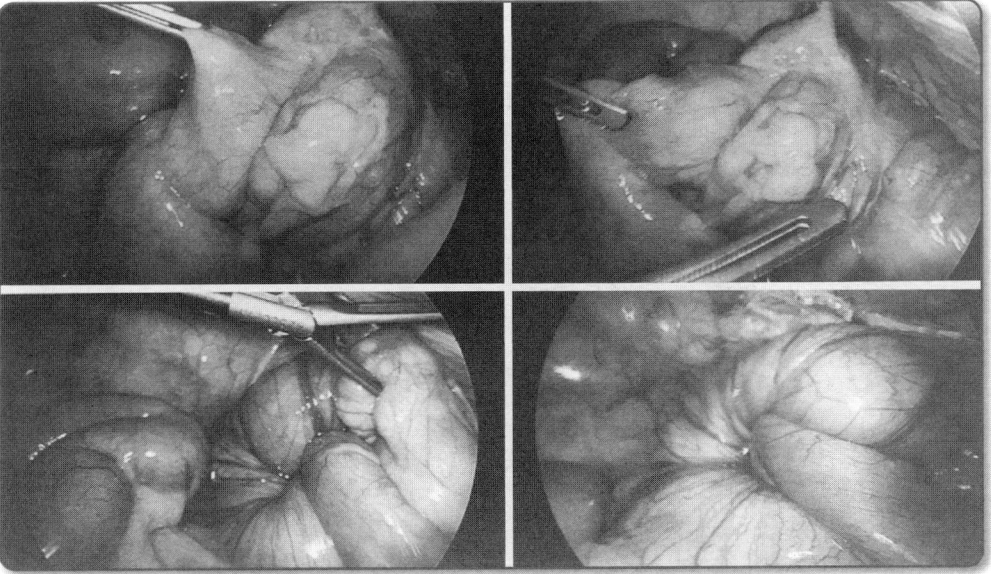

- Proceed to a resection without attempted reduction of the intussusception due to inflamed nature of the bowel. Also, as this patient is over 60 and there is an increased risk (50%) that the underlying cause could be malignant an oncological right hemicolectomy should be considered
- Laparoscopic/open mobilisation of the terminal ileum and right colon including the hepatic flexure will be performed along the avascular plane of Toldt
- Right hemicolectomy following oncological principles carefully protecting the duodenum at all times
- I would then perform a side-to-side anti-peristaltic stapled ileocolic anastomosis

If there was evidence of perforation/significant abdominal cavity soiling/poor nutritional state or use of inotropes an ileostomy could be brought out to avoid an anastomosis.

Q. 8.6 This is the resected specimen. What was the underlying cause of the intussusception?

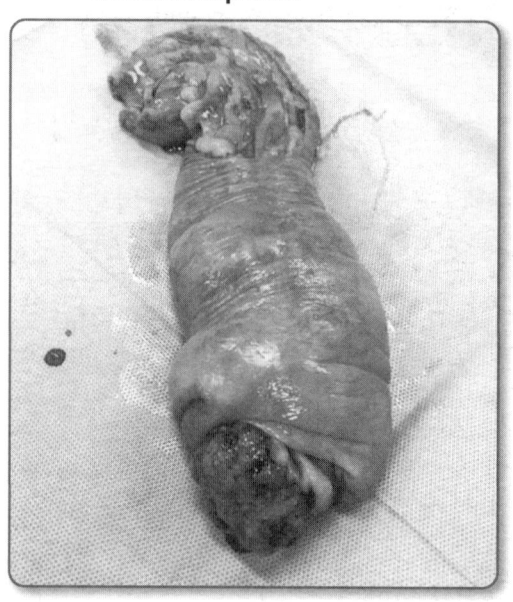

There is a small lesion of the caecal pole close to the ileocaecal valve that is the lead point of the intussusception. This is likely a small cancer in view of the surface appearance although a high-grade dysplastic polyp is a possibility.

Further reading

Begos DG, Sandor A, Modlin IM. The diagnosis and management of adult intussusception. Am J Surg 1997; 173:88–94.

Brayton D, Norris WJ. Intussusception in adults. Am J Surg 1954; 88:32–43.

Carter CR, Morton AL. Adult intussusception in Glasgow, UK. Br J Surg 1989; 76:727.

Gammeri E, Catton A, van Duren BH, Appleton SG, van Boxel GI. Towards an evidence-based management of right iliac fossa pain in the over 50-year-old patient. Ann R Coll Surg Engl 2016; 98:496–499.

Hadid T, Elazzamy H, Kafri Z. Bowel intussusception in adults: think cancer!. Case Rep Gastroenterol 2020; 14:27–33.

NELA. NELA Risk Calculator. [online] Available from https://data.nela.org.uk/riskcalculator. [Last accessed March, 2022].

Reijnen HA, Joosten HJ, De Boer HH. Diagnosis and treatment of adult intussusception. Am J Surg 1989; 158:25–28.

Royal College of Surgeons of England. (2014). Association of Surgeons of Great Britain and Ireland, Royal College of Surgeons of England Commissioning guide: Emergency general surgery (acute abdominal pain), 2014. [online] Available from https://www.rcseng.ac.uk/library-and-publications/rcs-publications/docs/emergency-general-guide/. [Last accessed March, 2022].

Scenario 9

Acute lower limb ischaemia

You are assessing an 80-year-old man in A&E who has attended with an acutely painful left leg. He has a background of hypertension and a 60-pack-year smoking history.

Q. 9.1 What would you do initially?

Take a focussed history, focussing on:
- Onset and nature of the pain
- Have there have been any previous episodes of pain especially on exercise?
- Is the pain worse on movement?
- Any recent surgery
- Any recent long journeys
- Any recent long-term inactivity

Focus on past medical history specifically looking at cardiovascular risk factors including:
- Smoking
- Ischaemic heart disease (IHD)
- Hypertension
- Hypercholesterolaemia
- Transient ischaemic attack (TIAs)/cerebrovascular accident (CVAs)
- Diabetes

I would then perform a focussed examination of both limbs:
- Listen to heart and check for irregular rhythm
- Palpate abdomen for AAA
- Check for peripheral pulses bilaterally (including hand-held doppler)
- Check capillary refill bilaterally
- Check for calf swelling/pain
- Check for any ulcers

Q. 9.2 Your examination findings show a left leg that is cool peripherally below the knee with a capillary refill of >5 seconds. Neurology is intact. What is your differential diagnosis and what initial investigations would you order?

- Acute limb ischaemia
- Bloods including:
  - FBC/U and Es/CRP/Clotting/G and S

- Electrocardiography (ECG)
- CT angiogram of the lower limb
- ECG

Q. 9.3 An ECG shows new onset of atrial fibrillation and CT angiogram shows a fresh 3 cm thrombus in the superficial femoral artery (SFA). What are your available management options?

- Start heparin infusion
- Thrombolysis
- Surgical embolectomy

Q. 9.4 Which management option would you choose in this patient and why?

- I would choose a surgical embolectomy
- The source is likely an acute embolus from new onset atrial fibrillation (AF), so embolectomy would be the best option in this situation. The limb is currently viable, and the surgery is time critical

Q. 9.5 Your consultant agrees to take the patient to theatre, talk me through what your approach would be?

- I would perform a femoral cut down to the common femoral artery (CFA)
- I would dissect the vessel out and gain proximal and distal control of the CFA/SFA/profunda arteries using vascular slings
- I would perform a transverse arteriotomy and check for viable inflow
- Ensure the patient receives 5,000 units of heparin
- Check for any back bleeding from SFA, if none is present then insert a 3F Fogarty catheter and remove and embolus/thrombus down to the level of the ankle
- Repeat this step multiple times until no more clot is removed
- Check for back bleeding from the profunda artery, if none is present then insert a 3F Fogarty catheter and remove and embolus/thrombus
- Close the arteriotomy vertically using 5/0 prolene

Q. 9.6 Would you routinely perform fasciotomies?

- Yes, due to the risk of compartment syndrome secondary to reperfusion syndrome and the resultant oedema

Q. 9.7 What other postoperative management is needed?

- Address all cardiovascular risk factors
- ECHO to rule out any mural thrombus
- Ensure AF is controlled

Further reading

Björck M, Earnshaw JJ, Acosta S, et al. Editor's Choice - European Society for Vascular Surgery (ESVS) 2020 Clinical Practice Guidelines on the Management of Acute Limb Ischaemia. Eur J Vasc Endovasc Surg 2020; 59:173–218.

Scenario 10

Acute pancreatitis

A 35-year-old female patient presents to A&E with a 24-hour history of sudden onset epigastric pain radiating to the back.

Q. 10.1 What are your differential diagnoses?

- Perforated peptic ulcer
- Acute pancreatitis
- Gastritis

Q. 10.2 What specific investigations would you like?

- Bloods especially amylase/LFTs
- Erect chest X-ray (CXR)
- Possibly a CT scan if the amylase and CXR are normal

Q. 10.3 What are the Atlanta criteria?

- This is the criteria to establish a diagnosis of acute pancreatitis, of which you must have two of the following:
  - Pain consistent with acute pancreatitis
  - Serum amylase greater than three times the upper limit of normal
  - CT evidence of pancreatitis

Q. 10.4 The patient's amylase returns at 1,300, with a bilirubin of 80, alkaline phosphatase (ALP) 400 and alanine transaminase (ALT) 80. What are the most common causes of pancreatitis and what is the likely cause in this patient?

- Given the deranged LFTs, the likely cause in this patient is gallstones
- The three most common causes are:
  - Gallstones
  - Excess alcohol intake
  - Drugs (e.g. steroids)

Q. 10.5 What scoring system are you aware of in acute pancreatitis?

The modified Glasgow score:

P	PO_2 <8 kPa	R	Renal (urea) >16 mmol/L
A	Age >55	E	Enzymes (LDH) >600 / AST >200
N	Neutrophils (WCC) >15 × 10^9/L	A	Albumin <32 g/L
C	Calcium <2 mmol/L	S	Sugar (glucose) >10 mmol/L
(LDH, lactate dehydrogenase; PO_2, partial pressure oxygen)			

A score of ≥3 indicates severe pancreatitis, and ITU should at very least be made aware of the patient.
   This is a predictive score for severity only.

Q. 10.6 This patient is currently scoring 2 for a WCC of 18 × 10^9/L and urea of 20 mmol/L. What is your initial management?

I would manage this patient conservatively in a level 1 ward ensuring the following:
- Adequate IV fluids
- Urinary catheter with hourly urine output measurement and strict fluid balance
- Analgesia

Q. 10.7 Would you start antibiotics in this patient?

- No
- There is no evidence for the routine use of antibiotics in pancreatitis
- The main indication for the use of antibiotics in pancreatitis is where there is evidence of infective necrosis

Q. 10.8 What further investigations would you like on this patient?

I would like an ultrasound scan of the abdomen to check for gallstones.

Q. 10.9 Ultrasound scan of the abdomen shows the presence of multiple gallstones in the gallbladder, with a normal calibre CBD. What would you do next?

Assuming that, the patient has no contraindications to an MRI scan, I would order an MRCP to check for the presence of any gallstones in the CBD

Q. 10.10 MRCP returns showing the presence of two small gallstones in the CBD, what would be your next step in management?

This patient requires an urgent ERCP ± stent insertion

Q. 10.11 When should a laparoscopic cholecystectomy be performed on this patient?

As per British Society of Gastroenterology (BSG) guidelines, either on the index admission or within 2 weeks of discharge

Further reading

Guyot A, Lequeu JB, Dransart-Rayé O, et al. Management of acute pancreatitis. A literature review. Rev Med Interne 2021; 42:625–632.

Goodchild G, Chouhan M, Johnson GJ. Practical guide to the management of acute pancreatitis. Frontline Gastroenterol 2019; 10:292–299.

Scenario 11

Oesophageal perforation

A 23-year-old male patient presents to A&E with sudden onset chest pain. The previous night he admits to drinking an excess amount of alcohol and he has been repeatedly vomiting since then. He is currently tachycardic at 130 bpm and has a temperature of 38.5.

Q. 11.1 What is the most likely diagnosis?

- The most likely diagnosis is Boerhaave's syndrome
- The patient is currently septic and needs to be treated as per the sepsis 6 urgently including antifungal treatment

Q. 11.2 What is Boerhaave's syndrome?

- This is a full-thickness rupture of the oesophagus secondary to profuse vomiting and/or retching in the absence of any oesophageal pathology
- It is caused by the sudden rise in abdominal pressure from the repeated vomiting and/or retching against a closed cricopharyngeus
- It most commonly occurs in the left lower posterolateral position just above the oesophagogastric junction (OGJ)

Q. 11.3 What is Mackler's triad?

- Vomiting
- Sudden onset chest pain
- Surgical emphysema

Q. 11.4 How would you confirm the diagnosis?

- CT chest and abdomen with oral contrast
- If this is not available, then an upper GI endoscopy

Q. 11.5 CT scan confirms a large perforation of the lower oesophagus with pneumomediastinum and left pleural collection. What are your management options?

- I would firstly seek advice from a tertiary oesophagogastric centre

- Given the age of the patient and CT findings, surgical intervention would be appropriate
- I would insert a chest drain in the first instance if surgery is delayed
- This would involve a thoracotomy and insertion of a T-tube or primary closure (if < 24 hours)
  - Primary closure can be performed in select cases with a history of <24 hours
- A feeding jejunostomy will be required for postoperative feeding

Q. 11.6 What are the other causes of oesophageal perforation?

- The most common cause is iatrogenic during a therapeutic upper GI endoscopy
- Other causes include:
  - Diagnostic OGD
  - Foreign body ingestion
  - Transoesophageal Echocardiogram (mainly during cardiac surgery)
  - Corrosive substance ingestion
  - Nasogastric (NG) insertion

Q. 11.7 If this had been a perforated cancer how would this change your management?

- Conservative management would be the approach used
- May consider the use of an oesophageal stent
- May still need chest drains to treat any collections

Further reading

National Institute of Health and Care Excellence. NICE guidelines oesophageal perforation. [online] Available from https://www.evidence.nhs.uk/search?q=Oesophageal+perforation. [Last accessed March, 2022].

Turner AR, Turner SD. Boerhaave Syndrome, in StatPearls. 2021, StatPearls Publishing Copyright © 2021. Treasure Island (FL): StatPearls Publishing LLC; 2021.

Scenario 12

Clostridium difficile infection

You are performing a ward round and come across an 80-year-old female patient who has been treated with broad-spectrum antibiotics for 5 days after an ultrasound scan showed acute cholecystitis. The nurse informs you she has developed severe diarrhoea over the last 12 hours.

Q. 12.1 what would be your management?

- This is a case of nosocomial diarrhoea in a patient who has been on broad-spectrum antibiotics for 5 days, thus *Clostridium difficile* must be assumed
- Ensure the patient is moved to a side room for isolation from other patients and all infection control guidelines adhered to including:
  - Gloves and apron to be worn
  - Strict handwashing with soap and water
  - Reduced number of staff to enter the room
- Urgent stool sample to be sent to the laboratory checking specifically for the presence of *C. difficile* toxins (PCR)

Q. 12.2 How would you classify *C. difficile* infection?

- *Mild/moderate*:
  - Loose stools ≤5 times per day
  - Abdominal pain
  - WCC <15 × 10^9
- *Severe*:
  - Loose stools >6 times per day
  - WCC ≥15 × 10^9
  - Fever > 38°C
  - Blood in stool
  - Tachycardia >90
  - Toxic megacolon/pseudomembranous colitis/perforation (rare)

Q. 12.3 What is *Clostridium difficile*?

- It is an anaerobic, gram-positive spore-forming bacillus
- *Toxin producing*:
  - Toxin A
  - Toxin B

- Toxins can trigger a severe systemic inflammatory response syndrome (SIRS) response

Q. 12.4 What are the causes of C. difficile colitis?
- *C. difficile* is colonised in 2–5% of the healthy adult population
- The use of antibiotics can alter gut flora, which in turn allows the proliferation of *C. difficile* and the release of toxins
- It is the toxins that cause symptoms not the colonisation

Q. 12.5 Which patients are at risk?
- Elderly patients
- Comorbid patients
- Any recent prolonged antibiotic use (≥5 days):
  - Beware even short course antibiotic therapy can cause *C. difficile* colitis

Q. 12.6 How would you treat C. difficile infection?
- Initial treatment is to stop the causative antibiotic
- Stop proton pump inhibitor (PPI) where possible
- Treatment is dependent on the severity of infection
- *Mild/moderate*:
  - Oral metronidazole
- *Severe*:
  - Oral vancomycin
- If a patient cannot tolerate oral antibiotics, then IV metronidazole is the choice as IV vancomycin is ineffective for the treatment of *C. difficile*

Q. 12.7 Should endoscopy be performed on a patient with C. difficile colitis?
No due to the high risk of perforation

Q. 12.8 Are there any specific risks you know related to the use of oral vancomycin?
This can lead to the development of vancomycin-resistant *Enterococci (VRE)*

Q. 12.9 Your patient recovers fully, are you aware of any governance issues that may arise from this case?
- Yes, this case must be reported and an incident form filled out
- There needs to be a serious incident requiring investigation (SIRI) undertaken
  - Root cause analysis performed

- All hospitals have an acceptable number of nosocomial *C. difficile* infections per annum set by the Department of Health

Further reading

National Institute of Health and Care Excellence. NICE guidelines for the management of *C. Difficile* colitis. [online] Available from https://cks.nice.org.uk/topics/diarrhoea-antibiotic-associated/management/diarrhoea-antibiotic-associated/. [Last accessed March, 2022].

Scenario 13

Abdominal compartment syndrome

You have performed a prolonged and difficult laparotomy with subtotal colectomy for a 50-year-old female patient with severe ulcerative colitis, toxic megacolon and perforation. It is now day 1 postoperatively and the patient remains intubated and ventilated on ITU.

Q. 13.1 What do you think is the cause of the patient's current clinical picture?

Given the complexity of the laparotomy with the rising ventilatory pressures, acidosis and reduced urine output despite adequate fluid resuscitation, I would be worried about abdominal compartment syndrome (ACS)

Q. 13.2 How would you classify intra-abdominal hypertension (IAP)?

- IAP is defined as a persistently raised abdominal pressure of ≥12 mmHg (normal range 5–7 mmHg):
  - Grade I (12–15 mmHg)
  - Grade II (16–20 mmHg)
  - Grade III (21–25 mmHg)
  - Grade IV (>25 mmHg)

Q. 13.3 How would you define ACS?

- An intra-abdominal pressure >25 with associated new organ dysfunction

Q. 13.4 How do you measure intra-abdominal pressure?

- This is performed in the supine position and requires the patient to have a urinary catheter in situ
- The bladder must be empty, and the catheter connected to a transducer that is then zeroed
- Up to 25 mL of sterile saline is inserted into the bladder, and the pressure is measured at the end of expiration
- This is usually performed in the ITU setting

Q. 13.5 What are the risk factors for developing ACS?

- Trauma (including laparotomy)
- Acute pancreatitis
- Peritonitis
- Perforation
- Intra-abdominal collection
- Volume-reducing surgery (large incisional hernia repair)
- Obesity

Q. 13.6 What are the sequalae of ACS?

- Decreased tidal volume
- Acute kidney injury
- Increased abdominal pressure leads to reduced venous return
- This in turn leads to reduced cardiac output
- The result is end-organ dysfunction and potentially multiorgan failure.

Q. 13.7 What are the treatment options?

- All measures aim to improve abdominal wall compliance
- *Conservative*:
  - Avoid excessive IV fluid administration
- *Medical*:
  - Neuromuscular blockade
  - Sedation
  - NG decompression
  - Prokinetic agents
- *Interventional*:
  - Drainage of any large collections
- *Surgical*:
  - *Laparotomy for decompression*:
    - Reserved only for severe refractory cases
    - Last resort

Further reading

Berry N, Fletcher S. Abdominal compartment syndrome 2012. [online] Available from https://academic.oup.com/bjaed/article/12/3/110/258792. [Last accessed March, 2022].

Scenario 14

Post-ERCP perforation

You are called to see a 30-year-old male patient on the ward 6 hours after having had an ERCP, removal of CBD stones and stent insertion. The patient is complaining of severe epigastric pain and has a temperature of 38.5. His heart rate is 120 bpm and he has a systolic BP of 90 mmHg.

Q. 14.1 What is your differential diagnosis?

- This patient has clear signs of sepsis. I would start first by resuscitating the patient in an ABC fashion and ensuring the sepsis 6 has been carried out
- *My differentials include*:
  - Post-ERCP pancreatitis
  - Post-ERCP perforation
  - Post-ERCP oesophageal perforation

Q. 14.2 How would you next like to manage this patient?

- I would like to order routine bloods including:
  - FBC/U and Es/LFTs/CRP/amylase
- Urgent CT AP with contrast

Q. 14.3 CT scan confirms a retroperitoneal duodenal perforation, what is your management?

- Retroperitoneal perforations are treated conservatively
- This would include:
  - Broad-spectrum antibiotics
  - Patient to be kept NBM and insertion of NG tube
  - Intravenous (IV) PPI treatment
  - IV fluid resuscitation.
  - Percutaneous drainage of any large collections

Q. 14.4 What is the most common risk factor for an iatrogenic ERCP duodenal perforation?

Presence of a duodenal diverticulum (D2)

Further reading

Stapfer M, Selby RR, Stain SC, et al. Management of duodenal perforation after endoscopic retrograde cholangiopancreatography and sphincterotomy. Ann Surg 2000; 232:191–198.

Scenario 15

Gunshot wounds

You are reviewing a 35-year-old male patient during a trauma call after he was shot in the abdomen with a shotgun. He is currently haemodynamically unstable.

Q. 15.1 What is your initial management?

- Follow ATLS guidelines and assess the patient in an ABC manner
- Begin major haemorrhage protocol:
  - Transfuse the patient with O negative blood
- If the patient has refractory shock, he needs an immediate laparotomy

Q. 15.2 The patient stabilises with fluid resuscitation and you manage to get a CT scan. This confirms a large amount of free fluid in the abdomen and free air. You decide to take the patient for a laparotomy, describe the steps you would take. On the way to theatre, the patient becomes haemodynamically unstable again.

- This is a damage control laparotomy
- Open the abdomen and release the falciform ligament
- I would proceed to pack all four quadrants of the abdomen including the pelvis
- Methodically check each quadrant of the abdomen and the pelvis for source of bleeding and perform haemostasis
- I would try to identify the source of perforation(s) and resect the affected areas and leave the stapled ends of bowel in the abdomen
- I would try to remove any obvious bullet fragments
- Leave the abdomen packed and use a temporary closure, e.g. negative pressure dressing or Bogota bag and send the patient to critical care with a planned relook laparotomy in 24–48 hours when the patient has stabilised

Q. 15.3 What are the two types of bullet injuries you are aware of?

1. *Low velocity*:
   - Speed <300 m/s
2. *High velocity*:
   - Speed >300 m/s

Q. 15.4 How do bullets cause injury?
- This is via the transference of kinetic energy from the bullet to the tissues
- Injury can be to any structure within the body including bone
- The presence of an exit wound reduces the chance of collateral damage by the bullet as there has been a lower transference of kinetic energy

Q. 15.5 Can bullet wounds be treated conservatively?
- They can in certain circumstances
- These include:
  - Presence of an exit wound
  - Imaging that confirms no injury to vital structures (e.g. blood vessels)
  - No evidence of neurological deficit
- They must be treated with washout and antibiotics

Q. 15.6 What is the main concern with a shotgun wound?
- Shotguns produce multiple pellets which can cause catastrophic damage in multiple areas within the body
- Patients require detailed examination and exploration on laparotomy for multiple injuries

Further reading

Cantú-Alejo DR, Reyna-Sepúlveda F, García-Hernández S, et al. Presentation, management and evolution of patients with abdominal gunshot wound. A decade of violence in Mexico. Cir Cir 2021; 89:39–45.

Klopper J, Moola H, Venter J, et al. Outcomes of patients with thoraco-abdominal gunshot wounds operatively managed at a district hospital in Cape Town, South Africa. Afr J Emerg Med 2021; 11:60–64.

Scenario 16

Haematemesis

You are reviewing a 35-year-old male patient in A&E who has been admitted following several episodes of haematemesis. He recently suffered an injury at the gym and has been taking non-steroidal-anti-inflammatory drugs (NSAIDs) for the past 2 weeks.

Q. 16.1 What is your initial management of this patient?

- Given the history I am concerned that this patient has a bleeding peptic ulcer
- Patient must be assessed in an ABC manner
- Major haemorrhage protocol should be initiated
- Two large-bore cannulas
- Transfuse O negative blood
- The patient needs an urgent OGD after initial resuscitation

Q. 16.2 You take the patient for an urgent OGD, and you find a bleeding duodenal ulcer. What would your management be?

- The patient would need control of bleeding using dual therapy from the following:
  - Adrenaline injection
  - Clips
  - Argon plasma coagulation
  - Heater probe

Q. 16.3 What is the most likely vessel causing the bleed?

Gastroduodenal artery (GDA)

Q. 16.4 How would you classify the risk of re-bleeding on endoscopy?

Forrest classification:

Stage	Characteristics on OGD	Risk of re-bleeding
Stage I: Active bleeding		
Ia	Arterial spurting	90%
Ib	Arterial oozing	80%

Continues opposite

Continued

Stage	Characteristics on OGD	Risk of re-bleeding
Stage II: Signs of recent bleeding		
IIa	Visible vessel	40–50%
IIb	Adherent clot	20–30%
IIc	Haematin covered lesion	5%
Stage III: Lesion with no evidence of recent bleeding		
III	Clean ulcer base	3–5%

Q. 16.5 Dual therapy OGD controls the bleed, and the patient is successfully resuscitated, how else will you manage the patient?

- Ensure the patient is on high-dose PPI
- Initiate *Helicobacter pylori* eradication therapy

Q. 16.6 What other scoring systems are you aware of for upper GI bleeds?

- Glasgow Blatchford score:
  - Risk stratifies patients with an upper GI bleed
- Rockall score:
  - Calculates the mortality risk secondary to an upper GI bleed

Rockall score:

Variable	Score = 0	Score = 1	Score = 2	Score = 3
Age	<60	60–79	>80	
Comorbidities	None		Cardiac failure IHD Any major comorbidity	Renal/liver failure Metastatic disease
Degree of shock	None	Pulse > 100 bpm	Systolic BP < 100 mmHg	
Initial score/7				
Additional score post-endoscopy:				
Source of bleed	Mallory–Weiss tear	All other diagnosis	Malignancy	
Recent stigmata of bleed	None		Adherent clot or spurting vessel	
Final score/11				
(BP, blood pressure; IHD, ischaemic heart disease)				

Rockall score mortality:

Score	Mortality
1–2	0%
3	5%
4–6	5–10%
≥7	10–35%

Q. 16.7 You are called to the ward the next day as the patient has had another two episodes of haematemesis, what are your current management options?

- Management would depend on the haemodynamic status of the patient:
  - Repeat OGD (if stable)
  - Interventional radiology – embolisation of GDA (if mildly unstable)
  - Laparotomy (if unstable)

Q. 16.8 The patient becomes severely haemodynamically unstable and you decide to perform a laparotomy, what operation would you perform and how?

- Under-running of the ulcer
- Via upper midline incision
- Transverse duodenotomy
- Four stitches at each quadrant of the ulcer to help control the haemorrhage
- Under-run the ulcer at the base
- Close the duodenum in opposite direction (vertically) to duodenotomy to reduce risk of stricture

Further reading

National Institute for Health and Care Excellence. NICE guidelines for the management of acute upper GI bleed, 2012. [online] Available from https://www.nice.org.uk/guidance/CG141. [Last accessed March, 2022].

Scenario 17

Head injury

You review an 80-year-old male patient in resus during a trauma call after he fell down the stairs and injured his head. He currently takes rivaroxaban for atrial fibrillation (AF).

Q. 17.1 What are the NICE guidelines for CT imaging in head injuries?

- Glasgow coma scale (GCS) < 13 on initial assessment
- GCS < 15 at 2 hours after initial assessment
- Suspected open or depressed skull fracture
- Suspected basal skull fracture
- Post-traumatic seizure
- Focal neurological defect
- More than one episode of vomiting

Any patients who have experienced any loss of consciousness or amnesia since the injury with any of the following risk factors:
- Age ≥ 65
- Bleeding/clotting disorders (including anticoagulant medications)
- Severe mechanism of injury [e.g. road traffic accident (RTA)]
- >30 minutes retrograde amnesia prior to trauma

Q. 17.2 What are the signs of a basal skull fracture?

- 'Panda/Racoon' eyes
- Battle's sign
- Cerebrospinal fluid (CSF) leakage from the nose

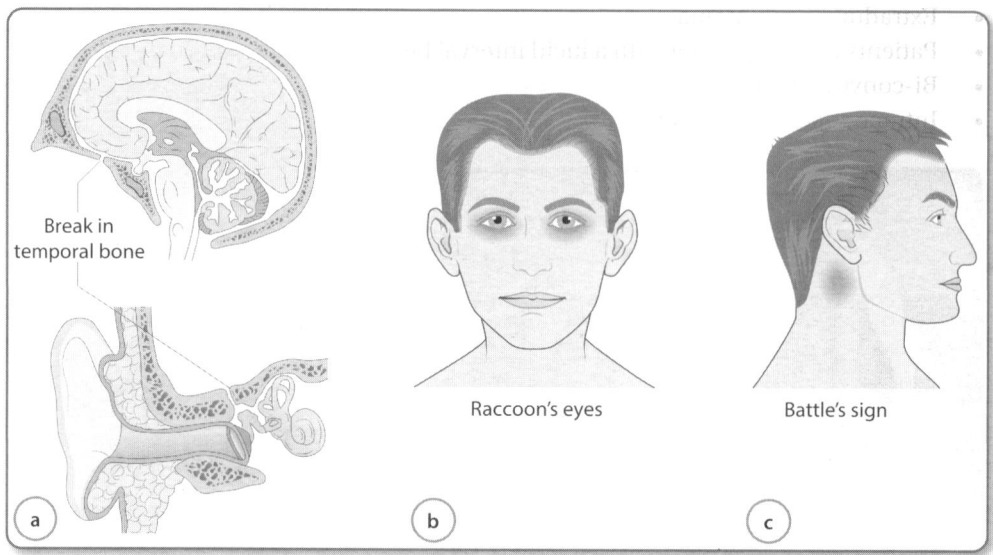

Source: Health Jade Team. Battle sign. [online] Available from https://healthjade.net/battle-sign/. [Last accessed March, 2022].

Q. 17.3 What are the different types of haemorrhagic brain injuries?
- Subdural haematoma
- Crescent shaped on CT

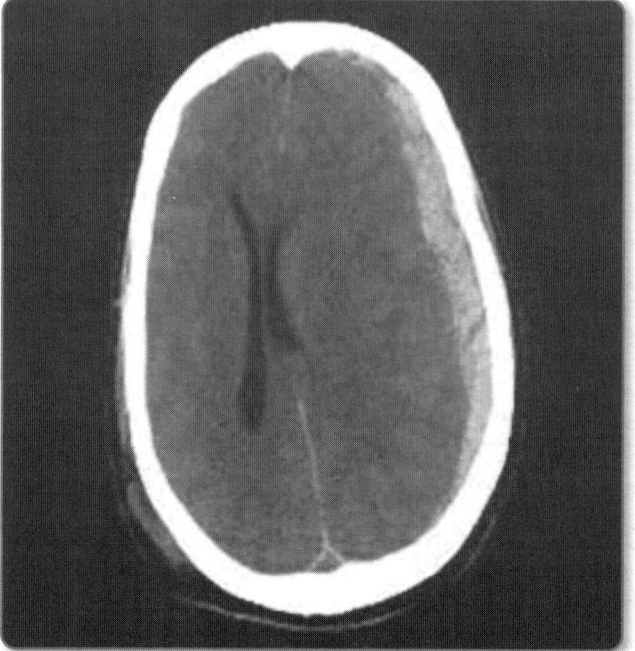

Source: ScienceDirect. Subdural Hematoma. [online] Available from https://www.sciencedirect.com/topics/neuroscience/subdural-hematoma. [Last accessed March, 2022].

- Extradural haematoma
- Patients usually present with a lucid interval before becoming confused again
- Bi-convex on CT
- Intracranial haemorrhage

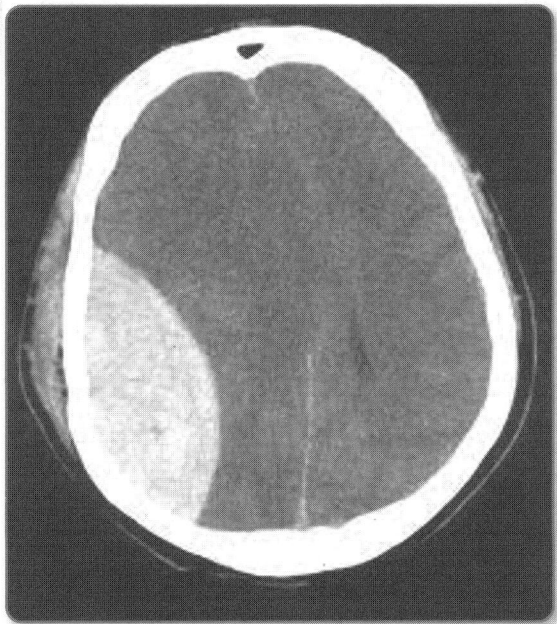

Source: Rasuli B. Extradural haemorrhage, 2021. [online] Available from https://radiopaedia.org/articles/extradural-haemorrhage. [Last accessed March, 2022].

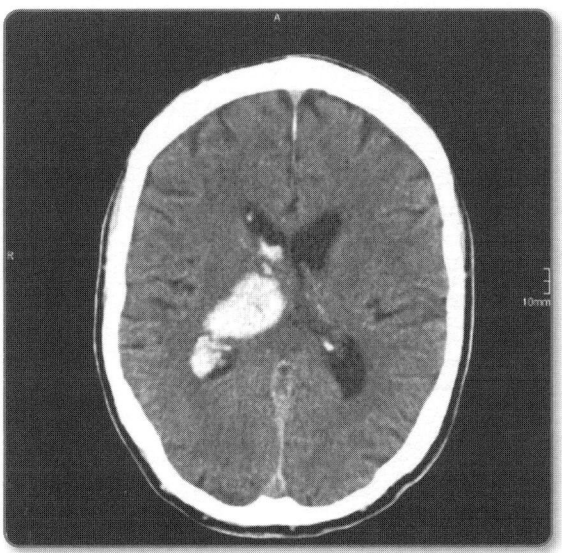

Source: Voss YL. (2016). Hyperacute intracerebral haemorrhage on MRI and CT. [online] Available from https://radiopaedia.org/cases/hyperacute-intracerebral-haemorrhage-on-mri-and-ct. [Last accessed March, 2022].

Q. 17.4 What is the Monro–Kellie Doctrine?

- This is a hypothesis that states the cranium is a fixed box, with the total volume of CSF, blood, and brain remaining constant
- CPP = MAP − ICP
  - CPP is cerebral perfusion pressure
  - MAP is mean arterial pressure
  - ICP is intracranial pressure
- Normal ICP is between 5 and 10 mmHg
- In cases of raised ICP:
  - Hypertension
  - Bradycardia

Q. 17.5 Why is permissive hypercapnia used in brain injuries?

- Used in ventilated patients with brain injuries
- By inducing hypercapnia:
  - Vasodilatation of cerebral arterioles
  - Reduce cerebral vascular resistance and increases cerebral blood flow
  - Reduces severity of brain injury

Q. 17.6 What medications can be used to reduce ICP?

- *Mannitol*:
  - Osmotic diuretic
  - Reduces brain fluid by creating an osmotic gradient
- *Furosemide*:
  - Known diuretic
  - Reduces brain fluid and CSF production

Further reading

National Institute for Health and Care Excellence. NICE guidelines on management of traumatic head injury. [online] Available from https://www.nice.org.uk/guidance/cg176. [Last accessed March, 2022].

Shih RY, Burns J, Ajam AA, et al. ACR Appropriateness Criteria® Head Trauma: 2021 Update. J Am Coll Radiol 2021; 18:S13–S36.

Scenario 18

Ingested foreign body

You are called to see a 12-year-old boy who has swallowed a button-shaped battery. A chest and abdominal plain film radiograph confirm the battery is lodged in the oesophagus.

Q. 18.1 What is your management?

- Button-shaped batteries pose a specific risk as they are highly corrosive especially when lodged in the oesophagus
- Therefore, they need urgent removal via an upper GI endoscopy and basket retrieval
- If retrieval is not possible, then the battery should be pushed into the stomach where it should pass spontaneously
- This is irrespective of whether the patient is symptomatic

Q. 18.2 What difference to your management would there be if the swallowed batteries were traditional AA or AAA?

- These batteries are not corrosive
- If the patient is asymptomatic then they will usually pass spontaneously

Q. 18.3 Where are the most common areas that ingested foreign bodies may become stuck?

- *Oesophagus*:
  - Cricopharyngeus
  - Aortic arch
  - Lower oesophageal sphincter
- Duodenum
- Ileocaecal junction
- Once an object has passed the duodenum, over 85% will then pass spontaneously
- Routine X-ray after 3 days if the patient has not passed the object is sufficient

Q. 18.4 What difference to your management would there be if the patient had swallowed bleach?

- This will likely cause a caustic injury to the oesophagus and stomach
- Would assess the patient in an ABC manner and ensure they have a secure and patent airway

- Start immediate high-dose PPI
- Would need an urgent OGD

Q. 18.5 How would you classify caustic injuries to the oesophagus?

Grade	Appearance
1	Superficial mucosal oedema
2	Mucosal/submucosal ulceration
3	Transmural ulceration with necrosis
4	Perforation

Q. 18.6 On OGD, there is evidence of grade 3 caustic injury with circumferential ulcers and necrosis, what would your management be?

- This would need urgent discussion with the local oesophagogastric unit
- As there is perforation, this would likely need surgery
- This would need an oesophagectomy ± colonic interposition dependent on the degree of injury to the stomach and duodenum

Further reading

Mathew RP, Sarasamma S, Jose M, et al. Clinical presentation, diagnosis and management of aerodigestive tract foreign bodies in the adult population: Part 1. SA J Radiol 2021; 25:2022.

Mathew RP, Liang TI, Kabeer A, Patel V, Low G. Clinical presentation, diagnosis and management of aerodigestive tract foreign bodies in the paediatric population: Part 2. SA J Radiol 2021; 25:2027.

Scenario 19

Paediatric trauma

You are called to resus for a trauma call involving an 8-year-old-boy who has been hit by a car during a road traffic collision. The child was a pedestrian and was struck at 30 mph.

Q. 19.1 How would you manage this patient?
- Manage as per ATLS protocol
- Immobilise C-spine
- ABC assessment
- Insertion of two large-bore cannulas

Q. 19.2 How would you fluid resuscitate a child?
- This would be based on ideal body weight:
  - Weight (kg) = 2 × (age + 4)
- Fluids should be given as:
  - 10–20 mL/kg

Q. 19.3 How would you assess the haemodynamic status of a child?
- Children will compensate far more than adults, and so assessment of heart rate and blood pressure alone is not reliable
- Hypotension is a very late sign and can be terminal
  - Acceptable systolic BP is 70 mmHg plus (age × 2)
- *More sensitive parameters*:
  - Capillary refill time
  - GCS

Q. 19.4 Why must you be more cautious in looking for injuries in paediatric trauma?
- Because children are smaller, there is a much larger force to mass ratio
- Therefore, the same impact is much larger on a child which can lead to much more serious injuries than expected in an adult ± polytrauma
- As children can haemodynamically compensate better than adults, there is always a risk of a false sense of security

Q. 19.5 What are the common injuries seen in children?

- *Chest*:
  - Uncommon as the chest wall in children is more compliant
- *Abdomen*:
  - Duodenal and pancreatic injuries are more common due to ongoing development of the abdominal cavity muscles and handlebar injuries
  - Bladder injuries are more common as it is more intraperitoneal in children
- *Limbs*:
  - Beware of spiral fractures as these can be a sign of non-accidental injury (NAI)
- *Eyes*:
  - Beware of retinal haemorrhages which can also be a sign of NAI

Q. 19.6 Why is temperature regulation important in children?

Children have a large body surface area to weight ratio and so lose heat much quicker than adults

Further reading

Birmingham Children's Hospital. Paediatric major trauma guidelines, 2012. [online] Available from http://kids.bch.nhs.uk/wp-content/uploads/2012/03/BCH-Major-Trauma-Guidelines-v7.pdf. [Last accessed March, 2022].

Scenario 20

Neck trauma

You are reviewing a 30-year-old male patient in resus who has presented with a stab injury to the left side of the neck.

Q. 20.1 How would you manage this?

- Ensure a trauma call has been put out
- Follow ATLS protocol
- There would be significant concern regarding the airway, the presence of a consultant anaesthetist is imperative to ensure that the airway is secure with a low threshold for intubation
- I would assess the patients breathing specifically looking for signs of tension pneumothorax or haemothorax
- If there is any obvious bleeding, I would try to control it with careful compression

Q. 20.2 Why is the neck so prone to serious injury?

- It is a conduit for many vital aerodigestive and vascular structures
- It does not have much overlying bony, muscle, or soft tissue protection thus making it vulnerable
- Penetrating trauma is the main mechanism of injury

Q. 20.3 What is the significance of penetrating platysma and sternocleidomastoid (SCM) with a neck injury?

- Injuries that do not penetrate platysma are *superficial*
- Sternocleidomastoid is the landmark that divides the anterior and posterior triangle and so the location of the injury in relation to SCM identifies what structures are most likely to be affected

Q. 20.4 What clinical features may be evident with penetrating injuries to the neck?

- *Vessels*:
  - Bleeding
  - Haematoma
- *Respiratory compromise*:
  - Respiratory distress
  - Stridor
  - Tension pneumothorax

- *Damage to structures*:
  - Odynophagia/dysphagia (oesophageal injury)
  - Surgical emphysema (tracheal/oesophageal injury/pneumothorax)
  - Bubbling/gurgling (tracheal injury)
  - Hoarseness (recurrent laryngeal nerve)
  - Cranial nerve deficits
  - Horner's syndrome (sympathetic chain)
  - Machinery bruit (AV fistula between IJV and carotid)

Q. 20.5 Can you tell me about the zones of the neck in relation to neck trauma?

There are three zones:

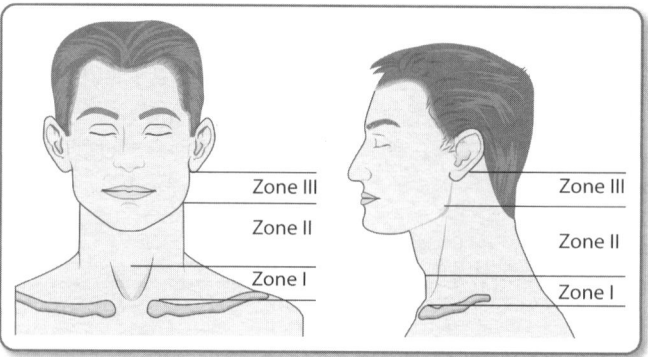

Source: Swaminathan A. (2018). Penetrating neck injuries. [online] Available from https://coreem.net/core/penetrating-neck-injuries/. [Last accessed March, 2022].

Zone	Anatomy	Major structures	Vessels	Nerves	Lymphatic structures
I	Clavicle to cricoid	Oesophagus Trachea Upper lung	Proximal carotid Subclavian artery Vertebral artery	Brachial plexus Spinal cord	Thoracic duct
II	Cricoid to angle of the mandible	Oesophagus Larynx Trachea	Carotid artery Vertebral artery Jugular vein	Spinal cord Vagus nerve Recurrent laryngeal	
III	Angle of mandible to base of the skull	Pharynx Parotid	Branches of external carotid Internal carotid Vertebral artery Internal jugular vein Facial vein	Cranial nerves	

- Zones I and III are relatively inaccessible to examination and rely upon radiological imaging

- Zone II is much more accessible and less reliant on imaging
- Penetrating injuries may extend for more than one zone

Q. 20.6 What are the triangles of the neck and what are their borders?

- *Posterior triangle*:
  - *Anterior*: Posterior border of the SCM
  - *Posterior*: Anterior border of trapezius
  - *Inferior*: Middle third of clavicle
- *Anterior triangle*:
  - *Anterior*: Midline
  - *Posterior*: Anterior border of SCM
  - *Superior*: Inferior border of mandible

Q. 20.7 Describe the contents of the anterior triangle of the neck.

Muscles	Suprahyoid and infrahyoid (strap) muscles
Vessels	Common carotid and bifurcation
Nerves	Facial nerve
	Glossopharyngeal
	Vagus nerve (in carotid sheath)
	Recurrent and external laryngeal nerves (from vagus)
	Hypoglossal nerve
	Ansa cervicalis
Other	Oesophagus
	Trachea
	Thyroid gland
	Parathyroid glands
	Submandibular gland

Q. 20.8 Describe the contents of the posterior triangle of the neck.

Muscles	Omohyoid – inferior belly crosses the posterior triangle splitting the triangle further into two
	Splenius capitis
	Levator scapulae
	Scalene muscles
Vessels	Subclavian artery
	External jugular vein
	Transverse cervical artery and vein
	Suprascapular artery and vein
Nerves	Accessory nerve (lies superficial and is vulnerable)
	Cervical plexus (within the muscles of the floor of the post-triangle)
	Phrenic nerve
	Brachial plexus trunks

Q. 20.9 What are the 'hard' and 'soft' signs of suggestive of major vascular or aerodigestive injury?

- *Hard*:
    - Airway compromise
    - Massive subcutaneous emphysema/air bubbling through wound
    - Expanding or pulsatile haematoma
    - Active bleeding
    - Shock
    - Neurological deficit
    - Haematemesis
    - Bruit or thrill
- *Soft*:
    - Dysphagia
    - Odynophagia
    - Dyspnoea
    - Pulse deficit
    - Venous oozing
    - Nonexpanding, non-pulsatile haematoma
    - Paraesthesia
    - Ipsilateral Horner's sign

Q. 20.10 How would you manage this patient?

- I would use a two-step approach as is advised by the Western Trauma Association Guidelines for penetrating neck injuries
    - *Step 1*: Are there any signs of a hard injury or haemodynamic instability?
    - *Step 2*: What is the zone of the injury?
- In the face of haemodynamic instability or hard signs:
    - Urgent surgery is indicated
    - This can only be delayed by securing an unstable airway or in an attempt to tamponade active bleeding
    - Operative exposure in these patients is determined by the anatomic zone of injury
- If the patient is HD stable and there are no hard signs:
- *Zone 1*:
    - CT angiography (CTA) of the chest and neck to evaluate both vascular and aerodigestive injuries
    - If CTA shows vascular injury, consider endovascular treatment using covered stents
    - If this is unavailable or failed, then surgery with proximal and distal vascular control
    - If CTA shows aerodigestive injury, then surgery is indicated
    - If CTA negative but concerning trajectory of penetrating injury, then consider:
        - OGD
        - Bronchoscopy

- *Zone II*:
  - *Presence of soft signs*:
    - Consider operative intervention with anterior SCM or cervical collar incision depending on the nature of the injury
    - If during surgery unable to completely assess oesophagus/trachea then consider on table OGD or bronchoscopy
  - *If there are no soft signs*:
    - CTA of the neck to evaluate both vascular and aerodigestive injuries
    - If CTA positive then surgery is indicated (due to easy access, definitive treatment, and no good evidence for stents for these injuries)
    - If CTA negative, then consider OGD/bronchoscopy
- *Zone III*:
  - CTA of the head and neck.
  - If CTA positive for arterial injury:
    - Consider embolisation if the vessel can be sacrificed
    - Consider covered stenting if vessel patency is required

Q. 20.11 What patterns of injury may be seen following blunt neck trauma?

- Can be subtle.
- *Mostly affects*:
  - *Carotids*:
    - Partial or complete occlusion
    - Pseudoaneurysm
    - Transection of carotid or vertebral
  - *Trachea*:
    - Subcutaneous emphysema
  - *Larynx*:
    - Fractures which may present with airway compromise as per penetrating injuries

Further reading

Coulter M, Mickelson RC, Dye JL, Myers EE, Ambrosio AA. Laryngotracheal and pharyngoesophageal traumatic injuries from US military operations in Iraq and Afghanistan, 2003-2017. BMJ Mil Health. 2021. Online ahead of print.

Sperry JL. Moore EE, Coimbra R, et al. (2013). Western trauma guidelines. [online] Available from https://www.westerntrauma.org/wp-content/uploads/2020/07/WTACriticalDecisionsPenetratingNeckTrauma.pdf. [Last accessed March, 2022].

Scenario 21

Renal trauma

A 62-year-old male patient is being reviewed in resus during a trauma call after suffering an assault. He has severe bruising over his right loin and frank haematuria.

Q. 21.1 How would you manage this patient?

- I would follow ATLS guidelines
- I would be worried about renal trauma
- Immobilise C-spine
- Primary survey and insertion of two large-bore cannulas
- Urgent CT scan given mechanism of injury

Q. 21.2 You perform a CT scan which confirms grade III right renal trauma. How do you classify renal trauma?

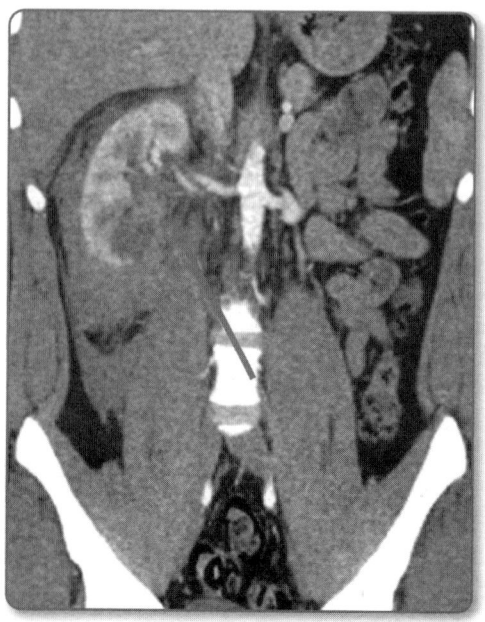

Source: Kelly ME. Renal Trauma: The Rugby Factor, 2015. [online] Available from https://www.researchgate.net/figure/Coronal-images-on-the-3-grades-on-renal-injury-in-this-series-according-to-AAST-OIS_fig1_283032127. [Last accessed March, 2022].

Grade	Type	Description
I	Contusion	Microscopic or frank haematuria with normal imaging
	Haematoma	Subcapsular, non-expanding without parenchymal laceration
II	Haematoma	Non-expanding per-renal haematoma confined to retroperitoneum
	Laceration	<1 cm in parenchymal depth or renal cortex with no evidence of urinary extravasation
III	Laceration	>1 cm in parenchymal depth or renal cortex with AND/OR evidence of urinary extravasation
IV	Laceration	Parenchymal laceration extending through renal cortex, medulla, and collecting system
	Vascular	Injury to main renal vessel(s)
V	Laceration	Shattered kidney
	Vascular	Avulsion of renal hilum with devascularised kidney

Q. 21.3 How would you manage renal trauma?

- The majority of cases do not need surgical intervention
    - IR and embolisation for control of bleeding
    - Ureteric stenting
- Surgical intervention is reserved for haemodynamically unstable patients and grade V injuries

Q. 21.4 What are the complications of renal trauma?

- Delayed bleeding
- Hypertension
- Urinoma
- Abscess formation

Further reading

European Association on Urology. European Association on Urology Trauma guidelines. [online] Available from https://d56bochluxqnz.cloudfront.net/documents/full-guideline/EAU-Guidelines-on-Urological-Trauma-2023_2023-03-20-083114_kgdg.pdf. [Last accessed March, 2022].

Scenario 22

Ruptured abdominal aortic aneurysm

You are assessing a 75-year-old male patient with severe left-sided loin to groin pain, and suspected renal calculi. He looks unwell and clammy, with a tachycardia of 130 bpm, and a systolic blood pressure of 85 mmHg.

Q. 22.1 How would you manage this patient?

- In a patient of this age and presentation, my first worry would be that this is a ruptured abdominal aortic aneurysm (AAA) until proven otherwise
- I would assess and treat the patient in an ABC manner
- Ensure two large-bore cannulas have been inserted
- Resuscitate the patient with permissive hypotension
- Initiate major haemorrhage protocol
- Organise an urgent CT aorta

Q. 22.2 How would you define permissive hypotension?

- Keep the systolic blood pressure at a level to maintain cerebral perfusion
  - Therefore, to keep the patient with a GCS of 15
- If you raise the blood pressure to high in this situation, you may dislodge any clot and release the tamponade effect which can result in mortality

Q. 22.3 What is the definition of a AAA?

- A dilatation of an artery involving all three layers to at least 1.5 times its normal diameter
- For the abdominal aorta:
  - Normal calibre 2 cm
  - Aneurysmal at 3 cm

Q. 22.4 You perform a CT aorta that shows a leaking AAA, what is your management?

- Urgent discussion with the on call vascular consultant/local vascular centre
- Continue resuscitation with permissive hypotension
- This is a time sensitive diagnosis and theatre should not be delayed under any circumstances

Q. 22.5 What is different about the anaesthesia for a ruptured AAA?

- Due to the hypotension that can occur on induction of anaesthesia, the patient is prepped and draped while awake
- Then induction of anaesthesia is performed, to lower the time between induction to clamp/balloon inflation (if an emergency EVAR is performed)

Q. 22.6 The vascular consultant attends and decides the aneurysm is not suitable for EVAR and performs an open AAA repair. After this has been performed, what else needs to be done in theatre?

- Thorough examination including Dopplers of both feet to check for evidence of any emboli that may have been thrown off from mural thrombus in the AAA sac
- If any distal pedal pulses are absent, femoral embolectomies ± fasciotomies may need to be performed

Q. 22.7 What do you know about aneurysm screening?

All men in the UK are offered a one-off ultrasound to check for a AAA at 65

Q. 22.8 How is the risk of rupture related to the size of the aneurysm?

AAA size (cm)	Risk of rupture per year (%)
<3	0
3–3.9	<0.5
4–4.9	1–3
5–5.9	5–10
6–6.9	10–20
7–7.9	20–40

Further reading

Chaikof EL, Dalman RL, Eskandari MK, et al. The Society for Vascular Surgery practice guidelines on the care of patients with an abdominal aortic aneurysm. J Vasc Surg 2018; 67:2–77.e2.

Scenario 23

Strangulated femoral hernia

You are called to A&E to see a 71-year-old female patient who has presented with a new painful lump in her left groin vomiting.

Q. 23.1 How would you manage this patient?

- I would be worried about an incarcerated/strangulated inguinal or femoral hernia
- Assess patient in ABC manner
- Focussed history
- Focussed examination paying close attention to groin:
  - Where is the lump in relation to the pubic tubercle?
  - Are there any skin changes?
  - Is the lump warm to touch?
  - Is it reducible?

Q. 23.2 You notice there is a firm irreducible lump below and lateral to the pubic tubercle, what is your diagnosis and management?

- This is a strangulated femoral hernia
- This patient requires an urgent CT scan

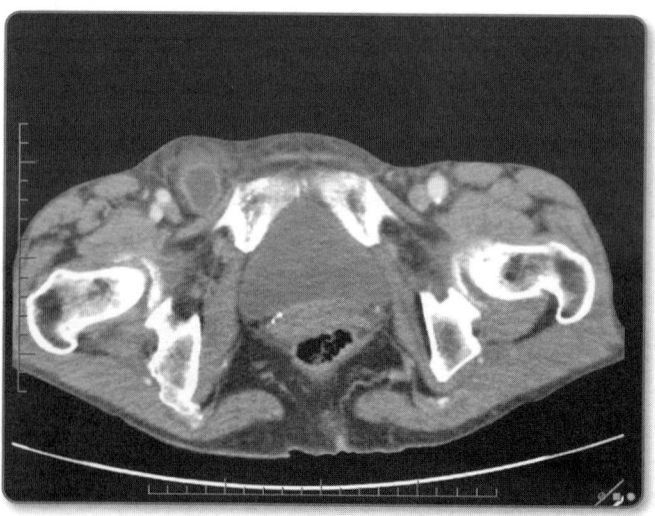

Source: O'Donnell C. Incarcerated femoral hernia with small bowel obstruction, 2012. [online] Available from https://radiopaedia.org/cases/incarcerated-femoral-hernia-with-small-bowel-obstruction. [Last accessed March, 2022].

Q. 23.3 Describe the surgical approach to this scenario.

- I would approach this using the modified McEvedy approach
- Transverse incision half-way between the umbilicus and pubic symphysis
- Preperitoneal approach, where you open the anterior rectus sheath and retract the rectus muscle
- Dissect toward the sac in the preperitoneal plane
- The sac is then opened, and contents inspected
- If the contents of the sac are difficult to reduce, the lacunar ligament may be divided
- If the bowel is necrotic or the contents are irreducible, then a 'laparotomy' can be performed at the level of the incision by incising the peritoneum and small bowel resection performed if necessary
- A suture repair of the hernia should be performed if there is any contamination, ensuring that you do not close the defect fully to allow for expansion of the femoral vein
- If there is no contamination, a plug mesh can be used

Scenario 24

Toxic megacolon

The gastroenterologists ask you to review a 21-year-old male patient who was admitted 5 days ago with a flare up of his known ulcerative colitis. He has been given infliximab and steroids but remains symptomatic. He is having bloody and loose bowel movements 5 times a day.

Q. 24.1 How would you assess this patient?

- I would take a focussed history specifically:
  - When this flare up began?
  - Is there any abdominal pain/distension?
  - Are the symptoms improving after treatment started?
  - Is his UC generally under good control?
  - When was his last colonoscopy?
- I would perform an abdominal examination looking for evidence of distension and peritonism
- I would review the patients notes:
  - Recent blood tests
  - Stool chart
  - Any recent imaging

Q. 24.2 Do you know of any criteria to classify a flare up of UC?

Truelove and Witts criteria:

	Mild	Moderate	Severe
Bloody stools per day	<4	4–6	>6
HR	<90	≤90	>90
Temperature	<37.5°C	37.5–37.8°C	>37.8°C
Hb	>11.5	≥10.5	<10.5
ESR	<20	≤30	>30
(ESR, erythrocyte sedimentation rate; Hb, haemoglobin; HR, heart rate)			

Q. 24.3 When you examine the patient, you note that he is tachycardic at 110 bpm with a systolic BO of 96 mmHg. He is distended and has epigastric tenderness. What would your management be?

- Asses in ABC manner with urgent fluid resuscitation
- I would be concerned that the patient has developed a toxic megacolon ± perforation
- I would organise an urgent CT AP

Q. 24.4 You organise a CT that shows toxic megacolon, how would you define this?

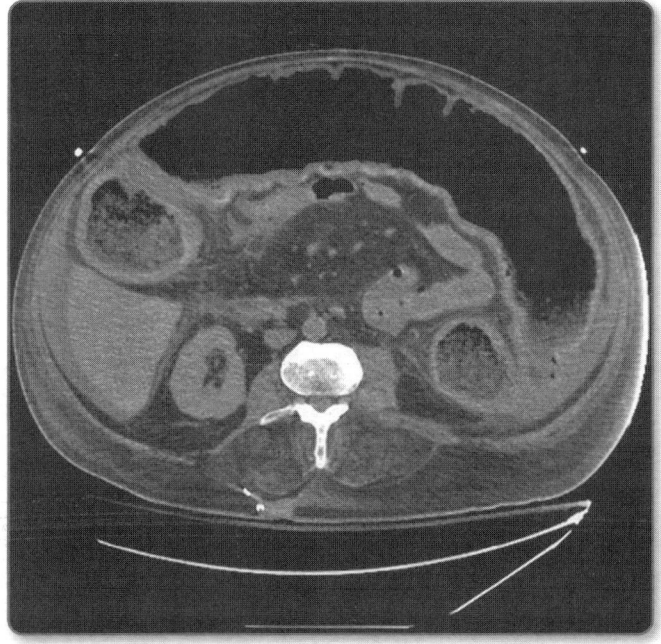

Source: Kusel K. Toxic megacolon, 2013. [online] Available from https://radiopaedia.org/articles/toxic-megacolon. [Last accessed March, 2022].

Toxic megacolon is defined as a non-obstructive dilatation of the colon, which can be segmental or total that is associated with systemic toxicity.

Q. 24.5 What is your management of this patient?

- This patient has toxic megacolon with systemic signs and so needs an urgent laparotomy
- This would be in the form of a subtotal colectomy and end ileostomy

Q. 24.6 What are the indications for emergency surgery in a patient with an acute flare up of UC?

- Intractable bleeding
- Toxic megacolon
- Perforation
- Severe symptoms (as per the Truelove and Witts criteria) refractory to treatment

Further reading

Fiorino G, Danese S, Giacobazzi G, Spinelli A. Medical therapy versus surgery in moderate-to-severe ulcerative colitis. Dig Liver Dis 2021; 53:403–408.

Scenario 25

Traumatic diaphragmatic rupture

A 35-year-old man presents as a trauma call after falling off a roof onto the edge of a brick wall. He is currently haemodynamically stable. He is complaining of epigastric pain and has bruising across his upper abdomen.

Q. 25.1 How would you manage this patient?
- I would follow ATLS guidelines
- Immobilise C-spine
- Primary survey and insertion of two large-bore cannulas
- Urgent CT scan given mechanism of injury

Q. 25.2 You perform a CT scan that shows a diaphragmatic rupture, how would you manage this?

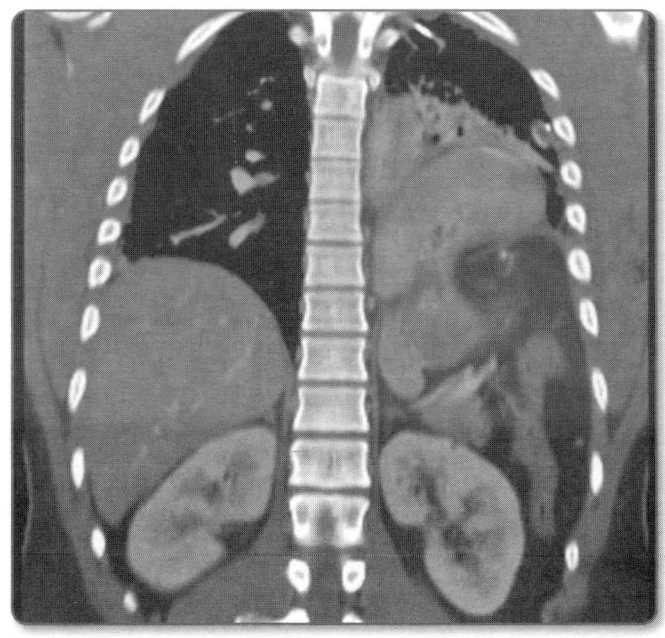

Source: El-Feky M. (2020). Diaphragmatic rupture. [online] Available from https://radiopaedia.org/articles/diaphragmatic-rupture. [Last accessed March, 2022].

- This requires urgent surgical fixation
- Early intubation of the patient with positive pressure ventilation should be considered to reduce collapse of the lung ± incarceration of the abdominal contents
- Repair is via a midline laparotomy and suture repair after reduction of the abdominal contents back into the abdominal cavity
  - Non-absorbable suture should be used
- If a pneumothorax persists then a chest drain should be inserted

Q. 25.3 Which side do diaphragmatic ruptures usually occur?

They usually occur on the left side due to protection from the liver on the right

Further reading

Haciibrahimoglu G, Solak O, Olcmen A, Bedirhan MA, Solmazer N, Gurses A. Management of traumatic diaphragmatic rupture. Surg Today 2004; 34:111–114.

Scenario 26

Trauma in pregnancy

You are attending a trauma call for a 25-year-old woman who has been involved in a road traffic collision. She is currently 32 weeks pregnant. She arrives on a spinal board with a C-spine collar and blocks in situ.

Q. 26.1 How would you manage this patient?
- I would manage this patient as per ATLS guidelines
- Ensure the obstetric team are present and involved in the care of the patient from the beginning
  - Need obstetric team to examine the patient following primary survey
  - CTG monitoring should be applied ASAP
- Urgent cross-match will need to be sent with rhesus status

Q. 26.2 Would you perform a CT on this patient?
- Yes, I would perform a CT on this patient, given the mechanism of injury
- The priority is to preserve the life of the mother
- In the third trimester, CT has a very small teratogenic effect:
  - Even if this was the 1st trimester, the patient would still require a CT scan with counselling and consent from the patient

Q. 26.3 Computed tomography (CT) shows a small bowel perforation, how would you proceed?
- This patient will need an urgent trauma laparotomy
- I would involve the obstetric and neonatal teams as if we are performing a trauma laparotomy in the 3rd trimester, ideally the obstetric team will need to deliver the baby intraoperatively during the laparotomy after control of sepsis
- The baby will be preterm and will likely require Neonatal Intensive Care Unit (NICU) support

Further reading
Jain V, Chari R, Maslovitz S, Farine D; Maternal et al. Guidelines for the management of a pregnant trauma patient. J Obstet Gynaecol Can 2015; 37:553–574.

Scenario 27

Pseudo-obstruction

You are asked to review a 77-year-old lady on an orthopaedic ward who is recovering after a dynamic hip screw for a fractured neck of femur. You are told that she has had absolute constipation for 2 days and is feeling nauseated. You are told that she has a 'virgin abdomen' but that her abdomen looks distended.

Q. 27.1 What are your differential diagnoses and how will you initially manage this patient?

Differentials:
- Constipation
- Colonic pseudo-obstruction, sometimes called Ogilvie syndrome
- Paralytic ileus
- Sigmoid volvulus
- Mechanical obstruction, either small or large bowel

Management:
- Full set of observations
- Full review of the notes and current drug chart
- Focussed history and examination (including PR)
- AXR (± CT abdominal dependant on local protocols)

Q. 27.2 Here is the AXR. How would you describe it?

This is a plain abdominal X-ray. This shows marked distension of the colon globally, from the caecum to the rectum. There is also some evidence of gas in the rectum and some scattered bowel contents throughout. The small bowel and stomach are unremarkable. This is therefore consistent with colonic pseudo-obstruction.

Q. 27.3 Tell me about pseudo-obstruction. How are you going to manage it in this patient?

- Pseudo-obstruction is a non-mechanical obstruction of the colon and rectum. There is no cutoff point identifiable radiologically to suggest a mechanical obstruction. It manifests as a gross, globally distended colon and rectum due to dysmotility (atony) causing symptoms of bowel obstruction. The most common causes can be categorised as either metabolic (e.g. hypokalaemia), drug induced

(e.g. opioids), neurological (e.g. multiple sclerosis), or post-trauma, surgery, or infection.
- Management of pseudo-obstruction is based on treating the underlying cause and symptom management for the patient. I would ensure that all electrolyte imbalances are corrected, and all opiate-based or unnecessary medications be stopped or altered where appropriate
- For symptom relief, if the patient is grossly distended and uncomfortable then passing a flatus tube can help to deflate the bowel and offer some relief (although distension is likely to recur). Similarly, endoscopic decompression can be considered (e.g. flexible sigmoidoscopy). If the patient is vomiting then an Ryles NGT may be passed; however, this will do little to treat the pseudo-obstruction itself (especially in the presence of a competent ileocaecal valve)

In rare, extreme cases, neostigmine may be considered; however, the patient should be on a cardiac monitor during treatment and this may not be feasible. Surgery is a last resort and should be reserved only for the most extreme, refractory cases or if caecal perforation is suspected (3–15%). If surgery is considered then the options include defunctioning stoma (ileostomy or caecostomy), segmental colonic resection or, if perforation is suspected or confirmed, subtotal colectomy ± primary anastomosis.

Q. 27.4 Can you tell me what the pathophysiology of colonic pseudo-obstruction is?

- The pathophysiology of colonic pseudo-obstruction is not clear. It may be due to an autonomic imbalance, with decreased parasympathetic tone or excessive sympathetic tone
- The parasympathetic supply to the gut is the vagus nerve to the splenic flexure, and the S2 to S5 sacral parasympathetic nerves (S2 to S5) supply the left colon, sigmoid, and rectum. Sympathetic stimulation reduces bowel motility and increases contraction of sphincters

Further reading

Miller AS, Boyce K, Box B, et al. The Association of Coloproctology of Great Britain and Ireland consensus guidelines in emergency colorectal surgery. Colorectal Dis. 2021;23:476–547.

Vogel JD, Feingold DL, Stewart DB, et al. Clinical practice guidelines for colon volvulus and acute colonic pseudo-obstruction. Dis Colon Rectum 2016; 59:589–600.

Valle RGL, Godoy FL. Neostigmine for acute colonic pseudo-obstruction: a meta-analysis. Ann Med Surg (Lond) 2014; 3:60–64.

Wells CI, O'Grady G, Bissett IP. Acute colonic pseudo-obstruction: a systematic review of aetiology and mechanisms. World J Gastroenterol 2017; 23:5634–5644.

Scenario 28

Ischaemic colitis

You are called to A&E resus to see a 56-year-old man who is acutely unwell with shortness of breath, generalised abdominal pain. He is clinically dehydrated. He is known to have chronic obstructive pulmonary disease (COPD), hypertension, and ethanol alcohol (ETOH) excess. There is no history of trauma.

Q. 28.1 How would you manage this patient?

I would initially resuscitate this patient as per sepsis-6 guidance (in the absence of a trauma history); however, if there were concerns regarding possible trauma, I would initiate ATLS principles:
- Full set of observations
- 15 L O_2 via non-rebreathe mask; IVI crystalloids; IV antibiotics (broad-spectrum)
- Catheterise; bloods for CRP, U and Es, LFTs, Lipase, Coagulation and Full Blood Count; Blood cultures
- Arterial blood gas (ABG)
- Ensure patient is haemodynamically stabilised with adequate fluid resuscitation.

When the patient is haemodynamically stable, I would then proceed for taking a focussed history and a full clinical examination.

His HR is 125, BP is 110/66, O_2 saturation is 97% on O_2 and his temperature is 38.2°C. His ABG shows a pH of 7.16, base excess – 12 and lactate of 5.4. His WCC is 13.7, CRP is 147 and creatinine is 424 (eGFR 16). His abdomen is generally tender, worse in the LIF but no guarding or rebound tenderness.

Q. 28.2 What is your next step?

- I would arrange for this gentleman to be urgently reviewed by the critical care team
- This patient will require an urgent contrast CT scan of his abdomen and pelvis. However, given his current acute kidney injury (AKI), there are significant risks involved with IV contrast. Discussion with critical care and radiology would be important. If the patient is suitable for renal replacement therapy (RRT) and critical care supportive, then directly to urgent CT. An alternative would be admission to a high-dependency unit (HDU) for further resuscitation with a view to performing the CT when his renal function improves
  I would also want an urgent urinary dipstick test and urine culture

Q. 28.3 What are your differential diagnoses?

- *Intra-abdominal sepsis*:
  - Perforated viscus
  - Bowel ischaemia
  - Diverticulitis/appendicitis
  - Infective enteritis/colitis
- Urosepsis
- Leaking AAA

Due to the uncertainty surrounding his diagnosis, he is admitted to HDU for resuscitation and monitoring.

Scenario 1

Q. 28.4 He improves with intravenous fluid resuscitation and his eGFR is now 40. What is your management?

I would arrange a contrast CT scan of his abdomen and pelvis.

Q. 28.5 The CT scan shows a poorly enhancing descending and sigmoid colon but there are patent mesenteric vessels. There is no evidence of diverticulosis or viscus perforation. How would you proceed?

This patient has symptoms and a CT scan consistent with ischaemic colitis. In light of the fact that he is improving clinically, I would continue with conservative/medical management by means of intravenous fluids, intravenous antibiotics, and bowel rest. I would consider early parental nutrition in this patient too. The caveat to this would be that if he clinically deteriorated then urgent laparotomy and bowel resection will be required.

Q. 28.6 If this gentleman eventually settles, are there any further investigations that you may want to arrange?

I would arrange a flexible sigmoidoscopy to assess the bowel in greater detail once his acute colitis has settled, no sooner that 6–8 weeks post-discharge.

I would also arrange vasculitis and thrombophilia screens, ECG and echocardiogram to investigate the potential underlying causes for his ischaemia.

Alternative scenario 2

He is moved to HDU for aggressive resuscitation. You get called to see him again a number of hours later as he develops PR bleeding and increased abdominal pain.

Q. 28.7 What are your concerns and what is your management in this scenario?

- I am concerned that this gentleman has acute colitis and that this is ischaemic in nature. I would like to get a full set of up-to-date observations and blood results. I would also re-review the patient in person, in particular to re-examine his abdomen
- I would then make a decision on whether or not to urgently CT this man with contrast (and then RRT if necessary thereafter) or proceed directly to an emergency laparotomy

Q. 28.8 When you re-review him, his temperature is 38.6°C, HR is 130, lactate 9, and eGFR is 20. Examining his abdomen shows signs of left-sided peritonism. The blood PR is a mixture of fresh red and altered blood but there is no active haematochezia and it is of relatively small volume. How will you proceed?

This gentleman clearly requires urgent surgical intervention by means of a laparotomy and bowel resection. The safest option is to proceed straight to surgery and perform a laparotomy, subtotal colectomy, and formation of end ileostomy.

There is still a case for performing a preoperative CT scan in terms of planning the extent of bowel resection. This should be considered if he is haemodynamically stable and the access to CT is quick. The CT would be able to ascertain the level of non-enhancement of the bowel wall which would guide me to performing either a segmental left haemicolectomy or sigmoid colectomy or proceeding directly to subtotal colectomy.

Q. 28.9 If, at operation, you found an infarcted descending and sigmoid colon, but the transverse colon and rectum look healthy with a palpable pulse in the mesentery, would you consider performing a primary colorectal anastomosis?

No, this would not be safe in this situation.

Further reading

Hung A, Calderbank T, Samaan MA, Plumb AA, Webster G. Ischaemic colitis: practical challenges and evidence-based recommendations for management. Frontline Gastroenterol 2019; 10:44–52.

Tilsed JV, Casamassima A, Kurihara H, et al. ESTES guidelines: acute mesenteric ischaemia. Eur J Trauma Emerg Surg 2016; 42:253–270.

Scenario 29

Intravenous drug user groin abscess

On the post-take ward round, you see a 40-year-old man who is an intravenous drug user (IVDU). He was admitted overnight after he self-presented to A&E with a left-sided groin swelling, left-sided sciatica, back pain, and some light headedness.

Q. 29.1 How would you manage this?

Initial management:
- Full history and clinical assessment:
  - Ensure patient is haemodynamically stable
  - Particularly looking for signs of sepsis (SIRS; qSOFA; and qSIRS scoring)
  - Always thinking about vascular involvement/bleed in light of symptoms of light-headedness
  - Examination – looking for signs of infection
  - Differentials – incarcerated hernia, pseudoaneurysm, and lymphadenopathy
- Primary investigations:
  - Bloods – in particular FBC, CRP; U and E; clotting; G and S (secondarily LFTs; viral screens)
  - Swab any sinus opening for culture and sensitivity
  - Coronavirus disease (COVID) swabs
  - Duplex USS of left groin/leg
  - Consider straight to CT/CT angiography if clinical suspicion of vascular involvement
- Initial treatment:
  - Keep NBM
  - Sepsis-6 protocol (IVI; IV antibiotics; O_2, etc.)
  - Do not take straight to theatre
  - Inform/discuss with local vascular team

After your initial resuscitation, he is treated as a subcutaneous abscess with intravenous antibiotics and an USS (non-duplex) is arranged. It reveals a large collection in the left groin, surrounding the left iliofemoral vessels and tracking up toward the retroperitoneal space. His WCC is 23.4, CRP is 320, and his Hb is 88.

Q. 29.2 What are your concerns and what are your next steps?

- Concerned that this patient has a vascular injury and subsequent bleed/ haematoma
- Also concerned about potential neurological involvement
- Keep NBM and maintain current treatment regimen
- Arrange urgent cross-sectional imaging (CT or MRI) of abdomen/pelvis ± angiography
- Discuss with local vascular team re: advice ± transfer if CT proves vascular involvement
- *Do not take straight to theatre for incision and drainage!*

You get a CT of his pelvis. See the picture below.

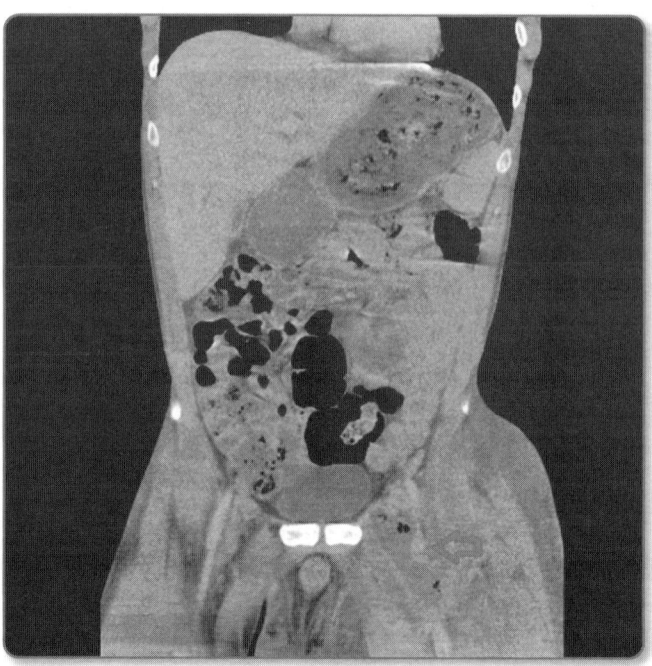

Q. 29.3 What do you think is going on here?

This is a coronal section of a contrast CT of the abdomen and pelvis. This shows a gas-containing collection in the left groin with distortion of the localised anatomy. It is difficult to tell on this image alone whether the Hounsfield units correlate with a haematoma or not, but given the presentation and this picture, my top differential would be an infected haematoma.

Q. 29.4 The radiologists confirm that this is a haematoma tracking retroperitoneally to involve the left psoas muscle. What are your definitive management options for this patient?

- Must involve local vascular team
- Also discuss with local interventional radiology team
- Options for management:
    - Conservative – watch and wait, bed rest, continue IV antibiotics as appropriate
    - Interventional – CT-guided drainage
    - Surgical – transfer to care of vascular team, but I would expect them to perform an open evacuation of the haematoma via a left-sided femoral cut down incision after isolating and controlling the femoral vessels with slings

Scenario 30

Appendicitis in pregnancy

During handover the night registrar tells you about a 34-year-old female patient who is 18 weeks pregnant. She was admitted under the obstetric team with a 4-day history of right sided abdominal pain and nausea. She is very anxious. Her white cell count is 14 and CRP is 30.

Q. 30.1 How will you manage her?

I would take a history regarding site, onset, and progression of abdominal pain. I would enquire about associated gynaecological symptoms including vaginal discharge and foetal movements. I will examine the patient. Because she has presented with RIF pain, my suspicion is that it could be appendicitis. I will organise an USS for the patient and continue with regular observation and keep her on clear fluids until the USS is complete. I will involve the obstetricians and gynaecologists to check foetal health as well.

Q. 30.2 After an USS the radiologist informed you that they were unable to see the appendix; however, noted some tenderness and free fluid in RIF. What will you do?

I would consider requesting an MRI as she is tender in RIF and with raised inflammatory markers. I will review the patient along with the gynaecologists. I will reassure the patient that based on the Royal College of Radiologists' report and many observational studies, there is no harm reported to the mother or foetus and it is safe to perform MRI in pregnancy. I would consider repeating blood tests to assess the trend.

Q. 30.3 The patient has agreed to go for an MRI and it shows uncomplicated appendicitis – what will you do?

I would discuss the management options with the patient, including conservative management with antibiotics and fluids or surgical intervention. Conservative management is an option in uncomplicated appendicitis in pregnancy but if it fails then there are increased risks of complication such as pre-term labour and termination of pregnancy. Laparoscopic appendectomy is deemed safe in pregnancy.

Alternative scenario: Patient is claustrophobic

Q. 30.4 The patient says that she does not want an MRI as she is claustrophobic. What will you do?

I will check with the radiologist whether they could do a 'leg first' MRI scan, so that her head can remain outside. If that is not possible, I will check with the patient whether she would like to try sedation. Other options include continued conservative management with antibiotics (explaining the risk of her appendicitis becoming complicated and threatening the foetus), perform a CT scan (the risk of CT scan induced teratogenicity and childhood cancer is minimal if it happens outside the 2–15 week window) or proceed with laparoscopic assessment.

All three options have their own risk and benefit. I will involve a colleague of mine and the obstetrics and gynaecology team.

Scenario 31

Perforated duodenum

You have been asked to review a 39-year-old builder in A&E who is peritonitic and tachycardic. He has had a CT scan which shows free air in the abdomen.

Q. 31.1 How will you manage this patient?

I will assess the patient in line with CCrISP protocol and ensure the patient has two large IV cannulas, IVF, analgesia, antibiotics, a nasogastric tube, and a urinary catheter. I will take a focussed history with regards to the duration of symptoms and any risk factors. I will include drug history, past medical history, social history, and family history. I will review the images with a radiologist to ascertain the most likely site of perforation. I will consent the patient and book him for an urgent laparotomy. After identifying the site of perforation if it is as expected in duodenum or stomach, I will perform Graham's patch repair after confirming the NGT position.

Graham's patch repair involves closing the perforation over plugged omentum using interrupted sutures.

I will place a 3-0 PDS suture going through both the edges of perforation.

I will patch the omentum over the sutures and tie over the omentum without excessive tension. I would assess the repair with an intra-operative leak test.

I will leave a drain adjacent to the closure in the sub-hepatic space. Postoperatively, I would continue antibiotics and start an intravenous PPI. The patient will require deep venous thrombosis (DVT) prophylaxis and appropriate analgesia. I would recommend sips of water only from day 1 and escalate the diet accordingly.

Q. 31.2 There was a 2 cm duodenal perforation that you repaired. The patient was recovering in the ward. During the ward round, you notice that the drain fluid is bilious in nature, and the patient is complaining of more discomfort, HR – 98, and RR – 30. What do you think is going on and how will you manage?

I suspect a postoperative leak from the repair site. As the patient is showing early signs of a systemic inflammatory response, I will keep the patient NBM and organise a CT with oral contrast.

Q. 31.3 The CT scan shows a large leak. The patient is now peritonitic. How will you proceed?

As the patient is peritonitic it is likely they will need a laparotomy, particularly if there is any evidence of decompensation or haemodynamic instability.

Q. 31.4 The patient is showing signs of sepsis and complains of worsening pain? UGI surgeons are not available. What will be your surgical plan?

Ideally this patient should be operated by UGI surgeons. However, in their absence, I will consent and book the patient for laparotomy. Consent will include laparotomy and T tube, venting gastrostomy, feeding jejunostomy, and placing large drains.

Intraoperatively, I will assess whether it is possible to safely redo the omental patch repair. If I could not establish a safe repair, then I would place a T tube in the perforation to create a controlled fistula. I will leave two large drains in the subhepatic and subphrenic spaces. I will also perform a venting gastrostomy and feeding jejunostomy.

I will continue to monitor the patient and involve the UGI team. Repeated oral contrast studies can be performed to assess any ongoing leak.

Further reading

Maghsoudi H, Ghaffari A. Generalized peritonitis requiring re-operation after leakage of omental patch repair of perforated peptic ulcer. Saudi J Gastroenterol 2011; 17:124–128.

Scenario 32

Blunt chest trauma

You are reviewing an 80-year-old lady with mild COPD who fell down her stairs yesterday. She has had a trauma series CT which revealed fractured ribs on the right (3–8) with a flail segment involving ribs 4–6. She complains of unbearable pain.

Her oxygen saturations are 93% on 2 L of oxygen, she has a respiratory rate of 25 breaths/min and a heart rate of 94 bpm.

Q. 32.1 How will you manage this patient?

I would assess and manage the patient in line with Advanced Trauma and Life Support (ATLS) principles. I will take a brief history focussing on presentation, COPD, medications, and her exercise tolerance. I will check baseline blood tests and an ABG. As she has a flail segment and considerable pain I will consider patient-controlled analgesia (PCA). I will ask the ITU outreach team to review the patient as she is at risk of respiratory failure. I will liaise with the anaesthetist to review pain management and consider thoracic epidural or paravertebral blocks.

Q. 32.2 The patient is commenced on a PCA. The ABG shows a PaO_2 of 8kPa on 4 L of oxygen and normal Pco_2. You have been informed by your juniors that she is struggling with pain and her oxygen saturation has dropped to 90% despite 15 L of O_2. The patient is becoming drowsy.

I am concerned that this patient is in type 1 respiratory failure. As she is drowsy, I will check for pupillary constriction to rule out opioid toxicity. I will also update the patient's relatives and discuss treatment escalation. I will refer her to the critical care outreach team for assessment and consideration of respiratory support.

Q. 32.3 The patient has been transferred to ITU and managed with continuous positive airway pressure (CPAP). ITU are struggling to ventilate her and manage her pain. They have organised a CT which has shown lung contusions and bilateral atelectasis. What will you do?

This patient may benefit from fixation of her ribs; therefore, I will have an MDT discussion involving the intensivists and cardiothoracic surgeons.

Q. 32.4 How do you define flail segment and flail chest?

- Flail segment is when three or more ribs are fractured in two or more places.
- Flail chest is when a segment of chest wall does not have bony continuity with rest of the thoracic cage leading to paradoxical movement of the segment

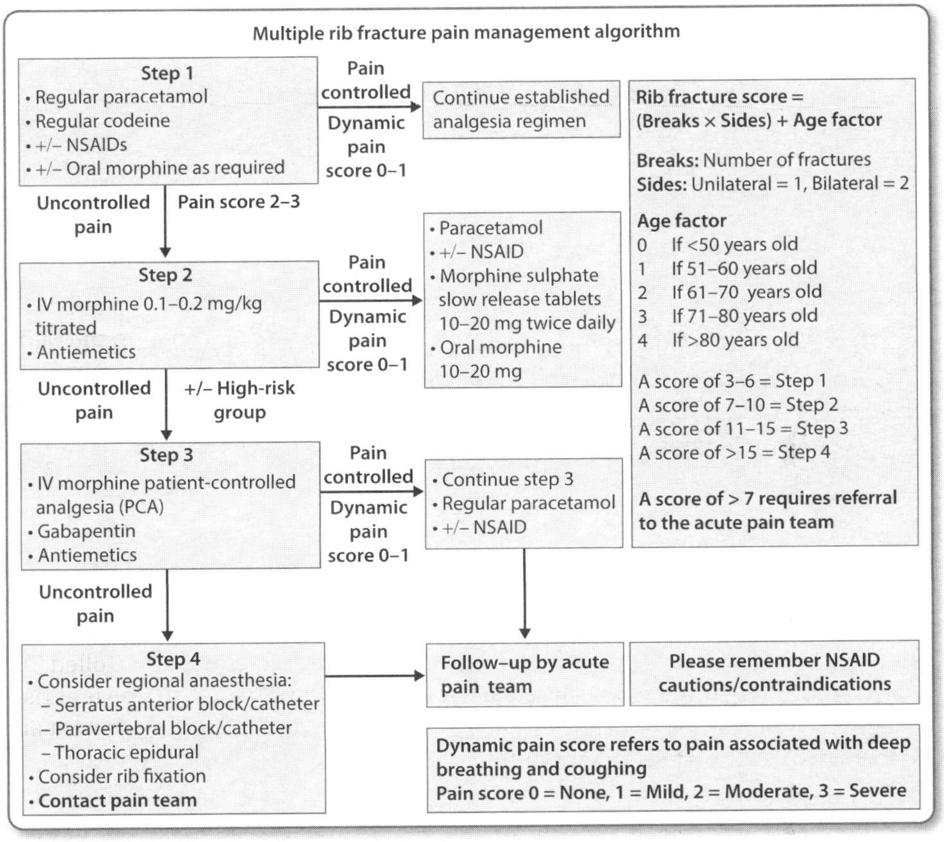

Scenario 32 Blunt chest trauma

Multiple rib fracture pain management algorithm

Step 1
- Regular paracetamol
- Regular codeine
- +/− NSAIDs
- +/− Oral morphine as required

Pain controlled, Dynamic pain score 0–1 → Continue established analgesia regimen

Uncontrolled pain | Pain score 2–3 ↓

Step 2
- IV morphine 0.1–0.2 mg/kg titrated
- Antiemetics

Pain controlled, Dynamic pain score 0–1 →
- Paracetamol
- +/− NSAID
- Morphine sulphate slow release tablets 10–20 mg twice daily
- Oral morphine 10–20 mg

Uncontrolled pain | +/− High-risk group ↓

Step 3
- IV morphine patient-controlled analgesia (PCA)
- Gabapentin
- Antiemetics

Pain controlled, Dynamic pain score 0–1 →
- Continue step 3
- Regular paracetamol
- +/− NSAID

Uncontrolled pain ↓

Step 4
- Consider regional anaesthesia:
  – Serratus anterior block/catheter
  – Paravertebral block/catheter
  – Thoracic epidural
- Consider rib fixation
- Contact pain team

→ Follow-up by acute pain team

Rib fracture score = (Breaks × Sides) + Age factor

Breaks: Number of fractures
Sides: Unilateral = 1, Bilateral = 2

Age factor
- 0 If <50 years old
- 1 If 51–60 years old
- 2 If 61–70 years old
- 3 If 71–80 years old
- 4 If >80 years old

A score of 3–6 = Step 1
A score of 7–10 = Step 2
A score of 11–15 = Step 3
A score of >15 = Step 4

A score of > 7 requires referral to the acute pain team

Please remember NSAID cautions/contraindications

Dynamic pain score refers to pain associated with deep breathing and coughing
Pain score 0 = None, 1 = Mild, 2 = Moderate, 3 = Severe

(NSAID, non-steroidal anti-inflammatory drug)
Source: May L, Hillermann C, Patil S. Rib fracture management. BJA Educ 2016; 16:26–32.

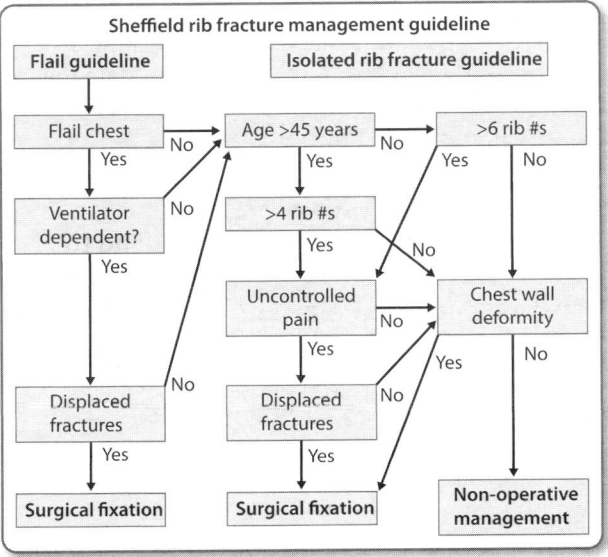

This is a non-validated tool that is being studied through Sheffield Multiple Rib Fractures Study (SMURFS) conducted by Mr J Edwards et al.

Scenario 33

Liver trauma

Your registrar informs you about a 42-year-old female patient brought in by ambulance after being trampled by a horse. She has undergone a primary survey and trauma series CT which revealed multiple right sided rib fractures and a grade 3 liver laceration with haematoma.

Other than tachypnoea her observations are normal.

Q. 33.1 How will you manage this patient?

I will review the images with the radiologist to know whether there is any active bleeding, the patient may require an urgent triple phase CT.

I would assess the patient as per the ATLS protocol. I will take a focussed history regarding comorbidities and any medications including anti-coagulants. I will inform the patient of the diagnosis. I will advise bed rest and start analgesia with a PCA. I will provisionally take her consent for laparotomy should she develop haemodynamic instability. I will also update her family and next of kin. I will make sure that the patient has received TXA and mechanical prophylaxis for DVT (such as intermittent pneumatic compression boots), avoiding chemical prophylaxis for now. I will check her bloods including Hb and cross-match, and replace any losses.

I will keep her NBM and catheterise and analyse her urine for β-hCG as well.

I will discuss with the hepatopancreatobiliary (HPB) surgeons and transfer images for their review and potential transfer of patient under their care. I would recommend close monitoring and she may require admission to ITU.

Q. 33.2 A triple phase CT has been performed; it does not show any evidence of active bleeding. The patient is on ITU. You get a call overnight that the patient is complaining of increasing pain and abdominal distension. The Hb has dropped to 70 from 100 g/dL, she is tachycardic and oliguric. Her blood pressure is now dropping despite all fluid challenges. How will you manage this?

I will ask my registrar to assess the patient urgently. I will call the anaesthetist and intensivist to prepare for a laparotomy. I would involve the HPB surgeons where possible. I will initiate the 'major haemorrhage' protocol.

I will assess the patient. As she is very haemodynamically unstable, Interventional Radiology embolisation may not be appropriate. I will book her for a laparotomy. During the brief I will request large packs, cell saver, wash, Omni-Tract, procoagulant adjuncts (Floseal, Tisseel, Surgicel, and KN unit), and warming blankets.

Q. 29.20 Take us through the steps of laparotomy.

I will make sure packs; cell saver and assistance are readily available. I will make a laparotomy incision through the midline.

I will pack all four quadrants of the abdomen with large packs starting from the right upper quadrant. Close communication with the anaesthetist is vital to ensure adequate simultaneous resuscitation.

Because the source of bleeding is likely to be the liver I will carefully remove the packs in a clockwise fashion starting from the left upper quadrant.

If there is bleeding from the liver I will inform the anaesthetist and perform 'sandwich packing' of the liver which can cause a drop in blood pressure. If it still bleeds, I will perform an intermittent pringle manoeuvre.

If there is minimal ooze then I would proceed to use the procoagulant adjuncts and pack the liver again to reassess.

Liver trauma: Pack and Pringle for non-specialist surgeons.

Management of liver trauma WSES, 2020 guidelines:

	WSES grade	AAST	Haemodynamic
Minor	1	1–2	Stable
Moderate	2	3	Stable
Severe	3	4–5	Stable
	4	1–5	Unstable

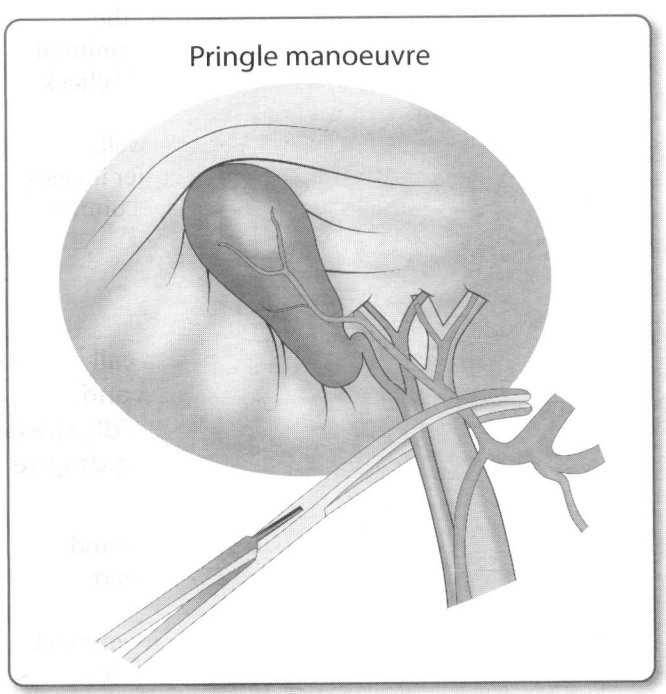

Pringle manoeuvre

Paula F, Ricardo F. Atlas of Trauma: Operative Techniques, Complications and Management, 8th edition. New Delhi: Springer Publication; 2019.

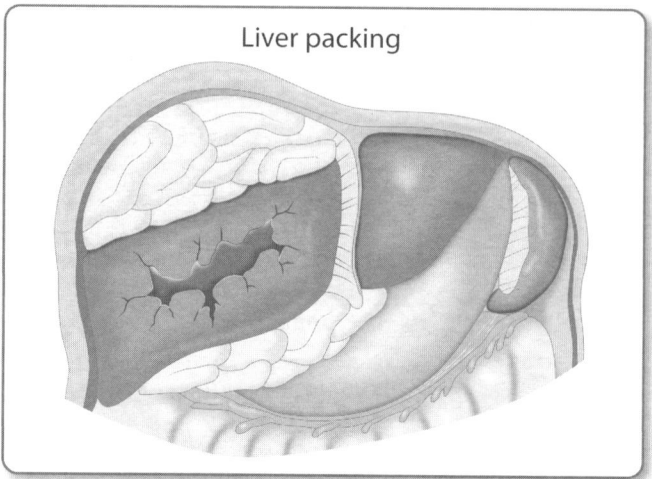

Paula F, Ricardo F. Atlas of Trauma: Operative Techniques, Complications and Management. New Delhi: Springer Publications; 2019.

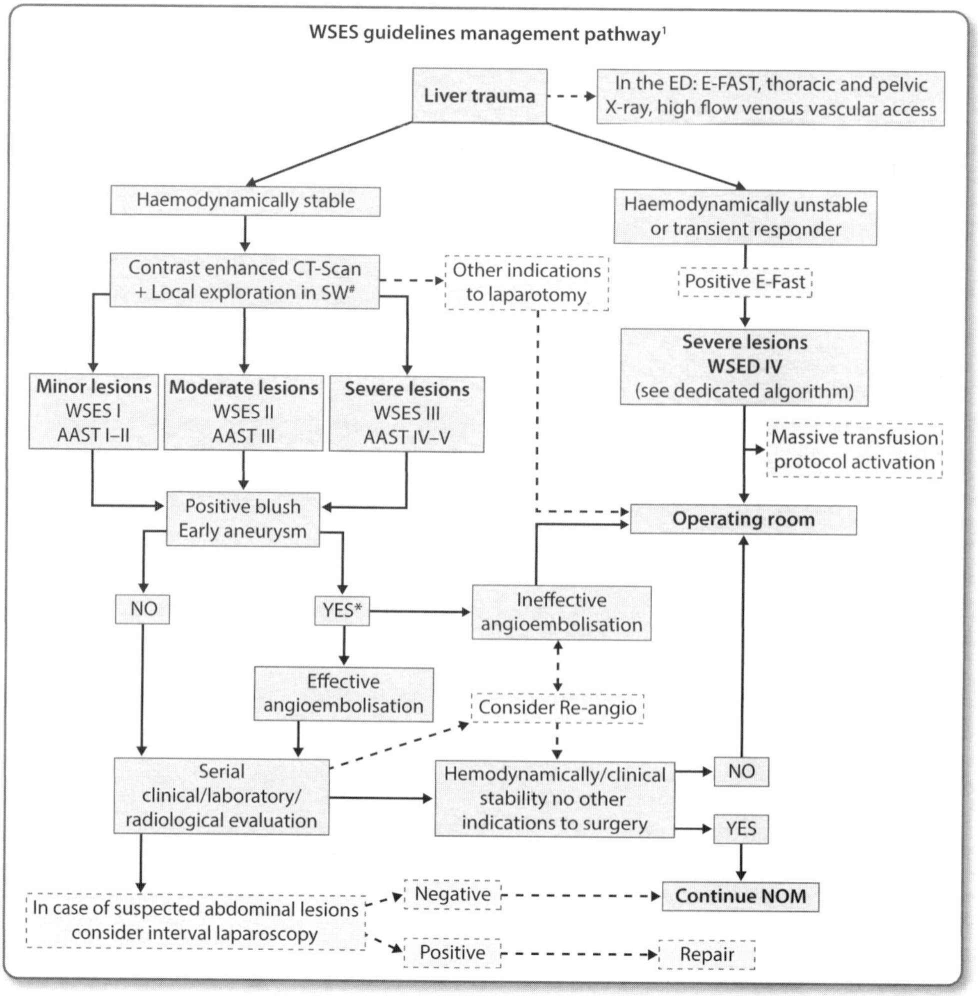

WSES guidelines management pathway[1]

```
Liver trauma ──▶ In the ED: E-FAST, thoracic and pelvic
                  X-ray, high flow venous vascular access
   │
   ├──────────────────────────┐
   ▼                          ▼
Haemodynamically stable    Haemodynamically unstable
                           or transient responder
   │                          │
   ▼                          ▼
Contrast enhanced CT-Scan ──▶ Other indications    Positive E-Fast
+ Local exploration in SW#    to laparotomy             │
   │                                                    ▼
   │                                            Severe lesions
   │                                            WSED IV
   │                                            (see dedicated algorithm)
   │                                                    │
   │                                                    ▼
   │                                            Massive transfusion
   │                                            protocol activation
   ▼
Minor lesions | Moderate lesions | Severe lesions
WSES I        | WSES II          | WSES III
AAST I–II     | AAST III         | AAST IV–V
   │              │                  │
   ▼              ▼                  ▼
        Positive blush
        Early aneurysm ◀───────┐
          │         │          │
         NO       YES*  ──▶ Ineffective
          │        │        angioembolisation
          │        ▼             │
          │   Effective           │
          │   angioembolisation   ▼
          │        │         Consider Re-angio
          ▼        ▼
        Serial
        clinical/laboratory/  ──▶ Hemodynamically/clinical ──▶ NO
        radiological evaluation    stability no other
          │                        indications to surgery  ──▶ YES ──▶ Operating room
          ▼
In case of suspected abdominal lesions  ─ ─ ▶ Negative ─ ─ ─ ▶ Continue NOM
consider interval laparoscopy           ─ ─ ▶ Positive ─ ─ ─ ▶ Repair
```

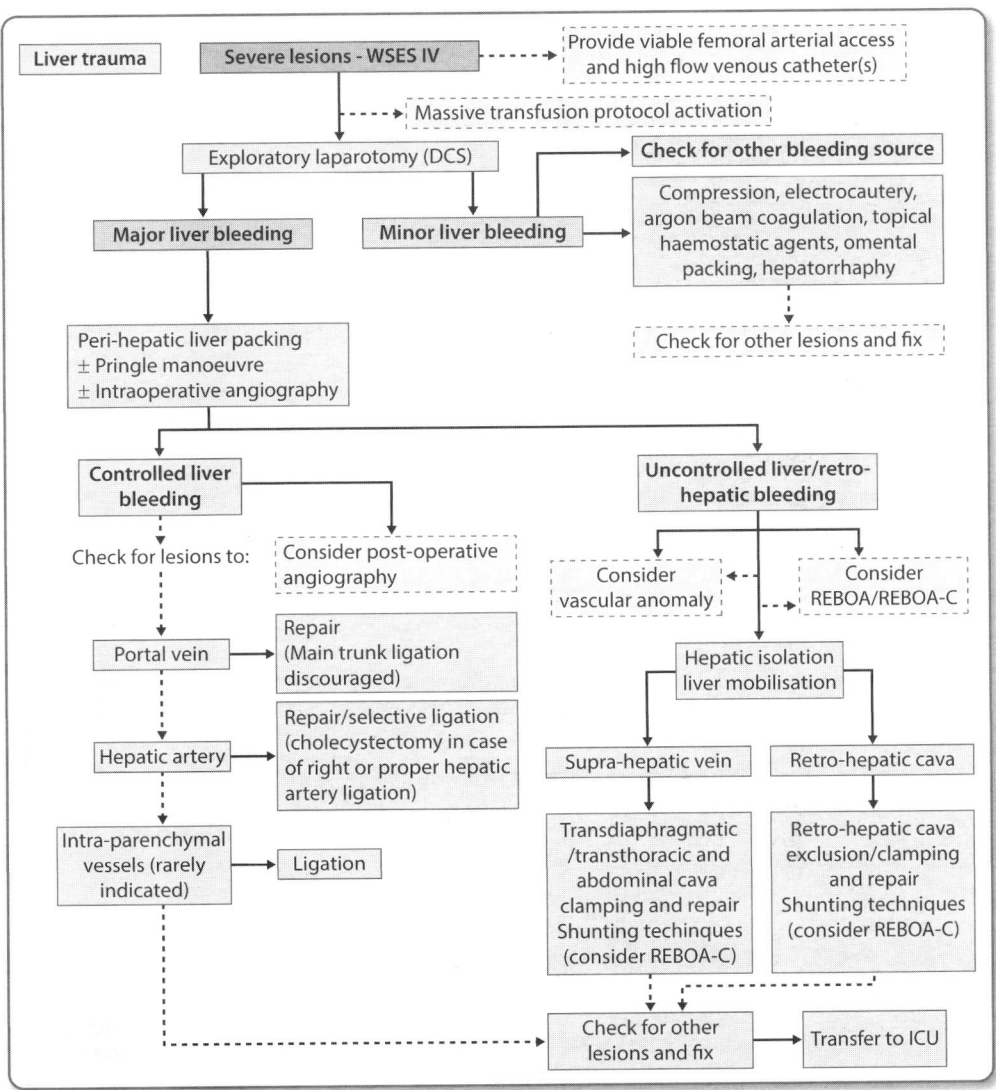

Further reading

Coccolini F, Coimbra R, Ordonez C, et al. Liver trauma: WSES 2020 guidelines. World J Emerg Surg 2020; 15:24.

Scenario 34

Biliary sepsis

You are asked to review a 68-year-old man who has a pacemaker for AF and takes warfarin. He has been in HDU on CPAP for pneumonia for the last 3 days. He is complaining of abdominal pain, and has been having rigors as well as raised inflammatory markers including a white cell count of 18 and CRP 180.

He also has deranged LFTs including a bilirubin of 52. He has acute kidney injury. A CT scan shows cholecystitis with a dilated common bile duct.

Q. 34.1 How will you assess this patient?

I will assess the patient in line with CCrISP principles. I will take a full history and examination. I would like to establish his exercise tolerance. I will review his bloods including clotting. I would like to know patient's international normalised ratio (INR) and his last dose of warfarin. I will catheterise the patient. I will let the patient know that he has got jaundice due to gallstones blocking the bile duct. I will advise him to stop warfarin and he may need an MRI scan to rule out common bile duct (CBD) stones. However, as he has a pacemaker, I will liaise with the radiologist and pacemaker team as we need to switch off the pacemaker during an MRCP.

Q. 34.2 The patient's INR is 3.5. MRCP shows two stones in bile duct. How will you proceed?

I will update the patient regarding the MRCP findings and counsel him for ERCP. I will organise an urgent ERCP in the next available list. Meanwhile, I will give 5 mg of vitamin K and recheck his INR in 6 hours, if it is still elevated I will repeat the dose of vitamin K. I will pre-emptively discuss with the haematologist to make sure prothrombin complex is available in an emergency situation.

Q. 34.3 The patient was observed in HDU. ERCP is not available until next week. You are the on-call consultant during the weekend and the patient deteriorates. How will you proceed?

The patient is cholangitic. He will need urgent biliary drainage. I will make sure that the clotting profile is normal. I will try to organise ERCP during the weekend. I will speak to my gastroenterology colleagues and if not available contact the regional centre for support.

Q. 34.4 No ERCP can be performed in your region during this weekend. His INR is 2.5. How will you manage?

The next option is cholecystostomy and further optimisation of his clotting. I will discuss with the interventional radiologists and plan for cholecystostomy as soon as possible; I will co-ordinate with the haematologists to administer prothrombin complex to the patient prior to the cholecystostomy.

Notes:
Tokyo guidelines 2018 for diagnostic criteria and severity of cholangitis:[1]

A: Systemic inflammation
    A-1: Fever and/or shaking chills
    A-2: Laboratory data: Evidence of inflammatory response
B: Cholestasis
    B-1: Jaundice
    B-2: Laboratory data: abnormal liver function tests
C: Imaging
    C-1: Biliary dilatation
    C-2: Evidence of the aetiology on imaging (stricture, stone, stent, etc.)

Suspected diagnosis: One item in A + One item in either B or C

Definite diagnosis: One item in A, one item in B, and one item in C

Note:
A-2: Abnormal white blood cell counts, increase of serum C-reactive protein levels, and other changes indicating inflammation
B-2: Increased serum ALP, r-GTP (GGT), AST, and ALT levels
    Other factors, which are helpful in diagnosis of acute cholangitis include abdominal pain (right upper quadrant or upper abdominal) and a history of biliary disease such as gallstones, previous biliary procedures, and placement of a biliary stent.
    In acute hepatitis, marked systematic inflammatory response is observed infrequently. Virological and serological tests are required when differential diagnosis is difficult.

Charcot's triad of fever, abdominal pain, and jaundice is noted to be highly specific but less sensitive, therefore absence of Charcot's triad does not exclude cholangitis.

Cholangitis – grades (Tokyo guidelines, 2018)

Grade III (severe) acute cholangitis:
'Grade III' acute cholangitis is defined as acute cholangitis that is associated with the onset of dysfunction at least in any one of the following organs/systems:
1. *Cardiovascular dysfunction*: Hypotension requiring dopamine ≥5 μg/kg per min, or any dose of norepinephrine
2. *Neurological dysfunction*: Disturbance of consciousness
3. *Respiratory dysfunction*: PaO_2/FiO_2 ratio <300
4. *Renal dysfunction:* Oliguria, serum creatinine >2.0 mg/dL
5. *Hepatic dysfunction*: Prothrombin time (PT)-INR >1.5
6. *Haematological dysfunction*: Platelet count < 100,000/mm^3

Grade II (moderate) acute cholangitis:
'Grade II' acute cholangitis is associated with any two of the following conditions:
- Abnormal WBC count (>12,000/mm^3, <4,000/mm^3)
- High fever (≥39°C)
- Age (≥75 years old)
- Hyperbilirubinaemia (total bilirubin ≥5 mg/dL)
- Hypoalbuminaemia (<0.7 lower limit of normal value)

Grade I (mild) acute cholangitis: 'Grade I' acute cholangitis does not meet the criteria of 'Grade III (severe)' or 'Grade II (moderate)' acute cholangitis at initial diagnosis.

Studies have identified 'percutaneous cholecystostomy' (PC) is a safe procedure to be performed in a cholecystitis/cholangitis patient. PC does not increase complication rate even if the patient needs cholecystectomy in future.

Further reading

Kiriyama S, Kozaka K, Takada T, et al. Tokyo Guidelines 2018: diagnostic criteria and severity grading of acute cholangitis. J Hepatobiliary Pancreat Sci 2018; 25:17–30.

Simorov A, Ranade A, Parcells J, et al. Emergent cholecystostomy is superior to open cholecystectomy in extremely ill patients with acalculous cholecystitis: a large multicenter outcome study. Am J Surg 2013; 206:935–941.

Treinen C, Lomelin D, Krause C, Goede M, Oleynikov D. Acute acalculous cholecystitis in the critically ill: risk factors and surgical strategies. Langenbecks Arch Surg 2015; 400:421–427.

Scenario 35

Haemothorax

You attend the trauma call for a 39-year-old male patient who fell from a 10 ft ladder onto his right side. He is complaining of pain during inspiration and he feels lightheaded.

He has oxygen saturations of 98% on 2 L of oxygen, a respiratory rate of 28 breaths/min, and a heart rate of 88 bpm.

A CT has shown a large right sided haemothorax.

Q. 35.1 How will you manage this patient?

I will review the patient urgently in line with ATLS principles. I will make sure he is on 15 L of oxygen, had 1g of TXA given and six units cross-matched. I will discuss with the patient regarding any medical history and allergies. I will check the patient's clotting and haemoglobin. I will consent the patient for a chest drain.

I will get the chest drain kit ready with under water seal prepared.

Under sterile precautions, I will provide liberal amount of local anaesthesia in the inter-costal space before making an adequate transverse incision over the skin and using blunt dissection slowly advance by opening and closing surgical clip such as Roberts or Spencer wells. Once reaching the pleura, I will enter the space bluntly and use finger dissection. I will clamp the proximal end of the chest drain and advance into the pleural space. Corresponding to the CT, I will expect to see some blood/fluid coming out. I will connect the tube to under water seal, release the clamp, and secure the chest drain in place. I will monitor the amount of blood coming out of the chest drain. I will check the observations to make sure they are stable.

Q. 35.2 The patient remains stable and you have moved them to a trauma ward. 6 hours later, you receive a call informing you that the patient's chest drain output over the last 6 hours has exceeded 600mL. The patient feels dizzy when he tries to sit up. HR: 90, SaO_2 92 on 4 L of oxygen, and RR 28.

I will ask the staff to initiate the major haemorrhage protocol and commence transfusion of blood products accordingly. I would commence 15 L of oxygen. I will inform the theatre anaesthetist that we have a patient in the ward who might need a thoracotomy. I will assess the patient and explain that he will need a thoracotomy to control the bleeding, I will refer him to a specialist centre urgently, but if the bleeding continues, he will need a thoracotomy locally.

Q. 35.3 While you are talking to the cardiothoracic surgeons, you have been informed by the nurse that patient's BP is now is in 60/40 mm Hg and HR is 160 bpm. What will you do?

I will book the patient for an urgent thoracotomy and inform the theatre staff and anaesthetist.

Q. 35.4 How will you perform a thoracotomy?

I will make sure that there is blood available, put the patient's arm out and prep and drape chest and abdomen. I will perform an anterolateral thoracotomy, making an incision just above the nipple. After dividing the intercostal muscles, I will apply the rib separator. Once in the thoracic cavity, I will pack the cavity and inform the anaesthetist regarding. Slowly taking the pack out, I will try to identify the bleeding point.

Q. 35.5 You have noticed some bleeding from the Intercostal blood vessel. How will you control it?

I will take figure of 8 stitches including the point of bleeding, if difficult, I will include one rib adjacent in the stitch.

Discussion

Indications of thoracotomy (ATLS manual, 9th edition):
- 1,500 mL of fluid is immediately evacuated.
- Volume of output and patient's physiologic:
  - <1,500 mL of fluid in initial evacuation but ongoing bleed
  - 200 mL/h for 2–4 hours

Scenario 36

Tension pneumothorax

You review an 18-year-old male patient who was struck by a car during a road traffic collision. He is stable with a GCS of 15. The car was travelling slowly so the trauma team performed plain film radiographs only.

While talking, the patient complains of chest tightness and difficulty breathing. He is unable to complete sentences.

Q. 36.1 What do you think is happening and how will you manage?

I suspect the patient has a tension pneumothorax, I would alert the trauma team and advise them to get a wide-bore needle and chest drain kit ready. I will insert a wide-bore needle in the triangle of safety. I will reassess the airway and breathing and set up for a chest drain to be inserted in the same location in the fifth inter-costal space just anterior to the midaxillary line under sterile precautions and connect it securely to an underwater seal drain. I will organise a trauma series CT to exclude any other injuries that may have been missed.

Q 36.2 The patient feels better and is moved to the ward. He remains stable. How will you manage further?

I will continue to observe on the ward. I will consider removing the chest drain after 48 hours provided the observations are stable, I would subsequently organise a chest X-ray.

Q. 36.3 After the patient is moved to the ward, you get a call saying the chest drain has stopped swinging, what will you do?

I will confirm the position of the chest drain. Once I have confirmed the position, I will attempt suction with 10–20 cm H_2O to release any blockage in the chest drain.

Q. 36.4 Now the chest drain is working. After 2 days, you remove the chest drain and the radiograph shows a pneumothorax. What will you do next.

I will re-site the chest drain.

Q. 36.5 The chest drain is re-sited, however the pneumothorax persists, what would you do?

I will make sure that the chest drain is completely inserted with no perforations outside the thoracic cavity and ensure the occlusive dressing is appropriate.

Q. 36.6 You have checked the drain and its dressing but still the patient has a persistent pneumothorax. How will you manage?

The possibilities include an isolated bulla appearing as pneumothorax or bronchoalveolar pleural fistula. I will organise CT chest and discuss with cardiothoracic surgeons as the patient may need further assessment.

Q. 36.7 What do you think cardiothoracic surgeons will do in the presence of a fistula?

Likely they will perform a VATS and inject sealant to occlude the fistula, and insert a new chest drain.

Scenario 37

Cholecystitis – necrotic gallbladder

You review a 46-year-old type 2 diabetic man with a BMI of 35 on the ward. He has developed sudden onset upper abdominal pain. He has a temperature of 37.6 and a heart rate of 90 bpm with otherwise normal observations.

Blood results are as follows: White cell count 16, CRP 58. LFTs are normal.

An ultrasound scan showed a thick-walled gallbladder with no evidence of free fluid.

Q. 37.1 How will you assess this patient?

I will take a history and examine the patient. I would like to know whether the patient is peritonitic. I will make sure that the patient has an ECG and erect CXR to rule out cardiac pathology or perforated viscera. I will take blood cultures and start the patient on antibiotics, and monitor his input and output. I would advise a normal diet as tolerated for the time being, with regular observation including blood sugar monitoring.

Q 37.2 You have managed the patient with antibiotics. 48 hours later his temperature is 38°C, HR: 102, urine output is 30 mL/h and blood sugar 20. What are your thoughts? How will you manage further?

The patient is showing signs of sepsis. I suspect he has developed a necrotic gallbladder with or without perforation/empyema. I will assess and resuscitate the patient as per CCrISP protocol, recheck his bloods, and perform an ABG. I will keep him NBM and start him on an insulin infusion and adequate analgesia. I will discuss with microbiology to escalate antibiotics, and organise an urgent CT AP.

Q. 37.3 You have organised a CT which shows a necrotic gallbladder, how would you manage this?

The patient will require a cholecystectomy, which is likely to be challenging. They would benefit from specialist UGI involvement. I will consent the patient for laparoscopic and open cholecystectomy and complications including bile leak, bile duct injury and sub-total cholecystectomy. I might also abandon the procedure if it is more complicated than I am able to manage (i.e. when risk of injury to the biliary tree and other organs outweighs the potential benefit from surgery) without access to a specialist UGI service. In such cases, abdominal drains would be left in situ, and the patient maintained on intravenous antibiotics according to specialist microbiology advice.

Q. 37.4 The UGI team are not immediately available. Take me through the steps of how you would proceed with the operation to achieve the 'critical view of safety'.

I will position the patient in supine. I will use standard four-port technique. I will dissect the hepatocystic triangle and attempt to obtain the critical view of safety. The three criteria required to achieve the critical view of safety are:
1. The hepatocystic triangle is cleared of fat and fibrous tissue. The hepatocystic triangle is defined as the triangle formed by the cystic duct, the common hepatic duct, and inferior edge of the liver. The common bile duct and common hepatic duct do not have to be exposed.
2. The lower one-third of the gallbladder is separated from the liver to expose the cystic plate. The cystic plate is also known as liver bed of the gallbladder and lies in the gallbladder fossa.
3. Two and only two structures should be seen entering the gallbladder.

Q 37.5 During the procedure you notice multiple necrotic patches in the gallbladder and Hartmann's pouch is thickened and necrotic. Calot's triangle seems inaccessible. How will you manage this?

This is a challenging scenario and likely to require the expertise of an UGI surgeon.

Q. 37.6 The UGI team is involved in a separate emergency and cannot attend. You have been advised to proceed in the manner you see most fit. What would you do?

I will open the gallbladder near the fundus, retrieve as many stones as possible, and perform a copious washout. I would leave drains in the subhepatic and subphrenic spaces.

However, given the findings, I do not think I would be able to achieve completion cholecystectomy even if I convert to open surgery. Therefore, the safest option for the patient is to leave the drains in situ. I would liaise with the UGI surgeons and gastroenterology team to organise an urgent ERCP.

Discussion

While performing emergency cholecystectomy, it is advisable to discuss all bailout options taking into account one's skillset, including abandoning the procedure.

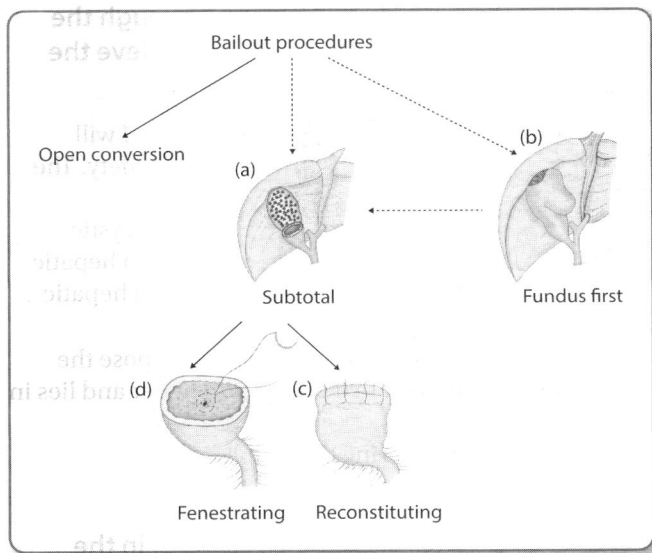

Bailout as advocated by Tokyo guidelines 2018. Detailed bailout procedures for difficult laparoscopic cholecystectomy: (a) subtotal cholecystectomy; (b) fenestrating (the GB is opened and the cystic duct is closed from inside); (c) reconstituting (closure of the remnant GB wall); (d) fundus first

Further reading

Wakabayashi G, Iwashita Y, Hibi T, et al. Tokyo Guidelines 2018: surgical management of acute cholecystitis: safe steps in laparoscopic cholecystectomy for acute cholecystitis (with videos). J Hepatobiliary Pancreat Sci 2018; 25:73–86.

Scenario 38

Right iliac fossa mass

A 54-year-old lady presented with a tender mass in the RIF for the last 10 days. She has had some diarrhoea and a fever. Bloods tests on admission show a raised white cell count of 18, with a CRP of 380. Her Hb is 100 with a mean corpuscular volume (MCV): 75.

Q. 38.1 How would you make your initial assessment and what is the differential diagnosis?

Initial assessment will be based around a thorough history and examination. Important points to cover are duration and progression of symptoms, red flag symptoms, family history of colorectal cancer or inflammatory bowel disease, foreign travel, unusual foods/takeaways, and previous surgical history.

Initial management includes intravenous fluids, analgesia, blood cultures, and intravenous antibiotics. Cross-sectional imaging will be required to ascertain a diagnosis; however, the differential includes:

- *Appendix mass:* A delayed presentation of acute appendicitis can result in an appendix mass which may be an inflammatory phlegmon. If there is significant fluid component (appendix abscess), this may be drained percutaneously
- Terminal ileitis may present with a right iliac fossa mass and diarrhoea. This may be due to inflammatory bowel disease e.g. Crohn's disease or an infective process (TB, actinomycosis, yersinia, salmonella, etc.). The presence of a mass might suggest local perforation or fistulation
- *Malignancy:* A tender mass in the right iliac fossa might be due to a locally advanced caecal cancer, particularly in the setting of altered bowel habit or iron-deficiency anaemia
- *Spigelian hernia:* An incarcerated Spigelian hernia may present with a tender mass in the RIF. Although this arises from the abdominal wall, it may be difficult to distinguish from intra-abdominal pathology in the obese patient

Q. 38.2 A CT scan is performed overnight which is reported as showing acute appendicitis and surrounding inflammatory phlegmon. There is a small fluid collection and a locule of free gas anterior to the caecum. You go to review the patient. How will you proceed?

At 10 days since the onset of symptoms and with radiological evidence of an inflammatory phlegmon, surgery is likely to be challenging. While laparoscopy could be attempted, the risk of an open operation would be significantly higher. The appendix itself may have disintegrated and not be identifiable and there would be a risk of inadvertent injury to the caecum or adjacent small bowel loops.

If the patient is stable with localised tenderness, conservative treatment with intravenous antibiotics would be preferable with close monitoring of her clinical condition and inflammatory markers. It would be reasonable to repeat the scan after an interval and if there is any fluid collection, percutaneous drainage may be considered.

Q. 38.3 You review the CT images with a specialist gastrointestinal radiologist who is concerned about some caecal thickening which could be reactive to the appendicitis but malignancy is a possibility. Would this alter your management plan?

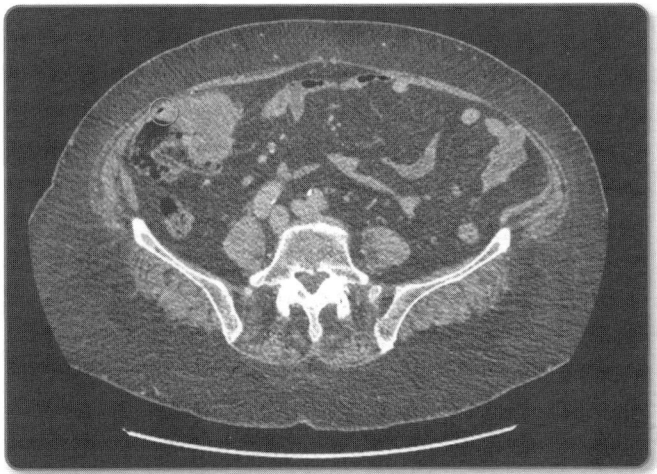

Management options:
- *Conservative treatment/deferred surgery*: If the patient is improving clinically and biochemically, conservative treatment with intravenous antibiotics (continued into the outpatient setting) might allow the acute inflammation to settle and would be the preferable course of action. This would then allow for repeat assessment with either CT at an interval of 4 weeks or a colonoscopy which would have the additional benefit of histological confirmation if malignancy is identified. This would also allow time for review in the colorectal MDT with completion of staging investigations and improved counselling and consent for surgery, which may be able to be performed laparoscopically without the need for a stoma. It is unlikely that this short delay would have any oncological sequelae
- *Early surgery*: If the patient is not improving with conservative treatment, emergency surgery is an option although this is likely to be an open operation/laparotomy. It can be difficult to make a firm diagnosis at operation and it is likely the patient would require a right hemicolectomy. If there is significant inflammation, an anastomosis may be considered unwise and would result in an ileostomy for the patient. This could be an overtreatment, if the ultimate pathology was found to be complicated appendicitis or an infective/inflammatory condition affecting the ileocaecal region

Scenario 39

Acute groin lump

A 43-year-old lady presents with a hot tender swelling in the right groin. It has been present for the last 48 hours and she has vomited twice. On examination, there is a 3 × 3 cm swelling in the groin with some overlying erythema.

Q. 39.1 What is the differential diagnosis and what information would you want to ascertain in the history?

- *Groin abscess:* Any history of diabetes or hidradenitis suppurativa
- *Infected pseudoaneurysm:* Any history of intravenous drug use
- *Incarcerated hernia (inguinal or femoral):* Was there a reducible lump at that site prior to presentation, any signs or symptoms of GI disturbance
- *Lymphadenopathy:* Any sign of infective or neoplastic process in lower limb, genitalia or perianal regions, any systemic signs such as fever, sweats, or weight loss to suggest lymphoma

Q. 39.2 What investigations would you request to reach a diagnosis?

If the lump is clearly a superficial abscess, no investigations are necessary and incision and drainage should be performed, either under local or general anaesthetic. If there is any concern regarding intravenous drug use or a deeper abscess surrounding the groin vessels, a duplex ultrasound scan or CT angiogram can determine if there is any evidence of a pseudoaneurysm, in which case, involvement of a vascular surgeon is required. For other nonreducible lumps in the groin, a CT scan can readily distinguish between an incarcerated hernia and tender lymphadenopathy.

Q. 39.3 A CT scan demonstrates this is an incarcerated femoral hernia containing a loop of small bowel with proximal dilatation. You consent the patient for urgent surgery on the emergency list. Please describe the surgical approaches for repair of a femoral hernia and state which you would use in this case.

The three open approaches for repair of a femoral hernia are:
- *McEvedy suprainguinal (high) approach:* The McEvedy approach describes a high, suprainguinal incision which allows reduction and repair of the hernia in the subcutaneous plane but also access to the peritoneal cavity to inspect or resect any involved small bowel. It is most useful for repair of a femoral hernia in the

emergency setting where there is a concern regarding strangulation or obstruction of the bowel. The original approach described a vertical paramedian incision; however, a transverse or oblique incision (Modified McEvedy) is cosmetically superior and allows the equivalent access to the peritoneal cavity
- *Lotheissen transinguinal approach:* This approach allows for repair of a synchronous inguinal and femoral hernia, but does disrupt the inguinal canal and is rarely used for to repair a femoral hernia in isolation
- *Lockwood infrainguinal (low) approach:* The low approach involves an incision over the lump and the hernia sac is dissected out and reduced. This is most suitable in the elective setting where the hernia usually contains extraperitoneal fat. The femoral canal can be obliterated with a mesh plug or interrupted sutures using a non-absorbable suture such as Ethibond or prolene. This incision does not give good access should bowel be involved as the femoral canal is particularly tight and a laparotomy might be required, if nonviable bowel is encountered. If there is a concern of strangulation or obstruction, a high approach should be utilised

Further reading

Sorelli PG, El-Masry N, Garrett WV. Open femoral hernia repair: one incision for all. World J Emerg Surg 2009; 4:44.

Scenario 40

Small bowel obstruction

A 66-year-old lady is admitted with bilious vomiting and constipation for the last 3 days. She has previously had a hysterectomy and a laparotomy for perforated duodenal ulcer in the past. She has had 2 episodes of adhesional small bowel obstruction, the last being 2 years ago which was managed conservatively.

Abdominal X-ray reveals evidence of small bowel obstruction.

Q. 40.1 What are the possible causes and how will you investigate and manage her initially?

Differential diagnosis:
- Adhesions
- Hernia – inguinal, femoral, or incisional
- Malignancy
- Volvulus/internal hernia
- Gallstone ileus
- Ischaemic bowel

Initial management for any patient with small bowel obstruction irrespective of underlying cause is fluid resuscitation and nasogastric decompression ('drip and suck'). I would insert a urinary catheter for hourly urine output monitoring - important to ensure adequate fluid replacement and correction of renal impairment.

I would request a CT scan to confirm the diagnosis of obstruction and this may identify a discrete transition point. It is also useful to rule out an obstructing mass lesion and give useful information regarding the quality of the bowel. Intravenous contrast is required to comment on enhancement of the bowel wall but the patient must be well hydrated to avoid contributing to acute kidney injury.

Q. 40.2 The CT scan reveals small bowel obstruction with a transition point in the mid-ileum. There is no hernia and no mass lesion and this is felt to be adhesional in nature. The bowel appears viable with no evidence of frank ischaemia on the scan. How will you proceed with her management? What features would prompt an early operation?

For adhesional obstruction, a period of conservative management is reasonable, particularly in the recurrent setting. With a period of drainage and bowel rest, a significant number of patients will settle. At 48 hours if the obstruction is not settling,

I would ask for a gastrografin study to clarify the degree and ongoing nature of obstruction. The decision of how long to wait for resolution can sometimes be difficult and depends on patients' comorbidities and operative risk, but should not usually exceed 72 hours.

Factors which suggest intestinal ischaemia [e.g. unremitting pain, elevated WBC count, high lactate, or CT evidence of ischaemia (poor enhancement or pneumatosis)] may prompt early surgical intervention. Patients with high-grade obstruction may be less likely to settle conservatively and early surgical intervention is preferred.

Q. 40.3 Can you tell me about any national audit data which might help to guide your decision making?

The National Audit of Small Bowel Obstruction (NASBO) – www.nasbo.com:
The NASBO report was published in 2017 and included snapshot audit data over an 8-week period from 131 hospitals. 2,434 patients with SBO were followed up for 30 days. The causes of SBO were adhesions (54%), hernia (19%) and cancer (10%), and other (17%). Inpatient referrals from other specialties often had delays in diagnosis and management.

About 24% were managed with early surgery within 24 hours of review. A further 24% underwent delayed surgery after a period of conservative management (3–64 days). Of these patients, 34% required a bowel resection and only 9% required a stoma. 49% had settled with conservative management. 3% had best supportive care as unfit for surgery or widespread malignancy.

The report highlights the significant morbidity and mortality associated with SBO (in-hospital mortality 8%). It stresses the need for careful fluid balance to correct acute kidney injury (present in 22%), early nutritional assessment and intervention, and pre-emptive involvement of critical care for moderate-/high-risk cases.

The main recommendations of the audit were:
- Early CT scan: CT scanning was used in 80% of patients, performed in average of 2.2 days from admission. AXR caused unnecessary exposure to ionising radiation
- Early use of water-soluble contrast in patients with adhesional obstruction who do not require immediate surgery (only used in a third of patients in this audit)
- Early nutritional assessment and intervention, particularly in the non-operative group (only 14% received PN and 26% received oral supplements)
- Operation within 72 hours if not settling with conservative treatment improves outcomes

National Emergency Laparotomy Audit (NELA) – www.nela.org.uk:
The NELA audit was commissioned by the Department of Health is response to the high mortality and wide variation in standards of care for patients undergoing emergency laparotomy. It is compulsory for all hospital trusts in England and Wales to submit data and annual report highlights specific areas for improvement. The main findings of the fifth annual report (2019) are:
- The 30-day mortality rate remains static at 9.6%
- Only 19% with suspected sepsis received antibiotics in the 1st hour
- Only 22.7% of patients had their preoperative risk documented

- Assessment of frailty is recommended for all patients >65 years. It is not routinely performed and only 36.9% had input from a geriatrician
- Patients with a predicted mortality >5% should have level 2 care (currently 77%)
- Importance of surgical and anaesthetic consultant input preoperatively and intraoperatively in high-risk cases

Scenario 41

Splenic trauma

A 60-year-old male patient is admitted following a road traffic collision. He was the driver in a head-on collision. He was wearing a seatbelt and the airbag was deployed. He is on clopidogrel for a previous TIA and has type 2 diabetes mellitus.

His heart rate is 125 bpm, BP 90/60 mmHg, saturations 96% on 15 L oxygen via non-rebreathe mask. He is complaining of left sided chest and abdominal pain.

Q. 41.1 How would you assess this patient?

I would assess the patient according to ATLS principles, paying attention to the airway and breathing first. With the patient immobilised, I would examine the chest for signs of bruising and palpate for broken ribs or surgical emphysema. I would auscultate for breath sounds and ensure the trachea is central to rule out pneumothorax. I would examine the abdomen looking for tenderness, distension, and bruising.

I would insert two large-bore cannulas and take blood for FBC, U and E, clotting profile, and crossmatch. I would give a litre of crystalloid and reassess for haemodynamic response.

Alongside my assessment, I would take an AMPLE history (Allergies, Medications, Past medical history, Last oral intake, and Events leading up to the incident).

I would arrange for a trauma CT with intravenous contrast within 15 minutes of arrival.

Q. 41.2 The CT scan suggests a splenic laceration with surrounding haematoma and a small amount of blood in the pelvis. After 1 L of crystalloid, his pulse is now 101 and BP 110/66 mmHg. How would you grade this splenic rupture and how would you manage the patient? What is the role of splenic artery embolisation and what are the risks?

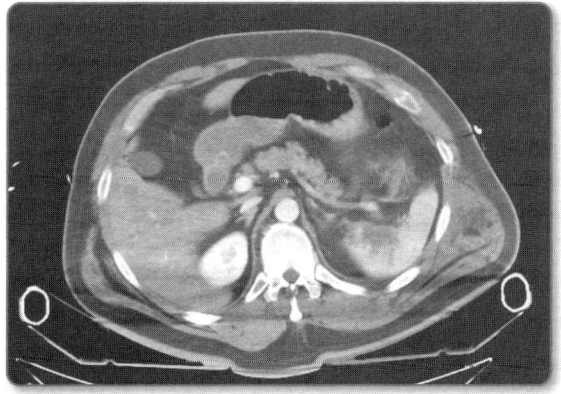

Grade of splenic injury:
The severity of splenic injury can be graded 1–5. Grades 1 and 2 are minor injury, grade 3 is moderate injury, and grades 4/5 are major injuries.
The American Association for the Surgery of Trauma (AAST) Splenic Injury Scale:
- Grade 1: Laceration <1 cm or subcapsular haematoma involving <10% surface area
- Grade 2: Laceration 1–3 cm or subcapsular haematoma involving 10–50% surface area
- Grade 3: Laceration >3 cm or subcapsular haematoma involving >50% surface area or ruptured subcapsular or parenchymal haematoma
- Grade 4: Segmental or hilar vascular injury causing >25% devascularisation of spleen
- Grade 5: Shattered spleen; major hilar injury

The patient has a grade 3 splenic injury. They have responded to initial resuscitation with crystalloid. I would liaise with the radiologist to see if there is any evidence of ongoing bleeding on the scan and if so, discuss with an interventional radiologist regarding embolisation of the splenic artery. If there is no active extravasation, a period of conservative management with close observation might be appropriate. I would arrange for the patient to be admitted to a major trauma ward or critical care environment.

I would liaise with a haematologist and whether they would advocate giving activated prothrombin complex or platelet transfusion should surgery be required.

Stage I and II splenic injuries may be managed conservatively with bed rest for 3 days. Splenic preservation with embolisation of the splenic artery is an option in higher grade injuries if the patient is haemodynamically stable. Embolisation is less likely to be successful if the patient is >55 years, significant haemoperitoneum >500 mL, concomitant solid organ injury or a vascular abnormality on the CT scan (Zarzour, 2017). Selective embolisation of a bleeding vessel might be appropriate; however, even in the absence of contrast blush embolisation of the proximal splenic artery in high-grade splenic injuries will reduce the perfusion pressure and can arrest bleeding. Potential complications include re-bleeding, splenic infarction and abscess, and local vascular injury.

Q. 41.3 The radiologist states there is no arterial extravasation so the patient is admitted for observation. At 10 PM, the patient becomes acutely unwell. There is no interventional radiology service overnight at your hospital. His BP drops to 70/45 mmHg and repeat haemoglobin is 66. You activate the major haemorrhage protocol and arrange to take him straight to theatre. Please explain how you would perform an emergency splenectomy.

Having prepared and draped the patient, I would perform a midline laparotomy. If there is significant haemoperitoneum, I would pack all four quadrants of the abdomen. I would medialise the spleen by dividing the lateral splenic attachments (gastrosplenic and lienorenal ligament). I would clamp the splenic artery and vein close to the hilum to avoid injuring the tail of the pancreas. Having resected the spleen, I would transfix the vessels and check for haemostasis. I would insert a tube drain to the splenic bed, close the abdomen, and return the patient to critical care.

Q. 41.4 What precautions are required post-splenectomy?

Asplenic patients are at risk of developing overwhelming sepsis and, therefore, require vaccination against *Haemophilus influenzae B, Meningococcus,* and *Pneumococcus.*

I would administer these vaccines 2 weeks postoperatively or on discharge. I would also prescribe lifelong prophylactic penicillin (penicillin V or amoxicillin). There is some evidence that this can be stopped after 2 or 10 years which is the highest risk period, but I would follow our local microbiology guidelines. I would explain the long-term susceptibility to infection and would advise the patient to seek urgent medical attention at the earliest indication of infection.

Further reading

Zarzour BL, Rozycki GS. An update on the nonoperative management of the spleen in adults. Trauma Sur Acute Care Open 2017; 2:1–7.

Scenario 42

Massive GI bleed

A 58-year-old man presents with 5 episodes of dark bleeding with clots from his rectum. He has collapsed and subsequently attended A&E. He has a history of peptic ulcer 20 years ago and haemorrhoids. He admits to drinking excess alcohol.

He is haemodynamically stable but his Hb is 71. He begins passing significant blood per rectum.

Q. 42.1 Please outline your initial management of this patient.

I would assess this patient according to CCrISP guidelines paying attention to his airway and breathing first. I would provide supplemental oxygen. I would insert a large bore cannula in each antecubital fossa and take blood for FBC, U and E, coagulation profile and crossmatch and begin fluid resuscitation. I would transfuse two units of blood initially and reassess. I would correct his coagulation if required and administer tranexamic acid 1 g intravenously and start a PPI infusion. If he became haemodynamically compromised,
I would initiate the major haemorrhage protocol. I would insert a urinary catheter to monitor fluid balance and have a low threshold for admission to critical care.

Q. 42.2 How will you investigate this patient and what are the differential diagnoses?

Initially, I will arrange for an OGD by an interventional gastroenterologist. If the patient is stable, this could be done in the endoscopy department, but if haemodynamically unstable, will be done in theatre with anaesthetic support. If a bleeding peptic ulcer is identified, dual modality endoscopic therapy can be performed (clip, injection, and heat).
If there is no evidence of blood in the upper gastrointestinal tract, the patient will need a CT angiogram to look for small bowel or colonic bleeding. Common causes include angiodysplasia, diverticular bleeding, colorectal malignancy, or Meckel's diverticulum.

Q. 42.3 The OGD is normal and CT angiogram does not show any active extravasation nor any other abnormality in the GI tract. The patient continues to bleed and requires a further four units blood transfusion. What further investigations would you consider?

Colonoscopy with irrigation is rarely successful in the acute setting but may identify angiodysplasia which could be treated with argon beam. It is also important to rule out haemorrhoidal bleeding.

Capsule endoscopy or a labelled red-cell scan (pertechnetate scan to rule out Meckel's diverticulum) can be helpful in a stable patient with ongoing occult bleeding but would not be relevant in the acute setting.

A CT angiogram is more sensitive than a mesenteric catheter angiogram for identifying the source of bleeding and, therefore, this is unlikely to add any further information.

If the patient continues to bleed, the only option is to repeat the CT angiogram or if unstable, perform a laparotomy with on table colonoscopy/enteroscopy. If no bleeding point can be identified, a right hemicolectomy with ileostomy is required to confirm whether bleeding is from the colon or small bowel.

Q. 42.4 The patient has attempted colonoscopy but this is impeded by altered blood coming from proximally and stool. The patient continues to bleed and becomes haemodynamically unstable so you repeat the CT angiogram. What does it show and how will you manage the patient?

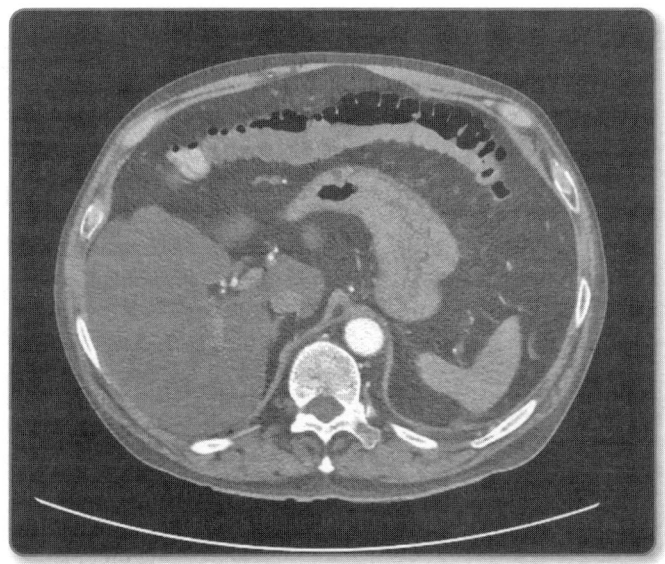

The CT angiogram shows active contrast extravasation at the hepatic flexure of the colon with no mass lesion. The likely cause is angiodysplasia or bleeding from a right-sided diverticulum. Either way, embolisation of the colon would risk local necrosis and perforation and many not be successful and, therefore, I would perform a laparotomy and perform a right hemicolectomy. Given his haemodynamic instability and diagnostic uncertainly, I would form an ileostomy rather than risk an anastomosis, which would also be diagnostically helpful if he was to continue to bleed.

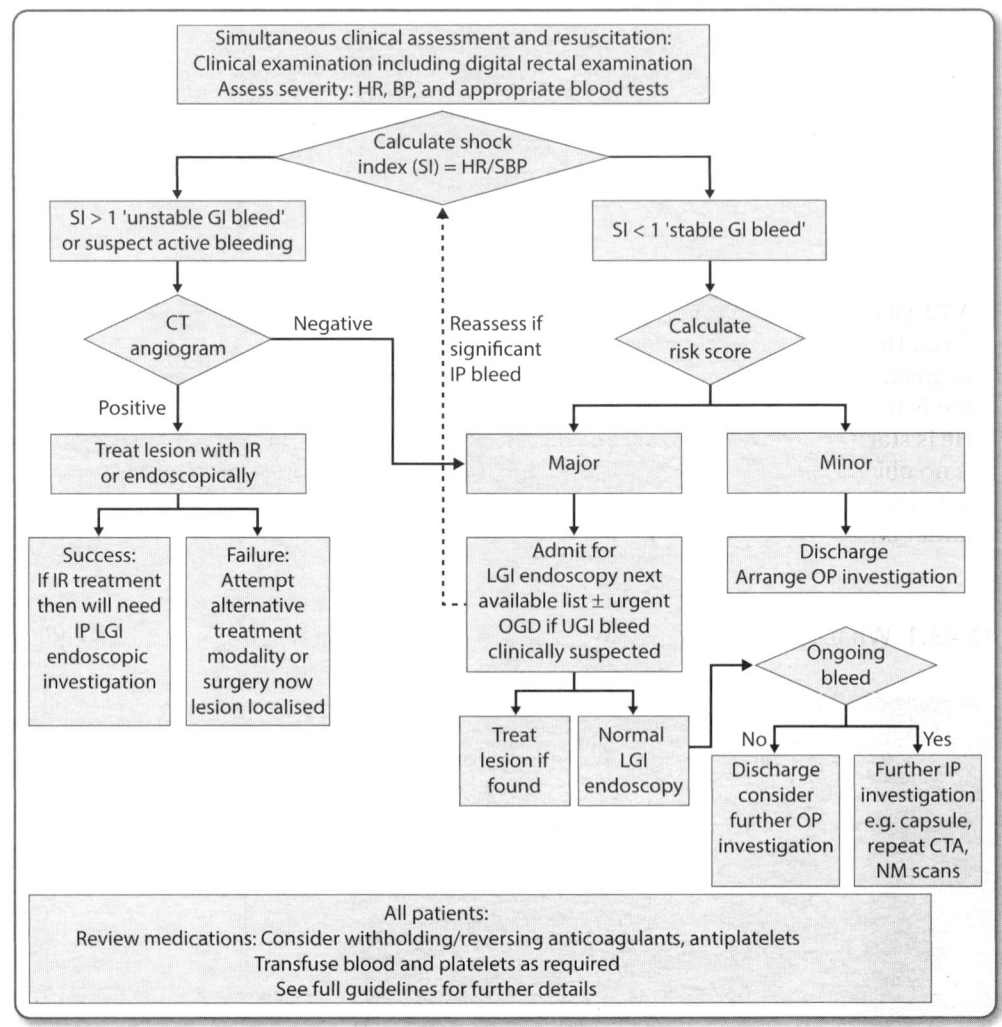

BP, blood pressure; CT, computed tomography; CTA, computed tomography angiography; GI, gastrointestinal
Source: Acute lower GI bleeding management algorithm (Gut, 2019).

Further reading

Oakland K, Chadwick G, East JE, et al. Diagnosis and management of acute lower gastrointestinal bleeding: guidelines from the British Society of Gastroenterology. Gut 2019; 68:776–789.

Scenario 43

Perianal sepsis

A 72-year-old unkempt gentleman presents with perianal pain, bleeding, and fever. He has a history of poorly controlled diabetes, alcohol excess, and self-neglect. He is clerked by the SHO on call who notes he has a temperature of 38.7°C but is too tender to examine. Blood tests show white cell count 18 and CRP 280. He is started on co-amoxiclav and is admitted. On the post-take ward round, there is no obvious abnormality in the perianal area but he cannot tolerate a digital rectal examination. An MRI scan is organised before considering examination under anaesthetic.

Q. 43.1 What does the MRI scan show and how will you manage this patient?

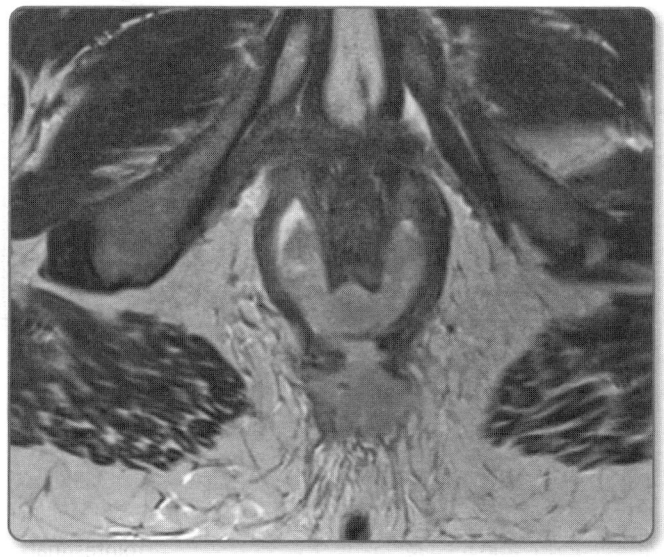

The MRI scan shows a horseshoe abscess in the intersphincteric plane with extension through the external sphincter at the 6 o'clock position with a further collection posteriorly.

This gentleman has signs of sepsis and having taken blood cultures, I would commence him on intravenous antibiotics and plan for urgent incision and drainage.

I would perform the procedure in lithotomy position and incise the abscess at the 6 o'clock position, making sure to adequately drain both limbs of the horseshoe collection.

I would thoroughly irrigate the cavity and place a corrugated drain in each limb. I would perform a rigid sigmoidoscopy to ensure there is no underlying rectal tumour or if a fistula is identified, I would insert a draining seton.

Q. 43.2 Unfortunately due to other emergencies, delays in theatre, and miscommunication at handover, the operation is not done and the patient is deferred till the next day. In the morning, he has deteriorated and is now drowsy, tachycardic, and hypotensive. On examination, he has a necrotic patch in the perianal region with erythema and crepitus extending over the perineum and scrotum. How will you manage this situation?

The patient has developed necrotising fasciitis extending to the scrotum (Fournier's gangrene). This is a surgical emergency and requires prompt drainage and debridement. I would ensure the patient is resuscitated with intravenous fluids and antibiotics. I would liaise with critical care and the on-call anaesthetist and book him for a Category 1 operation (within 1 hour). I would arrange a joint operation with the urology team to drain the perianal sepsis and debride all infected tissue from the perineum and scrotum, sending samples for culture and sensitivity. I would dress the wounds in betadine-soaked gauze and arrange for a second look in theatre in 24 hours. The patient would need intensive care postoperatively. This is a synergistic polymicrobial infection so I would liaise with the microbiologist to ensure that the adequate antibiotics were provided until cultures were obtained. This usually includes piperacillin–tazobactam and clindamycin.

Q. 43.3 At operation, you perform a wide debridement of perianal skin and scrotum. At EUA, you find he has a bulky rectal tumour which has perforated locally caused the sepsis. What is your ongoing management plan?

At second look EUA, I would debride any further devitalised tissue and irrigate the cavity. I would also perform a defunctioning sigmoid loop colostomy in order to avoid contamination of the wounds and promote healing. I would take biopsies of the tumour and refer him to the colorectal MDT with a CT scan to complete staging. I would liaise with the plastic surgery team, who may wish to consider skin grafts in due course.

Scenario 44

Ischaemic bowel

A 76-year-old lady presents with a 24-hour history of abdominal pain and vomiting. She has a history of previous CVA, myocardial infarction (MI), diabetes, stage 3 chronic kidney disease (CKD3), and claudication. On examination, her abdomen is soft with mild tenderness in the right iliac fossa but no peritonism. She is in fast atrial fibrillation (pulse 148 bpm, BP 101/69 mmHg) and looks clammy. Her blood tests show white cell count: 18, Hb: 148, CRP: 82, her lactate is: 4.2, and eGFR: 29.

Q. 44.1 How will you assess her?

I will resuscitate her with supplemental oxygen, intravenous fluids, and antibiotics and ensure monitoring is in place such as ECG and urinary catheter. I will take a history of her presenting complaint and also ascertain her general fitness and performance status.

Her history is concerning for ischaemic bowel where often the degree of pain is greater than the abdominal signs. This may be embolic from atrial fibrillation or thrombotic as she has widespread arterial disease.

I would arrange a CT scan with IV contrast despite her impaired renal function as without contrast, it is not possible to comment on the enhancement of the bowel.

I would ensure she was well hydrated and monitor her renal function closely. This would also rule out any perforation, obstruction, or malignancy.

Q. 44.2 The CT scan suggests there is a loop of distal ileum approximately 50 cm in length which is thick-walled and does not enhance. There appears to be clot within the superior mesenteric artery (SMA), although the vessel is small calibre and heavily calcified. How will you proceed?

I will calculate the patient's mortality risk (p-Possum) and liaise with the emergency anaesthetist and intensive care team to ascertain her fitness for surgery. I will counsel the patient regarding laparotomy and small bowel resection for ischaemic bowel, explaining that this would be a high-risk procedure with a significant risk to life and prolonged recovery. I would explain that we will remove any ischaemic bowel and she will likely require a small bowel stoma which could be high output and might require parenteral nutrition for a prolonged period.

I would liaise with vascular surgical colleagues and interventional radiology to see if they wish to explore the SMA and perform an embolectomy or thrombectomy on-table or bypass.

Q. 44.3 At operation, she has 50 cm of necrotic terminal ileum and caecum. The rest of the small bowel looks dusky. The vascular surgeon performs an SMA embolectomy and some of the small bowel pinks up. What is your operative plan?

I would resect any frankly ischaemic bowel and staple off the ends. If there is bowel of dubious viability, I would leave the abdomen open with a temporary covering (e.g. ABThera™ Open Abdomen Negative Pressure Therapy System or an alternative negative pressure temporary closure, Bogota bag, wound manager, or Opsite sandwich) and perform a second look laparotomy at 24 hours. This allows time for resuscitation and optimisation on intensive care with correction of electrolytes and control of arrhythmia. If the bowel is viable, I would then create stomas and close the abdomen. I would liaise with vascular colleagues about the need for a heparin infusion.

Q. 44.4 At second look laparotomy, the rest of the small bowel has infarcted up to 30 cm from the DJ flexure; however, the colon remains perfused. The patient is unstable and keeps dropping her blood sugar. What will you do?

This is an unsurvivable condition and the low blood sugar suggests global ischaemia. Resecting the remainder of the small bowel would subject her to lifelong TPN. I would close the abdomen and return to the patient to intensive care. I would speak with the family and involve palliative care services to begin end of life care.

Further reading

Bala M, Kashuk J, Moore EE, et al. Acute mesenteric ischemia: guidelines of the World Society of Emergency Surgery. World J Emerg Surg. 2017;12:38. doi:10.1186/s13017-017-0150-

Hung A, Calderbank T, Samaan MA, Plumb AA, Webster G. Ischaemic colitis: practical challenges and evidence-based recommendations for management. Frontline Gastroenterol 2019; 10:44–52.

Tilsed JV, Casamassima A, Kurihara H, et al. ESTES guidelines: acute mesenteric ischaemia. Eur J Trauma Emerg Surg 2016; 42:253–270.

Chapter 4

General surgery

Paul Wilson, Robin Som

Scenario 1

Female groin hernia

A 75-year-old female patient is referred by her general practitioner (GP) to your outpatient clinic with a symptomatic (painful) groin lump, which does reduce on lying supine.

Her body mass index (BMI) is 22 kg/m², she is hypertensive and a non-smoker.
On examination there is a: reducible non-tender groin lump – thought to be an inguinal hernia.

Q. 1.1 How would you manage the patient?

Clinical assessment: Hernia symptoms including reducibility, comorbidities including fitness for general anaesthesia (GA), previous abdominal surgery (? hostile abdomen for laparoscopy).

Careful clinical examination of the hernia – to assess site, reducibility, and tenderness.

If the abdomen is not 'hostile' for laparoscopy – list the patient urgently for diagnostic laparoscopy proceeding to laparoscopic repair ± bilateral repairs.

If the patient is unfit for GA – list urgently for local anaesthesia (LA) open repair via an inguinal approach – if on opening the inguinal canal no hernia is evident and a femoral hernia is diagnosed – repair via the posterior inguinal canal wall – middle approach and carry out inguinal repair on exiting.

If the abdomen is hostile for laparoscopy then carry out a similar open approach under GA or LA.

Q. 1.2 What investigations are appropriate?

Although ultrasound/MRI might be helpful in diagnosis – investigating the patient introduces further delay before surgery and increases the risk of strangulation if the hernia is femoral. The definitive investigation here is a diagnostic laparoscopy – proceeding to hernia repair.

The diagnostic accuracy of clinical examination and differentiation between femoral and inguinal hernia in females is poor (50–60%) even in experienced hands.

Because of the high risk of strangulation with femoral hernias (cumulative probability of strangulation was 22% at 3 months and 45% at 21 months following diagnosis) and their need for urgent treatment. All females with a groin hernia, irrespective of whether thought to be inguinal or femoral should be assumed to have a femoral hernia until proven otherwise at urgent diagnostic laparoscopy or by urgent open inguinal surgical approach.

There is also a high prevalence of bilateral femoral hernias in females (30–50%). Therefore, diagnostic laparoscopy will determine the bilateral nature of the hernias, and even if asymptomatic, the contralateral femoral hernia should also be repaired.

It is not uncommon also in females to have concomitant inguinal and femoral defects – which can be repaired at laparoscopy.

'To quantify the risk of obstruction in groin hernia, the cumulative probability of strangulation in relation to the length of history has been calculated for inguinal and femoral hernias in a study of 476 patients (439 inguinal and 37 femoral). There were 34 strangulations (22 inguinal and 12 femoral). After 3 months, the cumulative probability of strangulation for inguinal hernias was 2.8%, rising to 4.5% after 2 years. For femoral hernias, the cumulative probability of strangulation was 22% at 3 months and 45% at 21 months.'

Q. 1.3 What guidelines are available regarding the management of groin hernias?

There have been many published guidelines over the last two decades, including the National Institute of Clinical Excellence (NICE) guidelines, the European Hernia Society Guidelines, etc.

The most up-to-date guidelines are as follows:
- British Hernia Society – Groin Hernia Guidelines (ASGBI) 2013, updated in 2016
- The Hernia Surge Group. International guidelines for groin hernia management. Hernia 2018; 22:1–165

These guidelines recommend that females with a groin hernia should be referred urgently by their GP to a surgeon who should list for urgent diagnostic laparoscopy and hernia repair.

Q. 1.4 What are the boundaries of the femoral canal?

- *Anteriorly:* Inguinal ligament
- *Posteriorly:* Pectineal ligament
- *Medially:* Lacunar ligament
- *Laterally:* Femoral vein

Femoral canal anatomy – open and laparoscopic (see figures below)

Scenario 1 Female groin hernia

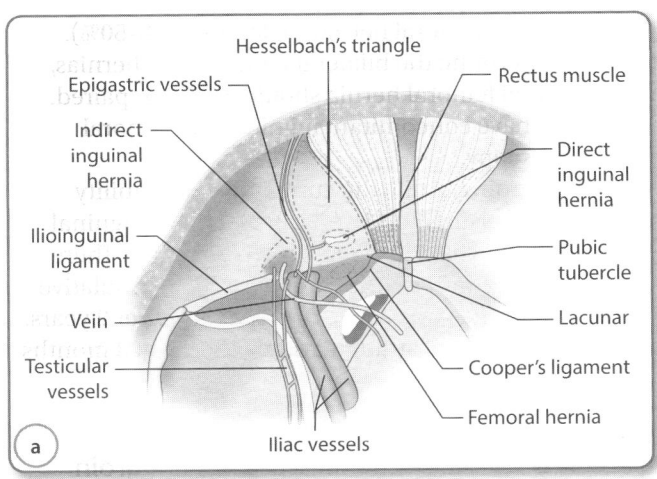

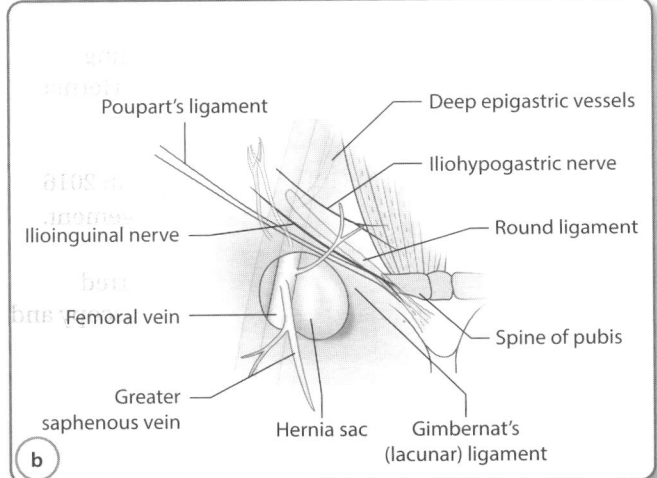

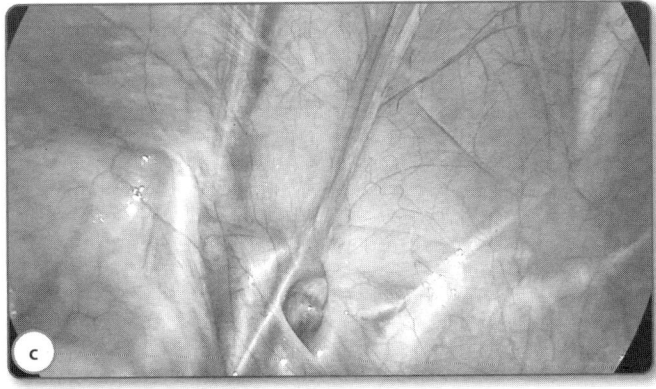

Further reading

Gallegos NC, Dawson J, Jarvis M, Hobsley M. Risk of strangulation in groin hernias. Br J Surg 1991; 78:1171–1173.

Scenario 2

Consent for inguinal hernia repair

A 47-year-old builder presents with a symptomatic inguinal hernia. He has no significant comorbidities and has no previous abdominal surgery.

Q. 2.1 How would you consent the patient with regard to management of his groin hernia?

Having established that the patient has capacity –
The consent process would involve:
- At the consent discussion, provide information on the procedure and its implications. In particular, you should discuss information about:
  - The patient's diagnosis and prognosis
  - Options for treatment, including non-operative care and no treatment
  - The purpose and expected benefit of the treatment
  - The likelihood of success
  - The clinicians involved in their treatment
  - The risks inherent in the procedure, however, small the possibility of their occurrence, side effects and complications. The consequences of non-operative alternatives should also be explained
  - Potential follow-up treatment

In relation to the patient's inguinal hernia an explanation as to the nature of the hernia and its natural history.

All options for treatment would include:
- Non-operative – conservative approach
- Surgical intervention – open versus laparoscopic versus endoscopic

Conservative approach

The risk of hernia strangulation with a watchful wait approach is relatively low (*after 3 months, the cumulative probability of strangulation for inguinal hernias was 2.8%, rising to 4.5% after 2 years*) and therefore, a conservative non-operative approach is a safe option.

The patient must be made aware of the risks of a non-operative approach – increasing size and discomfort within the hernia causing limitation in activities, irreducibility, obstruction due to incarceration, and strangulation – with its serious risk to life.

The patient should be made aware that with increasing symptoms – an operative approach may have to be considered if on a conservative pathway.

'To quantify the risk of obstruction in groin hernia, the cumulative probability of strangulation in relation to the length of history has been calculated for inguinal and femoral hernias in a study of 476 patients (439 inguinal and 37 femoral). There were 34 strangulations (22 inguinal and 12 femoral). After 3 months, the cumulative probability of strangulation for inguinal hernias was 2.8%, rising to 4.5% after 2 years. For femoral hernias, the cumulative probability of strangulation was 22% at 3 months and 45% at 21 months.'

Surgical intervention

The techniques of open surgical repair, laparoscopic repair (TAPP and TEP) should be explained and a detailed explanation of the risks of each procedure, including recovery after surgery.

The risks to discuss would also include an approximate incidence of the specific complication and the treatment that each complication might involve.

Risks to include:
- *General complications*: Venous thromboembolism (VTE), anaesthetic complications, respiratory problems

Specific complications related to hernia repair:

Significant complications associated with groin hernia repair
- *Self-limited neuralgia:* 10–20%
- *Chronic pain:* 10–12%
- *Haematoma:* 5–16%
- *Seroma:* 1–12%
- *Recurrence:* 1–5%/5 years
- *Urinary retention:* LA: 0.37%, GA: 2–3%
- *Wound infection:* 1–3% open, 0.32–0.65% lap
- *Testicular complication:* 0.5–1%
- *Bladder damage:* Uncommon, open/lap, 0.2%
- *Vas injury:* 0.3–2%
- *Mortality:* (same as general population) 0–0.02%
- *Mesh infection:* <0.5%
- *Numbness:* Less after lap

Complications specific to laparoscopic repair

Intestinal obstruction (TAPP): 0.07–0.4%; port site hernia: 1% intestinal/visceral injury: 0–0.21%; Vascular injury: 0.06–0.13

Further reading

Gallegos NC, Dawson J, Jarvis M, Hobsley M. Risk of strangulation in groin hernias. Br J Surg 1991; 78:1171–1173.

Scenario 3

Incisional hernia: Part 1

A 50-year-old male patient with no comorbidities undergoes an emergency laparotomy and Hartmann's procedure for perforated diverticulitis. After he is discharged, he re-attends a few weeks later with a tender swelling from the midline scar.

Q. 3.1 What measures can be taken to reduce the risk of incisional hernia occurrence?

- Patient factors
- Operative factors
- Perioperative factors

Patient factors (in elective, non-cancer patients):
- Obesity – weight reduction programmes. Aim to get BMI < 35 kg/m^2, and <30 if possible. Weight reduction of 25% body weight is possible. If not possible, consider Bariatric surgery for weight reduction prior to elective procedures
- *Smoking:* Smoking cessation
- *Type 2 diabetes mellitus:* Optimisation
- *Chronic obstructive pulmonary disease (COPD)/Asthma:* Optimisation
- *Prehabilitation programmes:* To improve exercise tolerance and nutritional state

Operative factors:
- Laparoscopic approach, if feasible
- Paramedian/non-midline approaches
- Midline closure suture techniques–suture length (wound to suture ratio 1:4), short stitch – bite and length (0.5 cm)
- Prophylactic mesh to augment midline closure (elective, low infective risk cases)
- Port-site closure devices in laparoscopic surgery
- Prophylactic mesh in stoma formation

Perioperative factors:
- Prophylactic antibiotics – reduction in surgical site infections (SSIs)
- Pre-/peri-/postoperative optimisation of nutrition
- Measures to reduce increased abdominal pressure:
    - Regional analgesia – epidural, TAP block, rectus sheath block/catheter infusion – to reduce opiate requirements

- Avoidance of constipation – laxatives
- Chest physiotherapy

Suture length to wound length ratio of at least 4, stitch length 10 mm versus longer length. 737 patients, incisional hernias: Long-stitch length 18%, short-stitch length 5.6%, $p < 0.001$.

Small bites suture technique (5 mm bites and 5 mm length) is more effective than the traditional large bites technique (10 mm bites and 10 mm length) for prevention of incisional hernia in midline incisions. 560 patients, 1-year follow-up, incisional hernias: Small bites 13%, large bites 21%, $p = 0.022$.

Elective abdominal aortic aneurysm (AAA) repairs. Prophylactic retromuscular mesh-augmentation of midline closure. 120 patients. 2-year follow-up. Incisional hernias: Non-mesh 28%, mesh-augmentation 0%, $p < 0.0001$.

Onlay mesh versus sublay mesh versus primary suture, elective AAA patients – 480, 2-year follow-up,

Incisional hernia:
- Onlay mesh: 13%
- Sublay mesh: 18%
- Suture: 30%

Meta-analysis of 11 randomised controlled trials (RCTs), 907 patients, concluded: Reinforcing elective stomas with mesh (primarily synthetic) reduces subsequent parastomal hernia rates, complications, repairs and saves money.

Further reading

Deerenberg EB, Harlaar JJ, Steyerberg EW, et al. Small bites versus large bites for closure of abdominal midline incisions (STITCH): A double-blind, multicentre, randomised controlled trial. Lancet 2015; 386:1254–1260.

Findlay JM, Wood CPJ, Cunningham C. Prophylactic mesh reinforcement of stomas: a cost-effectiveness meta-analysis of randomised controlled trials. Tech Coloproctol 2018; 22:265–270.

Jairam A, Timmermans L, Eker H, et al. Prevention of incisional hernia with prophylactic onlay and sublay mesh reinforcement versus primary suture only in midline laparotomies (PRIMA): 2-year follow-up of a multicentre, double-blind, randomised controlled trial. Lancet 2017; 390:567–576.

Millbourn D, Cengiz Y, Israelsson LA. Effect of Stitch Length on Wound Complications After Closure of Midline Incisions: A Randomized Controlled Study. Arch Surg 2009; 144:1056–1059.

Muysoms FE, Detry O, Vierendeels T, et al. Prevention of Incisional Hernias by Prophylactic Mesh-augmented Reinforcement of Midline Laparotomies for Abdominal Aortic Aneurysm Treatment: A Randomized Controlled Trial. Ann Surg 2016; 263:638–645.

Scenario 4

Recurrent umbilical hernia

A 42-year-old female with a, obese, BMI of 44 kg/m², has a background of type 2 diabetes mellitus. She is having intermittent obstructive symptoms – with vomiting and abdominal distension. On examination there is an irreducible, tender umbilical hernial with a large sac and a 5-cm diameter defect.

CT abdomen/pelvis shows a loop of small bowel within the hernial sac. The small bowel loop is well perfused with no signs of strangulation. The remaining small bowel is not distended.

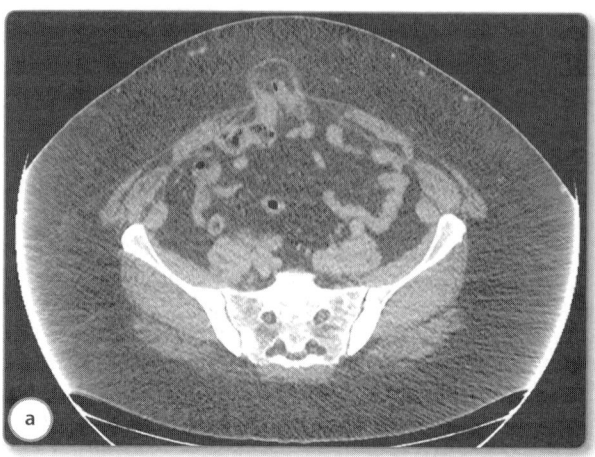
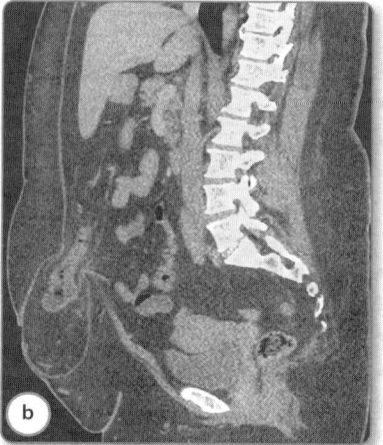

Q. 4.1 How would you manage the patient?

This patient is a 'high risk' patient related to morbid obesity, smoker, type 2 diabetes mellitus, recurrent nature of hernia, features of intermittent small bowel obstruction, tenderness on palpation, bowel loops within hernia sac confirmed on the CT scan, and the need for urgent surgery (lack of time for optimisation).

Despite these risks the patient does need urgent operative intervention as there is significant risk of strangulation.

A conservative approach would be high risk – strangulation requiring emergency surgery would carry a higher morbidity and mortality risk.

There is little time to wait to optimise the patient: Weight loss reduction/bariatric surgery, smoking cessation, diabetic optimisation.

Detailed assessment of cardiopulmonary function [cardiopulmonary exercise testing (CPET)] may be possible but the patient does need urgent surgery and will need a high-dependency unit/ITU bed postoperatively.

The same risk factors are predictive of a higher risk of postoperative complications for this patient:
- Respiratory problems
- Surgical site infections
- Seroma formation
- Hernia recurrence
- Mortality risk

Q. 4.2 What operative approach for this high-risk patient?

Laparoscopic versus open repair

- *Laparoscopic repair*: Intraperitoneal onlay mesh repair (IPOM) + − defect closure and intraperitoneal onlay mesh augmentation or E-TEP repair (laparoscopic Rives–Stoppa) with defect closure and retrorectus mesh augmentation
- *Open repair*: Sutured repair (Mayo) or sublay retrorectus mesh augmentation with defect closure

In favour of laparoscopic approach/against open repair:
- Recurrent hernia lower risk of recurrence in laparoscopic repair
- Reduced risk of SSI in laparoscopic repair
- Defect diameter is 5 cm – the laparoscopic approach is feasible with defect closure and intraperitoneal onlay mesh augmentation (IPOM+ associated with lower risk of seroma and recurrence)
- The defect is too large to carry out as an open technique under local anaesthesia

Against laparoscopic/in favour of open repair:
- GA/pneumoperitoneum associated with higher morbidity in high-risk patients
- Large hernial sac – difficult to excise laparoscopically – higher risk of seroma
- Contents of sac – small bowel may be difficult to dissect free laparoscopically – increased risk of small bowel injury requiring resection

Further reading

Henriksen NA, Montgomery A, Kaufmann R, et al. European and Americas Hernia Societies (EHS and AHS). Guidelines for treatment of umbilical and epigastric hernias from the European Hernia Society and Americas Hernia Society. Br J Surg 2020; 107:171–190.

Scenario 5

Spigelian hernia

An 83-year-old female presents with an uncomfortable left iliac fossa (LIF) lump which does not reduce when supine.
- She has a background of hypertension and high BMI, and has not had any previous abdominal surgery.
- On examination there is a vague, diffuse swelling in the LIF which is irreducible and non-tender

CT scanning confirms a LIF hernia containing a loop of small bowel. There are no features to suggest small bowel obstruction.

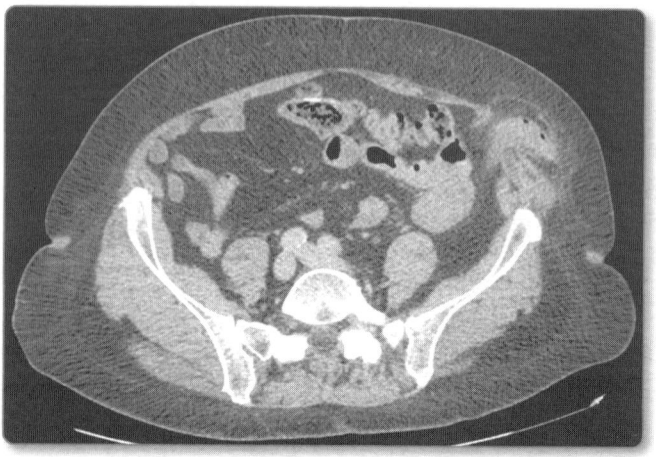

Q. 5.1 What is a spigelian hernia? What is the nature of the defect? How would you manage this patient?

A spigelian hernia (or lateral ventral hernia) is a hernia through the spigelian fascia, which is the aponeurotic layer between the rectus abdominis muscle medially, and the semilunar line laterally. Spigelian hernia occurs through slit-like defect in the anterior abdominal wall adjacent to the semilunar line. Most of spigelian hernias occur in the lower abdomen (below the arcuate line) where the posterior sheath is deficient. The hernia ring is a well-defined defect in the transversus aponeurosis. These are generally interparietal hernias, meaning that they do not lie below the subcutaneous fat but penetrate between the muscles of the abdominal wall; therefore, there is often no notable swelling.

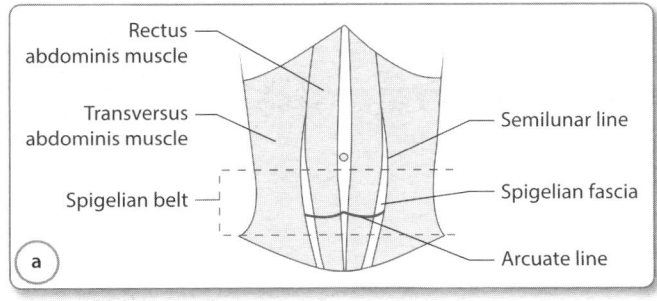

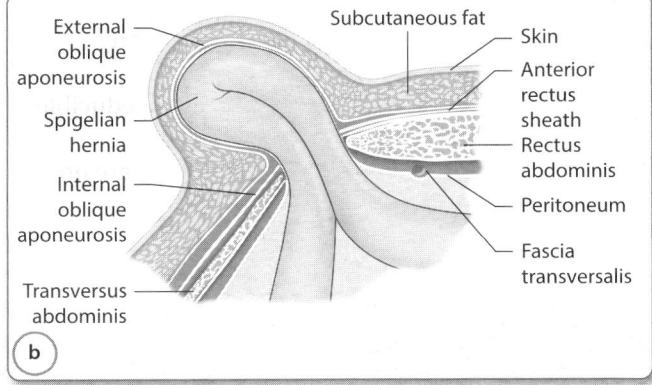

The patient is in high risk for surgery related to her age (83 years), obesity, irreducibility, and the presence of small bowel loop within the hernial sac.

However, spigelian hernias have a high risk of strangulation and this patient should undergo urgent surgery.

Laparoscopic versus open repair

Laparoscopic repair has the benefit of confirming the diagnosis and can be repaired with a preperitoneal prosthetic mesh placement without the need for defect closure via a transabdominal preperitoneal (TAPP) or totally extraperitoneal (TEP) technique. It can also be repaired with an IPOM technique.

Open repair can be carried out with a simple sutured repair with or without a sublay prosthetic mesh augmentation. It can be done under local anaesthetic in high-risk patients.

Morbidity and recurrence risk are lower for laparoscopic repair. Hospital stay is also reduced.

Further reading

Henriksen NA, Kaufmann R, Simons MP, et al. EHS and AHS guidelines for treatment of primary ventral hernias in rare locations or special circumstances. BJS Open 2020; 4:342–353.

Scenario 6

Incisional hernia: Part 2

A 68-year-old male presents with a symptomatic (painful) midline incisional hernia following a previous midline laparotomy in 2016 with small bowel resection for a strangulated umbilical hernia.
- *Comorbidities*: Current smoker, obese (BMI: 33 kg/m^2), sleep apnoea.
- *On examination*: There is a recurrent umbilical defect (measuring 7 cm in transverse diameter), and smaller epigastric incisional defects. All are reducible and non-tender.

CT scanning confirms multiple defects.

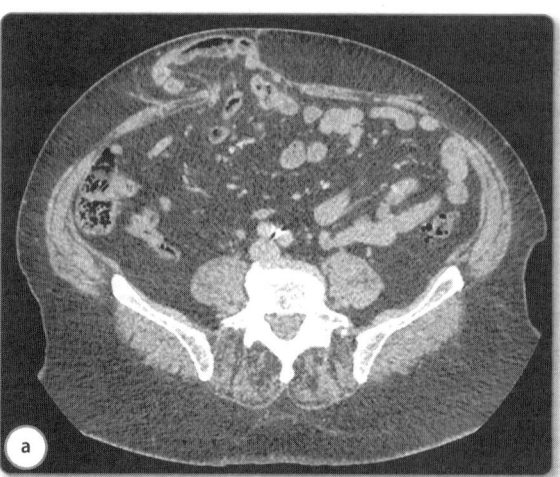
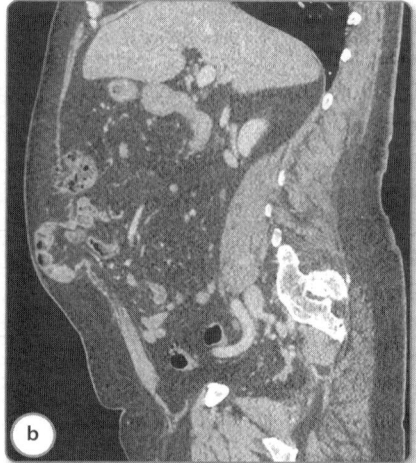

Q. 6.1 In the management of incisional hernias what measures can be taken to reduce tension and to allow closure of the midline defect?

- Weight reduction
- *Component relaxation:* Preoperative botulinum A toxin (BOTOX 400 IU) to lateral abdominal wall – ultrasound guided – 4 weeks prior to surgery
- Component separation – anterior (open/endoscopic) – external oblique release, posterior (open/laparoscopic) – transversus abdominis release (TAR)
- Progressive CO_2 pneumoperitoneum – 500 mL daily via laparoscopic port, as an in-patient – until target volume achieved – to increase the size of the abdominal cavity

Q. 6.2 How can this patient be optimised prior to surgery?

- Smoking cessation
- Weight reduction
- Exercise to improve cardiorespiratory function
- Continuous positive airway pressure (CPAP) (e.g. 4 hours per night for 3 months) preoperatively significantly improves perioperative respiratory function
- Anaesthetic assessment
- Cardiopulmonary exercise testing

Q. 6.3 What operative techniques are feasible for this patient?

Laparoscopic:
- IPOM augmentation
- IPOM+ (defect closure with IPOM)
- E-TEP [extra-peritoneal approach with defect closure and retrorectus mesh augmentation (laparoscopic Rives–Stoppa)]

Open:
- Sutured defect closure – sutured repair
- Mesh repair – defect closure with:
  - Retrorectus mesh augmentation (Rives–Stoppa)
  - Intraperitoneal sublay mesh augmentation
  - Onlay mesh augmentation

Further reading

Sanders DL, Pawlak MM, de Beaux AC, European Hernia Society incisional hernia guidelines. Br J Surg 2023; 110:343.

Scenario 7

Massive incisional hernia

A 73-year-old obese (BMI: 37 kg/m^2) female presents with a large symptomatic (uncomfortable) incisional hernia following a previous lower midline laparotomy for endometrial Ca in 2012.

The hernia does not reduce when supine.

The patient has had a previous admission for small bowel obstruction which was managed conservatively.

The patient is cancer-free and has recently had six stone weight loss – intentional.

CT scanning shows a large incisional hernia with defect dimensions of 9 cm transverse and 22 cm vertically.

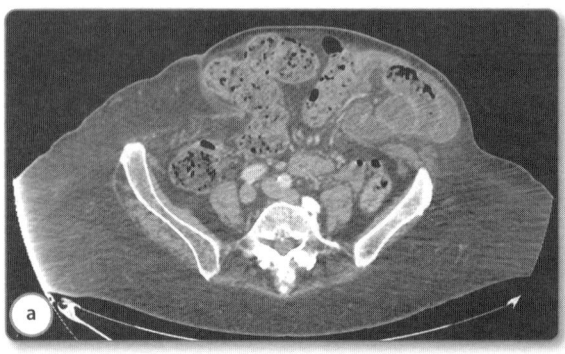
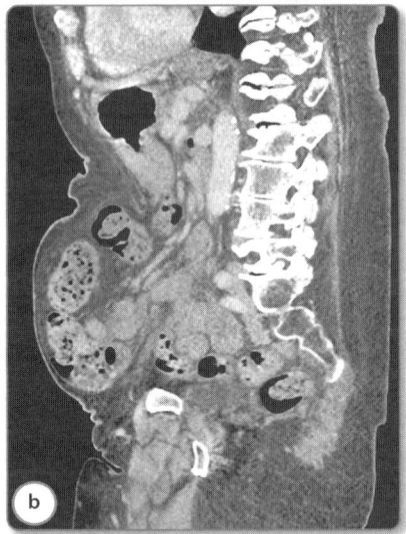

Q. 7.1 How would you manage this patient?

Factors to consider:
- The patient is high risk for surgery related to her age and obesity
- There is significant loss of domain with a large defect measuring over 9 cm in transverse diameter and 22 cm in vertical length
- The hernial sac is large and contains a significant amount of small intestine and colon

- The abdominal cavity is relatively small
- The patient has had a previous episode of small bowel obstruction and is therefore, at risk of further episodes and the need for emergency surgery

There is certainly indication for the patient to undergo surgery – because of her episode of obstruction, but the patient needs thorough preoperative assessment and optimisation.

The patient is at significant risk of respiratory problems postoperatively when the contents of the hernial sac are returned to the abdominal cavity due to diaphragmatic splinting.

The patient is at higher risk of SSI, seroma, and recurrence related to her obesity.

Preoperative requirements:
- Multi-disciplinary team (MDT) discussion
- Radiological measurement of hernial sac and abdominal cavity volumes
- Anaesthetic assessment
- Cardiopulmonary exercise testing – this will aid planning of immediate post-operative care (e.g. ward-based, or high-dependency unit/intensive care unit-based care)
    - Exercise tolerance assessment
    - Cardiac rhythm (ECG) and function (echocardiography) assessment
    - Pulmonary function testing (dynamic)
    - Anaerobic threshold measurement
- *Weight reduction:* 3–6-month trial

Preoperative botulinum A toxin (BOTOX 400 IU) to lateral abdominal wall – ultrasound-guided – 4 weeks prior to surgery – component relaxation.

Progressive CO_2 pneumoperitoneum – 500 mL daily via laparoscopic port, as an in-patient – until target volume achieved – to increase the size of the abdominal cavity.

Operative technique

- Not suitable for laparoscopic repair – defect size is too large
- Would require open repair with excision of the hernial sac, adhesiolysis, defect closure, and mesh augmentation (retrorectus/intraperitoneal sublay)
- Component separation would also be required bilaterally – TAR or anterior component separation (open/endoscopic)

High-dependency unit care:
- Thoracic epidural for postoperative analgesia
- Antibiotic prophylaxis
- Venous thromboembolism prophylaxis – chemical and mechanical

Further reading

Sanders DL, Pawlak MM, de Beaux AC, European Hernia Society incisional hernia guidelines. Br J Surg 2023; 110:343.

Scenario 8

Melanoma

A 43-year-old female consults her GP regarding a pigmented skin lesion on the back measuring approximately 8 mm × 14 mm, presents for 3 months, which appears to be enlarging.
The patient has had no previous such skin lesions.

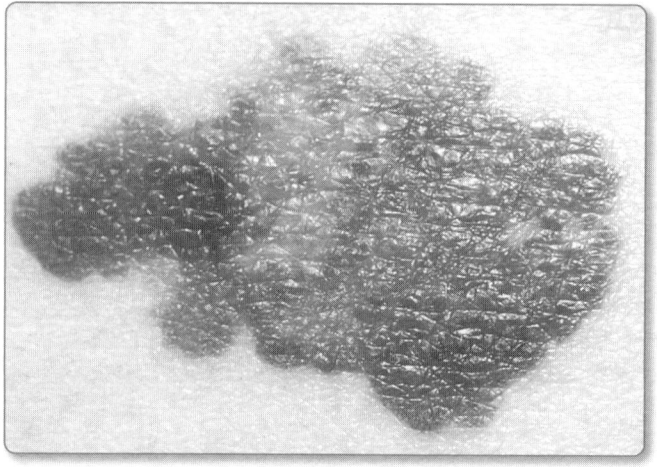

Q. 8.1 Describe the skin lesion.

Asymmetrical, irregular bordered, pigmented, and non-elevated skin lesion.

Q. 8.2 What is the likely diagnosis?

The lesion has the characteristic features of a malignant melanoma.

Q. 8.3 What differential diagnoses should be considered?

The following differential diagnoses should be considered:
- Atypical mole (Clark naevus or dysplastic naevus)
- Basal cell carcinoma
- Blue naevus

- Cherry haemangioma
- Cutaneous squamous cell carcinoma
- Dermatofibroma
- Halo naevus
- Keloid and hypertrophic scar
- Keratoacanthoma
- Lentigo
- Melanocytic naevus
- Seborrheic keratosis
- Spitz naevus
- Vitiligo
- Mycosis fungoides
- Benign melanocytic lesions
- Sebaceous carcinoma

Q. 8.4 How would you manage the patient?

Clinical assessment of regional lymph nodes – cervical, axillary, and inguinal
   Urgent excision biopsy with adequate surgical margins – Wide local excision

Breslow thickness	Excision margin
In situ	0.5 cm
<1 mm	1 cm
1–2 mm	1–2 cm
2–4 mm	2–3 cm
>4 mm	3 cm

Sentinel lymph node biopsy:
- CT/MRI brain, CT thorax, abdomen, and pelvis to detect nodal and distant metastasis (PET-CT) – Stage IIc/III/IV patients

Referral to specialist oncology unit/multi-disciplinary team
- Patient may require radical lymph node dissection (controversial)
- Patient may also require adjuvant treatment including chemotherapy, targeted therapy, immunotherapy, and radiotherapy

Q. 8.5 What types of melanomas occur?

Melanoma is divided into the following types:
- Lentigo maligna
- Lentigo maligna melanoma
- Superficial spreading melanoma
- Acral lentiginous melanoma
- Mucosal melanoma

- Nodular melanoma
- Polypoid melanoma
- Desmoplastic melanoma

Q. 8.6 How do we stage melanoma?

TNM staging

Also of importance are the 'Clark level' and 'Breslow's depth', which refer to the microscopic depth of tumour invasion.

Tumour describes the thickness of the melanoma. There are six main stages of tumour thickness in melanoma – Tis to T4.

- *Tis* means the melanoma cells are only in the very top layer of the skin surface. It is called *melanoma in situ*
- *T0* means no melanoma cells can be seen where the melanoma started (primary site)
- *T1* means the melanoma is 1 mm thick or less. It is split into T1a and T1b
- *T1a* means the melanoma is <0.8 mm thick and the skin over the tumour does not look broken under the microscope (not ulcerated)
- *T1b* means either:
  - The melanoma is <0.8 mm thick but is ulcerated.
  - The melanoma is between 0.8 mm and 1.0 mm and may or may not be ulcerated.
- *T2* means the melanoma is between 1 mm and 2 mm thick
- *T3* means the melanoma is between 2 mm and 4 mm thick
- *T4* means the melanoma is >4 mm thick

T2 and T4 melanomas are further divided into 'a' and 'b' depending on whether it is ulcerated or not. 'a' means without ulceration, and 'b' means with ulceration.

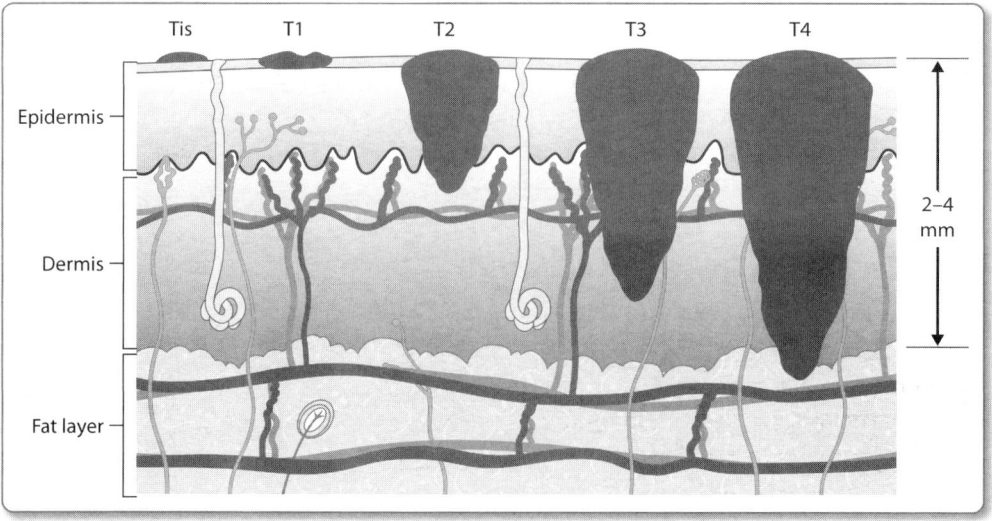

Regional metastasis:
- *N1*: Single positive lymph
- *N2*: Two-to-three positive lymph nodes *or* regional skin/in-transit metastasis
- *N3*: Four positive lymph nodes *or* one lymph node and regional skin/in-transit metastases

Distant metastasis
- *M1a*: Distant skin metastasis, normal lactate dehydrogenase (LDH)
- *M1b*: Lung metastasis, normal LDH
- *M1c*: Other distant metastasis *or* any distant metastasis with elevated LDH

Anatomic stage/prognostic groups

	Clinical staging				Pathologic staging		
Stage 0	Tis	N0	M0	0	Tis	N0	M0
Stage IA	T1a	N0	M0	IA	T1a	N0	M0
Stage IB	T1b	N0	M0	IB	T1b	N0	M0
	T2a	N0	M0		T2a	N0	M0
Stage IIA	T2b	N0	M0	IIA	T2b	N0	M0
	T3a	N0	M0		T3a	N0	M0
Stage IIB	13b	N0	M0	IIB	T3b	N0	M0
	T4a	N0	M0		T4a	N0	M0
Stage IIC	T4b	N0	M0	IIC	T4b	N0	M0
Stage III	Any T	>N1	M0	IIIa	T1–4a	N1a	M0
					T1–4a	N2a	M0
				IIIB	T1-4b	N1a	M0
					T1–4b	N2a	M0
					T1–4a	N1b	M0
					T1–4a	N2b	M0
					T1–4a	N2c	M0
				IIIC	T1–4b	N1b	M0
					T1–4b	N2b	M0
					T1–4b	N2c	M0
					Any T	N3	M0
Stage IV	Any T	Any N	M1	IV	Any T	Any N	M1

Q. 8.7 What factors affect the prognosis?

Factors that affect prognosis include:
- Tumour thickness in millimetres (Breslow's depth)
- Depth related to skin structures (Clark level)
- Type of melanoma
- Presence of ulceration
- Presence of lymphatic/perineural invasion
- Presence of tumour-infiltrating lymphocytes (if present, prognosis is better)
- Location of lesion
- Presence of satellite lesions, and
- Presence of regional or distant metastasis

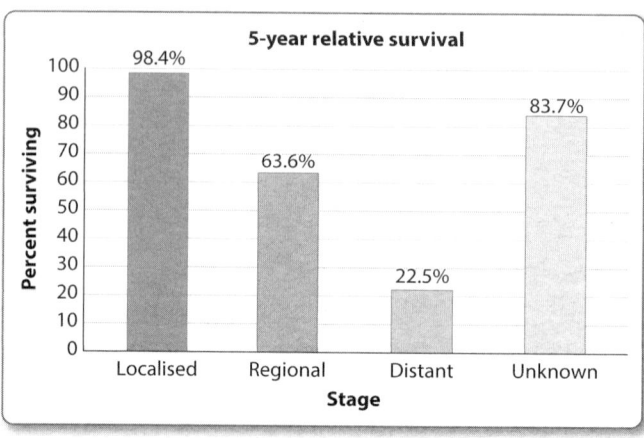

Further reading

National Collaborating Centre for Cancer (UK). Melanoma: assessment and management. London: National Institute for Health and Care Excellence (NICE), 2015.

Scenario 9

Lymphadenopathy

A 60-year-old male presents with non-tender, hard left supraclavicular lymphadenopathy. He has lost 1 stone in weight over a 4-month period. He is having drenching night sweats.

Q. 9.1 What clinical sign does this patient have?

Troisier's sign, which is the finding of an enlarged, hard Virchow's node (left supraclavicular node).

Q. 9.2 From where do the lymphatics drain into this lymph node?

The left supraclavicular nodes are the classical Virchow's node because they receive lymphatic drainage of most of the body (from the thoracic duct) and enters the venous circulation via the left subclavian vein.

Virchow's nodes take their supply from lymph vessels in the abdominal cavity, and are therefore sentinel lymph nodes of cancer in the abdomen, particularly gastric cancer, ovarian cancer, testicular cancer and kidney cancer, that have spread through the lymph vessels, and Hodgkin's lymphoma. Such spread typically results in Troisier's sign, which is the finding of an enlarged and hard Virchow's node.

Q. 9.3 What are the differential diagnoses to be considered?

- Lymphoma
- Infections – upper limb
- Breast cancer
- *Intraabdominal malignancies:* Gastric, ovarian, renal, and testicular

Q. 9.4 How would you investigate this patient?

- Clinical examination of cervical, axillary, and inguinal node areas
- Clinical examination of the abdomen – hepatic masses/enlargement, splenomegaly, palpable masses, testicular examination
- *Blood tests:* Carcinoembryonic antigen (CEA), human chorionic gonadotropin (hCG), alpha feto-protein (AFP), and cancer antigen-125 (Ca-125)
- Fine-needle aspiration (FNA) cytology/core needle biopsy
- Excision biopsy of the lymph node

- *CT:* Thorax/Abdomen/Pelvis
- Examination reveals left axillary lymphadenopathy, with no evidence of abdominal masses, or hepatosplenomegaly
- CT confirms iliac lymphadenopathy, but no other pathology
- Biopsy confirms the presence of multinucleated Reed–Sternberg cells (RS)

Q. 9.5 What is the diagnosis?

Hodgkin's lymphoma.

Q. 9.6 What is the stage of the disease?

Stage III – with lymphadenopathy on both sides of the diaphragm.
Staging in Hodgkin's lymphoma (Ann Arbor staging classification):
- Stage I is involvement of a single lymph node region (I) (mostly the cervical region) or single extra-lymphatic site (Ie)
- Stage II is involvement of two or more lymph node regions on the same side of the diaphragm (II) or of one lymph node region and a contiguous extra-lymphatic site (IIe)
- Stage III is involvement of lymph node regions on both sides of the diaphragm, which may include the spleen (IIIs) or limited contiguous extra-lymphatic organ or site (IIIe, IIIes)
- Stage IV is disseminated involvement of one or more extra-lymphatic organs

Q. 9.7 What pathological sub-types exist?

- Nodular sclerosing
- Mixed cellularity
- Lymphocyte rich
- Lymphocyte depleted

Nodular sclerosing: It is the most common sub-type and is composed of large tumour *nodules* showing scattered lacunar classical RS cells set in a background of reactive lymphocytes, eosinophils and plasma cells with varying degrees of collagen fibrosis/sclerosis.

Mixed cellularity: It is a common sub-type and is composed of numerous classic RS cells admixed with numerous inflammatory cells including lymphocytes, histiocytes, eosinophils, and plasma cells without sclerosis. This type is most often associated with Epstein–Barr virus (EBV) infection and may be confused with the early, so-called 'cellular' phase of nodular sclerosing classical Hodgkin lymphoma (CHL).

Lymphocyte rich: It is a rare sub-type, shows many features which may cause diagnostic confusion with nodular lymphocyte predominant B-cell non-Hodgkin lymphoma (B-NHL). This form also has the most favourable prognosis.

Lymphocyte depleted: It is a rare sub-type and composed of large numbers of often pleomorphic RS cells with only few reactive lymphocytes which may easily be confused with diffuse large cell lymphoma. Many cases previously classified within this category would now be re-classified under anaplastic large cell lymphoma.

Further reading

Eichenauer DA, Aleman BMP, André M, et al. Hodgkin lymphoma: ESMO Clinical Practice Guidelines for diagnosis, treatment and follow-up. Ann Oncol 2018; 29:iv19–iv29.

Follows GA, Barrington SF, Bhuller KS, et al. Guideline for the first-line management of Classical Hodgkin Lymphoma — A British Society for Haematology guideline. Br J Haematol 2022; 197:558–572.

Scenario 10

Venous thromboembolism

A 60-year-old male presents with left leg swelling. This developed somewhat suddenly over the last 48 hours, but now is tender and associated with redness from the calf to the knee.

He underwent a total hip replacement 3 weeks ago and has recovered well post-operatively.

Q. 10.1 What is Virchow's triad?

Virchow's triad or the triad of Virchow describes the three broad categories of factors that are thought to contribute to thrombosis.
1. Hypercoagulability
2. Haemodynamic changes (stasis and turbulence)
3. Endothelial injury/dysfunction

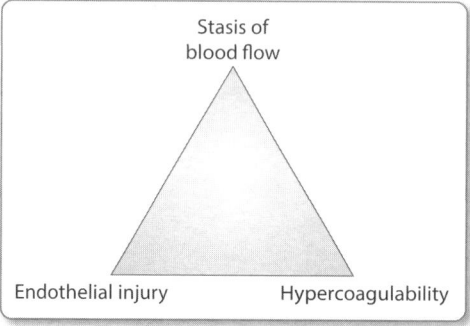

Stasis
These include venous stasis, long surgical operations, prolonged immobility (while on a long plane or car ride, bed bound during hospitalisation), and varicose veins.

Endothelial injury
Injuries and/or trauma to endothelium include vessel piercings and damages arising from shear stress or hypertension. This category is ruled by surface phenomena and contact with procoagulant surfaces, such as bacteria, shards of foreign materials, biomaterials of implants or medical devices, membranes of activated platelets, and membranes of monocytes in chronic inflammation.

Hypercoagulability

Alterations in the constitution of blood have numerous possible risk factors such as hyperviscosity, coagulation factor V Leiden mutation, coagulation factor II G2021A mutation, deficiency of antithrombin III, protein C or S deficiency, nephrotic syndrome, changes after severe trauma or burns, cancer, late pregnancy and delivery, race, advanced age, cigarette smoking, hormonal contraceptives, and obesity. All of these risk factors can cause the situation called hypercoagulability (excessively easy clotting of blood).

Q. 10.2 What measures can be taken to reduce the risk of perioperative VTE?

Preoperative:
- Smoking cessation
- Weight reduction
- Oral contraceptive pill – stopping 4–6 weeks prior to surgery
- Adequate hydration
- Low molecular weight heparin (LMWH) or fondaparinux sodium

Intraoperative:
- Antiembolism stockings – graduated compression stockings
- Intermittent pneumatic calf compression
- Adequate hydration
- Optimal oxygenation

Postoperative:
- LMWH or fondaparinux sodium – duration?
- Adequate hydration
- Early mobilisation and leg exercises
- Chest physiotherapy

Q. 10.3 What is the mechanism of action of heparin in the coagulation cascade?

Heparin binds to the enzyme inhibitor antithrombin III, causing a conformational change that results in its activation. The activated antithrombin III then inactivates thrombin, factor Xa and other proteases.

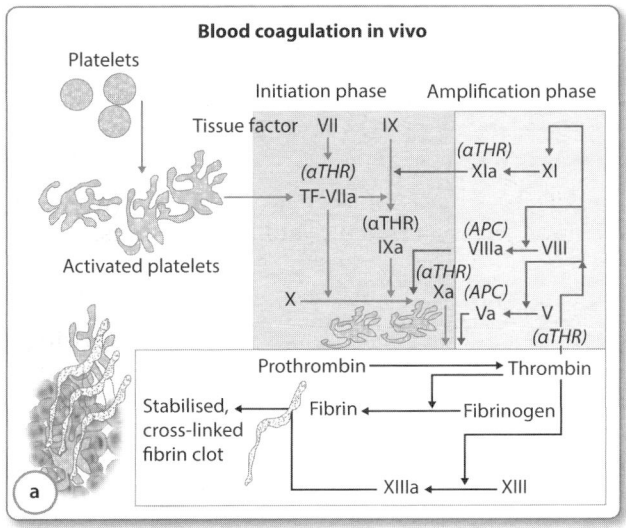

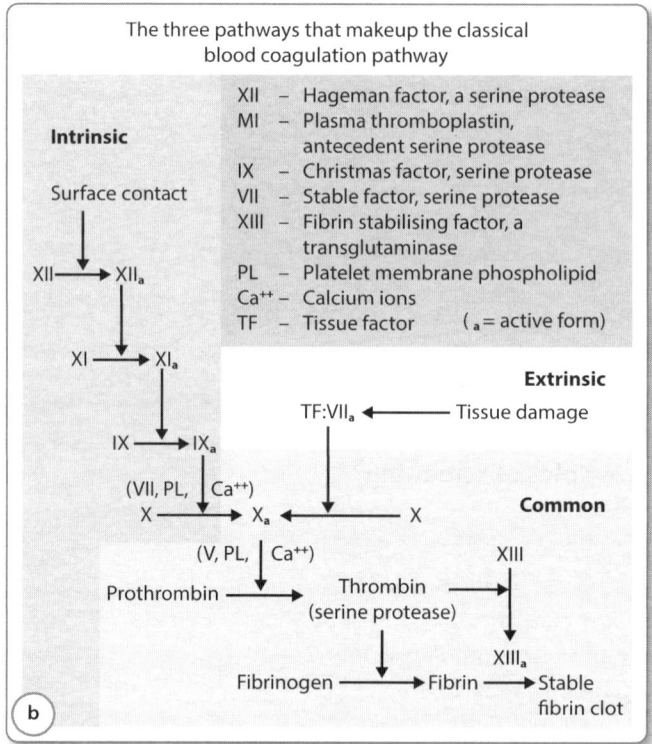

Q. 10.4 How can heparin be reversed?

Heparin reversal: Protamine sulphate 1 mg neutralises 100 units of heparin. Administer protamine up to a maximum of 50 mg in a single dose as slow IV infusion over 10 minutes (anaphylaxis has been reported). Avoid protamine in patients with allergies to fish or fish products.

Further reading

National Institute for Health Care and Excellence (NICE) guideline [NG89]. (2018). Venous thromboembolism in over 16 s: Reducing the risk of hospital-acquired deep vein thrombosis or pulmonary embolism. [online] Available from https://www.nice.org.uk/guidance/ng89 [Last accessed March, 2023].

Scenario 11

Screening

You see a 72-year-old male patient in clinic following a colonoscopy as part of the national screening program. He has had a polyp biopsied, and you are about to discuss the results with him.

Q. 11.1 What are the basic principles of screening?

The principles of screening:
WHO guidelines 1968:
- The condition should be an important health problem
- There should be a treatment for the condition
- Facilities for diagnosis and treatment should be available
- There should be a latent stage of the disease
- There should be a test or examination for the condition
- The test should be acceptable to the population
- The natural history of the disease should be adequately understood
- There should be an agreed policy on whom to treat
- The total cost of finding a case should be economically balanced in relation to medical expenditure as a whole
- Case-finding should be a continuous process, not just a 'once and for all' project

WHO modifications 2008:
- The screening programme should respond to a recognised need
- The objectives of screening should be defined at the outset
- There should be a defined target population
- There should be scientific evidence of screening programme effectiveness
- The programme should integrate education, testing, clinical services and programme management
- There should be quality assurance with mechanisms to minimise potential risks of screening
- The programme should ensure informed choice, confidentiality and respect for autonomy
- The programme should promote equity and access to screening for the entire target population
- Programme evaluation should be planned from the outset
- The overall benefits of screening should outweigh the harm

Q. 11.2 Describe an example of screening.

Examples of screening:
- *Cancer screening:*
  - Pap smear or liquid-based cytology to detect potentially precancerous lesions and prevent cervical cancer
  - Mammography to detect breast cancer
  - Colonoscopy and faecal occult blood test to detect colorectal cancer
  - Dermatological check to detect melanoma
  - Prostate specific antigen (PSA) to detect prostate cancer
- Purified protein derivative (PPD) test to screen for exposure to tuberculosis
- Beck Depression Inventory to screen for depression
- Brief form of the social phobia and anxiety inventory (SPAI-B), the Liebowitz Social Anxiety Scale and social phobia inventory to screen for social anxiety disorder
- Alpha-fetoprotein, blood tests and ultrasound scans for pregnant women to detect foetal abnormalities
- Bitewing radiographs to screen for interproximal dental caries
- Ophthalmoscopy or digital photography and image grading for diabetic retinopathy
- Ultrasound scan for AAA
- Screening of potential sperm bank donors
- Screening for metabolic syndrome
- Screening for potential hearing loss in newborns

Q. 11.3 What are the limitations of screening?

- Screening can involve cost and use of medical resources on a majority of people who do not need treatment
- Adverse effects of screening procedure (e.g. stress and anxiety, discomfort, radiation exposure, and chemical exposure)
- Stress and anxiety caused by prolonging knowledge of an illness without any improvement in outcome. This problem is referred to as overdiagnosis
- Stress and anxiety caused by a false positive screening result
- Unnecessary investigation and treatment of false positive results (namely misdiagnosis with type I error)
- A false sense of security caused by false negatives, which may delay final diagnosis (namely misdiagnosis with type II error)

Q. 11.4 What are type I and type II errors?

In statistical hypothesis testing:
- *Type I error*, also known as a *'false positive'*: The error of rejecting a null hypothesis when it is actually true. In other words, this is the error of accepting an alternative hypothesis (the real hypothesis of interest) when the results can be attributed to chance. It occurs when we are observing a difference when in truth there is none (or more specifically – no statistically significant difference)

- *Type II error*, also known as a *'false negative'*: The error of not rejecting a null hypothesis when the alternative hypothesis is the true state of nature. In other words, this is the error of failing to accept an alternative hypothesis when you do not have adequate power. It occurs when we are failing to observe a difference when in truth there is one

Further reading

Screening Programmes: A short guide. https://apps.who.int/iris/bitstream/handle/10665/330829/9789289054782-eng.pdf [Accessed 1st April 2023]

Scenario 12

Laparoscopy

35-year-old female patient with known gallstones presents with acute cholecystitis. She is booked on CEPOD for a laparoscopic cholecystectomy.

Q. 12.1 What methods are available to safely establish pneumoperitoneum in laparoscopic surgery?

- Open technique (Hasson) – direct vision – umbilical
- Closed technique (Veress needle) – umbilical (U), left upper quadrant – Palmer's point (P), midline upper abdomen – Lee-Huang point (L-H)
- Optical access technique – umbilical, Palmer's point, Lee-Huang point
- Safety tests (Veress) – Irrigation and aspiration test, hanging drop test, and gas insufflation test

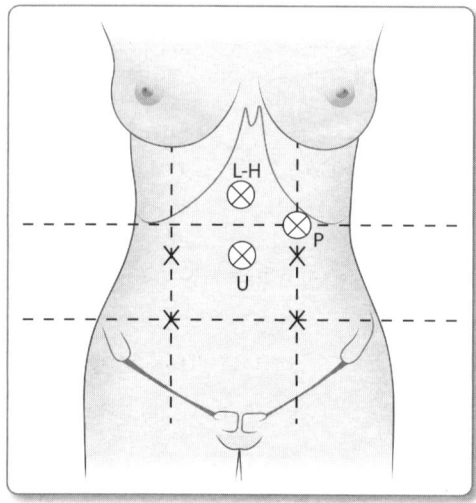

Q. 12.2 What complications can arise related to laparoscopic access?

Major: (1.4–5.7/1,000)
- Small bowel injury
- Colonic injury
- Bladder injury
- Gastric injury

- Vascular injury arterial and venous – aorta, IVC, iliac vessels (mortality rate 15%)
- CO_2 gas embolism (0.001%)
- Mortality
- Omental injury – bleeding

Minor:
- Inferior epigastric injury – bleeding
- Abdominal wall haematoma
- Wound infection
- Port site hernias (40%)

Q. 12.3 What physiologic effects occur during CO_2 pneumoperitoneum?

Systemic absorption of CO_2
- *Hypercapnia*: Cardiac arrhythmias, vasoconstriction of the pulmonary vessels, and a mixed response in cardiac function, autonomic nervous system stimulation leading to tachycardia and increased myocardial contractility
- *Acidosis*: Depressed myocardial contractility

Increased requirements for CO_2 elimination

Increased abdominal pressure
- *Haemodynamic changes and cardiac function*: Increased heart rate, increased mean arterial pressure, reduced cardiac output, increased systemic vascular resistance, increased central venous pressure
- *Hepatic function*: Decreased portal venous flow – hepatic hypoperfusion and acute hepatocyte injury – causing raised alanine transaminase (ALT) and aspartate transaminase (AST)
- *Pulmonary function*: Decreased respiratory compliance, increased airway pressure, increased respiratory rate, decreased tidal volume, increased minute ventilation
- *Renal function*: Decreased urine volume
- *Venous stasis*: Reduced femoral venous flow – compressive effect on iliac veins

Q. 12.4 How would you define a 'Hostile' abdomen for laparoscopic surgery?
- A 'hostile abdomen' is an abdomen that has either undergone previous surgical intervention, penetrating trauma, sepsis, or radiation
- This increases the amount of intraabdominal adhesion formation, which increases the risks of bleeding and bowel injury during laparoscopic access and surgery

Further reading

Holihan JL, Chen JS, Greenberg J, et al. Incidence of Port-Site Hernias: A Survey and Literature Review. Surg Laparosc Endosc Percutan Tech 2016; 26:425–430.

Krishnakumar S, Tambe P. Entry Complications in Laparoscopic Surgery. J Gynecol Endosc Surg 2009; 1:4–11.

Scenario 13

Nutrition

42-year-old alcoholic presents with profuse vomiting and epigastric pain. He is admitted to HDU, and an NG tube is inserted. He develops ARDS and delirium and pulls out his NG tube and requires a short stay on HDU.

After he returns to the ward the dietician notices that his nutritional intake has been very poor, and he looks malnourished.

Q. 13.1 What is re-feeding syndrome?

The re-feeding syndrome is a potentially fatal condition, caused by rapid initiation of re-feeding after a period of undernutrition.

It is characterised by hypophosphataemia, associated with fluid and electrolyte shifts and metabolic and clinical complications.

During starvation, intracellular electrolyte stores, particularly phosphate, are depleted despite normal serum concentrations. Feeding stimulates the cellular uptake of electrolytes and can lead to electrolyte disturbances with profound hypophosphataemia.

The syndrome is complex and may also feature abnormal sodium and fluid balance; changes in glucose, protein, and fat metabolism; thiamine deficiency; hypokalaemia; and hypomagnesaemia.

Clinical features usually develop within 4 days of re-feeding but are often non-specific – fatigue, weakness and confusion.

Later manifestations include rhabdomyolysis, cardiac failure, hypotension, arrhythmias, respiratory failure, seizures, coma and death.

Q. 13.2 What other complications can occur in patients receiving total parenteral nutrition (TPN)?

Central venous catheter complications:
- Infection
- Sepsis
- Pneumothorax
- Vascular injury
- Thrombophlebitis
- Deep vein thrombosis
- Pulmonary embolism
- Mortality

Hepatobiliary dysfunction:
- Hepatic steatosis
- Steatohepatitis
- Hepatic failure
- Cholestasis
- Cholelithiasis
- Biliary sludge

Metabolic complications:
- Re-feeding syndrome
- Overfeeding
- Hyperglycaemia
- Hypoglycaemia
- Ketoacidosis
- Hypertriglyceridaemia
- Hyperazotaemia
- Hypercalcaemia

Others:
- Fluid overload
- Coagulopathy
- Hypersensitivity
- Hunger

Classification of complications

Q. 13.3 What systems for classification of postoperative complications do you know of?

- The Clavien–Dindo classification
- The Accordion score

Q. 13.4 Can you describe them to me?

The Clavien–Dindo classification is outlined in the table below. Have a good grasp of these different grades, and know that there are *five*. Remember that:
- For grade I complications, some pharmacological treatments are allowed
- Grade III complications are further stratified into IIIa (surgical/endoscopic/radiological interventions not under general anaesthetic); and IIIb (interventions under general anaesthetic)
- Grade IV complications are stratified into IVa (single organ dysfunction) and IVb (multi-organ dysfunction)

\multicolumn{2}{|c|}{Classification of surgical complications}
Grade	Definition
Grade I	- Any deviation from the normal postoperative course without the need for pharmacological treatment or surgical, endoscopic, and radiological interventions - Allowed therapeutic regimens are – drugs as antiemetics, antipyretics, analgesics, diuretics, electrolytes, and physiotherapy. This grade also includes wound infections opened at the bedside
Grade II	- Requiring pharmacological treatment with drugs other than such allowed for grade I complications - Blood transfusions and total parenteral nutrition are also included
Grade III	Requiring surgical, endoscopic or radiological intervention
Grade IIIa	Intervention not under general anaesthesia
Grade IIIb	Intervention under general anaesthesia
Grade IV	Life-threatening complication (including CNS complications)* requiring IC/ICU management
Grade IVa	Single organ dysfunction (including dialysis)
Grade IVb	Multi-organ dysfunction
Grade V	Death of a patient
Suffix 'd'	If the patient suffers from a complication at the time of discharge (see examples in the next Table), the suffix 'd' (for 'disability') is added to the respective grade of complication. This label indicates the need for a follow-up to fully evaluate the complication

(CNS, central nervous system; IC, intermediate care; ICU, intensive care unit)
*Brain haemorrhage, ischaemic stroke, sub-arachnoidal bleeding, but excluding transient ischaemic attacks.
Source: With permission from Dindo et al. (2004).

The Accordion Score is outlined below:

Severity grade	Grading criteria
Mild complication	- Requires minor invasive procedures that can be done at bedside, e.g. catheter - Physiotherapy and following drugs are allowed–antiemetic, antipyretic, analgesics, diuretics, electrolytes
Moderate	Requires pharmacological treatment other than those allowed for minor complications, e.g. antibiotics, blood transfusion, TPN
Severe: Invasive procedure without general anaesthetic	For example, radiological guided drain under local anaesthetic
Severe: Operation under general anaesthetic	For example, closure of full thickness dehiscence of abdominal wound
Organ system failure	Applies to one or more organ system failure
Death	

Q. 13.5 A patient develops continuous blood per rectum on postoperative day 1 after an elective laparoscopic right hemicolectomy. Their haemoglobin is 69 g/L. The patient remains haemodynamically normal, but requires transfusion of 6 units of blood to keep their haemoglobin above 70 g/L over the next 24 hours. A CT angiogram is performed on postoperative day 2 and is normal. The patient continues to pass small amounts of blood, and requires another 6 units of blood. The surgeon decides to continue conservative management. By postoperative day 3, the bleeding has stopped, and the patient's haemoglobin is now 98 g/L. What grade or score of complication has this patient suffered?

- Clavien–Dindo grade II
- Accordion score 2

Q. 13.6 The patient's operating surgeon goes away on holiday on postoperative day 5. On postoperative day 6, the patient begins to pass blood per rectum again, but remains haemodynamically normal. The haemoglobin on this day is 64 g/L. The on-call surgeon decides to take them for a colonoscopy under general anaesthetic. What grade or score of complication does this patient now suffer? How does this example highlight a disadvantage of these classifications?

- Clavien-Dindo grade IIIb
- Accordion score 4

Different surgeons will take different approaches to complications. The patient's operating surgeon felt the bleeding would settle without intervention, whereas the on-call surgeon did not.

In spite of the detail, in practice the grades do not always appreciate the severity of complication – the patient in this scenario has required 12 units of bloods over a 48-hour period – although this cannot quite be defined as massive blood transfusion, it is a significant deviation from the expected postoperative course of an elective right hemicolectomy.

Further reading

Dindo D, Demartines N, Clavien PA. Classification of surgical complications: a new proposal with evaluation in a cohort of 6336 patients and results of a survey. Ann Surg 2004; 240:205–213.

Scenario 14

Diathermy

You are about to start an inguinal hernia repair under general anaesthetic. Your scrub staff and assistant are relatively junior and are uncertain about where the diathermy plate should be placed.

Q. 14.1 What are the principles of diathermy plate placement?

The plate should not be sited close to any *metal implants*. It should be as *close* to the area of surgery as is safely possible. The site of the plate should be *clean* and *free of hair* – the area should thus be shaved well if necessary; hairs can lead to diathermy plate burns. *Bony regions* and areas of *scar tissue* should also be avoided. There should be *good contact* between the patient and the plate, and the thus the plate should not be crumpled or folded. If in doubt, do not place the plate yourself.

Q. 14.2 In what circumstances monopolar diathermy is contraindicated?

The only absolute contraindication is use on *end-arterial organs/appendages,* i.e. fingers, ears, the nose and the penis. This is because if the main artery supplying these is thrombosed for whatever reason, use of monopolar diathermy will coagulate the rest of the vasculature to them, resulting in necrosis.

Q. 14.3 This patient has a pacemaker. Is the use of monopolar diathermy absolutely contraindicated? Explain your answer and how you would approach this situation.

Pacemakers and defibrillators are not absolute contraindications to monopolar diathermy, though the concerns are that the *diathermy can interfere with the pacemaker*; and that *energy can be transferred through the leads* of the device and cause heating of tissue.

There are *preoperative, perioperative* and *postoperative considerations.*

Preoperatively, one needs to ascertain the *indication*, and the exact *type of device*. Patients often carry *cards* with them that give information regarding the device, or this information can be found in the notes. Then inform a *cardiologist*, or a *cardiac technician*, and the *anaesthetist*. A joint decision can then be reached. Sometimes monopolar diathermy is contraindicated; however, some devices can be switched to safe mode.

During surgery, *extracardiac monitoring* may be needed; the team should ensure that they are ready to pace, or cardiovert should life-threatening arrythmias evolve – this might involve placing defibrillator pads on the patient's chest, or having pacing equipment on standby.

After surgery, cardiac technicians need to be informed to *switch the device back on, and test*. Cardiac devices do not preclude patients from having day case surgery or being cared for on a level one bed afterwards, but you should be guided by local protocols.

Q. 14.4 What methods of intraoperative haemostasis aside from diathermy do you know?

- Manual pressure
- Ultrasonic, e.g. harmonic scalpel
- Surgical clip application, e.g. Liga-clips, artery forceps, larger clips such as Roberts'
- Ligatures, i.e. hand ties
- Sutures
- Products, e.g. Surgicel

Further reading

Watson AB, Loughman J. The surgical diathermy: principles of operation and safe use. Anaesth Intensive Care 1978;6:310-21. doi: 10–321.

Scenario 15

Principles of consent

You are about to consent a 54-year-old gentleman with a right-sided inguinal hernia.

Q. 15.1 Talk me through how you would consent this patient?

When discussing consent, candidates usually focus on risks and complications. It is important to discuss the benefits and alternatives as well.

You should explain that the operation has *more benefits than risk*. The benefits of hernia surgery are primarily *prognostic* – to prevent incarceration or strangulation. If the patient has a painful hernia, there is also *symptomatic* benefit.

Discussing complications and risks in the format of early and late, specific and general is not necessarily the best way to start – the examiners will want to see that you know *the important, relevant risks of the operation*, and you should begin with these. Remember, the main risks of hernia are surgery present late. If you spend 30 seconds to a minute talking about early complications, you may run out of time and not get a chance to talk about the more relevant risks. It should also be noted that the consent process has changed slightly over the last decade to focusing on any complication, no matter how rare, that could be relevant to a specific individual. This means that the traditional view of stating complications > 1% or serious complications has been expanded.

The main risks that come with hernia surgery are *recurrence*, and *chronic pain*. You will be expected to quote recurrence rates – 1% for open surgery, and 2% for laparoscopic. The exact rates of chronic pain are not exactly known, but you could state that anecdotally, the rate is low. The chronic pain rate is lower with laparoscopic surgery.

Other risks can then be categorised into early and late; specific and general. Early, specific complications include visceral perforation, which is rare (but may be more relevant if the patient is having a laparoscopic transabdominal approach), urinary retention, acute pain, numbness around the incision and groin, scrotal swelling and bruising.

Early, general complications are bleeding and pain; and risks associated with general anaesthesia.

Late, specific complications are recurrence and chronic pain – which you should have already mentioned by now, as well as testicular atrophy, persistent numbness, and mesh infection. If the patient is having laparoscopic surgery, you should mention port site hernia.

The alternative is no surgery, with a watch and wait approach – you could invite the patient back from an annual review in clinic. You can offer the patient a truss. You should explain that without an operation, the hernia will always be present, and they are at risk of incarceration or strangulation. Though these carry significant morbidity, the life-time risk is low.

Q. 15.2 Imagine you are now seeing the patient in the emergency setting. The patient has severe learning difficulties. There is a scar over the groin already. His wife is present and confirms that he had a hernia in the right groin operated on over 10 years ago. She is his next of kin. While trying to consent him, you note that he does neither appear to be able to understand or retain the information you are giving him, nor can he weigh up the risks and benefits. Can his wife consent for him?

No, his wife cannot consent for him. In the UK, no adult can provide consent for another adult to undergo medical treatment. However, the wife should of course be involved in the discussion as much as possible, i.e. she should be told the risks and benefits of the surgery.

Q. 15.3 What would you do next in this setting with regard to consenting this patient?

- A 'type 4 consent' should be utilised
- A patient is considered competent to consent if they can *understand* the information they are given, *retain* the information they are given, and *weigh up* the risks and benefits of the treatment
- Type 4 consent is when the clinician goes ahead and consents a patient for medical treatment or surgery if they feel the patient is not competent to consent, and receiving the treatment is in their best interests
- The wife should not make this decision – it is the surgeon who needs to make the decision in the best interests of the patient. As above, the wife should still be included in the discussion, and she may also sign the consent form
- A second opinion should be sought for such cases. This can come in the form of a discussion between colleagues within the surgical team, i.e. the surgical registrar and the surgical consultant agreeing that type 4 consent is necessary

Q. 15.4 Imagine that you are seeing a male patient who is 14 years old and has presented with acute testicular pain to the accident and emergency (A&E) department. He is alone. Can he give consent? What is the principle used to guide clinicians for consenting children?

Yes, he can give consent. According to the UK law, individuals are deemed adults on their 18th birthday. Those aged 16 years or less need to be deemed '*Gillick competent*' to give consent.

Gillick competency arose from a court case in 1983. Victoria Gillick took her local health authority to court, challenging them for giving contraceptive advice to patients under 16 years of age without parental consent. The House of Lords eventually ruled that a doctor could give advice and treatment to patients <16 years of age if:

- The young patient has sufficient maturity and intelligence to understand the nature and implications of the treatment
- The young patient's physical or mental health is likely to suffer unless they received the treatment
- The advice or treatment is in the young patient's best interests

Q. 15.5 What are the Fraser guidelines?

The Fraser guidelines are frequently confused with the Gillick test. The Gillick test broadly refers to a young patient's capacity to consent, whereas the Fraser guidelines refer to a young patient's capacity to accept advice and treatment, specifically in relation to contraception. They adhere to the above principles and should help to provide guidance to clinicians when discussing contraception with young patients. According to the guidelines, clinicians should provide advice and treatment if:
- The young patient is likely to commence and continue sexual intercourse with or without contraception
- The young patient cannot be persuaded to tell her parents or allow the clinician to tell them
- It is in the patient's best interests to take contraception

Further reading

https://www.gmc-uk.org/ethical-guidance/ethical-guidance-for-doctors/0-18-years [Accessed 1st April 2023]

Scenario 16

Splenectomy and post-splenectomy management

You are seeing a 35-year-old woman who has been referred for consideration of splenectomy.

Q. 16.1 What are the indications for splenectomy?

The indications for splenectomy can be thought of as *emergency* and *elective*:

Emergency
- Traumatic rupture
- Spontaneous rupture

Elective
- *Haematological*:
  - Idiopathic thrombocytopenic purpura (ITP)
  - Autoimmune haemolytic anaemia
  - Hodgkin's disease
- *Non-haematological*:
  - During gastrectomy
  - During pancreatectomy

Q. 16.2 What will you tell her about the postoperative care she will require following a splenectomy?

You should explain that the spleen plays a role in protecting against infection. After the operation, she will receive *vaccinations* against three specific microbes – *pneumococcal, meningococcal* and *haemophilus influenzae* vaccinations.

She will require antibiotic tablets called *penicillin V,* every day for the rest of her life. This is to further protect her from infection. You should advise her that she is still at risk from a quite serious infection in her lifetime known as *overwhelming postsplenectomy infection (OPSI)*, although it is rare, with a risk of <1% every year. It starts as a flu-like illness that rapidly worsens with symptoms of migraine, abdominal pain, vomiting, nausea, myalgia, headaches and rashes. You should advise her to *carry an information card* with them in their wallet or purse, and also, if possible, an *alert bracelet* or pendant. When going abroad, she should ensure she has her penicillin V with her to take, and should be aware of the *infection risks of whichever country she visits,* e.g. is malaria prevalent, etc.

After discharge, she should *avoid contact sports* for 3 months.

Q. 16.3 She tells you that she is a Jehovah's witness and will not accept blood transfusion. Can you name some alternatives to blood transfusion that you can offer this patient?

Many patients who are Jehovah's witness will not accept the transfusion of allogenic and autologous blood. However, this is not the case for all Jehovah's witnesses, and a discussion about their wishes, and the risk of not having transfusion should still take place. Other options of maintaining blood levels during surgery are:
- Intraoperative cell salvage machine
- Tranexamic acid
- IV albumin
- IV iron

Erythropoiesis stimulating agents are of more use in the elective setting and are usually administered preoperatively. One should discuss these options with the patient, in case they are actually not acceptable to them.

Q. 16.4 She undergoes laparoscopic splenectomy, but it is converted to open. She is a little slow to mobilise post-surgery. She develops a fever (38.7°C) and tachycardia on postoperative day 5. What are your differentials for this?

Local causes
- Pancreatic leak/fistula
- Visceral perforation, e.g. stomach/colon/small bowel
- Collection

Non-local causes
- Pneumonia
- Line infection
- Urinary infection
- Wound infection
- Overwhelming postsplenectomy infection

Remember, OPSI is rare, but patients undergoing elective splenectomy – especially for haematological disorders – carry a higher risk than those undergoing emergency splenectomy. Though uncommon, it carries a high risk of mortality. It is thus important to consider other differentials.

Further reading

Update of guidelines for the prevention and treatment of infection in patients with an absent or dysfunctional spleen. Available at https://b-s-h.org.uk/media/16267/spleen_bjh_2002.pdf [Accessed 1st April 2023]

Scenario 17

Meckel's diverticulum

During an open appendicectomy, you discover that the appendix is normal. You assess the small bowel. Your findings can be seen in the photograph below.

Q. 17.1 What is this? Can you tell me the embryological origin of it?

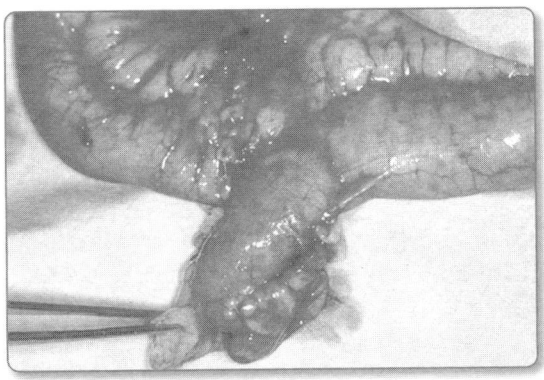

This is a Meckel's diverticulum. It is a remnant of the *omphalomesenteric (vitelline) duct*.

Q. 17.2 What rule of thumb should one use to help to locate one of these during surgery?

Use the rule of two – a Meckel's diverticulum is usually found *2 feet* from the ileocaecal valve; most commonly presents at *2 years of age*; and is *2 inches* in length.

Other components of the rule of two are that it is present in *2% of the population*; it is usually made up of *two types of tissue* (pancreatic and gastric); and affects males more commonly than females at *2:1 ratio*.

Q. 17.3 How does this usually present?

Although an important differential diagnosis for appendicitis, Meckel's diverticulum usually presents with *painless bleeding per rectum* in patients who are around 2 years of age. It should be considered as a differential in any patient with bleeding per rectum, where endoscopic and other investigations have been normal. It may also present with *inflammation* (Meckel's diverticulitis), *obstruction, perforation, intussusception* and *volvulus*.

It is, of course, also found incidentally.

Q. 17.4 You are seeing another patient with suspected Meckel's diverticulum; this time in out-patients. Your gastroenterology colleagues have referred the patient with bleeding per rectum; they have performed gastroscopy and colonoscopy, both which have been normal. What investigations will you consider?

A 'Meckel's scan' – this is *technetium-99m pertechnetate scintigraphy*. This is a nuclear medicine scan.

CT or *CTA* is more useful in the acute setting, where complicated Meckel's diverticulum is a differential.

In this brief scenario, it is also worth checking if the gastroenterologists have performed or are considering a *capsule endoscopy*.

Q. 17.5 What are the surgical options for resection?

The options are either *diverticulectomy* or *wedge/segmental resection*. The size of the diverticulum, how it appears at surgery, and the clinical picture it has caused will determine which approach is used. A segment of perforated or severely inflamed diverticulum should be resected as a wedge or a segment, and the healthy ends re-anastomosed.

Bleeding or simple diverticulitis can be treated with diverticulectomy. This usually involves stapling off the diverticulum.

Further reading

Spottswood SE, Pfluger T, Bartold SP, et al. SNMMI and EANM Practice Guideline for Meckel Diverticulum Scintigraphy 2.0 J Nucl Med Technol 2014; 42:163–169

Scenario 18

Anticoagulants

You are on call when an 84-year-old man with an obstructed inguino-scrotal hernia presents. He needs urgent surgery. He takes rivaroxaban for non-valvular atrial fibrillation.

Q. 18.1 What will you expect the haematologists to suggest for reversing the effect of the rivaroxaban; and what is the product made of?

Reversal agents for rivaroxaban can be considered as either *non-specific* or *specific*.

In this setting, for speed and ease of reversal, it is likely that the haematologists will suggest *prothrombin concentrate complex (PCC)*. The trade name for this is 'Beriplex'. It contains clotting factors II, IX and X. It is given intravenously.

Specific reversal agents include andexanet alfa and ciraparantag.

Vitamin K is not indicated here.

Q. 18.2 The surgery goes well and the patient returns to the ward on the same day. When will you re-start his rivaroxaban?

Tell the examiner what you would do, and be prepared to explain your rationale. Be guided by local protocols. Generally speaking, once you are satisfied that there is no evidence of ongoing bleeding, and the patient is no longer at risk of bleeding, you can re-start the patient's anticoagulation. Some surgeons prefer to withhold any anti-coagulant, including LMWH, while drains are still in.

Q. 18.3 Imagine you are in out-patients. You are about to see a patient who is on rivaroxaban; and has been referred to you for consideration of laparoscopic cholecystectomy. What things must you consider when planning how to manage his anticoagulation?

You should liaise with your haematology and anaesthetic colleagues, and use local guideline; but this alone not a sufficient answer in the examination. This can seem to be a complex task, but provided you ask yourself a structured set of questions, you can form an appropriate treatment plan:

Patient factors

- Indication for anticoagulation
- What anticoagulation are they on exactly, i.e. vitamin K antagonist, direct oral anticoagulant?

Surgical factors
- Major or minor procedure
- Risk of bleeding from procedure

Preoperative factors
- When to stop?
- Is there a need for bridging therapy?
- Will the patient need admission for bridging?
- What blood tests need to be taken prior to surgery?

Postoperative factors
- What are the risks of bleeding in the postoperative phase?
- Can you commence prophylactic doses of LMWH?
- When will you re-commence the anticoagulation and at what dose?

Further reading
Chen A, Stecker E, A Warden B. Direct Oral Anticoagulant Use: A Practical Guide to Common Clinical Challenges. J Am Heart Assoc 2020; 9:e017559.

Scenario 19

Clostridium difficile

You are referred an 89-year-old man with diabetes because he has developed cramping abdominal pain. He recently underwent debridement of an infected toe ulcer. During your review, you note that he has had 4 episodes of watery diarrhoea in the last 2 days. He looks dehydrated. His temperature is 37.7 and on examination his abdomen is distended but soft to palpation.

Q. 19.1 What is the likely diagnosis? What are your differential diagnoses?

As this patient almost certainly is on, or recently had antibiotics, one must suspect *Clostridium difficile*. Differentials include infectious (*Norovirus, Salmonella, Shigella*) and non-infectious (inflammatory bowel disease and diverticulitis).

Q. 19.2 Outline your management of this patient.

Conservative measures
- Stool sample to be sent
- Stool chart to begin
- Liaise with microbiology about stopping causative antibiotics
- Counsel patient and explain need for isolation
- Move to side room, ensure signs are up on the door and ensure gloves and aprons are provided to those who will come into contact with

Medical measures
- Check electrolytes and inflammatory markers
- Ensure the patient is well hydrated with IV fluids
- Order abdominal film to assess for mega colon
- Gauge severity and liaise with microbiology re: antibiotics for the *C. difficile*

Q. 19.3 What antibiotics will you give this patient for the *C. difficile*?

Currently, this patient appears to have mild-to-moderate disease. He should have *oral metronidazole*, 400 mg, three times a day.

Q. 19.4 Two days later, his white cell count goes up to 22, and the frequency of diarrhoea has gone up to 9 per day. Stool cultures confirm that he has *C. difficile*. What treatment should he receive now?

He should be commenced on *oral vancomycin*, 125 mg, four times a day.

Q. 19.5 The patient is significantly more tender on examination. He underwent a repeat abdominal film before your assessment. What are the radiological features you might expect?

An abdominal film may demonstrate *dilated large bowel >6 cm; thumb-printing, and loss of haustral markings*.

Q. 19.6 He is stable enough to undergo a CT scan, which is below. Please describe it.

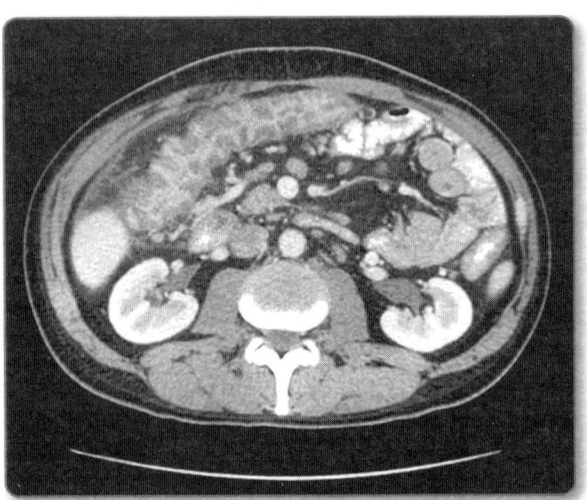

- There is colonic thickening, oedema and pericolonic stranding
- CT may also show free air or pneumatosis, indicating perforation

Q. 19.7 What are the indications for surgery?

- Megacolon
- Perforation
- Toxic colitis

Q. 19.8 What operation will you perform if the patient requires surgery?

Sub-total colectomy and end ileostomy

Further reading

Seltman AK. Surgical Management of *Clostridium difficile* Colitis. Clin Colon Rectal Surg 2012; 25: 204–209.

Scenario 20

Never events

You are supervising an ST3 during an endoscopy list and ask them to give a patient 3 mg of midazolam IV. The patients the procedure very well, and his observations are stable throughout. However, when the nurses check the vials of midazolam, they tell you that 6 mg has been given because a preparation of 2 mg/mL was used rather than the usual 1 mg/mL.

The patient remains well in recovery with normal observations and is able to go home later that day.

Q. 20.1 Is this a never event? Define a never event.

Yes, this is a never event. National Health Service (NHS) improvement has defined a never event as 'a serious incident that is entirely preventable because guidance or safety recommendations providing strong systemic protective barriers are available at a national level and should have been implemented by all healthcare providers.'

Note that no one has to have come to harm for this to have been a never event.

Q. 20.2 Can you list some never events?

National Health Service improvement have a full list of never events. They can be categorised as *surgical, medication, mental health,* and *general*. Examples are:

Surgical
- Wrong site surgery
- Retained foreign object post procedure

Medication
- Administration of drug through wrong route
- Mis-selection of high strength midazolam during conscious sedation

Mental health
Failure to install functional, collapsible shower or curtain rails

General
- Falls from poorly restricted windows
- Misplaced naso- or oro-gastric tubes

Q. 20.3 What should you do next?

Trusts will have a policy for reporting and dealing with never events. The principles and necessary steps are as follows:
- Firstly, check that *the patient is safe* and has come to no harm. In this setting, a longer period of observation might be a good idea, or perhaps even admitting the patient overnight. If the patient is at risk or unwell, you should take immediate steps to manage this
- Secondly, you have *a duty of candour* towards the patient, and should apologise and explain what has happened to them, and what the next steps are. The conversation should be documented, and it is sensible to have another clinical staff member who was not involved with you, e.g. nurse in charge
- Thirdly, the never event has to be *reported*. Most trusts have a system of reporting, e.g. online incident reporting

This will lead to an investigation and *root cause analysis*, so that learning can take place. A discussion with the clinical director of your department should take place. In this scenario, it is also important to *discuss what happened with your trainee*, perhaps after a few days have passed. The trainee should document their thoughts and feelings in their portfolio.

Further reading

NHS. (2023). Major plan to recover urgent and emergency care services. [online] Available from https://improvement.nhs.uk/documents/2266/Never_Events_list_2018_FINAL_v5.pdf [Last accessed March, 2023].

NHS. (2015). Revised Never Events Policy and Framework [online] Available from https://improvement.nhs.uk/documents/2265/Revised_Never_Events_policy_and_framework_FINAL.pdf [Last accessed March, 2023].

Scenario 21

Gynaecomastia

You are about to review a 59-year-old man in the breast clinic. He has been referred with an enlargement of breast tissue bilaterally over the last 3 months by the GP. They were also concerned that they could palpate a lump within the right breast.

Q. 21.1 Outline how you will assess this patient.

History
- Symptoms of breast disease, namely any lump that he has noticed, pain in the breasts; any nipple discharge; duration of symptoms; how he first presented to the GP
- Past medical history, namely any previous history of breast or other cancers, in particular lung, testicular or prostate cancers. Also take history for cardiac, liver and endocrine disease
- Drug history, namely use of spironolactone, histamine receptor blockers, steroids, therapy for prostate cancer
- Family history, i.e. any history of cancer, including breast cancer
- Social history, in particular alcohol history and cannabis use

Examination
Examine as you would for a breast lump. Remember to examine both sides, and assess both axillae. It is worth saying you would assess for any signs of liver or thyroid disease.

Imaging
- Either mammogram or ultrasound, with or without core biopsy depending on findings

The take home message of the above answer is to remember that male breast lumps need to be approached in the same way as female breast lumps – *triple assessment*. Here, the likely diagnosis is gynaecomastia, but breast cancer is an important differential.

Q. 21.2 Aside from the differentials mentioned in the previous answer, what other differential diagnosis is there?

Pseudogynaecomastia, which is weight gain around the breast area.

Scenario 21 Gynaecomastia

Q. 21.3 What are the causes of gynaecomastia?

You should categorise the causes as pathological and physiological.

Pathological
- *Endocrine*
    - Hyperthyroidism
    - Hypothyroidism
    - Congenital adrenal hyperplasia
    - Problems in androgen synthesis
- *Neoplastic*
    - Testicular
    - Lung
- *Systemic*
    - Liver cirrhosis
    - Renal failure

Physiological
- Age related – seen in puberty and in old age
- *Social:*
    - Alcohol use
    - Cannabis use
- *Drug induced:*
    - Cardiovascular drugs
        - Spironolactone
        - Digoxin
    - Psychiatric
        - Benzodiazepine
        - Antipsychotics
    - Endocrine
        - Steroids
        - Hormones for prostate cancer

Q. 21.4 There is no lump and the clinical findings are consistent with gynaecomastia. Discuss treatment options with the patient.

Conservative
Reassure and treat cause – discuss with patient and referring doctor which medications could be changed.

Surgical
- Liposuction
- Reduction mammaplasty
- Subcutaneous mastectomy

Further reading

https://associationofbreastsurgery.org.uk/media/65097/abs-summary-statement-gynaecomastia-2019.pdf [Accessed 1st April 2023].

Scenario 22

Neck lumps

You review a 22-year-old female patient in clinic with a neck lump.

Q. 22.1 You are in clinic about to see a 22-year-old female for a lump in the neck. Describe your approach to examining this lump.

Neck lumps are common in the examination, and may be relatively uncommon in your clinical practice, depending on your subspecialty. It is therefore, important to a have a thorough yet logical system.

When describing a lump, take a systematic approach. One should always adopt the approach of *looking, feeling, moving* and then performing *extra tests*. This basic approach can be applied to any aspect of clinical examination.

With regard to lumps, you can use the mnemonic, '*4 S*tudents and *3 T*eachers around a *CAMPFIRE*'.

Inspect for:
- Site, size, shape, and the surface

Feel for:
- Tenderness, temperature, transillumination

And feel and check:
- Consistency
- Appearance of patient
- Mobility
- Pulsation
- Fluctuation
- Irreducibility
- Regional lymph nodes
- Edge and extra tests

Q. 22.2 On examination, your patient has a lump in the midline of the neck. What extra tests can you do now?

Ask her to take a sip of water, and then ask her to swallow while you watch the lump. Then ask her to stick her tongue out, while watching the lump.

Q. 22.3 The lump moves up with protrusion of the tongue. What is the diagnosis? From what embryological remnant does it arise from?

A thyroglossal cyst. This is a classic examination question. It arises when a thyroglossal duct does not close.

Q. 22.4 How would you confirm the diagnosis and what is the operation of choice?

The diagnosis is a clinical one, but it is useful to do an ultrasound to assess the size of the cyst and exclude thyroid pathology.

The operation of choice is the *Sistrunk procedure*, where the cyst, some of the hyoid bone, and surrounding tissue in the midline are excised.

Q. 22.5 Can you tell me about any other congenital neck lumps?

- *Cystic hygroma*: A congenital lymphatic malformation at the root of the neck. It usually presents at birth, and the central clinical finding is that the lump transilluminates brilliantly
- *Branchial cyst*: A cyst that presents along the sternocleidomastoid muscle. The second, third and fourth branchial clefts usually obliterate; failure to do so lead to a branchial cyst. The most common site is the second branchial cleft (under the anterior border of sternocleidomastoid). The cyst can fistulate with the skin

Q. 22.6 List the borders of the anterior triangle of the neck. What lumps might present in the anterior triangle?

The superior border is the mandible; the medial border is the midline of the neck; the lateral border is the medial border of the sternocleidomastoid muscle. Think of the lumps that can present as:

Neoplastic
- Metastatic lymph node
- Thyroid cancer
- Chemodectoma
- Parotid lesion

Benign
- Thyroid nodule
- Reactive lymph node
- Submandibular gland

Congenital
- Branchial cyst
- Thyroglossal cyst

Q. 22.7 List the borders of the posterior triangle of the neck. What lumps might present in the posterior triangle?

The anterior border is the posterior border of the sternocleidomastoid; the posterior border is trapezius muscle; the inferior border is middle third of the clavicle.

Neoplastic
- Metastatic lymph node

Benign
- Pharyngeal pouch
- Reactive lymph node

Congenital
- Cystic hygroma

Further reading

https://cks.nice.org.uk/topics/neck-lump/diagnosis/assessment/ [Accessed 1st April 2023]

Scenario 23

Laparoscopic cholecystectomy

You see a 35-year-old patient on the ward round following an elective laparoscopic cholecystectomy the day before. He is in a significant amount of pain. He has a drain in situ which is empty.

Q. 23.1 Outline how you will assess this patient; and subsequent management.

In this scenario, one needs to work towards *excluding a bile duct injury*.

As with all patients you are meeting for the first time, begin with a *clinical assessment* – a history and examination; in particular, looking for peritonitis. Look at the observation charts, drug charts and drain chart – the drain is empty now, but check if it had drained earlier, and if the content was documented – have any of the nursing staff seen bile in the drain?

Once you are happy that the patient does not need immediate intervention, *look at the operation note*. Was the operation particularly difficult? Why was a drain left in? It may be worth ringing the surgeon who performed the operation.

Commence *non-operative measures* – antibiotics, analgesia, fluids, repeat bloods and venous or arterial gas.

In this scenario, you then need to decide whether this patient needs *observation* and analgesia; *further imaging, percutaneous drain* or to be taken back to *theatre*.

If the patient's observations are normal, and there is no significant tenderness, and settles with some minor adjustment to analgesia, they may be observed on the ward.

If there has been bile in the drain 24 hours after surgery, they should have imaging for a bile collection. The options are ultrasound or CT. CT so soon after laparoscopic surgery may not be helpful, but would pick up large volume collections. An ultrasound is operator dependent, and may also miss small leaks. Depending on the patient's condition and the findings on imaging, a percutaneous drain is an option.

If the patient has peritonitis, or is unwell, early re-look with a laparoscope is a good option for these patients; and do not forget important differentials – bleeding, visceral perforation, early port site hernia.

Q. 23.2 The patient's observations are normal and there has been no evidence of bile in the drain. The patient's abdomen is not peritonitic. You are unable to get through to the operating surgeon. The operation note indicates that the dissection was difficult, but a critical view was obtained. An hour later, the nurses report that his pain has increased, and he is tachycardic. You decide to take the patient

straight to theatre. Upon placing your laparoscope, you find that his abdomen is full of bile. The drain that was placed at first operation has kinked. Outline what you will do next in theatre.

Place the rest of the ports. Commence *washout* of the bile with saline. Try and *assess where the leak is coming* from in a systematic manner – start with the gallbladder bed for a *duct of Luschka* leak. Then assess the *cystic duct stump*. Check if there is a stone in the stump that may be driving the leak. With care, assess for *injury to the hepatic ducts or common bile duct*.

A clear leak from the duct of Luschka can be controlled with a stitch. If the leak is clearly from the cystic duct, then this can be controlled with a clip or an endo-loop. Unless you are a hepatobiliary surgeon, do not attempt repair of the hepatic ducts or common bile duct. If the leak is from here, you will need to discuss the patient with a hepatobiliary centre.

If the leak cannot be identified, perform a thorough washout of the abdomen, and leave a drain in the gallbladder fossa and the pelvis. Drains should still be left even if you are confident that you have identified and controlled the leak.

Post-surgically, ensure the patient is on antibiotics and analgesia, and has blood taken.

Q. 23.3 You were not able to identify the leak at surgery, so you performed washout and placed drains. After surgery, the patient is much improved, but there is still frank bile in the drain on Sunday. What will you do next?

An endoscopic retrograde cholangiopancreatography (ERCP) should be organised. This can help to identify the source of the leak. A stent can also be placed in the common bile duct – this will take pressure off a leaking cystic duct.

Q. 23.4 What is the critical view of safety?

This the view that needs to be achieved prior to any clipping and division during cholecystectomy. There are three aspects to the view:
1. The hepatocystic triangle must be clear of fat and areolar tissue
2. One must be able to see only two structures entering the gallbladder
3. The lower one-third of the cystic plate must be cleared

Further reading

https://www.nice.org.uk/guidance/cg188/ [Accessed 1st April 2023].

Scenario 24

Pyloric stenosis

You are assessing a 5-week-old boy with vomiting. The referring clinicians are suspicious of pyloric stenosis.

Q. 24.1 Describe your assessment of the patient, and what features in particular you are looking for.

History
- *Vomiting:*
  - Duration – usually presents with persistent vomiting at any point between 3 and 6 weeks of age.
  - Timing – soon after feeding
  - Appearance – milk stained; *ensure not bilious* – bilious vomiting is paediatric surgical emergency
  - Nature – usually projectile
- Appetite – the baby usually remains hungry
- Any weight loss
- Any symptoms of dehydration – lethargy, dry nappies

Examination
- *Systemic*: assess for dehydration – irritability, lethargy, dry mucous membranes, and sunken fontanelle
- *Focussed:*
  - Visible gastric peristalsis
  - Presence olive sized mass in the epigastrium

Biochemical
- Hypokalaemic, hypochloraemic, hyponatraemic metabolic alkalosis
- Acidic urine

Imaging
The diagnosis can be made clinically but imaging might be needed if other differentials are suspected. The options are ultrasound and contrast study.

Q. 24.2 Why does the aforementioned biochemical picture occur?

Try and think of the physiology in the *stomach* and the physiology in the *kidney*.
- When the baby begins to vomit, there is loss of hydrogen and chloride ions
- Loss of hydrogen drives the carbonic anhydrase reaction, leading to generation of bicarbonate, and metabolic alkalosis
- The kidney is a sodium preserving organ. It now has less chloride to undertake sodium absorption with, so exchanges hydrogen for sodium. This makes the urine acidic and worsens the alkalosis
- The vomiting and sodium preservation mechanisms continue to deplete hydrogen levels. The kidney then begins to perform sodium exchange with potassium, leading to hypokalaemia

Q. 24.3 What is the epidemiology of paediatric pyloric stenosis?

It is usually seen in first born males with an incidence of 4 per 1,000.

Q. 24.4 What is the operation of choice and describe how it is performed?

After correcting the biochemical and volume disturbances, the operation of choice is *Ramstedt's pyloromyotomy*. This is performed with an open or laparoscopic approach. For an open approach, the incision is a transverse one in the right upper quadrant. The thickened pylorus is identified and split until mucosa is clearly seen through the myotomy.

Further reading

https://www.ouh.nhs.uk/services/referrals/paediatrics/documents/pyloric-stenosis-guidelines.pdf [Accessed 1st April 2023].

Scenario 25

Enhanced recovery

> You see a 58-year-old female patient in clinic with a high rectal tumour. She will require an elective laparoscopic anterior resection. She would like to know more about enhanced recovery.

Q. 25.1 What is enhanced recovery?

Enhanced recovery is an approach to caring for patients having surgery. The overall goal is to help patients to recover from surgery quicker. You can think of enhanced recovery as having *four strategies* that inform the *three stages of operative care*. The four strategies underpinning this are:
1. Assessment, planning and preassessment prior to admission and surgery
2. Reducing the physical stress of surgery
3. Optimal perioperative management and immediate postoperative care
4. Early mobilisation

These are used to guide the patient's care at each of these stages:
- *Preoperative*: For example, patient education and engagement; management of pre-existing medical conditions; preoperative carbohydrate drinks; smoking cessation; assessing for barriers to discharge
- *Perioperative*: For example, minimising opioid use; use of laparoscopic techniques
- *Postoperative*: For example, good pain control; oral intake to start as early as possible; multi-disciplinary approach even during acute postsurgical phase

Q. 25.2 Which other healthcare professionals apart from surgeons and anaesthetists are involved in enhanced recovery?

Again, think of the patient journey – from before surgery to afterwards. Generally speaking, the same professionals are involved throughout. These include stoma nurses, dietician, physicians, e.g. POPS physicians (Perioperative medicine for Older People undergoing Surgery), physiotherapists, and speech and language therapists, pain specialists, and enhanced recovery clinical nurse specialists.

Q. 25.3 What are the benefits of enhanced recovery programmes?

There is evidence to show that patient's satisfaction is higher when going through enhanced recovery programmes as well as reduced length of stay, reduced complication rates and hospital costs.

Q. 25.4 Now imagine you are a new consultant. You have been tasked with establishing an enhanced care recovery programme for the general surgery department. Outline how you would achieve this.

There are three areas of focus:
1. *Staff training*: Use the latest evidence; educate to ensure staff have the right mindset; educate surgeons and anaesthetists
2. *Improve processes*: Plan what needs to happen to patients, and where exactly, e.g. what is to be done at the preassessment; when will they meet all important professionals, e.g. could this all take place in a one stop clinic?
3. *Protocols and procedure specific care plans*: These are day-by-day plans that inform patients and staff what will happen on each day, e.g. day 1 – commence free fluids, etc.

Further reading

NHS. (2023). Major plan to recover urgent and emergency care services. [online] Available from https://improvement.nhs.uk/documents/2111/enhanced-recovery.pdf [Last accessed March, 2023].

Scenario 26

Hydrocoele

You are teaching medical students with some volunteer patients in clinic. One of your patients is a 65-year-old man with a scrotal swelling.

Q. 26.1 What will you tell your medical students about how to differentiate between a hydrocoele and an inguinoscrotal hernia?

Clinically – which usually should suffice and *radiologically*.

From the history, the patient may report being able to *reduce the swelling* – this is consistent with a hernia.

Examination findings are key. If one can *get above the swelling*, this indicates a hydrocoele. One should try and see if the testicle is separate to the swelling – it usually is in hernias, but not in hydrocoele. *Transillumination* is brilliant, and this also is indicative of a hydrocoele, as is the presence of *fluctuance*.

One could also auscultate for bowel sounds – this would suggest an inguinoscrotal hernia.

If there is doubt over the diagnosis, or if there is suspicion of a malignant hydrocoele, an ultrasound is helpful.

Q. 26.2 Your volunteer patient does have a hydrocoele. One of the students asks about aspirating the fluid and sending it off. What will you tell her?

Aspiration is feasible, but not recommended, especially if there is a concern that a malignancy is causing the hydrocoele. This would cause seeding of malignant cells to the skin. A fistula may then also form. It is also likely that the fluid would simply re-accumulate.

Q. 26.3 What are the different types of hydrocoele?

There are several ways of thinking of hydrocoele. It is important to think of *primary* and *secondary* hydrocoeles, especially in adults. Primary hydrocoeles are idiopathic; pathologies causing secondary hydrocoeles include:
- Testicular cancer
- Infection, e.g. orchitis
- Trauma

One can also think of *which part of the cord or processus* is affected:
- Vaginal hydrocoeles – here, the processus is obliterated and fluid collects only around the testicle. This is the most common
- Infantile hydrocoeles occur when the processus vaginalis is patent from the deep inguinal ring distally. Do not be fooled by the name; these can present in adulthood
- Congenital hydrocoeles can occur when the processus vaginalis is patent all the way to the peritoneal cavity, i.e. there is a connection with the peritoneal cavity
- Hydrocoele of the cord is relatively uncommon and occurs when fluid is an isolated sac around the cord

Q. 26.4 What are the operative options for hydrocoele?

The *Jaboulay procedure* – a scrotal incision is made. The hydrocoele sack is opened and everted. Excess sack is excised, and the remnants are sutured together behind the cord.

The *Lord's procedure* – the sac is plicated at several points and sutured to the epididymo-testicular junction.

Q. 26.5 Imagine you are in a children's surgery clinic. You see a 15-month-old boy with a hydrocoele. What operation will you offer him and his parents?

None – surgery should only be offered to babies whose hydrocoele persists beyond 2 years, as most will resolve before then.

Further reading

https://cks.nice.org.uk/topics/scrotal-pain-swelling/management/hydrocele/ [Accessed 1st April 2023].

Scenario 27

Undescended testis

You are seeing an 18-month-old boy with his parents in clinic. The GP has referred him because on a routine checkup the left testicle was not palpable. On examination you can palpate the right testicle within the scrotum, but the left hemiscrotum is underdeveloped. There is a palpable lump in the left groin.

Q. 27.1 Will you offer surgery, and if so, why?

Yes, you should offer surgery. Babies with cryptorchidism should be offered surgery around the *age of 12 months*, depending on the exact clinical circumstances. In this case, unfortunately, the baby's cryptorchidism has gone undetected for some reason. The reason for surgery is that undescended testicles carry a significant *risk of malignant transformation*. Secondarily, bringing the undescended testicle down into the scrotum preserves its *ability to produce sperm*.

Q. 27.2 What important differential diagnosis do you need to exclude?

An important differential for a lump in a baby's groin is inguinal hernia. These have a high risk of strangulation.

Q. 27.3 What operation will you perform? What would you do in this case if the testis was impalpable?

In this particular case, an *inguinal approach* is taken. An incision in the left groin is made. The testicle is dissected out and mobilised. It is brought down into the scrotum. An incision in the scrotum is then made to facilitate orchidopexy to a sub-dartos pouch.

If the testis was impalpable, one then needs to start with an *examination under anaesthesia plus proceed to orchidopexy/laparoscopy/Fowler–Stephens procedure*. Under anaesthesia, assess if the testis is truly impalpable. If you can feel it, perform an orchidopexy with an inguinal approach as described. If it is truly impalpable, laparoscopy is warranted. At laparoscopy, if you find that there is an atrophied testicle in the abdomen (a testicular 'nubbin'), this should be removed to prevent malignant transformation. If there is a healthy intraabdominal testicle, a Fowler–Stephens procedure should be carried out.

A Fowler–Stephens procedure can be done in one stage, or in two. In a one-stage procedure, the testicular vessels are ligated and divided, and the testicle is brought down into the scrotum. In a two-stage procedure, the vessels are ligated and divided, and then the baby is left for 6 months. This allows collateral vessels to develop. Then, at 6 months, the testicle is brought down into the scrotum.

In this scenario, as the baby is already 18 months, everything should be done to bring the testicle down as soon as possible.

Q. 27.4 Can you outline the embryological descent of the testes?

- At *week 7*, the testes are in the retroperitoneum. Superiorly, the testes are attached by the caudal genital ligament; inferiorly, by the gubernaculum
- At *week 12*, the peritoneum evaginates, and the vaginal process grows towards the scrotal swelling. As it grows, a cavity involving all the layers of the abdominal is created, which leads to the formation of the inguinal canals. The shortening of the gubernaculum and intraabdominal pressure directs the direction of the testicles
- At *9 months*, the testes will have travelled through the inguinal canals into the scrotum. The caudal genital ligament will have regressed, and the gubernaculum will fix the testes in the scrotum

Further reading

https://cks.nice.org.uk/topics/undescended-testes/ [Accessed 1st April 2023].

Scenario 28

Antisepsis

You have completed the WHO sign out prior to starting an emergency laparotomy for a 58-year-old man with peritonitis. The scrub nurse asks you which agent you would like to prep with.

Q. 28.1 Define antisepsis.

Antisepsis is the process by which bacteria are removed from the surgical site.

Q. 28.2 How does it differ to sterilisation?

Sterilisation is the process by which all viable micro-organisms, including spores and viruses, are destroyed. One cannot sterilise a surgical site, as it is a process that destroys live tissue.

Q. 28.3 What antiseptic solutions do you know of? Can you list some facts that are important in their use?

- Chlorhexidine – bactericidal but not sporicidal, fungicidal or sporicidal; can be used when prepping delicate areas, e.g. the vagina.
- Alcohol – can be irritant to delicate areas and mucous membranes; must be careful to prevent pooling
- Povidone-iodine – is fungicidal

Q. 28.4 Do you know of any guidelines for antiseptic skin preparation? What do they say about the choice of antiseptic solution?

The National Institute for Health and Care Excellence (NICE) has guidelines on prevention and treatment of SSIs. In regard to the choice of antiseptic solution, *alcohol-based chlorhexidine is the first choice*, unless contraindicated, or if the surgical site is next to a mucous membrane. If the surgical site is next to a mucous membrane, aqueous solution of chlorhexidine should be used. Where chlorhexidine is contraindicated, the next choice is alcohol-based solution of povidone-iodine; and if both alcohol-based solution and chlorhexidine are unsuitable, aqueous solution of povidone-iodine should be used.

Q. 28.5 List some principles of how to use antiseptic solutions.
- Prep the surgical site first, unless it is dirty or contaminated, e.g. abscess – in such a setting prep last to avoid spread of micro-organisms to surrounding tissue
- Do not dip the sponge holder back into the prep once it has touched the surgical site
- If diathermy is being carried out, ensure prepped sites are dry and avoid pooling

Q. 28.6 What methods of sterilisation do you know of?
- Pressurised steam autoclaves – suitable for most surgical equipment; unsuitable for flexible endoscopes (which need to be disinfected)
- Dry heat sterilisation – cannot be used on rubber or plastic materials
- Ionising radiation – can be used on an industrial scale for single use items, e.g. swabs
- Ethylene oxide – a gas that can be used to sterilise heat sensitive equipment, e.g. rubber or plastic
- Low pressure steam combined with formaldehyde – useful for equipment that might be damaged by high temperature processes

Further reading

National Institute for Health and Care Excellence. (2020). Surgical site infections: prevention and treatment. [online] Available from https://www.nice.org.uk/guidance/ng125/chapter/Recommendations#antiseptic-skin-preparation [Last accessed March, 2023].

Scenario 29

Surgical site infection

You see a 58-year-old gentleman in A&E 6 weeks after an elective inguinal hernia repair, he is complaining of pain around the incision site. On examination, the incision site is cellulitis, swollen and tender. There is an opening at the medial aspect. On further examination, the wound dehisces, and frank pus is expressed.

Q. 29.1 Define a surgical site infection (SSI).

An SSI is defined as an infection-related to an operative procedure within *30 days of the procedure*, or *within 90 days where a prosthetic material* has been used during the procedure.

Q. 29.2 What types of SSI does this patient have?

This patient at least has a deep incisional SSI. The types of SSI are:
- *Superficial incisional*: This involves the skin or subcutaneous tissues around the incision. It can usually be treated with antibiotics alone
- *Deep incisional*: The infection affects the tissues down to fascia and muscles. Anatomic source control as well as antibiotics are required. Patients are likely to display signs of sepsis, e.g. pyrexia
- *Organ space*: The infection involves any body cavity related to or near the surgical site. Again, source control and antibiotics are needed. Patients are again likely to have signs of sepsis

It is likely that this patient has a deep incisional SSI, though imaging or surgical exploration is needed to definitively exclude organ space involvement.

Q. 29.3 How can SSI be prevented?

SSI can be prevented during all the operative phases:
- *Preoperative*:
  - Showering
  - Nasal decolonisation
- *Perioperative*:
  - Hair removal, only if needed; and if so, use electric clippers on the day of surgery
  - Patient and staff to wear appropriate clothing
  - Staff to perform appropriate hand washing prior to operating
  - Antibiotic prophylaxis where indicated

- Do not use diathermy to make skin incision
- Cover wound with appropriate dressing at end of procedure
- *Postoperative*:
  - Use aseptic technique to change dressings

Q. 29.4 What are the principles of anatomic source control?

- *Drainage* of infected liquid, i.e. placement of drain in intraabdominal abscess
- *Debridement* of infected tissue
- *Device removal* where needed
- *Definitive measures* to aid healing, e.g. use of vacuum assisted closure when sepsis is controlled

Q. 29.5 Define clean, clean-contaminated, contaminated and dirty operations.

- Clean – there is no infection, and the gastrointestinal (GI), genitourinary (GU) and biliary tracts are not opened
- Clean-contaminated – there is no infection, but the GI/GU/biliary tracts have been opened in a controlled fashion with no spillage of content
- Contaminated – the surgical field contains gross GI/GU/biliary content
- Dirty – presence of organised infection that has existed prior to operation

Further reading

National Institute for Health and Care Excellence. (2020). Surgical site infections: prevention and treatment. [online] Available from https://www.nice.org.uk/guidance/ng125/chapter/Recommendations#antiseptic-skin-preparation [Last accessed March, 2023].

Scenario 30

Day surgery

You are running an all-day list in main theatres with a mix of general surgery cases. Unfortunately, the list is overrunning. Your last case is a laparoscopic cholecystectomy for a 67-year-old lady. The original plan was for her to stay overnight but you have been informed there are no in-patient beds.

The bed manager has asked if the operation can be done in the day-case unit with a view to discharging the patient later that evening.

Q. 30.1 How will you approach this?

Patient factors
- Does the patient have an escort to take them home?
- Who does the patient live with?
- Is there anything in the medical history that will prevent same day discharge, e.g. re-establishment of anticoagulants?
- Is the patient willing to go home the same day, having been told they would stay in?

Surgical factors
- Is the operation likely to be high risk or challenging, e.g. is a difficult dissection anticipated, whereby the patient might need monitoring and observation postsurgery?
- Is the day-case unit suitable for this patient, e.g. what are the limits on BMI?

Anaesthetic factors
The decision should be made jointly with your anaesthetist – what is the patient's ASA; will they need a level 2/3 bed postsurgery?

Q. 30.2 The patient is willing to have the procedure done as a day case and is surgically and anaesthetically suitable. She can arrange an escort. However, she lives alone, and the escort cannot stay with her overnight. Should the procedure still be done as a day case?

Recent guidelines have suggested that while an escort is mandatory, the patient does not necessarily have to have someone with them overnight. In this case, it will depend on whether or not you truly think the patient will be safe by themselves overnight.

Q. 30.3 You have been asked to establish an urgent/emergency service day-case pathway, where patients seen during the on call can go home after surgery or go home before surgery and then come back for their procedure. Outline the principles behind how you would do this.

- *Patient selection*: Which type of conditions will you treat? You need to be sure that the condition can be managed safely at home
- *Pathways for conditions*: Establish clearly which patients are suitable which are not – some patients with appendicitis, for example, may be suitable. Criteria for this might include having normal observations, not living alone
- *Finding the right theatre*: Not all theatres are set up for laparoscopy, for example, and this will affect which conditions and patients you can manage
- *Providing clear preoperative information* for patients, including fasting instructions, where to turn up, what to do if unwell at home

Further reading

Bailey CR, Ahuja M, Bartholomew K, et al. Guidelines for day-case surgery 2019. Anaesthesia 2019; 74: 778–792.

Scenario 31

Haemorrhoids

You see a 27-year-old lady in outpatient clinic who has presented with painless bleeding per rectum. This began a year ago when she was pregnant.

Q. 31.1 Outline your assessment of her.

History – how often does she bleed; what is the volume of blood; what is the exact colour of the blood; does she notice it on wiping or in the pan; any other symptoms, especially any pain on defecation; has she noticed any lumps; does she suffer from constipation; how many children has she had; any symptoms of anaemia?

Examination – systemic assessment for anaemia; PR examination should involve inspection for external haemorrhoids, skin tags or fissure, or any other lesions. Perform gentle digital rectal examination and proctoscopy – proctoscopy will visualise internal haemorrhoids.

Q. 31.2 What investigations you will organise for her?

A *full blood count* to assess for anaemia. If there is no evidence of anal fissure, the patient should have *flexible sigmoidoscopy* to exclude a colorectal cause of her bleeding.

Q. 31.3 What are the risk factors for haemorrhoids?

Haemorrhoids are usually caused by anything that *increases the pressure in the rectum*:
- Obesity
- Pregnancy
- Constipation
- Sitting on toilet for long periods of time
- Weightlifting

Q. 31.4 What is the dentate line, and explain its relevance to assessment and management of haemorrhoids?

The dentate line divides the anal canal into *upper* and *lower* parts. The anal canal above the line is derived from the embryonic hindgut; below it, the ectoderm of the proctodaeum. The innervation is different – below the line, innervation is somatic and thus sensitive to pain.

Internal haemorrhoids originate above the dentate line, and so can be banded or injected in an out-patient setting, although often due to clinic pressures banding is preferred over injection and usually performed in an endoscopy unit.

External haemorrhoids originate below the line and are sensate. They should not be banded or injected.

Q. 31.5 Aside from internal and external haemorrhoids, how else can you classify haemorrhoids?

- First degree – internal, do not prolapse and usually only seen on proctoscopy
- Second – can prolapse, but reduce spontaneously
- Third – prolapse and need to be reduced manually
- Fourth – prolapse and cannot be reduced

Q. 31.6 Your patient comes back a few weeks later. You saw internal haemorrhoids only on your examination; her blood tests were reassuring, as was her flexible sigmoidoscopy. What will you tell her?

Haemorrhoids should be treated conservatively in the first instance, unless they are especially symptomatic. She should focus on avoiding straining on the toilet and changing her diet and losing weight if applicable. She could try stool softeners to help her with this. Bleeding in itself is not a cause for concern unless it is causing her to be anaemic, is not being caused by a malignant lesion, and is not disrupting her quality of life.

Q. 31.7 She then presents to the emergency department 8 months later with a painful, thrombosed external haemorrhoid. How will you manage her?

Conservatively, with analgesia and advice. She should take painkillers, including local anaesthetic gel, lay ice packs on it, and elevate her legs at home to help to reduce the oedema. Reassure her that the pain will resolve after 3 days usually. She should then be considered for elective haemorrhoid surgery.

The rationale for avoiding surgery is two-fold; firstly, the pain from haemorrhoid surgery is as significant, and can take longer to recover from than allowing the acute haemorrhoid to settle. Secondly, the risks of incontinence to wind and faeces are increased in the acute setting.

Further reading

van Tol RR, Kleijnen J, Watson AJM, et al. European Society of ColoProctology: guideline for haemorrhoidal disease. Colorectal Dis 2020; 22:650–662.

Scenario 32

Hidradenitis suppurativa

You are seeing a 29-year-old male patient in A&E. He has presented with an acute abscess in his right axilla. He tells you that he has a diagnosis of hidradenitis suppurativa.

Q. 32.1 How will you manage him? What are the clinical features of hidradenitis suppurativa?

An acute abscess in patients with hidradenitis suppurativa needs to be managed like any other abscess – so, *incision and drainage*. However, it is worth also checking with the patient if they have any other synchronous and acute abscesses. *Antibiotic therapy*, if needed, should be tailored to previous sensitivities. On discharge, they should be referred to a surgeon or physician with a specialist interest if they are suffering recurrent abscesses.

Clinically, patients complain of recurrent abscesses in the *groin, axillae* and *perianal* region. Risk factors include *smoking, diabetes* and *Crohn's disease*. On examination, there may be several *sinuses* and *tracts* in the aforementioned areas.

Q. 32.2 What are the stages of this disease?

The Hurley classification should be used:
- Stage 1 – single/multiple abscesses present; no sinus tracts or cicatrisation
- Stage 2 – recurrent abscesses with tracts and cicatrisation
- Stage 3 – entire anatomical area affected by tracts and cicatrisation

Q. 32.3 What are the non-surgical management options?

Management of risk factors
- Smoking cessation
- Weight loss
- Optimal management of diabetes

Lifestyle factors
- Avoid deodorants
- Avoid tight clothing

Medical options
- Long-term antibiotics
- Oral contraceptive pill for women where symptoms occur with periods
- Antiseptic wash
- Immunosuppressants, e.g. ciclosporin and methotrexate in the short term for severe disease

Q. 32.4 What are the surgical options in the elective setting?
- Laying open of tracts
- Surgical excision of entire affected area and healing by secondary intent ± VAC dressing
- Skin graft

Further reading
Ingram JR, Collier F, Brown D, et al. British Association of Dermatologists guidelines for the management of hidradenitis suppurativa (acne inversa) 2018. Br J Dermatol 2019; 180: 1009–1017.

Scenario 33

Lymphoedema

You see a 54-year-old female patient in clinic following a wide local excision of a breast tumour and axillary node clearance on the right side recently. She has a swollen right arm.

Q. 33.1 What is the likely diagnosis and what are the differential diagnoses?

The most likely diagnosis is lymphoedema. The differential diagnoses for unilateral arm swelling include:
- Recurrent breast cancer
- New malignancy of chest wall causing outflow obstruction
- Cellulitis
- Venous thrombosis
- 'Effort' venous thrombosis (Paget–Schroetter disease)
- Trauma

Q. 33.2 How will you assess her and confirm the diagnosis?

With her history of breast cancer, you would need to begin with *triple assessment* of the breasts – history, examination and imaging with a view to performing a biopsy of any breast lumps.

If there is no evidence of recurrent breast cancer, then this is almost certainly secondary lymphoedema, as a result of her surgery. *Lymphoscintigraphy* is not essential, but it should be considered in idiopathic or primary lymphoedema. However, it is still necessary to *duplex* the limb to exclude a deep vein thrombosis; and you should perform baseline bloods and include a D-dimer. Duplex is also the investigation of choice for Paget–Schroetter disease. It usually presents in younger patients and comes on after strenuous arm activity.

If there is suspicion of a chest wall malignancy causing subclavian vein obstruction, a *CT* will be necessary.

Cellulitis and trauma are diagnosed *clinically*. Any suspected fractures of course need to be *X-rayed*.

Q. 33.3 What are the surgical options in lymphoedema?

Surgery can be thought of as *bypass procedures* and *debulking procedures*:

Bypass procedures
- Lymphovenous anastomosis (LVA)
- Vascularised lymph node flap transfer (VLNFT)

Debulking
- Liposuction
- Homan's procedure
- Charles procedure

Q. 33.4 Do you know of any grading systems for lymphoedema?

There are two. The *Brunner* grading system, which is used by the International Society of Lymphology, and the *Cheng* system.

Brunner grading

Grade	Clinical features
0	Subclinical – there is impaired lymph drainage but no oedema present
I	Oedema pits on palpation and is dependent, i.e. disappears with elevation
II	Non-pitting oedema that does not disappear with elevation
III	Non-pitting with skin changes, e.g. fibrosis, hyperpigmentation, and warts

The Cheng system is more detailed:

Grade	Symptoms	Circumferential difference	Lymphoscintigraphy	Management
0	Reversible	<10%	Partial occlusion	Rehabilitation
I	Mild	10–19%	Partial occlusion	LVA, liposuction, rehabilitation
II	Moderate	20–29%	Total occlusion	Bypass surgery
III	Severe	30–39%	Total occlusion	Bypass surgery
IV	Very severe	>40%	Total occlusion	Bypass surgery + debulking

(LVA, lymphaticovenular anastomosis)

Further reading

Patel KM, Lin CY, Cheng MH. A Prospective Evaluation of Lymphedema-Specific Quality-of-Life Outcomes Following Vascularized Lymph Node Transfer. Ann Surg Oncol 2015; 22:2424–2430.

Chapter 5

Breast surgery

*Tracey Irvine, Pooja Padmanabhan, Rachita Mallya,
Shramana Banerjee, Carol Norman*

Scenario 1

Mastitis and breast abscess

A 33-year-old woman is referred to clinic by her general practitioner with a 3 day history of a hot painful swollen red breast.

Q. 1.1 What are key features in the history and examination?

The candidate needs to mention that this patient should be managed using the principles of triple assessment.

History

- The key features in this history are whether the patient is lactating/breastfeeding or not; and whether they have a history of smoking
- The candidate must take a breast history which includes family history
- Other conditions that predispose for infection must be explored such as diabetes, steroid use and recent breast intervention
- The candidate should demonstrate that the likely diagnosis is breast sepsis but inflammatory breast cancer needs to be ruled out

Examination

- The candidate should express a desire to have a chaperone present for the examination
- Salient points of the examination include assessment of regional lymph nodes, presence or absence of skin necrosis and evidence of an abscess that is pointing
- Systemic overview to assess for signs of sepsis, rapidly progressing symptoms, haemodynamic instability or immunocompromise

Imaging

- First-line imaging in a patient under the age of 40 years with a focal area of concern is US
- The treatment for breast abscess is repeated US and aspiration. Surgical drainage is rarely needed unless there is skin necrosis, the pus is too thick to drain, or the patient is systemically unwell
- The aspirated fluid should be sent for microscopy, culture and sensitivity (MC&S)
- A breast milk sample may be sent for MC&S if symptoms do not resolve with first-line management

Q. 1.2 How would you manage this patient in the breast clinic? What are the common causative organisms in mastitis?

Antibiotics

Breastfeeding/lactational abscess: Staphylococcus aureus is the most common causative organism; however, *Staphylococcus epidermidis* and *Proteus mirabilis* can also be implicated. Antibiotic treatment involves a 10–14-day course of empirical treatment with flucloxacillin, erythromycin or clarithromycin in penicillin allergy; co-amoxiclav is recommended as a second-line treatment if no response to initial antibiotics after 48 hours. These antibiotics are considered acceptable and safe during breastfeeding. Tailor antibiotic treatment to pus/breastmilk MC&S where available.

Non-lactational: This is usually caused by periductal mastitis due to smoking and treatment involves broad spectrum antibiotics to cover anaerobes. Treat with co-amoxiclav for 10–14 days; a 10–14-day course of erythromycin or clarithromycin plus metronidazole can be given in penicillin allergy.

Arrange for the patient to be brought back for review – if pus has been aspirated, they should be booked for repeat US and aspiration within a week.

Arrange a hospital admission if there are signs of sepsis, rapidly progressing symptoms, haemodynamic instability or immunocompromise. The infant should be admitted with the mother to allow breastfeeding to continue.

Cause-dependent advice

In lactational mastitis: Advise the patient to continue to express milk or continue breastfeeding from the affected breast, maintain good breastfeeding technique and hygiene. Nipple soreness and cracking should be treated. Consider simple oral analgesia for symptom relief – paracetamol/non-steroidal anti-inflammatory drugs (NSAIDs).

In non-lactational mastitis: Advise the patient about smoking cessation, good hygiene and identify and manage any predisposing factors for mastitis (e.g. diabetes, immunocompromising conditions, long-term steroid intake, etc.).

If it is an ongoing or recurrent problem, also think about chronic causes of mastitis such as chronic granulomatous mastitis and treat accordingly.

Further reading

Dixon J, Khan L. Treatment of breast infection. Br Med J 2011; 342:d396.
NICE Guidelines: Mastitis and breast abscess – Management of Mastitis and breast abscess in lactating women. [online] https://cks.nice.org.uk/mastitis-and-breast-abscess#!scenario [Last accessed February, 2023].
World Health Organisation. (2000). Mastitis: Causes and management. [online] Available from https://www.who.int/publications/i/item/WHO-FCH-CAH-00.13 [Last accessed February, 2023].

Scenario 2

Tumours of the breast

A 65-year-old female patient presents to the breast clinic as a 2-week-wait referral with a 2 cm lump in the right breast.

Q. 2.1 How would you manage this patient in the breast clinic?

The candidate needs to mention that this patient should be managed using the principles of triple assessment. This should include a full history that covers past medical history, relevant comorbidities, risk factors associated with breast cancer [hormone replacement therapy (HRT)/oral contraceptive pills (OCP) use, age of menarche and menopausal status, etc.] and family history, followed by a consented, chaperoned bilateral breast and axillary examination with assessment of regional lymph nodes. This patient would also have mammography and USS evaluation of the breast and axilla followed by image-guided core biopsy of the lump.

Q. 2.2 Examination reveals a P5 lump in the right upper inner quadrant. What does this imaging show?

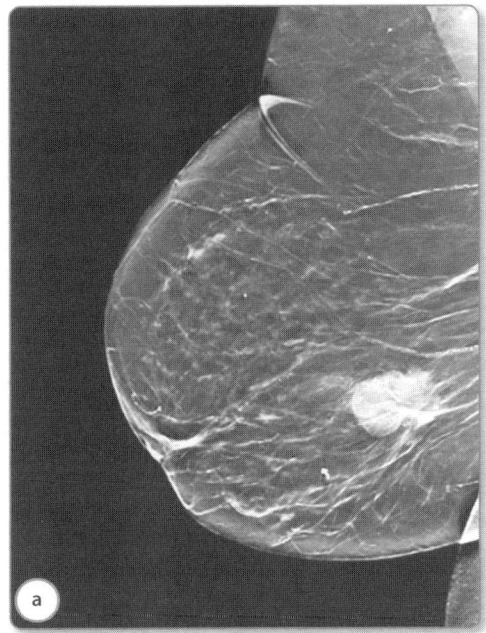
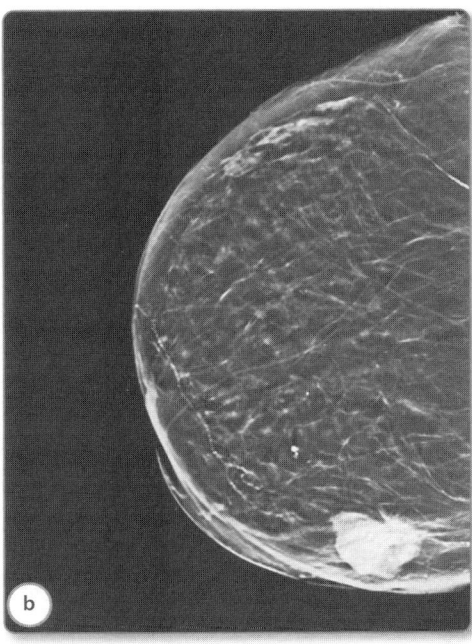

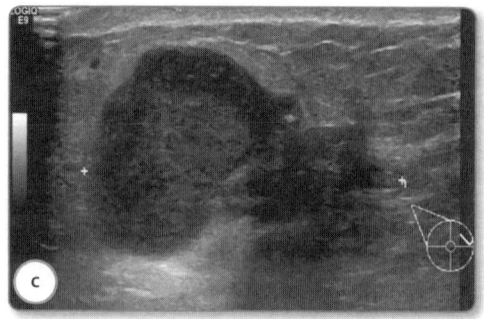

Mammogram and ultrasound images of the lady with symptomatic right breast upper inner/inner central lump – M5U5 irregular spiculate mass with microcalcifications.

Q. 2.3 The core biopsy confirms this as grade 3 invasive ductal carcinoma with high-grade ductal carcinoma in situ (DCIS). This is oestrogen receptor-8 (ER8) progesterone receptor-8 (PR8) human epidermal growth factor receptor-2 (HER2) negative. Axillary US is normal. How would this patient be managed?

The candidate should mention that the patient needs to be discussed at the breast multidisciplinary team (MDT) and should be supported by a breast care nurse.

Surgical treatment planning should be discussed with the patient and breast-conserving surgery (BCS) with wide local excision may be considered dependent on patient's choice. This will also include staging of the axilla using sentinel lymph node biopsy. This patient will need to be counselled on the role of adjuvant breast radiotherapy following the BCS and the potential need for further surgery to secure margins (~20%).

Q. 2.4 The patient has a wide local excision and sentinel node biopsy (SNB). This confirms a 20-mm G3 IDCA ER8/PR8/HER2. What adjuvant therapies would you consider for this patient within the MDT?

The next treatment plans are made once the surgical histopathology report confirms clear margins for the lumpectomy. According to recent ABS guidelines 1 mm margin for invasive cancer with or without DCIS and 2 mm margin for pure DCIS without any invasive disease, is recommended.

National Institute for Health and Care Excellence (NICE) guidance recommends the use of the PREDICT tool to estimate prognosis/eligibility for tumour profiling and the absolute benefits of adjuvant therapy for women with invasive breast cancer. Following MDT discussion, the recommended adjuvant therapies that may be considered for this patient include:
- According to NICE guidance this patient is eligible for genomics for tumour profiling. Chemotherapy should be offered according to results of tumour profiling – in line with NICE guidance and is the next line of treatment after surgery. This is then followed by breast radiotherapy. (NICE guidance recommends offering

whole – breast radiotherapy to women with invasive breast cancer who have had BCS with clear margins)
- *Endocrine treatment:* As this is an ER/PR + breast cancer and this patient is postmenopausal; an aromatase inhibitor may be considered as initial endocrine therapy
- Baseline dual energy X-ray absorptiometry (DEXA) scan to assess bone mineral density (BMD) prior to commencing aromatase inhibitors, is recommended.
- Bisphosphonates – NICE guidance recommends *consideration* for postmenopausal women and a high risk of recurrence; this must include a risk/benefit discussion with the patient

Q. 2.5 What are the types of endocrine treatment that you know of and what are the side effects of endocrine treatment?

Endocrine treatment involves administration of selective oestrogen receptor modulators (SERM), or aromatase inhibitors (AI) and the selection of treatment is based on menopausal status and assessment of relevant comorbidities and risk factors.
- Tamoxifen – SERM; may be used in both postmenopausal and premenopausal women. The main side effects are hot flushes and menopausal symptoms. Other common side effects include alopecia, anaemia, constipation, embolism and thrombosis, fatigue, fluid retention, headache, hot flushes, hypersensitivity, nausea and vaginal bleeding. Prompt investigation of abnormal vaginal bleeding must be undertaken in those receiving or having had tamoxifen due to an increased risk of endometrial cancer. Tamoxifen also increases the risk of thromboembolism during/immediately after major surgery and/or immobility and interrupting tamoxifen treatment must be considered
- The aromatase inhibitors – can only be used in postmenopausal women or premenopausal women with oestrogen suppression

Non-steroidal

- Letrozole (Femara): First-line treatment in postmenopausal women with hormone-dependent advanced breast cancer
- Anastrozole (Arimidex)

Side effects include alopecia, arthritis, asthenia, bone pain, carpal-tunnel syndrome, gastrointestinal (GI) side effects – vomiting/nausea/decreased appetite, osteoporosis and vaginal bleeding.

Steroidal

- Exemestane (Aromasin)

Side effects include alopecia, decreased appetite/constipation/diarrhoea/vomiting/nausea, arthralgia, asthenia, carpal-tunnel syndrome, depression, headache, hot flushes, leucopenia, osteoporosis and thrombocytopaenia.

Q. 2.6 What is the difference in tumour profiling tools?

As per the NICE guidance, EndoPredict, Oncotype DX and Prosigna are recommended as options for guiding adjuvant chemotherapy with ER positive, HER2 negative and lymph node negative disease (including micrometastasis) and low volume lymph node positive disease.

The EndoPredict test is used to predict the risk of distance recurrence of early-stage, ER/PR positive, HER2 negative breast cancer that is either node negative or has up to three positive lymph nodes.

The Oncotype DX is a genomic test that assesses the activity of 21 genes and is used to predict risk of cancer recurrence in early-stage ER positive breast cancer and outlines predicted benefit from adjuvant chemotherapy.

The Prosigna Breast Cancer Prognostic Gene Signature Assay (PAM50) is used to predict the risk of distant recurrence for postmenopausal women within 10 years of diagnosis of early stage, ER/PR positive disease with up to three positive lymph nodes after 5 years of endocrine therapy.

Of note, NICE guidance does not recommend the MammaPrint or IHC4+C profiling tools due to cost ineffectiveness and uncertain analytical validity, respectively.

Q. 2.7 Which patients would you consider extended endocrine therapy on?

NICE guidance (2018) recommends *offering* extended therapy (total duration of ET >5 years) with an AI for postmenopausal women with ER-positive breast cancer who are at medium or high risk of disease recurrence and who have been taking tamoxifen for 2–5 years. This may also be *considered* in women of this group who are at low risk of disease recurrence.

NICE guidance (2018) recommends *consideration* of extended duration of tamoxifen for longer than 5 years may be considered in premenopausal and postmenopausal women with ER-positive breast cancer.

Q. 2.8 What are the steps involved in management of optimal bone health?

NICE guidance recommends offering a baseline DEXA scan to assess BMD in women with invasive breast cancer who are not receiving bisphosphonates as adjuvant therapy and who are due to start treatment with an AI. Optimal bone health may be achieved through Ca/vitamin D supplementation, a recommendation for maintaining BMD through weight-bearing exercise and consideration of bisphosphonate treatment.

Q. 2.9 Would your management differ if this patient was 85 instead of 65?

Not necessarily. This patient should be treated in line from the recommendation of the National Audit of Breast Cancer in Older Patients. This highlighted that treatment of early invasive breast cancer must involve consistent assessment and recording of associated comorbidity and frailty in breast clinics (using a frailty score), shared decision making and medical optimisation of women with ER-positive early invasive disease to maximise potential for their suitability for surgery and adjuvant treatments. Counselling on the benefit and risks of adjuvant chemotherapy and/or radiotherapy following an objective assessment of patient fitness rather than chronological age alone should be undertaken.

Further reading

Rigby K, Wyld L, Cox K, et al. Association of Breast Surgery Guidelines – The management of radial surgical margins in relation to breast conserving surgery for invasive breast cancer 2024.

National Institute for Health and Care Excellence: Guidelines. Early and locally advanced breast cancer: diagnosis and management. London: National Institute for Health and Care Excellence (NICE); 2018.

National Institute for Health and Care Excellence: Guidelines. May 2024 Evidence-based recommendations on tumour profiling tests (EndoPredict, ICH4+C, MammaPrint, Oncotype DX and Prosigna) to guide adjuvant chemotherapy decisions in early breast cancer. (Available online at Overview | Tumour profiling tests to guide adjuvant chemotherapy decisions in early breast cancer | Guidance | NICE).

Scenario 3

Breast disorders related to pregnancy and lactation

A 35-year-old lady in her second trimester (16/40 weeks pregnant) present with a lump in her left breast.

Q. 3.1 How will you manage this case?

The candidate needs to mention that this patient should be managed using the principles of triple assessment.

History
- Past history of any breast problems
- History of any recent onset systemic symptoms
- Obstetric and ongoing pregnancy related history.
- Family history of breast/ovarian cancer

Examination
- The candidate should express the desire of having a chaperone for examination
- Salient points of examination include both breasts and regional lymph nodes with description of the lump and any other changes in the breasts such as erythema, peau d'orange, etc.

Radiological investigations

USG breast + axilla: US-guided core biopsy if the lump is a new solid lump, irrespective of its BI-RADS category. Inform rare possibility of milk fistula formation. Inform pathologists that breast biopsy is of a pregnant patient.

Q. 3.2 What breast lumps can occur in pregnancy?

Galactocele and Lactating adenomas. Pre-existing fibroadenomas associated with pregnancy induced changes like hyperplasia, infarction. Inflammatory conditions such as mastitis, abscess and granulomatous mastitis also need to be kept in mind.

Scenario 3 Breast disorders related to pregnancy and lactation

Q. 3.3 The ultrasound is suggestive of 25 mm U3/4 lump with normal appearing lymph nodes in the axilla. The core biopsy of the lump shows G3 invasive ductal carcinoma ER-/PR-/HER2- (TNBC). How would you manage this further?

- Complete radiological assessment of the breasts by performing bilateral breast mammograms with abdominal shielding
- Discuss in multi-disciplinary meeting (MDM) – management is based on same principles as in non-pregnant women
- See the patient in clinic in presence of a breast care nurse. Discuss with patient if keen on continuing pregnancy and if so reassure that this is possible. Termination of pregnancy does not improve maternal prognosis.
- Liaise with obstetrician to inform about recent diagnosis, treatment plan and confirm baseline assessment of the foetus
- Ideally, keeping in mind that it is TNBC, primary treatment would be systemic (with chemotherapy)

Q. 3.4 What else would you like to discuss with the patient?

- Genetic testing as young patient with triple negative cancer
- Insertion of marker coil in the lump prior to chemotherapy

Q. 3.5 What would be the ideal treatment plan for this lady?

She should start her treatment with NACT during her second trimester under close supervision of medical oncology and obstetric team. The last cycle of the chemotherapy is generally planned such that it is safe for her to deliver at about 35–36 weeks when foetal lung maturity is attained, and it is safe to deliver the baby. Since she is 16 weeks at diagnosis, she will probably be able to finish all her NACT just in time. She can then be planned for surgery and radiotherapy and continue with her targeted therapy based on response to NACT. She will be advised not to breastfeed due to ongoing treatment.

Q. 3.6 How can you define pregnancy associated breast cancer?

Breast cancer occurring during pregnancy or within 1 year postpartum. Incidence of 1 in 3,000 pregnancies.

Q. 3.7 What can and cannot be safely offered during pregnancy as a part of investigations and treatment of breast cancer?

	First trimester	Second trimester	Third trimester
MRI with contrast	Gadolinium contrast used for breast MRI is better avoided during pregnancy as it can cross the placental barrier. Its effects of foetus are unknown if MRI is needed; approved contrast agents include gadobenate dimeglumine (approved by the European Medicines Agency and US Food and Drug Administration) and gadoterate meglumine (approved by the European Medicines Agency). If MRI is needed, approved contrast agents include gadobenate dimeglumine (approved by the European Medicines Agency and US Food and Drug Administration) and gadoterate meglumine (approved by the European Medicines Agency)		
Staging scans	Bone scan and CT scan are contraindicated during pregnancy. Metastatic investigations for breast cancer during pregnancy include chest radiograph, liver ultrasonography, and a non-contrast skeletal MRI. Indications for staging are same as in non-pregnant women		
General anaesthetic	Surgery is safe at any time and during the first trimester as well, but breast conservation performed during a very early gestational age is associated with a long delay in postoperative radiotherapy		
Sentinel node biopsy	Sentinel node assessment using radioisotope scintigraphy does not cause significant uterine radiation, but blue dye is not recommended as the effect upon the foetus is unknown		
Anthracyclines Taxanes	Chemotherapy is contraindicated in first trimester	Chemotherapy can be given in second trimester and should be stopped around the 35th week of gestation to allow for a 2–3-week chemotherapy-free interval prior to delivery and to allow for a term delivery (>37th week). Children exposed to chemotherapy in utero seem to have no adverse outcome when compared to age-matched children	
Trastuzumab	Trastuzumab is contraindicated during pregnancy due to risk of causing oligohydramnios and spontaneous abortions		
Methotrexate 5-FU	Methotrexate is contraindicated during pregnancy due to risk of malformations and 5-FU is teratogenic, hence avoided		
Tamoxifen	Tamoxifen is contraindicated during pregnancy. Case reports indicative of development of ambiguous genitalia		
Radiotherapy	Radiotherapy is contraindicated during pregnancy due to risk of radiation exposure to the foetus		

During pregnancy, weekly chemotherapy regimens are preferred with strict maternal and foetal monitoring.

After birth, chemotherapy can be used as standard, but infant cannot be breastfed due to transfer of drugs into the breast milk.

Further reading

Amant F, Deckers S, Van Calsteren K, et al. Breast cancer in pregnancy: recommendations of an international consensus meeting. Eur J Cancer 2010; 46:3158–3168.

Amant F, Loibl S, Neven P, et al. Malignancies in pregnancy II. Lancet 2012; 379:570–579.

Amant F, Van Calsteren K, Halaska MJ, et al. Long-term cognitive and cardiac outcomes after prenatal exposure to chemotherapy in children aged 18 months or older: an observational study. Lancet Oncol 2012; 13:256–264.

Azim HA Jr, Metzger-Filho O, de Azambuja E, et al. Pregnancy occurring during or following adjuvant trastuzumab in patients enrolled in the HERA trial (BIG 01-01). Breast Cancer Res Treat 2012; 133:387–391.

Barthelmes L, Gateley CA. Tamoxifen and pregnancy. Breast 2004; 13:446–451.

Duncan PG, Pope WDB, Cohen MM, Greer N. Fetal risk of anesthesia and surgery during pregnancy. Anesthesiology 1986; 64:790–794.

Greenup R, Buchanan A, Lorizio W, et al. Prevalence of BRCA mutations among women with triple negative breast cancer in a genetic counselling cohort. Ann Surg Oncol 2013; 20:3254–3258

Kanal E, Barkovich AJ, Bell C, et al. ACR guidance document for safe MR practices: 2007. AJR Am J Roentgenol 2007; 188:1447–1474.

McCollough CH, Schueler BA, Atwell TD, et al. Radiation exposure and pregnancy: when should we be concerned? Radiographics 2007; 27:909–917.

Pereg D, Lishner M. Maternal and fetal effects of systemic therapy in the pregnant woman with cancer. Recent Results Cancer Res 2008; 178:21–38.

Sabate JM, Clotet M, Torrubia S, et al. Radiologic Evaluation of Breast Disorders Related to Pregnancy and Lactation. Radiographics 2007; 27:S101–S124.

Spanheimer PM, Graham MM, Sugg SL, et al. Measurement of uterine radiation exposure from lymphoscintigraphy indicates safety of sentinel lymph node biopsy during pregnancy. Ann Surg Oncol 2009; 16:1143–1147.

Scenario 4

Breast implants

A 43-year-old female patient with extensive DCIS presents to the breast clinic. Following MDT discussion, she is being worked up for a skin-sparing mastectomy and immediate reconstruction with implant. Her current bra size is 34B.

Q. 4.1 What are key points to go through while consenting this patient for implant-based reconstruction?

All patients should be consented in line with the National Health Service (NHS)/General Medical Council (GMC) guidelines; this should include a discussion of alternative options, specific complications discussed should include infection, extrusion, capsule formation, rupture, silicone granuloma, silicone bleed, implant malposition, implant loss – immediate or early postoperative period, further revisional surgery, BIA-ALCL and other implant associated malignancies and the risks and benefits of using ADM and other implanted products should also be discussed if appropriate, including absence of long-term data.

Consented medical photography to document preoperative baseline should be undertaken.

The patient should be informed about addition to the breast and cosmetic implant registry (BCIR); however, specific patient consent is no longer required.

Q. 4.2 This patient expresses concerns with anxiety around the safety of breast implants. She has looked into the composition of breast implants and has questions about the structure of the implant, materials involved and safety profile of silicone implants. What is silicon?

Silicon is a crystalline metalloid element found abundantly in minerals. Silicone is a manmade polymer made from silicon, oxygen and other elements.

Q. 4.3 What is the structure of a breast implant?

The outer layer (shell) is made of silicone, or polyurethane in some cases. Inside this, there is either silicone gel or saline.

Q. 4.4 What types of implants do you know?

Implants vary by:
- *Filling type/Material:* Silicone or saline
- *Shape/Projection:* Round breast implants (typically achieve a fuller upper pole), anatomical/teardrop-shaped implants (gentle sloping profile), and shaped implant
- *Texture:* Smooth breast implants, textured breast implant, micro-/nano-textured breast implants
- *Size/Volume:* Tissue expanders versus fixed volume, size ranges from 150 to 800 mL or larger

Q. 4.5 What is gel bleed and how is this diagnosed?

Microscopic diffusion of silicone gel through an intact semi-permeable breast implant elastomer shell. The patient may present with a lump – siliconoma or enlarged axillary nodes. The symptoms should be assessed using the principles of triple assessment. Although US is first-line imaging to assess implant integrity, MRI is better and is usually used second line if clinical or ultrasound concern.

Q. 4.6 What are the different grades of capsular contracture?

The Baker grading system is used to measure the degree of capsular contracture:
- Grade I: The breast is soft and looks natural
- Grade II: The breast is slightly firm but looks normal
- Grade III: The breast is firm and looks abnormal
- Grade IV: The breast is hard, painful and looks abnormal

Q. 4.7 What are the causes of capsular contracture?

Capsular contracture can be precipitated by an immune-mediated contracture/scarring around implant, presence of biofilm, postoperative complications such as haematoma/seroma and postoperative radiotherapy. An increased incidence is noted with smooth implants and sub-glandular implant placement.

Q. 4.8 What is biofilm?

A biofilm is where bacteria are adherent to an implant surface, encased by a protective layer of glycoprotein. Difficult to treat, this can lay dormant for years. BIA-ALCL tumour cells are theorised to result from a sustained T-cell immune response to the bacterial antigen in biofilm.

Q. 4.9 What is BIA-ALCL?

Breast implant associated large cell lymphoma (BIA-ALCL) is a rare sub-type of T-cell non-Hodgkin lymphoma. BIA-ALCL is one of four sub-types of ALCL which has been found in associating with breast implants. This sub-type is always both CD30 positive and ALK negative. The current estimated incidence of BIA-ALCL, based on confirmed cases where surgery occurred in the UK, is 1 per 16,500 implants sold.

- *Association*: Commonly associated with textured implants (including micro-polyurethane) but can occur independently of filler material, possible lower incidence with smooth implants
- *Presentation*: Swollen breast caused by formation of a delayed (>1 year since implant placement) unilateral idiopathic seroma occurring between the implant surface and the capsule. USS may detect seroma, with free floating debris. Rarely, a mass or a cutaneous nodule may also be present in the absence of a peri-prosthetic fluid collection in associated with severe capsular contraction. Bilateral BIA-ALCL can occur but is rare
- *Management*: Breast + haematology MDT discussion and input is essential, USS-guided aspiration cytology ± breast MRI, PET-CT to exclude regional or systemic spread if confirmed diagnosis
- *Diagnostic pathology*: CD30-positive cytokeratin-negative, ALK negative malignant cells infiltrating the luminal side of the peri-prosthetic capsule or within seroma/effusion
- *Management*: Varies by stage of BIA-ALCL – Treatment may be surgical and curative, by complete removal of capsule and implant along with targeted chemotherapy

Further reading

Association of Breast Surgery. (2012). ABS Guidelines: Oncoplastic Breast Reconstruction – Guidelines for best practice. [online] Available from https://associationofbreastsurgery.org.uk/media/1424/oncoplastic-breast-reconstruction-guidelines-for-best-practice.pdf [Last accessed February, 2023].

Association of Breast Surgery. (2020). ABS Guidance Platform for Aesthetic/Oncoplastic/Reconstructive Surgery. [online] Available from https://associationofbreastsurgery.org.uk/media/252043/oncoplastic-reconstructive-surgery-v5.pdf [Last accessed February, 2023].

Association of Breast Surgery. Summary Statement. Breast Implant Associated-Anaplastic Large Cell Lymphoma. ABS Guidelines: BIA-ALCL. [online] Available from https://associationofbreastsurgery.org.uk/media/64198/final-alcl.pdf [Last accessed February, 2023].

Vase MØ, Friis S, Bautz A, et al. Breast implants and anaplastic large-cell lymphoma: a Danish population-based cohort study. Cancer Epidemiol Biomarkers Prev 2013; 22:2126–2129.

MHRA Updated data for incidence of BIAALCL Breast Implant Associated Anaplastic Large Cell Lymphoma (BIA-ALCL) – GOV.UK (www.gov.uk).

Scenario 5

Nipple discharge

A 50-year-old female patient is referred to the breast clinic with a history of unilateral blood-stained nipple discharge.

Q. 5.1 What are the features of pathological nipple discharge?

- Single duct discharge (versus multiduct)
- Bloodstained or clear
- Spontaneous, e.g. on bra/night clothes rather than only present when she squeezes her nipple

Q. 5.2 She underwent triple assessment, and a core biopsy confirms that there is a B3 papilloma with no atypia, which is adjacent to the right NAC. How should this patient be managed?

Vacuum-assisted excision (VAE) may be considered for a papilloma with no evidence of atypia; however, this scenario states that the lesion is close to the nipple so surgical excision biopsy will be required.

Q. 5.3 Following MDT input, this patient is worked up for an excision biopsy however you get a call from your radiologist on the day of surgery as an US to localise the area demonstrates multiple areas of change in the breast with similar appearance – what would you do?

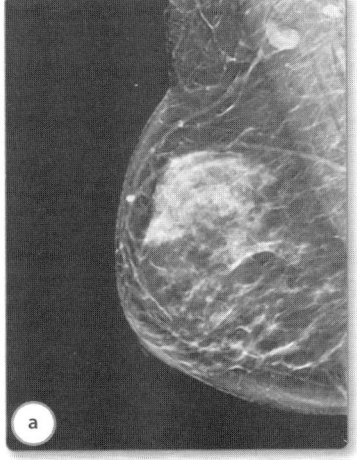
a

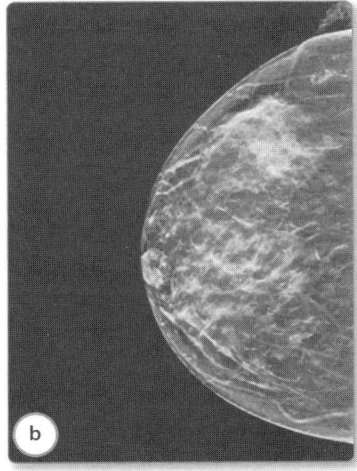
b

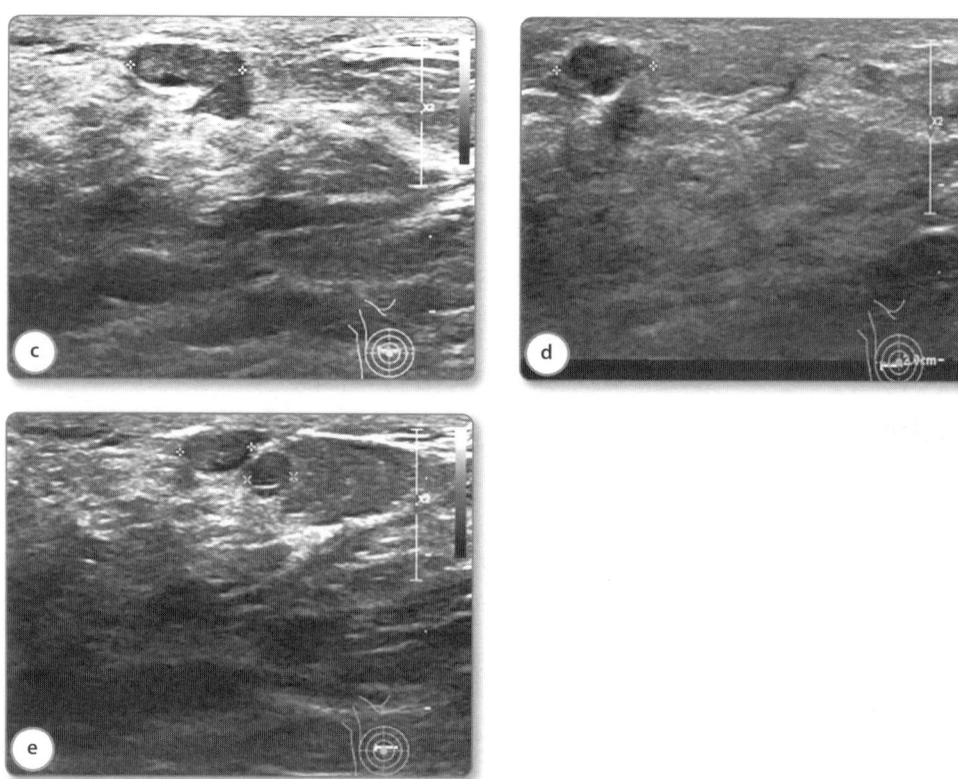

Ultrasound and mammogram images suggestive of multiple hypoechoic lesions largest one in the retro-areolar area, core biopsy of which was suggestive of a papilloma B3.

Confirm that the largest lesion/lesions or lesions with more concerning features are sampled by core biopsy. Defer surgery to another day. Rediscuss the case in MDM with the team in light of new findings, to plan further management.

On the day of operation consider biopsy of the most concerning lesions on imaging prior to MDT discussion.

This patient is symptomatic so at some point will need surgery for removal of the symptomatic lesion as planned +/− any other lesions that are of concern on biopsy. She would then be considered for longer term monitoring.

Q. 5.4 What are the different B3 lesions you know of?

B3 lesions include atypical intra-ductal epithelial proliferation (AIDEP); non-pleomorphic/classical lobular (in situ) neoplasia (LN); flat epithelial atypia (FEA); radial scar/complex sclerosing lesion – with or without epithelial atypia; papillary lesion – with or without epithelial atypia; cellular fibroepithelial lesion where a phyllodes tumour cannot be excluded; mucocoele-like lesion' other rare abnormalities such as spindle-cell lesions.

Q. 5.5 What does the upgrade rate depend on?

This depends on representative sampling volume, e.g. 14-G core versus VAE; associated epithelial proliferation/atypia, stromal atypia, architectural atypia, association of DCIS ± focus of invasive cancer.

Q. 5.6 What is the upgrade rate for radial scar?

This is heavily dependent on presence of associated atypical epithelial proliferation. Brenner et al. reported a 28% upgrade for radial scar with atypia and 4% without epithelial atypia.

Further reading

Brenner RJ, Jackman RJ, Parker SH, et al. Percutaneous core needle biopsy of radial scars of the breast: when is excision necessary? AJR Am J Roentgenol 2002; 179:1179–1184.

NHS: Public Health England. (2016). NHS Breast Screening Programme Clinical guidance for breast cancer screening assessment. ABS Guidance on the Management of B3 lesions. [online] Available from https://associationofbreastsurgery.org.uk/media/1414/nhs-bsp-clinical-guidance-for-breast-cancer-screening-assessment.pdf [Last accessed February, 2023].

Pinder SE, Shaaban A, Deb R, et al. NHS Breast Screening multidisciplinary working group guidelines for the diagnosis and management of breast lesions of uncertain malignant potential on core biopsy (B3 lesions). Clin Rad 2018; 73:682.

Scenario 6

Breast cancer risk assessment

A 38-year-old lady is referred by her general practitioner (GP) with complaints of breast pain. Her examination is normal but you notice in the history her mother had ovarian cancer at the age of 40 and both of her maternal aunts had breast cancers at ages 45 and 53.

Q. 6.1 Do you think this family history is of any significance? Why?

Yes, the family history is of significance. One first-degree relative with ovarian cancer and two second-degree relatives with breast cancer under the age of 60 years, means this lady may have a hereditary genetic mutation which puts her at a higher risk of developing breast/ovarian cancers.

Q. 6.2 Based on family history, how can the risk be evaluated?

Based on the family history (relation – first-/second-/third-degree, maternal/paternal side, type of cancer/cancers, age at diagnosis, any specific ancestry, number of unaffected relatives and their current age, etc.) one can use carrier probability calculation methods to assess the risk in a particular individual. Those that are acceptable and recommended by the NICE guidelines are for BRCA1 and 2 mutations are – BOADICEA and the Manchester scoring system.

Manchester score	
Cancer, age at diagnosis	**Score**
♀ Breast cancer, <30	11
♀ Breast cancer, 30–39	8
♀ Breast cancer, 40–49	6
♀ Breast cancer, 50–59	4
♀ Breast cancer, >59	2
♂ Breast cancer, <60	13
♂ Breast cancer, >59	10
Ovarian cancer, <60	13
Ovarian cancer, >59	10
Pancreatic cancer	1
Prostate cancer, <60	2
Prostate cancer, >59	1

Q. 6.3 How do we manage the varying risks?

Based on the risk scores from the above methods individuals can be classified into following groups:
- *Population risk:* Less than 17% life-time risk; 10-year risk; <3% aged 40–49 years. These individuals are managed in primary care
- *Moderate risk:* 17–30% life-time risk; 10-year risk 3–8% aged 40–49 years. These are referred to secondary care
- *High risk:* More than 30% life-time risk; 10-year risk >8% aged 40–49 years. These are referred to a tertiary care centre

Q. 6.4 Do you know of any other risk models? Can you describe them?

- *Gail model*: One of the oldest models. The major limitation of this model is that it considers only first-degree relatives, underestimating the risk of development of cancer.
- *Claus model and its expansion or modification:* This incorporates more relatives, and the extended version adds for bilateral breast cancer, ovarian cancer and three or more affected relatives. It does not include non-hereditary factors.
- *BRCAPRO model*: It includes information on affected and unaffected relatives. The drawbacks of this model are that it does not include any non-hereditary factors and only assess breast cancer related risk.
- *Tyrer–Cuzick model*: This includes all hereditary as well as non-hereditary factors such as exposure to exogenous hormones, BMI, etc. The family history incorporated is also much more extensive than the other models.
- The Breast and Ovarian Analysis of Disease Incidence and Carrier Estimation Algorithm (BOADICEA) or its' web interface, CanRisk, is a risk prediction model that is used to compute the probabilities of carrying rare loss-of-function variants in the breast or ovarian cancer susceptibility genes *BRCA1*, *BRCA2*, *PALB2*, *CHEK2*, and *ATM*

Q. 6.5 Which genes are associated with development of breast cancer?

- High-incidence high-penetrance genes: *BRCA1, BRCA2*
- Low-incidence high-penetrance genes: *PALB B2, Tp53, PTEN*
- Low-incidence low-penetrance genes: Check 2, *ATM, NAT 1/2/4*, cytochrome P450, GST family genes, etc.
- Rare association of breast cancer with following hereditary syndromes: Tp53 mutation in Li Fraumeni syndrome, ATM mutation in ataxia telangiectasia, *PTEN* mutation in Cowden syndrome

Q. 6.6 Which cancers are associated with *BRCA1* and *2* mutations? How frequently can they occur?

BRCA1: Lifetime cancer risks
- *Breast cancer:* 60–80%
- *Ovarian cancer:* 40–50%

- *Male breast cancer:* Twice population risk
- *Pancreatic cancer:* Two to three times population risk

BRCA2: Lifetime cancer risks
- *Breast cancer:* 40–85%
- *Ovarian cancer:* 10–25%
- *Male breast cancer:* 6%
- *Pancreatic cancer:* Three to four times population risk

Q. 6.7 What guidelines do we use for screening patients with hereditary mutations associated with high risk of developing breast cancer? Can you describe them?

The guidelines we used for screening women with high risk of development of breast cancer are the NICE guidelines. They are as follows:
- BRCA1/2 mutation carriers – annual MRI (30–49 years), annual mammograms (30–69 years)
- TP53 mutation carriers – annual MRI (20–69 years), no mammograms (RT induced risk of development of cancer)

High risk family history with >30% lifetime risk:
- Less than 30% chance of *BRCA/TP-53* gene mutation – annual mammogram age 40–59 years
- More than 30% chance of *BRCA* gene mutation – annual mammogram age 40–59 years, annual mammogram 40–69 years in known *BRCA1/2* mutation carriers, annual MRI age 30–49 years. If >30% chance of TP53 mutation – no mammograms, but annual MRI 20–49 years

Moderate risk family history (17–30% lifetime risk): Annual mammogram 40–49 years and NHSBSP programme over 50 years.

Q. 6.8 What options can be offered to the women for mitigating their risks of developing cancer?

- Surveillance as above helps in early detection. It does not reduce the risk and does not reduce mortality rates; however, it reduces morbidity associated with breast cancer treatment by early detection
- Chemoprevention: Tamoxifen/Raloxifene can be offered to women with high risk for 5 years and can be considered in women with moderate risk
- Risk reducing breast surgery: It reduces the risk of development of breast cancer by about 95%. It requires a team approach comprising of a geneticist, psychologist, breast and plastic surgeons and breast care nurses
- Risk reducing surgery for ovarian cancer (bilateral salpingo-oophorectomy): Offered to women over the age of 35 years. It reduces ovarian risk and also breast cancer risk in *BRCA2* mutation carriers
- Lifestyle modification: Healthy BMI, avoid smoking, reduce alcohol intake, avoid OCPs/HRT

Q. 6.9 How can you approach a lady who is known to have *BRCA1* mutation on surveillance and then develops breast cancer?

- Treatment of the cancer takes priority
- For the first 10 years, mortality is linked to the cancer rather than development of a new breast primary in the future, so prognosis of the index cancer needs to be borne in mind in any discussions
- Risk reducing surgery can be offered simultaneously as the surgery for the cancer, bearing in mind to minimise any delays in the cancer treatment
- There might be a possibility of addition of certain chemotherapeutic agents keeping in mind *BRCA1* mutation
- Consider offering bilateral salpingo-oophorectomy in premenopausal women

Further reading

De Jong MM, Nolte IM, te Meerman GJ, et al. Genes other than BRCA 1 and BRCA 2 involved in breast cancer susceptibility. J Med Genet 2002; 39:225–242.
Evans GR, Howell A. Breast Cancer risk assessment models. Breast Cancer Res 2007; 9:213.
https://www.nice.org.uk/guidance/cg164

Scenario 7

Advanced breast cancer

You are seeing a 56-year-old lady in clinic who was treated for breast cancer 4 years ago. This was a 3 cm G3 IDC with 4/20 positive lymph nodes. ER8+/PR8+/HER2 negative.

She has breast conserving surgery followed by adjuvant chemoradiotherapy. She has been on letrozole since. She has developed worsening lower back over the last few weeks.

Q. 7.1 How will you approach this case?

- *History:* Complete history of past treatment and current symptoms. History of any other systemic symptoms such as loss of appetite, nausea, vomiting, headaches, weight loss, chronic cough, etc. History of comorbidities especially those that can cause any neurological symptoms.
- *History of trauma:* The candidate needs to specifically ask about radiation of pain, change in sensation and any history of urinary or faecal incontinence
- *Examination:* In supine position
  - Candidate should express the desire of having a chaperone for examination
  - Salient points of examination include both breasts and regional lymph nodes
  - Detailed neurological examination with examination for other likely sites of metastasis
  - A rectal examination should be performed to assess anal tone and look for saddle anaesthesia

Q. 7.2 On further questioning, she mentions she has had few episodes of urinary incontinence over the past few days and feels her legs lack strength. What do you think is the likely diagnosis?

The signs and symptoms are suggestive of cord compression
- This patient needs to be admitted for urgent investigation and management
- Radiological investigations – MRI whole spine with contrast ASAP

Q. 7.3 What does this MRI show?

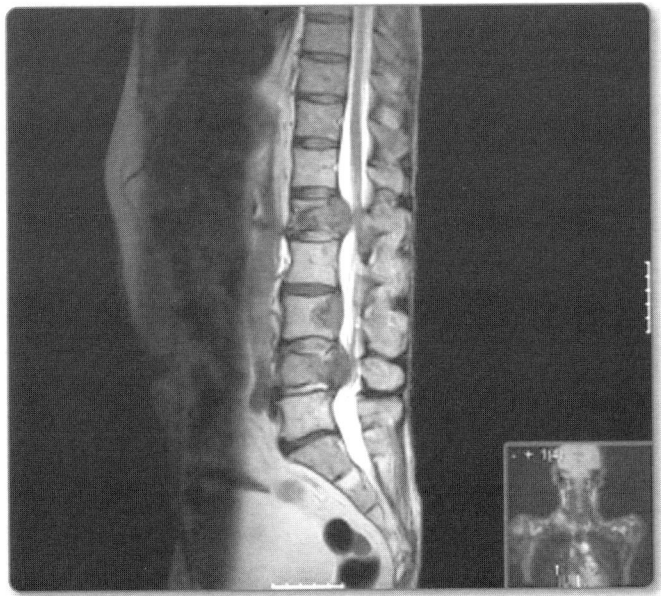

- Multiple spinal metastases with impingement on the spinal cord at L1 and L4
- *Routine blood tests*: FBC, kidney function, liver function, calcium, alkaline phosphatase (ALP), and tumour markers
- *Scans for further staging:* CT thorax/Abdomen and pelvis + MRI brain or PET-CT + MRI brain based on local policy and previously done scans for comparison

Q. 7.4 What should constitute her immediate treatment?

- Urgent referral to MSCC team
- Nurse in supine position
- Effective analgesia
- *Corticosteroids with gastric protection:* Steroids help with the pain and reduce vasogenic oedema to help to improve symptoms
- *Other supportive care:* Catheterisation, bowel care, prevention of pressure sores, and prevention of deep venous thrombosis
- *Bisphosphonates:* To reduce pain and risk of vertebral fracture/collapse

Q. 7.5 What treatment options can be offered to this patient?

Treatment is based on extent of disease within the spine and elsewhere in the body, degree of neurological instability and general health of the patient thereby implying life expectancy. Various scoring systems have been used for this. All the cases should be discussed urgently in the MSCC MDMs.

Radiotherapy usually given as 30 Gy in 10 fractions.

Depending on staging, surgery can include decompression of neural structures, pain relief, debulking or removal of tumour mass and spinal stabilisation to prevent deformity and allow mobilisation.

Indications for surgery include the following:
- Presence of solitary spinal lesion
- Progressive neurologic deficit before, during, or after radiation therapy
- Intractable pain unresponsive to conservative treatment
- Need for histologic diagnosis
- Radioresistant tumour histology
- Spinal instability (i.e. vertebral collapse)

Apart from all these local treatment options, the patient should be offered systemic treatment based on results of whole-body staging scans and continuation of bisphosphonates.

Q. 7.6 Which endocrine therapy drugs can this patient be prescribed, now that she has progressed on letrozole?

Selective oestrogen receptor down-regulator such as fulvestrant or irreversible oestrogen receptor blocker such as exemestane + CDK4/6 inhibitor is now the first-line medication approved in this setting.

Q. 7.7 Are you aware of any other medications that can be used to overcome endocrine resistance?

Medications to overcome endocrine resistance:
- *CDK4/6 inhibitors*: Combinations of AI or fulvestrant with CDK4/6 inhibitors (Palbociclib) are the current FDA approved standard of care for first-line treatment of HR + metastatic breast cancer
- *mTOR inhibitors*: Everolimus + Exemestane have shown to improve progression free survival in ER+/HER2-negative breast cancer patients with metastatic disease as compared to exemestane alone on progression on an AI
- *PIK3CA inhibitors*: Buparlisib, a pan-PI3K inhibitor, plus fulvestrant improved progression free survival but also increased toxicity compared with fulvestrant and placebo among women with hormone receptor (HR)-positive, HER2-negative, advanced *breast cancer*
- *ESR1* mutation targeting agent – under investigation – Lasofoxifene

Further reading

Baselga J, Im SA, Iwata H, et al. Buparlisib plus fulvestrant versus placebo plus fulvestrant in postmenopausal, hormone receptor-positive, HER2-negative, advanced breast cancer (BELLE-2): a randomised, double-blind, placebo-controlled, phase 3 trial. Lancet Oncol 2017.

Bhatt A, Schuler JC, Boakye M. Current and emerging concepts in non-invasive and minimally invasive management of spine metastasis. Cancer Treat Rev 2013; 39:142–152.

Criscitiello C, Andre F, Thompson AM, et al. Biopsy confirmation of metastatic sites in breast cancer patients: clinical impact and future perspectives. Breast Cancer Res 2014; 16:205.

National Institute for Health and Care Excellence. Advanced breast cancer: Diagnosis and Treatment. Updated NICE guidelines 2017. [online] Available from https://www.nice.org.uk/guidance/cg81. [Last accessed February, 2023].

National Institute for Health and Care Excellence. Spinal Metastases and Metastatic Spinal Cord Compression. NICE guideline [NG234]. Published September 6, 2023. Available from: https://www.nice.org.uk/guidance/ng234 [Last accessed June, 2024].

Turner NC, Slamon DJ, Ro J, et al. Overall Survival with Palbociclib and Fulvestrant in Advanced Breast Cancer. N Engl J Med 2018; 379:1926–1936.

Yardley DA, Noguchi S, Pritchard KI, et al. Everolimus Plus Exemestane in Postmenopausal Patients with HR+ Breast Cancer: BOLERO-2 Final Progression-Free Survival Analysis. Advances Ther 2013; 30:870–884.

Scenario 8

Oncoplastic breast reconstruction

A patient with extensive high-grade ductal carcinoma in situ is considered for a mastectomy and reconstruction. Her bra size is 36E.

Q. 8.1 What are the indications for a mastectomy?

There are relative (size dependent) and absolute indications to be considered.
- Diffuse suspicious or malignant-appearing microcalcifications on mammography and ductal carcinoma in situ (DCIS), i.e. >4 cm in area (relative)
- Breast cancer in pregnancy requiring radiotherapy depending on tumour profile and timing of surgery
- Patients with large tumours or multi-centric disease that cannot be locally excised with a satisfactory cosmetic result
- Positive pathological radial margins (invasive breast cancer or DCIS at margins <1 mm) following BCS where further excision would impact on cosmetic result
- Locally-advanced breast cancer
- Risk-reducing mastectomy
- Inflammatory breast cancer (IBC), i.e. responsive to neoadjuvant chemotherapy
- Paget's disease of the breast
- Recurrence with a history of previous whole breast radiation
- Patients who choose to have mastectomy over BCS or wish to avoid DXT

Q. 8.2 This patient has expressed a desire for a reconstruction following mastectomy. What types of reconstruction do you know?

Immediate versus delayed breast reconstruction (BR) options should be discussed with all women having a mastectomy, even if this is not available locally (NICE guidelines). If contraindications to BR present, this should be discussed fully with the patient and documented in the medical notes.

Commonly used surgical techniques for reconstruction are two-staged tissue-expander-to-implant, one stage direct-to-implant with or without biologic or synthetic mesh, LD myocutaneous flap with or without implant, free or pedicled flaps using lower abdominal tissue (TRAM and DIEP), free flap reconstruction using the thigh (TUG) and buttocks SGAP and IGAP.

Q. 8.3 What are the key features in history and examination while assessing this patient for reconstruction?

This patient should not require any other adjuvant therapies after surgery that need to be considered for reconstruction planning.

Salient preoperative history features should cover: Past medical/surgical history, medical comorbidities associated with poor/delayed wound healing, current medication, over-the-counter medication, smoking status, work, hobbies, hand dominance and family history.

Salient examination features: A consented, chaperoned bilateral breast and axillary examination; assessment of regional lymph nodes, detailing the shape of the breast, position of scars, breast and chest wall asymmetry and skin elasticity, soft-tissue thickness and overall body habitus.

Documentation needs to include the dimensions (base width, base height, sternal notch to nipple distance and nipple to IMF distance), volume and medical photographs should be taken.

If delayed breast reconstruction is planned, the scar should be sympathetic to this and a low scar with preservation of the IMF is best. A flap-based reconstruction is the most common type of delayed breast reconstruction and this is inset at the IMF. Contralateral symmetrisation surgery should be considered and can help patients feel less unbalanced, and if desired, can be performed at the same time as the mastectomy.

The patient must also be counselled about NAC reconstruction and nipple tattooing following index reconstructive surgery if the nipple is to be removed.

Q. 8.4 What are the main pros and cons of implant based versus autologous reconstruction?

Implant
Pros:
- No donor site issues
- Shorter operation and recovery
- Available if patient has no autologous options

Cons:
- Definite need for implant replacement down the line
- Least natural
- Risk of capsular contracture
- Shape does not change if patient puts on/loses weight
- Risk of BIA-ALCL

Autologous
Pros:
- More natural – softer and warmer
- Flexibility with shaping during inset

- May need minor adjustments but should not need revision for long-term
- Size will alter if patient puts on/loses weight

Cons:
- Major surgery
- Donor site issues
- Low risk of partial/complete flap loss

Further reading

Association of Breast Surgery. Oncoplastic Breast Reconstruction: Guidelines for Best Practice. London: ABS, BAPRAS, 2012.

NICE guideline [NG101]. Early and locally advanced breast cancer: diagnosis and management 2018. [online] Available from https://www.nice.org.uk/guidance/ng101/chapter/Recommendations#breast-reconstruction [Last accessed February, 2023].

Silverstein M, Mai T, Savalia N, et al. Oncoplastic breast conservation surgery: the new paradigm. J Surg Oncol 2014; 110:82–89.

Woerdeman LA, Hage JJ, Hofland MM, Rutgers EJ. A prospective assessment of surgical risk factors in 400 cases of skin-sparing mastectomy and immediate breast reconstruction with implants to establish selection criteria. Plast Reconstr Surg 2007; 119:455–463.

Scenario 9

Breast screening programme

You review a 60-year-old lady in clinic after a mammogram has revealed a suspicious mass within the left breast.

Q. 9.1 Tell me about the NHS breast screening programme.

This is a national screening for early detection of breast cancer in women, started in 1987–1988, based on the Forrest report of 1985. The two main trials: This report was based on are the US HIP trial and the Swedish two-county trial which suggested a 30% reduction in breast cancer mortality in women over the age of 50 years.

The programme began screening 50–64 years with single view mammography and the time interval of screening every 3 years was based on the Swedish two-county trial which had same benefit in mortality compared to other trials screening at shorter intervals. The Breast Screening Frequency Trial Group compared 3-yearly screening with annual screening in a randomised controlled trial (RCT) in 2002 and found no difference in the projected breast cancer related mortality rates.

The UK age trial randomised women in the age group of 39–41 to 48 years to screening versus no screening and found no benefit in mortality at 10 years possibly due to low incidence of breast cancer in this age group and less sensitivity of mammograms in younger population.

Extended follow-up of the Swedish two-county trial published in 2002 suggested ongoing benefit in women up to 70 years. From 2003 NHSBSP introduced two view mammography and now screens women from the age of 50 years to their 71st birthday 3 yearly.

Some women are currently being offered screening from 47–49 and 71–73 as part of the age extension trial. In 2020 as a result of the COVID-19 pandemic the extension trial was closed along with other screening services to allow the NHS to concentrate resources. After the pandemic the trialists did not resume randomisation with the trial closing prematurely. However, electronic data accrual continues on the randomised patients to date.

Q. 9.2 What principles are screening programmes based on?

The principles of screening are based on:
1. The characteristics specific to the test
    - There should be a suitable test, e.g. high specificity and sensitivity
    - The test should be acceptable to the population
    - Screening can be repeatable at intervals
    - The results of the test should facilitate diagnosis, and treatment should be available
    - Chance harm should be less than chance benefit

2. The characteristics of condition which
    - A significant health problem
    - The natural history should be understood
    - There should be an early or latent stage
    - Treatment of the early or latent stage should be more benefit than if started at a later stage and improves outcome.

Q. 9.3 Do you know of any biases that can influence screening programmes?

The following biases can influence apparent improvements in breast cancer survival in screening programmes:
- *Lead time bias:* The apparent improvement in survival because the screening test allows diagnosis to be made earlier in the patient's life without affecting the actual time of death so that the diagnosis is known for a longer period of time without there being any improved longevity of life
- *Length time bias:* Diagnosis of increased volume of less aggressive cases without improving the diagnosis of more aggressive rapidly growing cancers which present symptomatically in the interval between screens
- *Selection bias:* Attendees for screening are generally more aware of health issues and are generally healthier compared to those who decline screening so will have better outcome regardless of screening.

Q. 9.4 Are there any controversies associated with the NHSBSP?

Overdiagnosis: This means diagnosis of a condition/disease that will never cause a symptom of lead to death of the patients in their lifetime. A Cochrane review of the RCTs on screening revealed 15% reduction in breast cancer related mortality, with false positive rate of 10% over 10 years and 30% overdiagnosis.

For every 2,000 women screened for 10 years, one life is prolonged, 10 are overtreated and 200 experience psychological distress due to false positive results. Updated analysis of the Forrest report utilising quality adjusted life years reported that harms offset gains up to 10 years but thereafter gains increase.

The Marmot report is an independent review of breast screening chaired by Professor Sir Michael Marmot. It concluded that breast cancer screening resulted in absolute 20% benefit in breast cancer mortality. One death is prevented for every 235 women invited or about 180 women screened for 20 years. This translates to 1,300 lives saved per year in the UK. However, for each death prevented, three are over-diagnosed. The panel concluded that breast screening should continue but women should receive more information to make an informed decision.

Q. 9.5 How is the quality of the screening programme assured?

Minimum NHS standard for coverage is 70%. Regional Quality Assurance Reference Centres (QARCs) monitor standards in all disciplines (radiology, surgery, pathology, etc.). Screening units have regular QA visits.

Q. 9.6 What are interval cancers? What do you understand by the term "duty of candour"?

Interval cancers are an inevitable part of the breast screening programme. They are cancers that are diagnosed in between routine screening episodes.

There are three types of interval cancer.
1. Newly detectable cancers that have developed since the last screening appointment (common)
2. Cancers that were visible at the last screen but not recalled for further tests because the signs of cancer were very subtle and thought to be normal (less common)
3. Cancers that were visible at the last screen but not recalled for further tests because the signs were missed (rare)

Interval cancers occur in around three in every 1,000 women screened. The majority of these cancers were not seen at the previous screen. When a woman is diagnosed between screens (symptomatically), it is important that the screening service is informed so a review of the previous screening images can be undertaken as soon as possible (within 6 months of cancer diagnosis). The review compares the diagnostic mammogram with the previous screening mammogram. Women can ask for the results of an interval cancer review.

In a very small number of cases, duty of candour will apply. Within the screening programme, in cases where duty of candour applies, the screening service should write to the woman to ask if she would like to know the outcome of her interval cancer review. It is her choice whether she accepts this offer.

Further reading

Breast Screening Frequency Trial Group. The frequency of breast cancer screening: Results from the UKCCCR randomised trial. United Kingdom Co-Ordinating Committee on Cancer Research. Eur J Cancer 2002; 38:1458–1464.

Forrest APM. Breast Cancer screening. Report to the Health Ministers of England, Wales, Scotland and Northern Ireland by a working group chaired by Sir Patrick Forrest. London: HMSO. (http://www.cancerscreening.nhs.uk/breastscreen/publications/forrest-report.pdf).

Gotzsche PC, Nielsen M. Screening for breast cancer with mammography. Cochrane database Syst Rev 2009; 359:909–919.

Mahase E. Trial to extend breast cancer screening won't resume randomization after pandemic. BMJ. 2020;370

Marmot MG, Altman DG, Cameron DA, et al. The independent UK panel on breast cancer screening. The benefits and harms of breast cancer screening: An independent review. Br J Cancer 2013; 108:2205–2240.

Moss SM, Cuckle H, Evans A, et al. Trial management group. Effect of mammographic screening from age 40 years on breast cancer mortality at 10 years. Follow up: A randomised control trial. Lancet 2006; 368:2053–2060.

Public health of England. Population screening programme. NHSBSP Breast Screening: Interval cancers and duty of candour, 2018.

Raftrey J, Chorozoglou M. Possible net harms of breast cancer screening: updated modelling of Forrest report. BMJ 2011; 343:d7627.

Shapiro S. Periodic screening for breast cancer: The hip randomised control trial. Health insurance plan. J Nat Cancer Inst 1997; 22:27–30.

Tabar L, Vitak B, Chen HH, et al. The Swedish two county trial twenty years later. Updated mortality results and new insights from long term follow up. Radiol Clin North Am 2000; 38:625–651.

UK Government. Breast screening: interval cancers and duty of candour toolkit [Internet]. London: UK Government; [cited 2024 Jun 18]. Available from: https://www.gov.uk/government/publications/breast-screening-interval-cancers-and-duty-of-candour-toolkit/

Wilson JMG, Jungner G. Principles and practices of screening for disease. Geneva: World Health Organization; 1968.

World Health Organization. Report no. PHP 34. Geneva: World Health Organization; 1968.

Scenario 10

Ductal carcinoma in situ

A 60-year-old woman presents to the clinic with right breast pain. She underwent a mammogram which was normal on the right but revealed an area of calcification in the left lower outer quadrant. This was 15 mm in diameter and assessed as M3.

Q. 10.1 How should this patient be managed?

The candidate needs to mention that this patient should be managed using the principles of triple assessment.

History
- The candidate must take a breast history which includes a history of previous screening imaging and most recent mammography of co-morbidities, HRT use and family history
- History of previous breast cancer surgery, exposure to radiation or occupational risk needs to be explored

Examination
- The candidate should express a desire to have a chaperone present for the examination
- The candidate must indicate that they would assess the breast size, scars and symmetry and presence of a lump or nodularity occult to mammography
- Examination of regional lymph nodes should be performed

Imaging
- Comparison of previous mammography would need to be performed to identify if this is a new area or previously investigated. Different patterns of calcifications have been identified which may be suggestive of DCIS. Multiple clusters of fine microcalcifications are typically seen in low-grade DCIS, while linear, continuous, often branching, coarse calcifications are seen with high-grade disease. Magnified views are performed following identification to assess extent
- Ultrasound of the area identified on mammogram and the ipsilateral axilla should be performed
- Ultrasound of the axilla should be due to potential for invasive ductal carcinoma (IDC) associated with HG DCIS
- MRI not routinely used and does not improve outcome, NICE recommendation for use if there is a discrepancy between clinical and radiological findings

Management
Stereotactic core biopsy of the area should be performed

Q. 10.2 In the MDT the histopathology showed the presence of DCIS is all of the cores. Two cores showed IG DCIS and two cores showed HG DCIS. What will be the likely recommendation by the MDT and what factors affect the surgical plan?

In this case of a unifocal site of HG DCIS the surgical plan would be breast conserving surgery with an image-guided wide local excision.

Q. 10.3 The patient had breast conservation surgery with an oncoplastic approach with tissue displacement glanuloplasty. The histopathology of the specimen was as follows: HG DCIS total diameter 20 mm IG DCIS 10 mm superior margin: 6 mm from HG DCIS, inferior margin 0.2 mm lateral margin 0.5 mm, and medial margin 2 mm. Lobular neoplasia was seen 1 mm from medial margin. What are the likely MDT recommendations for this patient and which margins are considered clear and which are close?

- All margins ≥2 mm are considered as negative margins by current NICE/ABS/NCCN guidelines for DCIS
- The inferior and lateral margins are <1 mm. ABS guidelines would recommend further excision, and NICE would recommend consideration of further excision. The candidate must be clear which margin policy they follow and what they would do for this patient
- Incidental lobular neoplasia does not require further excision
- Once margins are clear then adjuvant radiotherapy is indicated followed by consideration for endocrine therapy depending on the receptor status

Q. 10.4 What is the pathology of DCIS? What is the significance of the Van Nuy's score?

- The candidate should be able to describe the salient differences as a spectrum of changes to cell size, morphology, mitosis and orientation in ductal epithelial cells. DCIS is classified as low intermediate or high grade
- The candidate should mention that classification assesses best treatment options using age, tumour size, tumour grade, and margins and categories patients in low-risk score (4–6), intermediate risk (7–9) and high risk (10–12)

Q. 10.5 What are the side effects of radiotherapy following surgical treatment for DCIS?

- Common adverse side effects include skin changes following radiotherapy which include loss of skin elasticity and firmness of the breast tissue resulting in a loss of ptosis in comparison to the contralateral breast

- Less commonly but recognised effects include skin discolouration with erythema effecting part or entire treated breast
- Radiotherapy related lung and cardiovascular injury have been historically reported but these are uncommon using current radiotherapy hypofractionation regimens
- Late side effects can also include osteonecrosis of the ribs, neuralgia and rarely angiosarcoma

Q. 10.6 What do you know about the LORIS trial?

- This patient would not meet the inclusion criteria because of the presence of high-grade DCIS
- Inclusion criteria for the trial non high-grade DCIS in women aged 46 years or above with screen detected microcalcifications
- *Exclusion criteria*: Mass component, nipple discharge, strong family history of breast cancer (two or more 1st or 2nd degree relatives) or previous history of invasive breast cancer or ipsilateral DCIS
- The trial compares outcome from surgical intervention versus active monitoring of low-risk DCIS
- This trial is now closed. Other similar trials include the LORD and COMET trials. Problems of recruitment to trial were related to randomisation to the observation arm where patients perceived being offered nothing versus something.

Q. 10.7 Is endocrine therapy indicated? Discuss the evidence base for its use.

Endocrine therapy may result in a modest additional benefit following breast-conserving surgery with radiotherapy but needs to be weighed against side effects of endocrine therapy which often result poor long-term compliance. The candidate should mention the NSABP-35 trial, IBIS II trial findings.

Further reading

Association of Breast Surgery. (2023). NICE guidance for DCIS. ABS guidance for DCIS. https://associationofbreastsurgery.org.uk/professionals/clinical/guidance-platform/cancer surgery13.2 [Last accessed February, 2023].

Scenario 11

Blue dye and allergic reactions

You have started operating on a fit 63-year-old patient due to have a wide local excision and sentinel node biopsy. You have located the sentinel node and as you place your instrument around the node the anaesthetist mentions the patient's neck appears flushed and the blood pressure begins to drop.

Q. 11.1 What do you do?

- The candidate should recognise that the patient is suffering from an anaphylactic reaction most probably due to the patient blue dye
- The candidate should recognise that surgery needs to stop and the immediate treatment of anaphylaxis should be initiated
- The first step should be to call for senior additional anaesthetic assistance to resuscitate and stabilise the patient. This should include administration of adrenaline, intravenous hydrocortisone, antihistamines and fluids
- Circulating theatre staff should be asked to contact the theatre co-ordinator and intensive care needs to be made aware of the event and postoperative care in a high dependence setting will be required

Q. 11.2 Tell me about the blue dye and allergic reactions and treatment?

The candidate should mention the following points:
- Patent blue is a dye manufactured for the purpose of identification of sentinel nodes following its injection into the subdermal plexus of lymphatic vessels. It travels first to the sentinel node before other regional lymph nodes. It may be administered by diluting 2 mL with saline to make 5 mL for injection
- The extent of reaction varies from development of a rash (grade I reaction) to life-threatening anaphylaxis (grade III) with airway and cardiovascular compromise and cardiac arrest (grade IV). The risk of a reaction is 1% but a serious allergic reaction occurring in 1:200–1:1,000
- Patients must be informed of the use of blue dye and its allergic potential as part of the consent process, and the risk documented on the consent form
- Patients with a history of food dye allergy can be offered blue dye. Skin *prick* testing with patent V blue dye *should not* be used as a pre-surgery screening tool but *may be* used to confirm the cause of anaphylaxis following SLNB
- Government advice for surgeons using blue dyes is to remain aware of the risk of serious allergic reactions, including anaphylaxis competent personnel and emergency facilities should be available for at least 1 hour after administration of blue dye because delayed reactions may occur

- *Treatment for adverse reaction is supportive and while patient is unstable surgery is discontinued:* The patient should be intubated during anaphylaxis to maintain the airway, fluid resuscitation to combat hypotension as well as intravenous adrenaline. The patient will need to be transferred to the intensive care unit and remain ventilated until the anaphylactic reaction has resolved. In less severe cases without airway compromise IV hydrocortisone as well as antihistamines should be given

Q. 11.3 The consultant anaesthetist and intensivist arrive in theatre and they quickly administer adrenaline and fluids and after 5 minutes the patient becomes normotensive and bronchospasm improves. What are the next steps?

- Once patient is stabilised with treatment for anaphylaxis, provided the anaesthetic team are in agreement surgery should be completed
- Postoperatively, the patient will required close monitoring in a high-acuity setting such as HDU or ICU
- The reaction must be reported to the Committee of Safety in Medicines (Yellow card scheme)
- Patient with suspected blue dye anaphylaxis must be investigated by allergy testing performed by specialist unit. Elevated tryptase is a sign of mast cell degranulation and will remain elevated for more than 6 hours so may be checked initially to confirm the diagnosis of anaphylaxis. (A list of these centres can be found on the Association of Anaesthesia website http://www.aagbi.org/safety/allergies-and-anaphylaxis)

Q. 11.4 Anything else that could cause anaphylaxis in surgery?

Candidates should be able to list the following with examples: Muscle relaxants (e.g. succinyl chlorine), latex, antibiotics, chlorhexidine, opioids, and colloids

Q. 11.5 What type of allergic reaction is it?

- The candidate should be able to identify this as type 1 immediate hypersensitivity
- *Type 1 should be described:* Type I reactions (i.e. immediate hypersensitivity reactions) involve immunoglobulin E (IgE)-mediated release of histamine and other mediators from mast cells and basophils. Examples include anaphylaxis and allergic rhinoconjunctivitis

Further reading

Barthelmes L, Goyal A, Newcombe RG, et al. Adverse reactions to patent blue V dye – The NEW START and ALMANAC experience. Eur J Surg Oncol 2010; 36:399–403.

Medicines and Healthcare products Regulatory Agency. (2012). Blue dyes: risk of serious allergic reactions. [online] Available from https://www.gov.uk/drug-safety-update/blue-dyes-risk-of-serious-allergic-reactions [Last accessed February, 2023].

NHS. (2019). Patient safety review and response report April to September 2018: A summary of how we reviewed and responded to the patient safety issues you reported. [online] Available from https://associationofbreastsurgery.org.uk/professionals/clinical/guidance-platform/-cancer surgery [Last accessed February, 2023].

Scenario 12

Ductal cancer

A 57-year-old patient who presented with a breast lump in the left breast has been diagnosed with a 12 mm grade 2 IDC ER+/PR8+ breast cancer and ultrasound examination of her axilla did not identify any pathological nodes.

Q. 12.1 She is coming to see you for her treatment planning session. What would you do during this session? What are the likely surgical options for the management of the axilla?

- The candidate should indicate that a breast CNS should be present during the interview
- The candidate should indicate that the results of the triple assessment would be explained to the patient and that the recommendation would be breast conservation surgery with surgical assessment of the axilla
- The candidate should indicate that a review if the medical history of the patient and clinical examination of both breasts and axilla in the presence of a chaperone should be done
- The candidate should identify that a sentinel node biopsy is required to assess the axilla as a diagnostic procedure

Q. 12.2 What types of sentinel node localisation are you aware of?

The candidate should be able to identify that there are several techniques in use for sentinel node localisation including dual agents technetium-99 with patient blue dye, superparamagnetic iron oxide combined with a magnetic probe (senti-mag), radioactive seeds, indocyanine green

Q. 12.3 What information will you give the patient regarding how you will perform the sentinel biopsy and what they could expect?

- The candidate should be able to describe a dual agent technique is the method of choice; patient will have undergone localisation using technetium-99 within 24 hours of surgery and after anaesthesia injection subdermally 2 mL of patent blue diluted with sodium chloride to a volume of 5 mL in the periareolar region
- All "hot" and blue nodes should be identified and removal of these nodes will involve making a skin crease incision in the axilla and using a gamma probe

the nodes would be localised with minimal dissection of the axilla. They should mention usually 1 on average 1–2 nodes are biopsied but up to 4 nodes may be taken. The results from the biopsy analysed through histopathology a process that will take up to 2 weeks. The results would be discussed at MDT additional treatment recommendations would be made at that time

- Administration of patent blue agent carries a risk of adverse reaction and this can range from a mild-to-severe reaction requiring emergency treatment to treat this and would require being admitted overnight if it occurred
- The procedure is associated with minimal morbidity with in terms of numbness in the axilla, arm stiffness or lymphoedema rarely occurs (1–5%)
- The patient should receive written information regarding sentinel node biopsy

Q. 12.4 The patient is due to have a sentinel node biopsy with a lymphoscintigram. Preoperatively when you view the lymphoscintigram there is no evidence of localisation only evidence of the index injection. What do you do next?

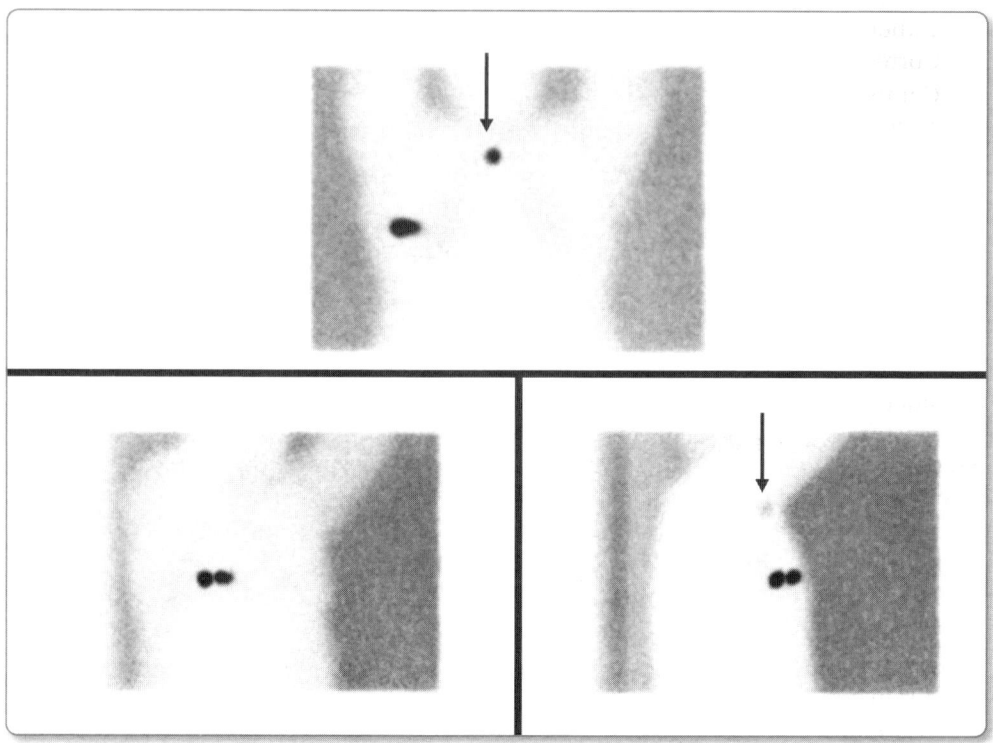

- The patient should be informed that a dual technique could not be used as planned
- A delayed scan may be appropriate depending on theatre timings

- The candidate should offer patient the option of having sentinel node biopsy with a single agent technique (patent blue) explaining that its sensitivity in detecting sentinel nodes is slightly less accurate compared to the dual technique. Alternatively, the patient could be offered axillary node sampling when a minimum of four nodes would be biopsied
- The default investigation should be axillary node sampling if the blue dye also fails to localise the sentinel node

Q. 12.5 Fortunately, the blue dye localises the node and there is a signal with the gamma probe so SLNB can be carried out at surgery. Two weeks later, you are at the MDT, the histopathology result is presented. There is a 14-mm G2 IDCA ER8/PR8/HER2 negative. The margins are clear but 1 out of 2 nodes contain macro-metastases. How would you manage this patient?

The patient will need DXT and endocrine therapy.

There are a number of options for managing the axilla according to the current ABS guidelines. The candidate has been asked what they would do and so must clearly state one rather than give a synopsis of current options.

Correct answers for this patient include (current ABS guidance 2018):
- Completion axillary node clearance
- Axillary radiotherapy – the candidate should mention the AMAROS trial
- No further treatment – ACOSOG Z0011

Q. 12.6 After discussion the patient is booked to have axillary clearance. What information must be included as a part of informed consent specific to this procedure?

The candidate should mention that the patient needs to be aware of the risk of shoulder stiffness, lymphoedema, numbness in the axilla due to neuropraxia to the intercostobrachial nerve, potential for damage to the long thoracic nerve causing winging of the scapula, injury to the thoracodorsal pedicle limiting its use in reconstruction.

Q. 12.7 What is your approach to axillary clearance?
- The candidate should demonstrate a logical approach to dissection and should clearly state the order in which they would identify the anatomy
- A skin crease incision in the axilla incorporating sentinel biopsy scar
- *Technique*: Open clavipectoral fascia and using combination of bipolar diathermy, pledgets and scissors dissect the lymph node packet from structures of the medial and lateral walls of the axilla. Superficially, this will involve identifying and preserving the intercostobrachial nerve if possible. More deeply and medially staying away from the fascia of pectoralis major to avoid damage to the long thoracic nerve and laterally using bipolar to dissect away from the

thoraco-dorsal pedicle. The apex of dissection will be to the level of the axillary vein and care needs to be taken to avoid tearing small tributaries often cause significant bleeding. Specimen kept intact delivered as a lymph node packet or as each level
- *Indications for extent*: Based on risk benefit. Most patient will have level 2 after positive sentinel node biopsy while radiologically clinically positive axilla will have level 2–3

Further reading

Association of Breast Surgery. (2018). ABS guidance 2018: Smart Function Implementation. [online] Available from https://ww2.eagle.org/content/dam/eagle/rules-and-guides/current/other/304-gn-smartfunctionimplementation-2018/smart-functions-gn-nov18.pdf [Last accessed February, 2023].

Association of Breast Surgery. (2018). ASCO guidance 2018. [online] Available from https://associationofbreastsurgery.org.uk/professionals/clinical/guidance-platform/cancer surgery [Last accessed February, 2023].

Scenario 13

Neoadjuvant chemotherapy

You are seeing a 42-year-old lady recently diagnosed with a 25 mm G3 IDC ER+/PR-/HER2+ breast cancer. Ultrasound of the axilla revealed 1 abnormal lymph node which was biopsied and revealed metastasis. The rest of the axilla appeared normal.

Q. 13.1 How will you approach this case?

This lady should be seen in clinic to inform her regarding her diagnosis in the breast clinic in the presence of a breast care nurse, once her results are discussed in MDM.

Check she has had a complete history – past breast related issues, family history of breast/ovarian malignancies, menstrual and obstetric history, family history of breast/ovarian malignancies, comorbidities.

This patient has a T2N1 HER-2 positive breast cancer, her first line of treatment would be neoadjuvant chemotherapy with targeted therapy.

To be able to offer breast and axillary conservation after NACT, the primary tumour and the lymph node in the axilla should be marked with a marker clip.

Q. 13.2 What are the indications for neoadjuvant chemotherapy?

To downstage:
- Inflammatory breast cancer
- Inoperable breast cancer/locally advanced disease: T4, N2/3
  - If postmenopausal ER positive/HER2 negative consider NET

To guide postoperative therapy based on pathological response:
- HER2 positive (TDM1) and TNBC (capecitabine)

Where chemotherapy will definitely be given adjuvantly, consider NACT to:
- To try to facilitate BCS +/- downstaging axilla
- To allow germline genetic testing
- To plan autologous reconstruction
- To facilitate participation on clinical trial

Q. 13.3 What are the patterns of response to NACT can be seen in the breast?

Patterns of response to neoadjuvant chemotherapy. Ref: Association of Breast Surgery. Neoadjuvant chemotherapy: multidisciplinary guidance 2023.

pCR
- No clinical abnormality
- Imaging-normal or residual mass that may be fibrosis alone
- Surgery: Smaller WLE around clip
- Pathology – no cancer – specimen should contain marker and show evidence of chemo response

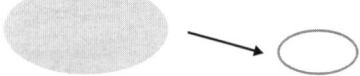

Concentric shrinkage
- Examination-smaller mass
- Imaging – smaller residual mass or may be normal
- Surgery: WILE around clip
- Pathology – smaller lesion, well - margins clear, may be downgraded

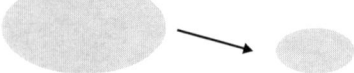

Honeycomb effect
- Examination – normal
- Imaging – may be normal or residual mass
- Surgery – smaller WLE around clip
- Pathology – cancer cells throughout specimen
- In this scenario consideration needs to be given to excising the original footprint. Re-iterate to the patient that this is still a response to chemotherapy

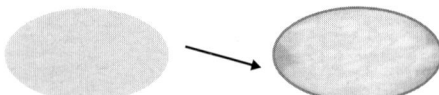

No response or progression - less than 3%
- Examination - larger mass
- Imaging - same or larger
- Pathology - larger lesion
- Should pick up on monitoring during chemo
- Usual to switch chemo, may need to operate sooner, poorer prognosis

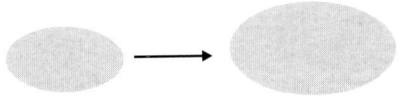

Scenario 13 Neoadjuvant chemotherapy

These are her pre- and postchemotherapy mammograms – what do they show?

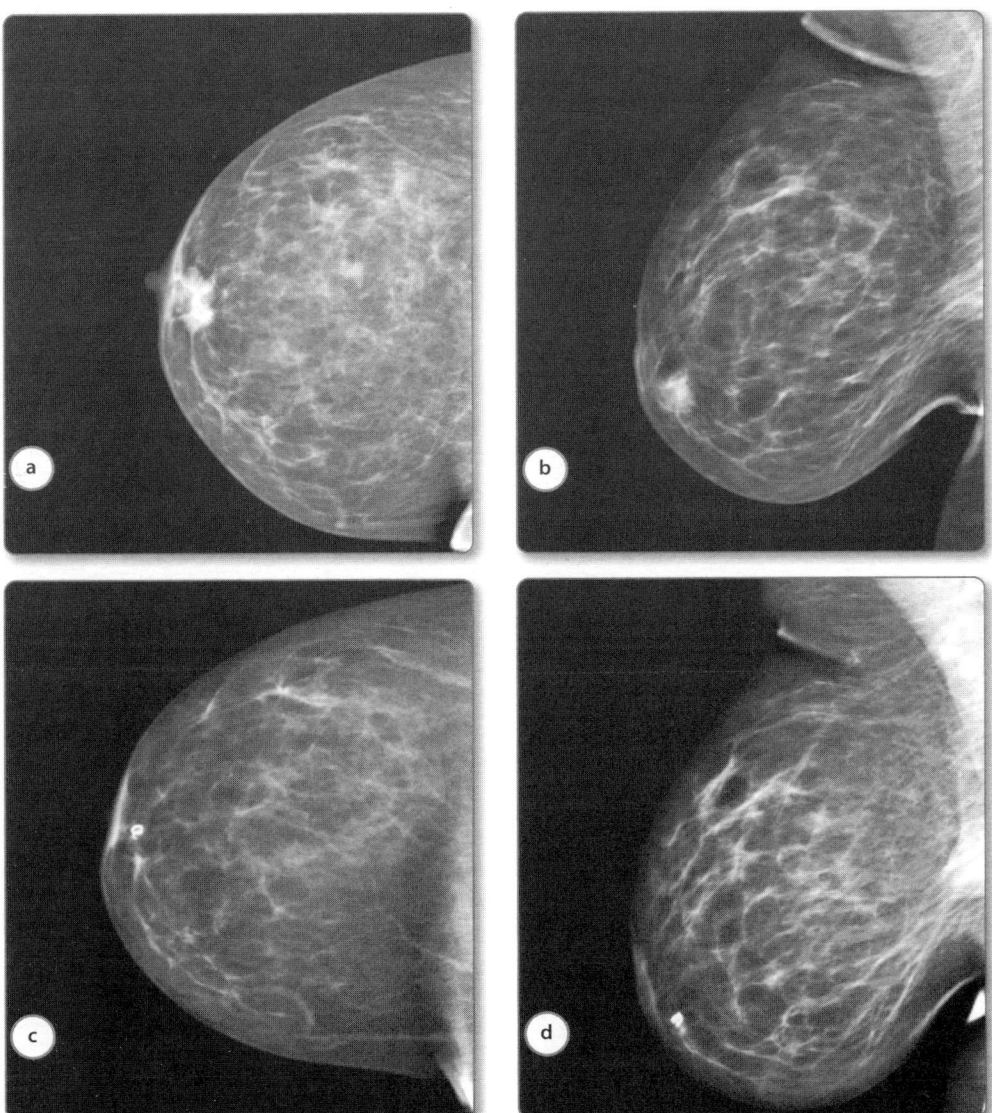

Pre-NACT images suggestive of M5U5 lesion posterior to the nipple areola complex.
Post-NACT images suggestive of good response to NACT in breast with no mass seen around the marker clips.

Q. 13.4 The axillary US is now normal. What is the recommended approach to surgery for her axilla in this setting? How will you support your argument?

The candidate must state what *they* would do.
Traditional approach to treating node positive axilla has been an axillary clearance.

This would be an acceptable answer. The candidate may then be asked for evidence for alternative approaches.

This lady has low volume axillary involvement prior to NACT (N1) and could be considered for axillary conservation based on her response to NACT.

The lymph nodes in her axilla appear normal on ultrasound after chemotherapy and the node is clipped so she can safely be offered sentinel node biopsy.

Two main trials that have looked at management of axilla post-NACT include the ACOSOG Z1071 and the SENTINA trials.

Further reading

Association of Breast Surgery. Neoadjuvant chemotherapy: multidisciplinary guidance [Internet]. 2023 [cited 2023 Jan 11]. Available from: https://associationofbreastsurgery.org.uk/media/515633/neoadjuvant-chemotherapy-manual-v1.pdf

Balasubramanian R, Morgan C, Shaari E, et al. Wire guided localisation for targeted axillary node dissection is accurate in axillary staging in node positive breast cancer following NACT. Eur J Surg Oncol 2020; 46:1028–1033.

Boughey JC, Suman VJ, Mittendorf EA, et al. Sentinel Lymph nodes biopsy after neoadjuvant chemotherapy in patients with node positive breast cancer – The ACOSOG Z1071 (Alliance) Clinical Trial. JAMA 2013; 310:1455–1461.

Caudle AS, Yang WT, Krishnamurthy S, et al. Improved Axillary Evaluation Following Neoadjuvant Therapy for Patients With Node-Positive Breast Cancer Using Selective Evaluation of Clipped Nodes: Implementation of Targeted Axillary Dissection. J Clin Oncol 2016; 34:1072–1078.

Gandhi A, Coles C, Makris A, et al. Axillary Surgery Following Neoadjuvant Chemotherapy: Multidisciplinary Guidance From the Association of Breast Surgery, Faculty of Clinical Oncology of the Royal College of Radiologists, UK Breast Cancer Group, National Coordinating Committee for Breast Pathology and British Society of Breast Radiology. Clin Oncol 2019; 31:664–668.

Kuehn T, Bauerfeind I, Fehm T, et al. Sentinel lymph node biopsy in patients with breast cancer before and after neoadjuvant chemotherapy (SENTINA): a prospective multicentre cohort study. Lancet Oncol 2013; 14:P609–P618.

Woods RW, Camp MS, Durr NJ, et al. Review of options for localisation of axillary lymph nodes in the treatment of invasive breast cancer. Acad Radiol 2019; 26:P805–P819.

Scenario 14

Fibroadenoma

A 20-year-old patient has been referred with a painless marble-sized right breast lump she noticed 3 months ago. She has attended the breast clinic.

Q. 14.1 How would you manage this patient?

The candidate needs to mention that this patient should be managed using the principles of triple assessment.

History

The candidate should take a full breast history that includes a history of the lump in terms of its change in size, fixity, its relationship to the menstrual cycle and use of oral contraceptives

Examination
- Full breast examination should be performed with a chaperone
- The examination includes assessing mobility, fixity to underlying structures and presence of locoregional lymph nodes

Imaging

This patient is under the age of 40 years and should have an ultrasound scan

Q. 14.2 Examination reveals a 15 mm P2 smooth very mobile round mass. Ultrasound shows a 15 mm U2 mass suggestive of a fibroadenoma. How would you manage this patient?

Core biopsy does not need to be performed to confirm the diagnosis in this young patient with P2U2 assessment suggestive of fibroadenoma.

She should be reassured that fibroadenomas are benign lesions that do not require removal. The majority will stay the same size of get smaller.

The size should be documented, and she should be advised to seek further referral if it increases in size.

The patient does not require follow-up.

A patient information booklet explaining the information in writing should be given to the patient.

Q. 14.3 A 45-year-old patient also presents with a 15-mm P2 mobile lump she became aware of her lump 6 months earlier. Will her management differ and if so in what way?

The patient should have bilateral mammograms in addition to an ultrasound of the lesion. A core biopsy should be performed in this case regardless of imaging results.

Q. 14.4 The core biopsy from this patient shows atypical epithelial changes suggestive of a Phyllodes tumour. What recommendations will the MDT likely to make?

- The MDT will recommend surgical excision of the lesion
- The lesion will require complete excision with the capsule intact

Q. 14.5 If the final histology shows a malignant phyllodes tumour what are the principles in subsequent management?

- Discussion in local sarcoma MDT
- Excisions with adequate margins >1 cm
- No need for axillary surgery
- Staging
- Radiotherapy and chemotherapy may be considered in certain cases
- Review family history to see if eligible for genetic testing for TP53 as under 46

Further reading

Association of Breast Surgery. ABS Summary Statement on Management of Fibroadenomas. Association of Breast Surgery; 2019 [cited 2024 Jun 19]. Available from: https://associationofbreastsurgery.org.uk/media/64950/abs-summary-statement-fibroadenomas-v1.pdf

Yu CY, Huang TW, Tam KW. Management of phyllodes tumor: A systematic review and meta-analysis of real-world evidence. Int J Surg.2022; 107:106969.

Scenario 15

Breast cancer in men

A 76-year-old man presented with left breast nodularity and tenderness to the breast clinic. It has been present for approximately 2 months and has been intermittently painful.

Q. 15.1 What is the management of this patient?

History
- The candidate must take a breast history including family history of breast or ovarian cancer
- History of medications and OTC preparations and recreational drugs in order to identify potential drug related gynaecomastia
- History of testicular symptoms/lumps
- History of weekly alcohol intake
- History of co-morbidities specifically liver disease

Examination
- The candidate should express a desire to have a chaperone present for the examination
- On inspection, the candidate should look for stigmata of liver disease and obesity
- The candidate must indicate that they would assess the breast size, scars and symmetry and presence of a lump with assessment for skin tethering, ulceration and fixity
- Examination of regional lymph nodes should be performed
- Testicular examination should be performed

Imaging/Investigations
- Imaging investigation of choice is US with mammography recommended for men suspected of having breast cancer
- Ultrasound of the axilla is warranted for indeterminate or clinical or radiological suspicious lesions
- U3/M3 or more suspicious lesions should undergo core biopsy

Blood tests
- 9AM Testosterone, thyroid function tests, liver function tests, α-fetoprotein, β-human chorionic gonadotrophin

- *If testosterone is abnormal:* Luteinizing hormone, follicle stimulating hormone, sex hormone binding globulin, albumin, oestradiol, prolactin
- *Testicular ultrasound scan if any of the following abnormal blood results are noted:* Raised β-hCG, raised α-fetoprotein

Management

The candidate should mention that likely diagnosis is commonly gynaecomastia. Differential diagnosis apart from male breast cancer, infection breast abscess, lipoma, pseudoangiomatous stromal hyperplasia (PASH), pseudogynaecomastia/lipomastia and haemangioma. Other non-breast cancer primary tumours such as sarcomas. Fibroadenomas are rare.

Q. 15.2 Imaging confirmed bilateral gynaecomastia, more pronounced on the left. You are due to see the patient in clinic what will you tell the patient?

- Explain to the patient that gynaecomastia is a benign change that occurs physiologically at his age due to relative hormonal imbalance in the breast tissue but also has other causes and explore how much and what way this is affecting his life
- Check that no underlying endocrine abnormality has been identified that requires specialist referral. If none found reassure the patient regarding this
- Review medication list to identify any drugs that may be exacerbate the development of gynaecomastia balancing the risk of withdrawing this with the persistence of gynaecomastia. If alternative medication can be given, this should also be considered
- If excess alcohol intake has been identified, then abstinence should be advised
- Symptomatic treatment by simple analgesics if not contraindicated

Hormonal Treatment

- The patient must be informed that this treatment is off-licence. It is most effective for recent onset gynaecomastia, i.e. before gynaecomastia becomes fibrotic, and alleviates mastalgia, not always regression of the mass
- *Tamoxifen 10 mg PO OD:* 3-9 months
- *Anastrozole 1 mg PO OD:* 3 months

Surgical Treatment

Dependent on local guidelines

Q. 15.3 If triple assessment had confirmed the diagnosis of a left 25 mm G2 IDCA ER8/PR8/HER2 negative breast cancer with no axillary nodal involvement. What would be treatment plan?

- Mastectomy or breast conserving surgery based on breast size – mastectomy is most likely surgical option due to smaller breast size in men

- He will need sentinel node biopsy
- He will require endocrine therapy postoperatively
- He should be considered for gene profiling postoperatively depending in results but it needs to be borne in mind that these studies were predominately performed on women

Q. 15.4 What is the incidence and life-time risk of male breast cancer and what factors increase this risk?

- The incidence of male breast cancer is much less common than in women accounting for <1% of all breast cancers
- The general population life-time risk is 1:1,000 compared to 1:8 in women. The average age at diagnosis is 5 years older compared to women
- Risk factors identified as increasing the chance of developing breast cancer in men include increasing age, black race, family history of breast cancer, radiation exposure, specific genetic mutations (*BRCA2, BRCA1, CHEK2* and *PALB2*). Additionally, conditions predisposing to excess oestradiol exposure (gynaecomastia, liver disease and obesity) as well as chromosomal (Klinefelter's syndrome-XXY) and testicular abnormalities also have been associated
- *BRCA2* carriage increases the risk to 7%. Fewer men with breast cancer carry *BRCA1* mutation (0–4% vs. 5–10%) *BRCA2* carriage is 4–16%

Q. 15.5 Is there a role for endocrine therapy in male breast cancer?

The use of endocrine therapy in men is recommended. Tamoxifen may be used unless contraindicated. Alternatively, aromatase inhibitors (AIs) may be used in combination with gonadotrophin-releasing hormone (GnRH) inhibitors due to less oestrogen suppressive effect of AIs in men compared to women when used alone. Dual agent therapy is also favoured.

Further reading

Association of Breast Surgery. ABS Summary Statement on Investigation and Management of Gynaecomastia in Primary & Secondary Care. Association of Breast Surgery; 2021 [cited 2024 Jun 19]. Available from: https://associationofbreastsurgery.org.uk/media/337465/abs-summary-statement-gynaecomastia-v3.pdf

Giordano SH. Breast cancer in men. N Engl J Med 2018; 378:2311–2320.

Giordano SH. A review of the diagnosis and management of male breast cancer. The Oncologist 2005; 10:471–479.

National Institute for Health and Clinical Excellence (NICE). (2018). NICE guidelines for diagnosis and management of breast cancer. [online] Available from https://www.nice.org.uk/guidance/ng101 [Last accessed February, 2023].

Scenario 16

Inflammatory breast cancer

A 44-year-old woman presents to your 2-week wait breast clinic. She has several weeks' history of a swollen thickened erythematous whole right breast, and 3 weeks of antibiotics have made no difference.

Q. 16.1 How would you initially manage this patient? What are your differentials?

The candidate should describe the steps of triple assessment.

History

The full 2-week wait history should be taken. Salient points will include the duration/rapidity of symptoms, any associated pain, systemic symptoms, management to date, breast feeding or pregnancy, smoking, a history of immunosuppression, and a past breast history including cancer.

Examination

A chaperone should be present. Bilateral breast, axillae and regional lymph node are examined. The extent of change should be documented including signs of infection, palpable lumps/abscess/collection, skin lesions, peau d'orange or skin thickening, breast asymmetry compared to the contralateral breast, nipple change/distortion and any systemic signs.

Investigations

Mammogram/tomogram, ultrasound (US) breast and axilla, with US-guided core biopsy or aspiration as required, and punch biopsy.

Differentials

Mastitis (lactational, non-lactational and granulomatous), related skin or breast infection with abscess, inflammatory breast cancer, non-inflammatory breast cancer involving the skin, breast lymphoma and radiation dermatitis.

Q. 16.2 She undergoes triple assessment. Her imaging returns as M5 U5 (oedema) with multiple abnormal lymph nodes. Her breast and axillary core biopsies return as a triple negative invasive breast cancer with axillary involvement. What are you specifically looking for in histology specimens? What are the next steps of management?

The candidate should be concerned that this is an inflammatory breast cancer.

If no skin samples were taken at US-guided biopsy, she will require punch biopsy of the skin which may reveal dermal lymphatic invasion of tumour cells/micro-emboli with E-cadherin overexpression.

Staging investigations are required (unit dependent) including CT thorax abdomen and pelvis with whole body nuclear medicine bone scan or 18F-fluorodeoxyglucose (FDG) positron emission tomography (PET) CT. Consider an MRI scan taking into consideration extent of disease and density of breast tissue.

The candidate should state that they would offer genetic testing. The National Institute for Health and Care Excellence (NICE) guidelines (2018) state that women under 50 years (including those without a relevant family history) with triple negative breast cancer should be offered genetic testing for at least BRCA1 and 2 mutations. They may be further questioned and should be aware of other breast cancer related genetic tests such as TP53 or CHEK-2 and panel testing.

The candidate should differentiate between the management of non-metastatic versus metastatic disease.

With non-metastatic disease standard treatment would be neoadjuvant chemotherapy followed by surgery, post-mastectomy radiotherapy and additional adjuvant therapy as required. In this case there is no role for endocrine therapy.

With metastatic disease primary systemic therapy is the management of choice to achieve optimal response.

Q. 16.3 What would be your specific surgical management if non-metastatic?

Mastectomy and axillary clearance. Candidates should state that immediate breast reconstruction should generally be avoided due to the importance of timely radiation to the skin in this disease process and need to remove involved skin.

Q. 16.4 What do you understand as the definition of locally advanced breast cancer?

Locally advanced breast cancer is defined as stage 3 disease. A spread to tissues surrounding the breast including the skin and chest wall and to lymph nodes but with no distant metastases.

Q. 16.5 Your registrar reports that she has been called to the ward to review an 84-year-old patient (WHO performance status 3) with multiple medical co-morbidities including dementia. She has been admitted after a fall and found to have a left breast malodorous large lesion. How should this scenario be managed?

The principles of triple assessment apply. A focused symptomatic history as well as a full exploration of her co-morbidities and treatment status is essential. Examination points should include an estimation of size of the lesion, skin/chest wall fixation, and ulceration, associated infection – wet/dry gangrene and associated regional lymph node involvement. Generalised clinic examination is required including the abdomen and spine, if accessible.

As the patient is bed bound and frail imaging access may be limited. Mammogram and ultrasound are considered 'gold standard' but a bedside clinical core biopsy using an aseptic technique and local anaesthetic may be more appropriate first-line management. Wound care is optimised in a fungating infected likely breast cancer with metronidazole gel and charcoal dressings. Ward and/or community staff attending the patient should be informed of this.

Q. 16.6 At MDT assessment her core biopsy returns as a grade 2 invasive ductal carcinoma, which is ER4, PR0 and Her-2 -negative. What are your options?

This patient would be a candidate for staging if complaint.

As she has dementia a best interest meeting should be held and it should be explored if someone has power of attorney for health. Emphasis should be given when planning care on her quality of life and unless staging reveals severely life limiting disease surgery would be part of improving her quality of life if feasible.

The candidate should be aware that the majority of locally advanced breast cancers in post-menopausal women would be hormone receptor positive and first-line management would therefore be primary endocrine therapy in the form of an aromatase inhibitor.

However, in a case with a frail elderly co-morbid effectively triple negative patient, symptom management is priority. High-risk anaesthetic opinion should be sought. If inappropriate for a general anaesthetic, local anaesthetic methods are a consideration. Palliative excision whether a limited wide local excision or simple mastectomy are possibilities dependent on disease extent and breast size. This is without axillary surgery.

In those appropriate for a general anaesthetic a palliative (toilet) mastectomy can be considered with or without axillary surgery for symptom control. The candidate should be aware that the question of closure is essential. A simple mastectomy may be possible, but in cases with extensive disease alternatives may be required. Rotational flaps, pedicled flaps (e.g. Latissimus dorsi resurfacing) and skin grafting are optional techniques.

Further reading

National Institute for Health and Care Excellence (NICE) guidelines. (2018). Early and locally advanced breast cancer: diagnosis and management. NICE guideline (NG101). [online] Available from https://www.nice.org.uk/guidance/ng101 [Last accessed July, 2023].

Chippa V, Barazi H. (2023). Inflammatory Breast Cancer. [online] Available from https://www.ncbi.nlm.nih.gov/books/NBK564324/ [Last accessed July, 2023].

Manjee K, Jorns J. (2023). Breast cancer inflammatory. [online] Available from https://www.pathologyoutlines.com/topic/breastmalignantinflamcar.html [Last accessed July, 2023].

National Institute for Health and Care Excellence (NICE) Guidelines. (June 2013, update 2019). Familial Breast Cancer: Classification and care of people at risk of familial breast cancer and related risks in people with a family history of breast cancer (CG164). [online] Available from https://www.medicinesresources.nhs.uk/en/Medicines-Awareness/Guidance-and-Advice/Guidance/Familial-breast-cancer-classification-care-and-managing-breast-cancer-and-related-risks-in-people-with-a-family-history-of-breast-cancer--6362579622/ [Last accessed July, 2023].

Scenario 17

Level 2 oncoplastic techniques – therapeutic mammoplasty

You are reviewing a patient in clinic with a 20 mm G3 IDC ER+/PR8+/HER2 negative right sided breast cancer. She would like to conserve as much breast tissue as possible and is anxious about the appearance of her breasts postoperatively.

Q. 17.1 What do you understand by the term level 2 oncoplastic technique?

The field of oncoplastic breast surgery has developed from the use of plastic surgery aesthetic principles to re-shape or re-create the breast immediately after resection. This can either be after breast conservation surgery (BCS) or mastectomy.

The candidate should be able to differentiate between level 1 and 2 oncoplastic techniques which focus on patients undergoing BCS:

- *Level 1:* <20% breast tissue loss – requiring a standard wide local excision with glandular mobilisation, with no skin loss ± nipple recentralisation as required
- *Level 2:* 20–50% breast tissue loss – requiring the use of volume displacement, therapeutic mammoplasty (TM), techniques with skin reduction/loss and nipple re-positioning often on a pedicle
- Partial breast reconstruction – using chest wall perforator flaps (e.g. LICAP/MICAP/AICAP/TDAP) or random flaps (e.g. anterior abdominal wall advancement flap) are alternate option with large volume excisions. These are volume replacement rather than displacement techniques in BCS. The candidate would be expected to focus their explanation primarily on level 2 oncoplastic techniques.

Q. 17.2 Which are the key selection considerations in level 2 oncoplastic surgery?

- *Excision volume:* The need for 20–50% breast volume loss for an oncological safe excision with clear margins
- *Tumour location:* The specific level 2 procedure used will depend on the quadrant or quadrants involved (see table below for a further explanation)
- *Glandular density:* The BIRADS density of the breast will determine the suitability of its use. For example, a dense glandular breast can undergo extensive undermining compared to a low density (BIRADS1/2) which conversely would mean a level 2 oncoplastic technique would be more suitable for the former
- *Breast size and grade of ptosis*

Scenario 17 Level 2 oncoplastic techniques – therapeutic mammoplasty 381

Q. 17.3 Which patient groups would be unsuitable for a therapeutic mammoplasty?

There are a variety of ways that this can be answered.
Looking at specific contraindications:
- *Absolute*: Inflammatory breast cancer, very large or unfavourable tumour to breast size ratio which would mean poor cosmesis, progression after neoadjuvant chemotherapy, recurrent breast cancers with previous radiotherapy (RT)
- *Relative:* No tumour free margins, multi-centricity

Or, as another example the use of a triple assessment model:
- *History:* Multiple medical co-morbidities, high-risk anaesthetic patients requiring a shorter length of general anaesthetic time, smoking (relative), the immunosuppressed patient (relative), recurrent breast cancers with previous RT, etc.
- *Examination/Investigation:* Inflammatory breast cancer, morbid obesity with high BMIs, very large tumour to breast ratio (>50% as standard), IMF or general breast chronic dermatological disorders (e.g. psoriasis, intertrigo), multi-centric disease on examination and imaging (relative)

The essence of answering any similar question is to have a system of classification that can be easily recalled during the pressurised examination setting.

Q. 17.4 Your patient has been diagnosed with a left 6-cm G3 ILCa, ER/PR positive and Her-2-negative. Imaging reveals unifocal involvement but from the 1–5 o'clock position, in a large DD cup grade-3 ptotic breast. Her US is node negative. As per MDT recommendation, the patients accept a therapeutic mammoplasty and SNB. Which TM technique would you use?

To answer succinctly the candidate should describe the incision and pedicle required dependent on grade of ptosis, breast size and quadrant(s) involved.
The most common incisions are:
- The wise pattern (inverted T) generally used when a larger proportion of skin excision is required to form the skin envelope
- The vertical scar (Lejour) used generally when less skin excision is required, i.e. less ptotic patients

The following table (Reproduced from the further reading section references) gives a non-exhaustive guide to technique choice:
 Level 2 oncoplastic/therapeutic mammoplasty techniques by quadrant and breast size.

Breast quadrant	Breast size		
Left	Small	Medium ± ptosis	Large/ptotic
12 o'clock (upper pole)	• Round block • Batwing	• Round block • Inferior pedicle • Batwing	• Inferior pedicle • Round block
1–2 o'clock (upper outer)	• Round block	• Round block • Racquet mammoplasty • Inferior pedicle	• Inferior pedicle • Supero-medial pedicle • Round block
4–5 o'clock (lower outer)	• Modified Grisotti • Comma mammoplasty	• Superior pedicle • Super-medical pedicle • Supero-inferior • J mammoplasty • Comma mammoplasty • Central mound	• Superior pedicle • Super-medial pedicle • Supero-inferior • J mammoplasty • Central mound
7–8 o'clock (lower inner quadrant)	• Modified Grisotti	• Superior pedicle/V scar • Central mound • Modified Grisotti	• Superior pedicle • Supero-inferior • Central mound
9–11 o'clock (upper inner)	• Round block	• Round block • Batwing • Inferior pedicle	• Inferior pedicle • Batwing • Round block • Supero-inferior
Central (dependent on involvement of NAC)	• Benelli • Modified batwing	• Grisotti • Benelli • Inferior pedicle • Modified batwing	• Inferior pedicle (wise pattern or V mammoplasty with NAC resection) • Grisotti

(NAC, nipple-areolar complex)

Therefore, in this situation, when there is both UOQ and LOQ involvement in a large ptotic breast, the candidate should offer a wise pattern (inverted T) supero-medial pedicle mammoplasty.

Q. 17.5 Please draw the incision and flap for a wise pattern supero-medial pedicled therapeutic mammoplasty. Describe the technique.

Specialist candidates are expected to be able to draw a variety of incisions, the pre-operative mark up and pedicles and therefore it would be wise to practise prior to the examination.

Scenario 17 Level 2 oncoplastic techniques – therapeutic mammoplasty

Incision examples:
- Wise pattern – anchor shape
- Vertical scar – lollipop shape without horizontal incision

Pre-operative mark up:
- Medial/central mark from sternal notch to umbilicus, sternal notch to nipple distance, nipple to IMF distance, IMF, breast base, breast meridian, vertical limbs, horizontal limbs, new nipple position (measured at IMF)
- The new areolar shape can be formed as a dome at this time or using a nipple marker intra operatively
- Map out the tumour and likely pedicle shape prior to surgery

General description for wise pattern pedicle technique:
- Define all incisions with a scalpel including peri-areolar
- Skin mark (clips or sutures) meridian and key vertical and horizontal corners
- De-epithelialisation
- Raise skin flaps in mastectomy plane to the breast base
- Perform wide local excision (bracketed localisation may be required) skin to pectoralis fascia
- Define and mobilise pedicle (NAC undermining may be required) glandular flap closure to fill defect
- Check closure (skin clips/suture) with patent sitting. Is there an appropriate skin envelope and acceptable aesthetic appearance? Debulk as required to avoid congestion and poor aesthetic outcome, check for kinking.
- Nipple areolar complex repositioning and delivery
- Final dermal and skin closure avoiding tension at the T junction and vertical scar junction with the areolar

Q. 17.6 Consent the above patient for the risks of therapeutic mammoplasty.

General breast surgery risks:
- Infection, bleeding/haematoma, seroma, scarring, pain, numbness, deformity, asymmetry, re-excision of margins, general anaesthetic risks, and venous thromboembolism risks

Specific mammoplasty risks:
- Skin flap necrosis/loss, nipple-areola complex necrosis/loss, fat necrosis, oil cysts, delayed or poor wound healing with wound dehiscence, reduced or enhanced nipple sensation, inability to breastfeed from the ipsilateral breast, nipple asymmetry and contralateral symmetrisation

Q. 17.7 Are you aware of any studies related to the use of the therapeutic mammoplasty technique?

TeaM – an international multicentre prospective cohort study exploring the practice and short-term outcomes of therapeutic mammoplasty published in 2018. This included 889 therapeutic mammoplasties at 50 centres. Its conclusion was that therapeutic mammoplasty is a safe and effective alternative to mastectomy or standard breast-conserving surgery.

ANTHEM feasibility study – extended to 2024 the overall aim is to assess the feasibility of undertaking a large-scale multicentre prospective cohort study to compare the clinical and cost effectiveness of oncoplastic breast conserving surgery as a safe and effective alternative to mastectomy ± immediate breast reconstruction.

Further reading

Clough KB, Kaufman GJ, Nos C, et al. Improving Breast Cancer Surgery: A classification and Quadrant per Quadrant Atlas for Oncoplastic Surgery. Ann Surg Oncol 2010; 17:1375–1391.

Fitzal F, Schrenk P. Oncoplastic Breast Surgery: A Guide to Clinical Practice, 1st Edition. New York, Austria: Springer Wien, 2010.

Gilmour A, Cutress R, Gandhi A, et al. Oncoplastic breast surgery: A guide to good practice. Eur J Surg Oncol. 2021 Sep;47(9):2272-2285. 2021; 47:2272-2285.

O'Connell R, Baker E, Trickey A, et al. Current Practice and short-term outcomes of therapeutic mammoplasty in the international TeaM multicentre prospective cohort study. Br J Surg 2018; 105:1778–1792.

Chapter 6

Colorectal surgery

*Nick Lees, Adam Rees, Muhammad Rafay Sameem Siddiqui, Faddy Kamel,
Tim James Royle, Kapil Sahnan, Rachael Coates*

Scenario 1

Obstructing colon cancer

A 65-year-old woman who smokes 10 cigarettes a day and has a history of chronic obstructive pulmonary disease (COPD) and a myocardial infarction (MI) 4 years earlier presents to an accident and emergency (A&E) with abdominal pain, distension, and no bowel movements for a week.

Q. 1.1 How would you assess the patient?

History and examination

I would take a detailed history and thorough examination focussing on the symptoms and signs of possible bowel obstruction.

My history would centre on whether there were any risk factors for adhesional small bowel obstruction (SBO), any features suggesting cancer (colorectal or other), or a past history of/risk factors for volvulus or pseudo-obstruction.

My history would establish fitness for operative and nonoperative treatment options given that she appears to be an ASA (American Society of Anaesthesiologists) 3, any operative morbidity and mortality is likely to be higher than other less morbid patients.

My examination would include establishing the presence or absence of abdominal hernias, distension, abdominal or rectal masses, tenderness, guarding, or rebound. I would personally perform a digital rectal examination (DRE).

My assessment would also determine the presence or absence of sepsis and/or peritonitis.

Q. 1.2 The patient has an elevated respiratory rate, slight confusion, and a BP of 110 mmHg. How would you initially manage her?

She is demonstrating signs of sepsis according to the 'Could this be sepsis' screening criteria and quick sequential organ failure assessment (Q-SOFA); she requires immediate management in the form of the sepsis 6.

Sepsis 6 involves giving three things and taking three things. The three medical interventions include oxygen, IV fluids, and antibiotics which should be administered ideally within an hour of presentation. The three items that should be taken or measured include urine output, blood and blood cultures, and lactate.

Q. 1.3 Would you take this patient straight to theatre or perform any other investigations?

This patient has bowel obstruction but we do not know the cause. It is likely that she will need surgical intervention but depending on the cause the operative options are considerable ranging from resection to washout and defunction stoma. She is also currently stable with a blood pressure of 110 mmHg and therefore, a definitive CT scan with an anaesthetic and surgical escort would be the most appropriate course of action. If there was suspicion of cancer, a CT chest could also be organised at the same time.

A CT also has the added advantage of including an assessment of bowel viability and for cancer information useful for formal staging.

The CT scan shows an obstructing T3/4 cancer of the descending colon without perforation or ischaemia.

Q. 1.4 Tell me about your management options and which you would choose.

In each surgical condition my options would include a gamete of surgical and non-surgical options.

My main nonsurgical option would include a self-expanding metal stent as bridge to surgery.

This would have the advantage of converting an emergency into a potentially elective procedure including discussion on a role for neoadjuvant chemotherapy.

Stenting reduces the likelihood of a stoma [CREST (Colorectal Endoscopic Stenting Trial)].

Neoadjuvant chemotherapy is well tolerated, with no increase in perioperative morbidity and a trend toward fewer serious postoperative complications.

A majority show histological regression and there are some pathological complete responders, with reduced risk of incomplete resection. This results in a nonstatistically significant trend to improvement in tumour free recurrence/persistence 2-year failure rate (FOxTROT).

The main emergency surgical options include a segmental colectomy with manual decompression or irrigation and defunctioning ileostomy, a subtotal colectomy if the caecum was compromised or a Hartmann's procedure.

Q. 1.5 Which option would you choose for this woman?

I would choose a colonic stent in a view to decompression, converting operative surgery into an elective procedure after discussion at multidisciplinary team (MDT). She is an ASA 3 and it would give us time to optimise any medical conditions that she has. Furthermore, there are no concerning signs on the CT scan.

Q. 1.6 There is no expertise for colonic stents at your centre. Which surgical option would you choose?

I would follow the recommendations set out by The World Society of Emergency Surgeons Guidelines which state that in the absence of caecal compromise or other ischaemia a primary resection with anastomosis and possibly a covering ileostomy would be the most preferable option. If the patient became anaesthetically labile, a Hartmann's procedure would be the option of choose.

Further reading

Hill J, Kay C, Morton D, et al. CREST: randomised phase III study of stenting as a bridge to surgery in obstructing colorectal cancer—results of the UK ColoRectal Endoscopic Stenting Trial (CREST). J Clin Oncol 2016; 34:3507–3509.

Pisano M, Zorcolo L, Merli C, et al. 2017 WSES guidelines on colon and rectal cancer emergencies: obstruction and perforation. World J Emerg Surg 2018; 13:36.

Seymour MT, Morton D, and on behalf of the International FOxTROT Trial Investigators. FOxTROT: an international randomised controlled trial in 1052 patients (pts) evaluating neoadjuvant chemotherapy (NAC) for colon cancer. J Clin Oncol 2019; 37:3504.

The SCOTIA Study Group. Subtotal colectomy versus on-table irrigation and anastomosis. Single-stage treatment for malignant left-sided colonic obstruction: a prospective randomized clinical trial comparing subtotal colectomy with segmental resection following intraoperative irrigation. Br J Surg 1995; 82:1622–1627.

Scenario 2

Acute appendicitis

A 23-year-old woman with a body mass index (BMI) 40 presents to the emergency department with a 24-hour history of right iliac fossa (RIF) pain? She is otherwise fit and well.

Q. 2.1 How would you assess this patient?

History and examination

I would take a careful and thorough history and examination focussing on the symptoms and signs of appendicitis and main differential diagnoses including an ovarian torsion, ovarian cyst rupture, pelvic inflammatory disease, ectopic pregnancy, ureteric colic, and pyelonephritis or urinary tract infection.

My history would centre on whether there were risk factors for appendicitis and the differentials. I would enquire regarding sexual intercourse without contraceptives, missed or relation to her period, urinary symptoms, family history of appendicitis (RR > 3 in patients with three relatives who have had appendicitis previously), and any urinary symptoms.

My examination would establish the precise position of the pain and whether any rebound existed. I would examine the renal angle to elicit any tenderness suggesting ureteric colic or pyelonephritis.

The patient has rebound right iliac fossa tenderness, a temperature of 38.5°C, and begins to vomit.

Q. 2.2 What initial investigations would you want before making a decision on management?

I would request blood tests in particular a white cell count, urine, and pregnancy tests.

Her urine has a trace of leucocytes and blood and her pregnancy test comes back as negative. The white cell count is 16 and neutrophil count is 10.

Q. 2.3 How would you classify her risk of having appendicitis?

Appendicitis is largely a clinical diagnosis although there are some scoring systems that may be used to help in classifying the risk of having appendicitis. A well-known scoring system is the ALVARADO score and in her case the score would be seven indicating a likely appendicitis [migratory abdominal pain, anorexia, nausea/vomiting, tenderness in right iliac fossa, rebound, elevated temperature, leucocytosis, and shift to left (neutrophils)].

Q. 2.4 How accurate is the ALVARADO score and do you know of any other scoring systems?

The sensitivity and specificity of the ALVARADO ranges significantly from reports of 60% to 90% and affected by whether it is used in the context of an adult or child and a man or woman. This makes it an adjunct rather than a definitive tool for clinical decision making.

An alternative score is the appendicitis inflammatory response score which has been shown in some studies to be better than the ALVARADO score but still has variable sensitivity and specificities. It incorporates parameters such as C-reactive protein (CRP) and an assessment of degree of tenderness. It should still be regarded as an adjunct to clinical decision making.

You review her in the emergency department and note she has a pulse rate of 110 bpm after analgesia and some initial IV fluids.

Q. 2.5 Would you immediately take her to theatre?

I would not immediately take her to theatre. There are a range of alternative diagnoses and a known negative appendicectomy rate especially in women.

The RIFT (Right Iliac Fossa Pain Treatment) study has shown that the negative appendicectomy rate approaches 30% in women and 12% in men and is partly due to the reduced usage of imaging such as CT scans. Surgery is not risk free and there should be a move towards the use of scoring systems and imaging to reduce the need for unnecessary surgery.

I would therefore perform an urgent CT scan to see if this was a perforated appendix warranting urgent surgery or an alternative diagnosis warranting involvement from other specialities such as the gynaecologists. An ultrasound may be useful in some circumstances but in the context of an obese patient with signs of inflammatory response (raised pulse rate) it is unlikely to be beneficial.

Q. 2.6 Would your management have differed if she was found to be 6 weeks pregnant?

The main concern is that she is unwell with a raised pulse rate. Her main differential is an ectopic pregnancy. In this circumstance, a transvaginal ultrasound (TVUS) would exclude this but would not exclude a perforated appendicitis. It may be that a TVUS may be used in conjunction with another imaging modality but if another modality is going to be used then the need for a TVUS is unnecessary and potentially delays the management.

My main options for imaging are an MRI scan or a CT scan. Although no evidence exists that MRI scans cause miscarriages in the first trimester, many MRI units will still refuse to perform them. This would mean that a CT scan is the best option to image given that it a perforated appendix is potentially life-threatening. The risk of teratogenicity and long-term cancer risk in a foetus should be discussed with the patient and although perception is that this risk is high, the risk is unlikely to be significant. A CT typically delivers radiation at 30 mGy and the risk of foetal abnormalities is associated with radiation above 50 mGy.

Q. 2.7 Would your management change if she looked comfortable and her pulse rate was 85 bpm?

I would admit this lady and observe her for a period of 8–12 hours and sequentially reassess her to elicit whether there has been any progression of her symptoms. The World Society of Emergency Surgeons have stated that in patients who are of intermediate risk according to scoring systems or in some cases high risk should be admitted and observed in a view to performing an ultrasound scan at the earliest opportunity.

Depending on the ultrasound scan findings, I would then discuss surgical options with her if it was positive. The most appropriate surgical option would be a diagnostic laparoscopy and proceeding to a laparoscopic appendicectomy. Other options would include treatment with antibiotics and this is something that has recently been highlighted with the COVID-19 situation. Historically there is a concern regarding recurrence with appendicitis treated with antibiotics and careful consideration needs to be made regarding this. If a patient is treated with antibiotics, she should be followed up for a discussion regarding an interval appendicectomy.

Q. 2.8 What would influence your decision to perform an interval appendicectomy?

The World Society of Emergency Surgery does not recommend a routine interval appendicectomy; however, this is in the context of an appendiceal phlegmon or abscess that is treated with appendicitis. I would perform an interval appendicectomy if there was the presence of a faecolith at the time of presentation. Other factors to consider are recurrent symptoms or suspicion of an underlying neoplasm.

You take this lady for a laparoscopic appendicectomy and when you enter the abdomen and look at the appendix it appears lilywhite.

Q. 2.9 What would you do next?

I would complete my diagnostic laparoscopy including looking for any evidence of pelvic inflammatory disease, ovarian pathology evidence of endometriosis, or inflammatory bowel disease (IBD). In the absence of any other alternative diagnosis, I would follow the World Society of Emergency Surgery guidelines and remove the appendix.

I would remove the appendix because sometimes there can be microscopic rather than microscopic disease, there may not be inflammation but rather appendiceal colic related to faecoliths or there may be an underlying neoplasm that is not immediately obvious.

Further reading

Alvarado A. A practical score for the early diagnosis of acute appendicitis. Ann Emerg Med 1986; 15:557–564.

Andersson M, Andersson RE. The appendicitis inflammatory response score: a tool for the diagnosis of acute appendicitis that outperforms the Alvarado score. World J Surg 2008; 32:1843–1849.

Di Saverio S, Birindelli A, Kelly MD, et al. WSES Jerusalem guidelines for diagnosis and treatment of acute appendicitis. World J Emerg Surg 2016; 11:34.

Di Saverio S, Sibilio A, Giorgini E, et al. The NOTA study (nonoperative treatment for acute appendicitis) prospective study on the efficacy and safety of antibiotics (amoxicillin and clavulanic acid) for treating patients with right lower quadrant abdominal pain and long-term follow-up of conservatively treated suspected appendicitis. Ann Surg 2014; 260:109–117.

Gorter RR, Eker HH, Gorter-Stam MA, et al. Diagnosis and management of acute appendicitis. EAES consensus development conference 2015. Surg Endosc 2016; 30:4668–4690.

Li HM, Yeh LR, Huang YK, et al. Familial risk of appendicitis: a nationwide population study. J Pediatr 2018; 203:330–335.e3.

National Surgical Research Collaborative. Multicentre observational study of performance variation in provision and outcome of emergency appendicectomy. Br J Surg 2013; 100:1240–1252.

Ratnapalan S, Bona N, Chandra K, et al. Physicians' perceptions of teratogenic risk associated with radiography and CT during early pregnancy. Am. J. Roentgenol 2004; 182:1107–1109.

Royal College of Surgeons and Association of Surgeons of Great Britain and Ireland. Commissioning guide 2014: emergency general surgery (acute abdominal pain). London, 2014. [online] Available from https://www.rcseng.ac.uk/-/media/./commissioning-guide-egs-published-v3.pdf [Accessed on 1 Jan 2017].

Scenario 3

Stomas

You operate on a 68-year-old man with an obstructing rectal cancer and during the operation are unable to perform an anastomosis. You decide to perform an end colostomy.

Q. 3.1 How you fashion an end colostomy in a Hartmann's procedure?

I would perform an end colostomy for this man. It will be a permanent stoma and the initial decision is whether to perform an intraperitoneal or extraperitoneal technique.

The advantages of an extraperitoneal technique are the potential reduction of a parastomal hernia versus the risk of obstruction.

I do not have (or do) much experience in the extraperitoneal technique and therefore I would perform an intraperitoneal technique.

Q. 3.2 Do you know any types of intraperitoneal techniques?

The main approaches to an intraperitoneal technique are transrectus, lateral to the rectus, and transoblique. In my experience, the transoblique is a bit too lateral often and lateral to rectus techniques may predispose to more parastomal hernias. I would therefore perform a trans-rectus stoma with a cruciate incision in the rectus sheath allowing two fingers to pass through.

If this man presented as an emergency and you wanted to perform a defunctioning colostomy.

Q. 3.3 What options would you consider?

My options for formation include an open and laparoscopic technique. I would perform an open trephine technique with a cruciate incision.

In an emergency setting, the priority is usually the preservation of life and the technique adopted for formation of the colostomy should be that which provides an adequately vascularised colostomy, with minimal risk of postoperative obstruction in the quickest and the safest manner.

Q. 3.4 Are you aware of any evidence regarding the size of the trephine or incisions in the rectus sheath?

The aperture size I would use is normally about 2.5 cm but the Association of Coloproctology of Great Britain and Ireland (ACPGBI) position statement states there is insufficient evidence on this as well as the incision in the anterior sheath and whether a cruciate or circular incision is better.

Q. 3.5 How would you council him regarding the long-term complications of an end colostomy?

The main complications include a parastomal hernia which can be up to 50% in some studies. These herniae can present with or without associated incarceration, obstruction, or strangulation. In addition, the stoma can retract or prolapse.

There are also dermatological complications such as irritation from the stoma content and repeated changes.

Q. 3.6 Are there any techniques that you know of that may help prevent a parastomal hernia?

By virtue of making an incision within the sheath or fascia there is a near universal development of some parastomal bulge which may or may not then develop into a formal hernia.

Although there are conflicting results from trials of the use of prophylactic mesh, the ACPGBI position statement states that prophylactic synthetic nonabsorbable mesh may be used when constructing an elective permanent end colostomy for cancer only to reduce the risk of parastomal hernia development.

Q. 3.7 How would you assess a parastomal hernia?

I would perform a full history and examination of the patient. Salient points within the history include the size and onset of the hernia as well as the impact it has on daily living or work activities. I would examine the hernia to ascertain whether it was a true hernia or a bulge and whether it was reducible or not. In some cases, a CT scan will help to delineate the anatomy and degree of herniation.

Q. 3.8 Are there any classification systems you know of?

The European Hernia Society has developed a classification system which includes whether there is a concomitant incisional hernia, whether the peristomal hernia is less than or greater than 5 cm and whether it is primary or recurrent.

Q. 3.9 How would you manage his hernia?

The main factors to decide on management are related to symptoms and quality of life. Operative management often has poor results with a high recurrence rate and in a patient where symptoms are not significant; these hernias can be managed non-operatively, with stoma care nurse support.

If an operative approach is considered, the ACPGBI evidence-based position statement strongly asserts that suture repair should not be used for elective repair of parastomal hernias unless appropriately counselled, because results with mesh reinforcement have been superior in trials. There is insufficient evidence to favour one mesh type over another. There is a trend towards higher recurrence rates when mesh is placed as an onlay, compared with other sites of mesh placement.

In an emergency setting, suture repair may still be appropriate because of the need for time-limited surgery. Relocation of a stoma is associated with high rates of parastomal hernia at the new site and incisional hernia at the old site.

Q. 3.10 What is the incidence of incisional hernia after reversal of colostomy and how can you avoid it?

It is 30% from several studies. The ROCSS (Reinforcement of Closure of Stoma Site) trial showed a reduction of symptomatic incisional hernia at 2 years when using biological mesh compared with suture repair only.

Further reading

ACPGBI Parastomal Hernia Group. Prevention and treatment of parastomal hernia: a position statement on behalf of the Association of Coloproctology of Great Britain and Ireland. Colorectal Dis 2018; 20:5–19.

Bhangu A, Nepogodiev D, Futaba K, et al. Systematic review and meta-analysis of the incidence of incisional hernia at the site of stoma closure. World J Surg 2012; 36:973–983.

Brandsma HT, Hansson BM, Aufenacker TJ, et al. Prophylactic mesh placement during formation of an end-colostomy reduces the rate of parastomal hernia: short-term results of the Dutch PREVENT-trial. Ann Surg 2017; 265:663–669.

Hansson BM, Slater NJ, van der Velden AS, et al. Surgical techniques for parastomal hernia repair: a systematic review of the literature. Ann Surg 2012; 255:685–695.

Odensten C, Strigård K, Rutegård J, et al. Use of prophylactic mesh when creating a colostomy does not prevent parastomal hernia: a randomized controlled trial—STOMAMESH. Ann Surg 2019; 269:427–431.

Schreinemacher MH, Vijgen GH, Dagnelie PC, et al. Incisional hernias in temporary stoma wounds: a cohort study. Arch Surg 2011; 146:94–99.

Scenario 4

Rectal prolapse

A 30-year-old man presents to your colorectal clinic complaining of a small amount of bleeding from the back passage straining and he has recently noticed a lump that protrudes out of his anus which requires manual reduction.

Q. 4.1 How would you assess the patient?

History and examination

I would take a thorough history and conduct a careful examination, including DRE and rigid sigmoidoscopy.

I would establish whether there are any red flag symptoms or signs. Salient points of the history would include sexual history and any prior history of perianal surgery.

Q. 4.2 How would you like to investigate this man?

Rectal prolapse in men is relatively uncommon and can be as low as 10% in some studies. The work up should be similar to that of women though to ensure that the correct surgical procedure or indeed non-operative option is chosen.

Given that this patient is a young man and in the absence of red flags I would perform a flexible sigmoidoscopy to exclude any proximal lesion and to exclude haemorrhoids as a potential diagnosis. I would also perform a defecating proctogram and anorectal physiology tests.

The pathophysiology of rectal prolapse includes intussusception in the early stages and part of this may be due to straining and raised intra-abdominal pressure. It is also therefore important to consider performing a CT scan to ensure that there is no intra-abdominal cause such as a mass. A CT scan also allows preoperative planning if one would perform an abdominal repair.

All his investigations confirm a full thickness rectal prolapse.

Q. 4.3 How would you approach his management?

I do not have specific experience in advanced specialist pelvic floor surgery and therefore I would initially consult the regional or local pelvic floor MDT to decide on the best option for this man.

Q. 4.4 What operative procedures do you know for rectal prolapse?

Operative procedures can be broadly divided into perineal and abdominal techniques.

Perineal procedures include a Delorme's procedure and an Altemeier's procedure. A Delorme's procedure does not involve resection of the rectum and can be performed in smaller prolapses generally between up to 10 cm beyond the anal verge. It involves reduction of the rectum by concertinaing of the rectal muscle after stripping the mucosal layer. An Altemeier's procedure generally involves resection of the prolapsed rectum and is useful in circumstances where the prolapse is large.

Perineal approaches are generally reserved for those who need a quicker operation due to anaesthetic concerns in particular elderly patients. The main disadvantage of a perineal approach is the risk of recurrence which can be up to 30% in both techniques.

Abdominal procedures include the choice between laparoscopic and open. The technique can be suture rectopexy with or without resection. The PROSPER trial showed that although a rectopexy with resection had lower recurrence rates at this did not achieve significance.

Q. 4.5 What are the main risks of repairing a rectal prolapse using an abdominal approach?

In a young man such as this, there are risks regarding the pelvic nerves which may result sexual or bladder dysfunction. There are risks of mesh erosion and chronic pain although this is considered less when using biologic mesh and recurrence of prolapse.

There is, however, a lack of evidence favouring one option over another and a Cochrane review (2015) as well as the prospect trials has shown no difference. The challenge in establishing evidence in rectal prolapse is related to the heterogeneity of patient population and degree of prolapse. Future studies considering in-depth sub-classifications of different techniques for different degrees of prolapse and different patient populations may help with clarifying which technique is best for which population demographic.

There is evidence to suggest that division of the lateral ligaments was associated with less recurrent prolapse but more postoperative constipation. As in previous studies comparing laparoscopic and open procedures, laparoscopic rectopexy was associated with fewer postoperative complications and shorter hospital stay.

Bowel resection during rectopexy was associated with lower rates of constipation. In the PROSPER trial although quality of life improved when using any of the techniques for repair there were no differences between the different kinds of prolapse surgery.

Further reading

Senapati A, Gray RG, Middleton LJ, et al. PROSPER: a randomised comparison of surgical treatments for rectal prolapse. Colorectal Dis 2013; 15:858–868.

Tou S, Brown SR, Nelson RL. Surgery for complete (full-thickness) rectal prolapse in adults. Cochrane Database Syst Rev 2015; CD001758.

Scenario 5

Bowel ischaemia

A 70-year-old man presents with severe abdominal pain. He has a history of an MI and a smoker.

Q. 5.1 How would you assess and initially manage this patient?

I would take a thorough history and conduct a careful examination. This man sounds unwell and so I would approach the management using CCrISP (Care of the Critically Ill Surgical Patient) principles.

In particular, I would ascertain whether his pain was disproportionate to his clinical findings which would suggest bowel ischaemia or infarction. I would ensure on going resuscitation with IV fluids, antibiotics, and oxygen.

Q. 5.2 How would you investigate this man?

The main purpose of investigation is to establish a diagnosis and ascertain suitability for theatre if required. As I am suspecting bowel ischaemia I would want to perform a CT scan. I would therefore perform a CT of the abdomen and pelvis or a CT angiogram to establish the diagnosis.

He has had a previous MI and it may be that he has concomitant atrial fibrillation as a cause of multiple emboli.

The CT scan is reported as widespread small bowel ischaemia with gas in the mural wall along with oedema.

Q. 5.3 How would you definitively manage this man?

This man is elderly and focus needs to be on whether the pathology is survivable and if so an assessment of general fitness for possible life-saving surgery, assessment of quality of life.

In this man a formal assessment of frailty should be performed. The recent emergency laparotomy and frailty (ELF) study showed that frailty was associated with an odd of three times greater mortality. Having said this in this gentleman the bowel is profoundly ischaemic and likely to be unviable. This means that any operative intervention would be futile and therefore careful discussion should be had with the patient and his family about their wishes and the possibility of palliative care as a definitive management option.

NELA showed a mortality of 40% of those operated on. Schoots et al showed an overall in-hospital mortality of 74% considering all-comers (operated on or not).

Involvement of coeliac axis and/or more than one of celiac axis (CA), superior mesenteric artery (SMA), and inferior mesenteric artery (IMA) territory associated with mortality.

Q. 5.4 Do you know of any evidence related to bowel ischaemia and infarction?

The world Society of Emergency Surgeons developed some guidelines in relation to bowel ischaemia. They advise that in a patient with bowel ischaemia and peritonitis a laparotomy should be performed and that there are potential roles for endovascular techniques in certain cases or continuous heparin infusions. In the case of nonobstructive mesenteric ischaemia then the mainstay of treatment is management of the underlying cause such as heart failure or sepsis.

Further reading

Bala M, Kashuk J, Moore EE, et al. Acute mesenteric ischemia: guidelines of the World Society of Emergency Surgery. World J Emerg Surg 2017; 12:38.

Parmar KL, Law J, Carter B, et al. Frailty in older patients undergoing emergency laparotomy: results from the UK observational emergency laparotomy and frailty (ELF) study. Ann Surg 2021; 273:709–718.

Royal College of Surgeons of England. 2023. Care of the Critically Ill Surgical Patient (CCrISP). https://www.rcseng.ac.uk/education-and-exams/courses/search/care-of-the-critically-ill-surgical-patient-ccrisp/

Schoots IG, Koffeman GI, Legemate DA, et al. Systematic review of survival after acute mesenteric ischaemia according to disease aetiology. Br J Surg 2004; 91:17–27.

Scenario 6

Small bowel obstruction

A 73-year-old woman with a history of an open right hemicolectomy 30 years earlier for a large benign polyp and a caesarean section presents with a 4-hour history of abdominal distension and vomiting.

Q. 6.1 How would you assess the patient?

History and examination

I would take a thorough history and conduct a careful examination. Symptoms of constipation, abdominal bloating, nausea and vomiting, and abdominal pain suggest bowel obstruction.

Past abdominal surgical history a risk factor for adhesions. Multiple previous operations, pelvic operations, and past presentation with adhesional small bowel obstruction (SBO) are risk factors for SBO.

Given her history of previous cancer, I would want to exclude a cancer although recurrence this late would be unusual. I would check for hernias and examine her groin regions but also consider the differential of an obturator hernia.

Pseudo-obstruction may also be a possibility given her age.

On examination, the patient's abdomen does not show signs of peritonism, but the patient has a high respiratory rate of 24 breaths per minute.

Q. 6.2 How would investigate and manage this woman?

I would initiate resuscitation according to CCrISP protocols. My main concern is SBO and as such I would want to confirm the diagnosis and the cause for the obstruction. I would do this by ensuring a CT scan was performed. If this confirms our diagnosis of SBO, I would want to assess the patient for suitability for early or delayed operative intervention if her condition required it.

The CT scan confirms an adhesional SBO with a suggested cut-off in the mid-ileum. Her abdomen is not peritonitic, and she is comfortable after a passage of a nasogastric (NG) tube.

Q. 6.3 What would your management be?

This lady is comfortable and has no signs that would indicate immediate surgery is required. I would follow the Bologna guidelines and initiate a period of conservative management and use of water-soluble contrast via the NG tube. I would make serial clinical assessments over the next 24 hours and obtain an abdominal X-ray to see if the contrast has gone through into the colon. If this is the case then I would continue my watch and wait policy for up to 72 hours.

Q. 6.4 Do you know of any evidence to suggest how successful or not this approach is?

The National Audit of Small Bowel Obstruction has shown that about two-thirds of patients who undergo conservative management resolve without operative intervention.

During your assessment over the initial 24 hours, she develops pain and her CRP increases to over 90.

Q. 6.5 What would you do?

These findings would indicate a failure in conservative management and she needs to go to theatre. The Bologna guidelines have stated that if a patient develops signs of peritonitis, CRP of over 75, a WCC >10, intraperitoneal fluid > 500 mL (on a CT), persistent obstruction or greater than 500 mL of NG drainage per day after 72 hours constitutes failure of nonoperative management.

The NASBO has reported values of 8% mortality despite management and so timely intervention and regular assessment is essential.

Q. 6.6 What would your surgical approach be to this lady and what is your major concern when undertaking an operation for SBO?

I would undertake an open adhesiolysis on this lady. She has had two previous abdominal and pelvic operations which although suggest the risk of enterotomy is lower than if she had had more, it is one of the main concerns. Small bowel injuries can occur in up to 20% of reported cases and should be avoided to prevent unnecessary morbidity. Where patients have had more than two laparotomies bowel injury can be as high as 50% in cases.

I would perform a careful sharp dissection of the adhesions to avoid injury. I would avoid finger dissection and meticulously handle oedematous tissues to avoid rupture. I would then ensure that I have examined the entire small bowel from the duodenojejunal (DJ) flexure to the ileocaecal valve and take time to examine the contents of the abdomen to ensure that another cause has not been missed such as a large bowel tumour.

Q. 6.7 Is there a role for laparoscopic adhesiolysis?

There is a role for a laparoscopic approach but only in select cases. These cases are usually when there is a suspicion of a band adhesion, fewer than three laparotomies, and absence of a mid-line incision. In these cases, the risk of bowel injury is less but still present and cases need to be chosen based upon the experience of the surgeon performing them and the suitability of this approach such as available space within the abdomen.

You complete the operation and are about to close up.

Q. 6.8 Are there any agents that can be used to prevent adhesion formation?

The two main agents that are available are a physical film to help prevent adhesion formation and a liquid which is infused and left in the abdomen. Although there is evidence to suggest these work the results in everyday clinical practice are variable and have not gained widespread acceptance. I have limited experience of using these agents and so I would not use them in my practice.

Further reading

ACPGBI. [online] Available from https://www.acpgbi.org.uk//content/uploads/2017/12/NASBO-REPORT-2017.pdf [Last accessed March, 2022].

Van Der Krabben AA, Dijkstra FR, Nieuwenhuijzen M, et al. Morbidity and mortality of inadvertent enterotomy during adhesiotomy. Br J Surg 2000; 87:467–471.

WJES. (2018). [online] Available from https://wjes.biomedcentral.com/articles/10.1186/s13017-018-0185-2 [Last accessed March, 2022].

Scenario 7

Advanced colorectal cancer

An 83-year-old reasonably fit man is discussed in the colorectal MDT and is determined to have a T2N0M1 mid-rectal cancer. He has a solitary metastasis in the liver.

Q. 7.1 How would you assess the patient?

History and examination

I would take a thorough history with particular focus on symptoms of obstruction and bleeding and assessment of fitness for treatment. I would undertake a formal assessment of frailty given that morbidity increases with increasing frailty as shown by the recent ELF study.

Q. 7.2 What are your management options for this man?

Although this man has an early tumour, it has become metastatic.

In the immediate term, I would ascertain whether the tumour requires emergency management in the case of obstruction or excessive bleeding. If after assessment he appears suitable for surgical intervention then my options would be a sigmoid loop colostomy or a low Hartmann's procedure. If he is deemed too high risk for surgical intervention then I would use a supportive care approach for him in the emergency setting.

After the emergency situation has passed my management options would include nonoperative and operative options provided he was fit with a performance status of two or less. His tumour is a T2 lesion and in some centres transanal resection may be performed. Formal surgical options would include an elective low Hartmann's procedure, a restorative anterior resection with a defunctioning ileostomy or an abdominoperineal (AP) resection depending on distance from the anal verge.

The complicating factor is that this is metastatic. He needs to be discussed carefully at the MDT. The broad decision making is related to whether the metastases are resectable or not and whether the primary tumour is symptomatic or not.

If metastases are resectable, there are three main potential options:
1. Metastasectomy first then rectal resection
2. Resection of the rectum and then metastasectomy
3. Chemoradiotherapy to rectum and during the post-CRT period (usually 6 weeks but can be 12 weeks), to perform the liver resection

In the case of a T2 tumour, CRT may or may not be used and therefore only options 1 and 2 would be feasible.

Palliative chemotherapy may be used if metastases are unresectable, surgery then chemotherapy or a combination of both depending on individual cases and circumstance.

Q. 7.3 What chemotherapeutic options could you use in this man when administering palliative chemotherapy?

The standard chemotherapy agents used in rectal cancer are oxaliplatin and capecitabine. In this man, it would be useful to find out if the histology was KRAS-wild type or mutant. In the case of wild type, cetuximab can be used in metastatic disease.

Q. 7.4 How would your management approach differ in someone with a T3M1N0 mid-rectal cancer?

The two main areas to consider are the more advanced nature of the tumour and the location of the tumour. The T3 nature of the tumour would favour administration of chemoradiotherapy first then metastasectomy in the 6/12 weeks interval with subsequent rectal resection provided both metastases and tumour were considered resectable.

The surgical options are low anterior resection with or without defunctioning ileostomy. If I was concerned about poor function postoperatively or was unable to perform a primary anastomosis, I would consider either a low Hartmann's procedure or an intersphincteric abdominoperineal resection. These two techniques are subject to a recent study in the form of the HIP study and outcomes are awaited.

Further reading

Cancer Research, UK. [online] Available from https://www.cancerresearchuk.org/about-cancer/find-a-clinical-trial/a-study-comparing-2-operations-for-people-with-rectal-cancer-hip-study [Last accessed March, 2022].

Fowler H, Clifford R, Sutton P, et al. HiP collaborators. Hartmann's procedure versus intersphincteric abdominoperineal excision (HiP Study): a multicentre prospective cohort study. Colorectal Dis 2020; 22:2114–2122.

Pfeiffer P, Gruenberger T, Glynne-Jones R. Synchronous liver metastases in patients with rectal cancer: can we establish which treatment first? Ther Adv Med Oncol 2018; 10:1758835918787993.

Scenario 8

Rectal cancer

A 65-year-old man who has an ASA of 2 comes to the endoscopy unit after a history of weight loss and rectal bleeding. When performing the colonoscopy, you see a suspicious lesion within the mid-rectum.

Q. 8.1 How would you assess the patient?

I would perform a thorough history and examination. I would ensure that I take at least six biopsies from the lesion to ensure adequate tissue sampling. I would complete staging by CT chest, abdominal, pelvis and MRI of the pelvis scanning and then add him to the MDT for discussion.

The results from your staging suggest a T3 mid-rectal tumour with no evidence of metastases.

Q. 8.2 What would your management strategy be?

T3 tumours are a heterogeneous group and can be divided into T3a and b or T3c and d. These two groups can be summarised as T3 tumours which have less than 5 mm invasion beyond the muscularis propria and those that have more than 5 mm.

Some studies have shown that T3a and b tumours behave in a similar way to T2 tumours whereas T3c and d behave more aggressively and have poorer survival.

I would give patients who are T3c/d long course chemoradiotherapy followed by a low anterior resection with covering ileostomy. For patients with T3a and b I would weigh up the risk benefit of going either straight to surgery or giving short course radiotherapy followed by surgery.

Q. 8.3 What radiotherapy protocol would you give in short or long course radiotherapy and would you give them chemotherapy too at the same time?

Traditionally long-course radiotherapy is given in small doses such as 2–3 Gy on a daily basis over 4–6 weeks amounting to 45–54 Gy in total. In long-course radiotherapy a sensitising chemotherapy agent is often used to allow the radiotherapy to have a greater effect. The chemotherapy agent used is capecitabine however it is a much lower dose than that used in an adjuvant setting.

Short-course radiotherapy is given usually within 5 days and a dose of 5 Gy is given per day. A chemotherapy agent is not used in this case because of the short-time period not allowing adequate sensitisation.

Q. 8.4 Would you give radiotherapy to a patient with a T2 tumour?

The National Institute for Health and Care Excellence (NICE) guidelines suggest that if a patient is fit and is node positive radiotherapy should be considered but has no role in T1/2 tumours with node negative disease except in the context of a trial.

Q. 8.5 Do you know of any on-going trials that is looking into the management of early rectal cancers?

The STAR-TREC study, he is currently looking at the role of radiotherapy for patients with early rectal cancer and they included patients with a T3b tumour without nodal or distant metastases. These results are currently awaited.

Q. 8.6 How would your approach to management differ in a 72-year-old man who is a Jehovah's Witness with a T4N0M0 obstructing cancer of the splenic flexure?

I would initially take a thorough history and examination and institute early management according to the CCrISP protocols.

This is a high-risk case and an advanced tumour. It is likely that he will need extensive surgery if a resection were to be considered given that this is a T4 tumour. My options for an obstructing tumour are primary resection, defunctioning stoma, or stent.

Given that he is a Jehovah's Witness a major primary resection would not be the most appropriate option given that there is a risk of bleeding and major morbidity especially in the context of a T4 tumour. I would consider a temporising measure such as a stoma or stent to be the most appropriate option.

With the recent results from the FOxTROT study, there is a strong argument for performing a stent and then giving neoadjuvant therapy in an attempt to downstage the tumour which may then become more amenable to surgery. The CREST showed that stenting as a bridge to definitive surgery reduces the risk of stoma formation. Stenting is not risk-free and may not always be appropriate depending on the degree of luminal obstruction from the actual tumour in which case a defunctioning loop transverse colostomy may be the best option.

In either case of stoma or stenting, it would give time to consider our further options in the form of optimisation of management in Jehovah's Witness such as advanced directives, use of cell savers, or fractions of whole blood.

Further reading

ClinicalTrials.gov. [online] Available from https://clinicaltrials.gov/ct2/show/NCT02945566 [Last accessed March, 2022].

Foxtrot Collaborative Group. Feasibility of preoperative chemotherapy for locally advanced, operable colon cancer: the pilot phase of a randomised controlled trial. Lancet Oncol 2012; 13:1152–1160.

Hill J, Kay C, Morton D, et al. CREST: randomised phase III study of stenting as a bridge to surgery in obstructing colorectal cancer—Results of the UK ColoRectal Endoscopic Stenting Trial (CREST). J Clin Oncol 2016; 34:3507.

NICE. (2020). Colorectal cancer. [online] Available from https://www.nice.org.uk/guidance/ng151/resources/colorectal-cancer-pdf-66141835244485 [Last accessed March, 2022].

Siddiqui MRS, Simillis C, Bhoday J, et al. A meta-analysis assessing the survival implications of subclassifying T3 rectal tumours. Eur J Cancer 2018; 104:47–61.

Scenario 9

Anal cancer

A 63-year-old man is referred to the out-patient clinic by his General Practitioner with troublesome 'haemorrhoids'. He complains of several months' history of progressive peri-anal pain and bleeding. Of note his clothes feel looser over recent weeks.

Q. 9.1 How would you assess this patient?

I would take a thorough history and conduct a careful physical examination. Within the history I would like to pay attention to any 'red flag' symptoms, such as the bleeding, if there is any change in bowel habit and the weight loss. I would also like to know if the patient can feel a lump in the peri-anal region.

With the patient's weight loss and 'haemorrhoids' it would be important to consider anal carcinoma as a potential differential diagnosis and this it is important to note key risk factors for developing anal carcinoma, including a history of immunocompromise, e.g. HIV infection, postorgan transplantation, etc. and social factors, e.g. receptive anal intercourse. I would also screen for medical co-morbidities and make an initial assessment of fitness looking at the patients' performance status.

During my examination, I would perform a DRE if the patient tolerates and palpate for inguinal lymphadenopathy, which is the most common site of lymph node metastases after peri-rectal nodes.

Q. 9.2 What is AIN and how is it managed?

AIN stands for anal intraepithelial, neoplasia; it has now been superseded by the terms low-grade squamous intraepithelial lesion (LSIL) and high-grade squamous intraepithelial lesion (HSIL). HSIL lesions refer to the old classification of AIN II and III. HSIL can represent carcinoma in situ.

These are premalignant conditions and have a risk of progressing to anal carcinoma, especially with HSIL lesions. These lesions must be biopsied to ascertain histologically the grading, it is not a clinical diagnosis.

Treatment for LSIL lesions is with 6 monthly clinical follow-up. If there is any recurrence of lesions then examination under anaesthesia (EUA) and anal mapping is required. Medical treatment includes topical agents such as 5FU and imiquimod. The evidence is available, is limited to the follow-up and treatment of these lesions, each trust will follow its own guidelines.

Q. 9.3 What are the anatomical variants of anal cancer?

There are two main ways anal cancer can be classified anatomically:
1. Anal canal
2. Anal margin (within 5 cm)

The importance here is that small anal canal cancers are not completely excised to sphincter involvement, and the increased chance of incontinence associated and so biopsies are the main stay of treatment for small anal canal lesions.

Q. 9.4 What is the TNM staging of anal cancer?

T staging	Description	Nodal status	Description
1	<2 cm	0	No regional lymph nodes
2	>2 cm	1	Metastasis in perirectal lymph nodes
3	>5 cm	2	Metastasis in unilateral internal iliac and/or inguinal lymph nodes
4	Invading deep structures (vagina, urethra bladder. NOT sphincters)	3	Metastasis in perirectal and inguinal lymph nodes and/or bilateral internal iliac nodes and/or inguinal lymph nodes

M0 – no distant metastasis
M1 – distant metastasis
Upon physical examination you find this.

Q. 9.5 How will you manage this patient?

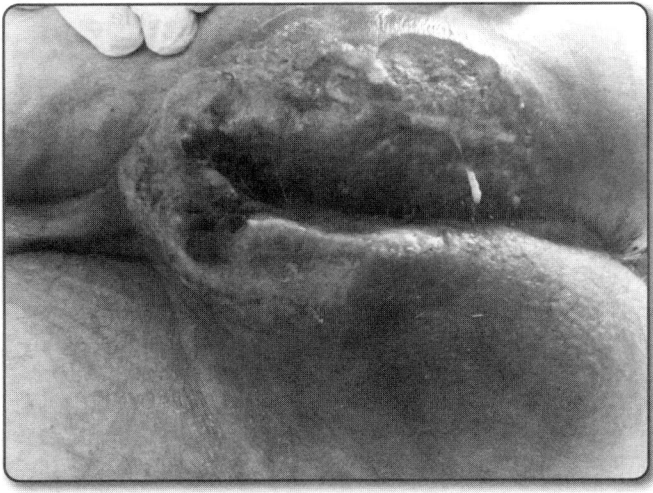

I am concerned that this patient may have an anal cancer. I would start by taking a full history and examination. Following this the patient would require an examination under anaesthesia and biopsy. Given the size of the lesion a defunctioning stoma should be considered.

The patient will require full staging including a CT of the chest, abdomen, and pelvis and MRI of the pelvis. Consideration should also be given to HIV testing after appropriate patient counselling.

In female patients, screening for cervical intraepithelial neoplasia (CIN) and vulvar intraepithelial neoplasia (VIN) should be considered given the size of the lesion in this case.

Upon completion of staging I would arrange for his case to be discussed at the specialist regional anal cancer MDT.

Q. 9.6 What is definitive therapy likely to involve?

Initial treatment is in the form of chemoradiotherapy (*chemotherapy:* 5FU + mitomycin, *radiotherapy:* 50.4 Gy in 28 daily fractions).

Q. 9.7 Is there any role for surgery?

Yes, there is a role for surgery in certain cases. These include:
- Local excision for small T1 tumours
- Salvage AP resections for failed chemoradiotherapy
- Salvage AP resection for recurrent disease
- Surgery to manage complications of chemoradiotherapy (faecal incontinence, fistulae etc.)

Further reading

Geh I, Gollins S, Renehan A, et al. Association of Coloproctology of Great Britain & Ireland (ACPGBI): Guidelines for the management of cancer of the colon, rectum and anus (2017)–anal cancer. Colorectal Dis 2017; 19:82–97.

James RD, Glynne-Jones R, Meadows HM, et al. Mitomycin or cisplatin chemoradiation with or without maintenance chemotherapy for treatment of squamous-cell carcinoma of the anus (ACT II): a randomised, phase 3, open-label, 2× 2 factorial trial. Lancet Oncol 2013; 14:516–524.

Lynne-Jones R, Nilsson PJ, Aschele C, et al. Anal cancer: ESMO-ESSO-ESTRO clinical practice guidelines for diagnosis, treatment and follow-up. Eur J Surg Oncol 2014; 40:1165–1176.

UKCCCR Anal Cancer Trial Working Party. UK Co-ordinating Committee on Cancer Research. Epidermoid anal cancer: results from the UKCCCR randomised trial of radiotherapy alone versus radiotherapy, 5-fluorouracil, and mitomycin. Lancet 1996; 348:1049–1054.

Scenario 10

Perianal sepsis/fistula

A 37-year-old man presents on the emergency general surgical take complaining of severe perianal pain and swelling for 3 days. He admits feeling feverish intermittently over the last 24 hours.

Q. 10.1 How would you manage him?

I would begin by assessing the patient in an ABCDE fashion, and given the patient is feverish I would implement the sepsis 6 bundle. I would then take a focused history concentrating on the salient points including the duration of this episode of pain, any peri-anal discharge, and previous episodes.

I would also enquire about any past medical history of IBD (Specifically Crohn's) and diabetes.

I would perform a thorough examination which would include a DRE. I would look for signs of anorectal sepsis, e.g. swelling, erythema, etc. I would note the presence of any scars from previous surgery. I would palpate for underlying fluctuance.

Your assessment reveals evidence of a 7 cm perianal abscess that is exquisitely tender which limits your overall assessment.

Q. 10.2 How would you proceed?

This patient needs to go to theatre for an EUA of the rectum and incision and drainage of the abscess. I would gain informed consent from the patient, discuss with the Confidential Enquiry into Perioperative Deaths (CEPOD) anaesthetist and ensure the patient is booked onto the CEPOD list. If there are any signs of sepsis, I would ensure that the surgery is performed without delay. I would start antibiotics prior to surgery.

Q. 10.3 Describe what you would do in theatre?

In theatre, following completion of the World Health Organization (WHO) checklist, I would place the patient in the lithotomy position. I would perform a thorough assessment noting the position and extent of induration, health of the overlying skin, and the presence of any internal/external openings or fistula tracts. I would perform a thorough EUA of the rectum using an Eisenhammer retractor, looking for an os in the anal canal or evidence of internal fistula opening. I would then proceed to drain all the pus in the cavity ensuring my incision is over the area of the greatest fluctuance.

If I discovered an obvious fistula, there are two options I would consider:
1. Not to treat surgically at the time, as over 50% of these will heal after drainage of the sepsis.
2. Place a loose draining set on.

You review the patient in the out-patient department 3 months later. Although the wound healed well initially, he now complains of persistent intermittent discharge.

Q. 10.4 How would you proceed?

This history would raise the suspicion that the patient has developed a fistula-in-ano. I would proceed to take a full history and examination of the patient, paying specific attention to any areas of induration around the anal margin and fistula openings. Up to 50% of patients who present with perianal sepsis will develop fistula-in-ano.

If there are obvious signs of a fistula then I would book the patient for an elective EUA +/- insertion of seton +/- laying open of fistula tract. If there was no obvious fistula opening, or if the patient was a female or there was any history of IBD I would then organise for the patient to have an MRI scan of the pelvis to look for a fistula tract and delineate the anatomy.

Q. 10.5 What is the pathophysiology behind the formation of a fistula-in-ano?

This is the cryptoglandular theory. In normal circumstances, the sphincter muscles act as a barrier to infection passing from the bowel lumen into the surrounding area. In an abscess, infection arises in the cryptoglandular epithelium which can occur from the crypts of Morgagni in the upper anal canal.

Q. 10.6 How would you classify fistula-in-ano?

Parks classification

Type	Anatomy	Percentage occurrence
1	Intersphincteric	45%
2	Transsphincteric	30%
3	Suprasphincteric	20%
4	Extrasphincteric	5%

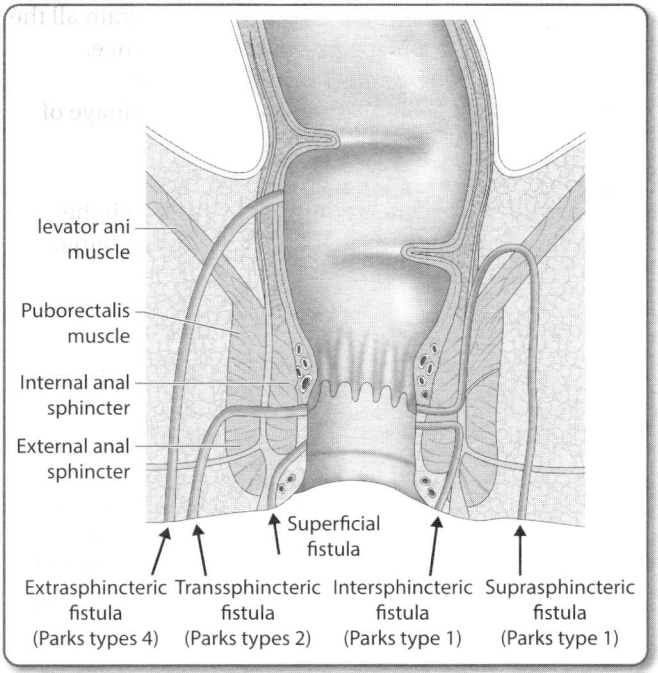

Q. 10.7 What is Goodsall's rule?

This states that if the fistula lies anteriorly then it will open directly into the anal canal in that position. If the fistula lies posteriorly, then it will track downwards and open in the midline posteriorly.

Q. 10.8 What are the surgical management options for fistula-in-ano?

The management options would depend on the Park's classification of the fistula, the amount of sphincter muscle involved, and whether the patient was male or female.
Simple fistulae (No involvement of external sphincter of puborectalis)
- Drainage setons
- Fistulotomy
- Fistulectomy
- Fistula plugs
- Ligation of the intersphincteric fistula tract (LIFT) procedure

Complex fistulae (involvement of over 1/3 of the external sphincter, multiple tracts, IBD related, suprasphincteric or high transsphincteric)
- Cutting seton
- Advancement flap
- Diversion stoma

Care must be taken in female patients to preserve sphincter function, and thus anal physiology should be performed prior to any surgery that may damage the sphincter muscle.

Further reading

Jayne DG, Scholefield J, Tolan D, et al. Anal fistula plug versus surgeon's preference for surgery for trans-sphincteric anal fistula: the FIAT RCT. Health Technol Assess 2019; 23:1–76.

Malik AI, Nelson RL, Tou S. Incision and drainage of perianal abscess with or without treatment of anal fistula. Cochrane Database syst Rev 2010(7).

Malik AI, Nelson RL, Tou S. Incision and drainage of perianal abscess with or without treatment of anal fistula. Cochrane Database Syst Rev 2010;Cd006827.

Quah HM, Tang CL, Eu KW, et al. Meta-analysis of randomized clinical trials comparing drainage alone vs primary sphincter-cutting procedures for anorectal abscess-fistula. Int J Colorectal Dis 2006; 21:602–609.

Scenario 11

Haemorrhoids

A 34-year-old lady is referred to the colorectal clinic with painless bright red rectal bleeding.

Q. 11.1 What would your initial assessment entail?

I would take a focused history and perform a detailed examination. I would establish the presence or absence of 'red flag' symptoms suggestive of any serious underlying aetiology, e.g. malignancy, IBD, and any relevant personal/family history.

My examination would include a careful DRE. I would look for any signs of previous scarring around the anal margin, the presence of any skin tags or prolapsing haemorrhoids.

Q. 11.2 How would you classify haemorrhoids?

Haemorrhoids can be classified based on the Goligher's classification system, namely:
- *Grade 1:* Bleeding anal cushions with no prolapse
- *Grade 2*: Prolapse of haemorrhoidal tissue on straining that reduces spontaneously
- *Grade 3:* Prolapse of haemorrhoidal tissue on straining that requires manual reduction
- *Grade 4:* Haemorrhoidal tissue that is constantly prolapsed

On a practical level the grade of haemorrhoid will guide the most appropriate management.

Q. 11.3 What are the management options for grade 3 haemorrhoids?

Firstly, all patients who have haemorrhoids should be treated conservatively to ensure they avoid constipation and straining. This includes dietary advice such as a high-fibre diet and adequate fluid intake. Laxatives may also be prescribed.

Surgical management of haemorrhoids is dependent on how symptomatic a patient is with the disease. There are various surgical management options:
- Rubber band ligation
- Haemorrhoidal artery ligation (HALO/THD)
- Excisional haemorrhoidectomy
- There is also the newer technique called the Rafaelo technique involving radiofrequency ablation although this is generally not offered on the NHS at present.

Stapled haemorrhoidectomy is seldom used nowadays. In general, rubber band ligation and haemorrhoidal artery ligation can be used in up to grade 3 haemorrhoids depending on surgical preference. (In an exam situation you need to tell the examiner what YOU would do based on your previous experience)

Excisional haemorrhoidectomy can be used for grade 3 or 4 haemorrhoids, has the lowest recurrence rates but a lot of postoperative pain.

Q 11.4 What trials do you know regarding haemorrhoid surgery?

HubBLe trial:
- Haemorrhoidal artery ligation versus rubber band ligation for the management of symptomatic second-degree and third-degree haemorrhoids
- There was a higher recurrence rate at 1 year in the rubber band ligation (RBL) group (49%) compared to the haemorrhoidal artery ligation (HAL) group (30%)
- Pain scores at 1 day were lower in RBL group
- No difference in pain scores at 21 days or 6 weeks
- Haemorrhoidal artery ligation suffered more complications

eTHoS trial:
- Comparison of stapled haemorrhoidectomy with traditional excisional surgery for haemorrhoidal disease
- Open label, multicentre, parallel group RCT
- In adults for grade 2–4 haemorrhoids
- Stapled haemorrhoidopexy was less painful in short-term
- Similar complication rates between the groups
- Quality of life was better in first 6 weeks for stapled
- After that excisional was better at 2 years
- No significant difference in complications

Further reading

Brown SR, Tiernan JP, Watson AJ, et al. Haemorrhoidal artery ligation versus rubber band ligation for the management of symptomatic second-degree and third-degree haemorrhoids (HubBLe): a multicentre, open-label, randomised controlled trial. The Lancet 2016; 388:356–364.

Watson AJ, Hudson J, Wood J, et al. Comparison of stapled haemorrhoidopexy with traditional excisional surgery for haemorrhoidal disease (eTHoS): a pragmatic, multicentre, randomised controlled trial. The Lancet 2016; 388:2375–2385.

Scenario 12

Diverticular disease

Q. 12.1 What does this CT scan show?

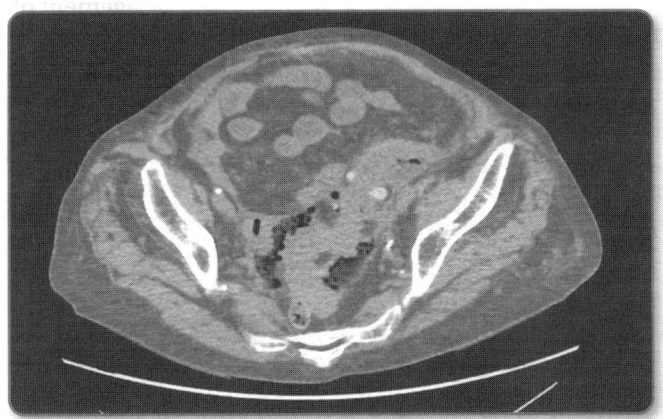

This is a CT scan of the abdomen and pelvis, it shows evidence of acute diverticulitis. There is no evidence of any localised perforation or abscess formation.

Q. 12.2 How is diverticulitis classified?

The Hinchey classification is a system used to classify the severity of acute diverticulitis.

Modified Hinchey classification	
Stage Ia	Confined pericolonic inflammation or phlegmon
Stage Ib	Pericolic or mesocolic abscess
Stage II	Pelvic abscess
Stage III	Generalised purulent peritonitis
Stage IV	Generalised faecal peritonitis

Q. 12.3 How would you manage somebody with Hinchey III diverticulitis?

Initially I would assess and manage the patient using an ABCDE approach. I would resuscitate the patient accordingly and initiate the 'sepsis 6' bundle. I would organise a CT to confirm the clinical diagnosis. During my initial assessment I would establish the patient's fitness for surgical intervention.

In general, for a patient with Hinchey III diverticulitis, surgical management is needed. This can be in the form of:
- Hartmann's procedure
- Sigmoid colectomy with primary anastomosis +/– defunctioning loop ileostomy
- Laparoscopic lavage +/– defunctioning stoma

The Ladies trial has shown in haemodynamically stable, immunocompetent patients younger than 85 years, primary anastomosis is preferable to Hartmann's procedure as a treatment for perforated diverticulitis (Hinchey III or Hinchey IV disease). Caution should be used when patients are requiring ionotropic support.

Laparoscopic peritoneal lavage and drainage are another option resulting in shorter operative times in unwell patients and the avoidance of colostomy. However, this management strategy remains controversial. Of note, the LaparOscopic Lavage (LOLA) arm of the Ladies trial was closed early due to a high re-intervention rate in the laparoscopic group. Caution is still advised when considering laparoscopic lavage as a management option although recently, the 3-year results of the LOLA trial have shown patients who had a lavage are more likely to be stoma free at the expense of recurrent episodes of diverticulitis (although recurrences are less frequent after 12 months).

Further reading

Angenete E, Thornell A, Burcharth J, et al. Laparoscopic lavage is feasible and safe for the treatment of perforated diverticulitis with purulent peritonitis: the first results from the randomized controlled trial DILALA. Ann Surg 2016; 263:117.

Ceresoli M, Coccolini F, Montori G, et al. Laparoscopic lavage versus resection in perforated diverticulitis with purulent peritonitis: a meta-analysis of randomized controlled trials. World J. Emerg. Surg 2016; 11:42.

Campana JP, Mentz RE, González Salazar E, et al. Long-term outcomes and risk factors for diverticulitis recurrence after a successful laparoscopic peritoneal lavage in Hinchey III peritonitis. Int J Colorectal Dis. 2023; 38: 18.

Lambrichts DP, Vennix S, Musters GD, et al. Hartmann's procedure versus sigmoidectomy with primary anastomosis for perforated diverticulitis with purulent or faecal peritonitis (LADIES): a multicentre, parallel-group, randomised, open-label, superiority trial. Lancet Gastroenterol Hepatol 2019; 4:599–610.

Schultz JK, Yaqub S, Wallon C, et al. Laparoscopic lavage vs primary resection for acute perforated diverticulitis: the SCANDIV randomized clinical trial. JAMA 2015; 314:1364–1375.

Vennix S, Musters GD, Mulder IM, et al. Laparoscopic peritoneal lavage or sigmoidectomy for perforated diverticulitis with purulent peritonitis: a multicentre, parallel-group, randomised, open-label trial. The Lancet 2015; 386:1269–1277.

Scenario 13

Ulcerative colitis

A 27-year-old woman presents with generalized abdominal pain and diarrhoea on a background of known ulcerative colitis.

Q. 13.1 How would you manage this patient?

- I would firstly assess this patient in an ABCDE fashion ensuring appropriate resuscitation is started. I would then take a focused history paying attention to the frequency of stools, presence of any blood in the stool, and previous episodes. I would also like to ask about recent foreign travel, and any associated viral symptoms
- Family history of IBD
- I would perform a general abdominal examination looking for signs of distension and peritonism

Q. 13.2 What investigations would you get?

- I would perform routine bloods including full blood count (FBC)/urea and electrolytes (U&E)/liver function test (LFT)/CRP/amylase
- I would send stool cultures
- I would request a CT AP

Q. 13.3 What criteria do you know of in assessing patients with acute flare ups of UC?

Truelove and Witts criteria

	Severe
Bloody stools per day	>6
Pulse	>90
Temperature	37.8°C
Anaemia	<10.5
CRP	>30

Travis criteria
If a patient has stool frequency of >8 per day or 3–8 bowel movements per day and a CRP of >45 after 3 days of treatment, there is an 85% chance the patient will require emergency surgery.

Q. 13.4 How would you manage a patient with an acute flare up of UC?

Initial management of such patients is best undertaken in an MDT fashion involving the gastroenterology team. Antibiotics should be started, and steroids should be avoided unless with gastroenterology input.

Rescue therapy may be started by the gastroenterology team.

Q. 13.5 What are the indications for emergency surgery in a patient with UC?

- Intractable PR bleeding
- Toxic megacolon
- Perforation
- Failure of medical therapy

You make the decision to take the patient to theatre.

Q. 13.6 What procedure will you perform?

The operation of choice in an emergency setting for a patient with UC is a subtotal colectomy with an end ileostomy.

Q. 13.7 How would you deal with the rectal stump?

There are various options in this scenario, depending on the length of rectal stump left and how diseased the rectum is:
- Leave rectal stump in situ
- Leave rectal stump open with a drain at the stump site
- Fix the stump to the rectus sheath
- Create a mucous fistula

Potential complications of leaving the rectal stump in situ are that of a stump blowout.

The patient makes a good recovery from surgery and attends clinic 6 months later asking for a pouch.

Q. 13.8 How would you counsel her and what are the practical considerations?

I would counsel the patient for the following:

Surgery:
- Risk of damage to pelvic nerves leading to bladder and sexual dysfunction
- Good pouch function will entail 6 motions per day
- The patient will still require a loop ileostomy to begin with
- Anastomotic leak
- Anastomotic stricture

Pouch:
- Pouch failure rate is roughly 10%
- Defined as need for a diversion stoma or taking the pouch down
- 30% of patients will suffer from recurrent pouchitis

Further reading

NICE Guideline NG130. Ulcerative colitis: management. 2019 [Accessed 1st April 2023].
Travis SP, Farrant JM, Ricketts C, et al. Predicting outcome in severe ulcerative colitis. Gut 1996; 38:905–910.
Waljee A, Waljee J, Morris AM, et al. Threefold increased risk of infertility: a meta-analysis of infertility after ileal pouch anal anastomosis in ulcerative colitis. Gut 2006; 55:1575–1580.
Weston-Petrides GK, Lovegrove RE, Tilney HS, et al. Comparison of outcomes after restorative proctocolectomy with or without defunctioning ileostomy. Arch. Surg 2008; 143:406–412.

Scenario 14

Enterocutaneous fistula

You are called to the ward to see a 30-year-old female patient who has had an ileocaecal resection for Crohn's disease 10 days ago. She has a temperature of 38.2°C and a HR of 110 beats per minute.

Q. 14.1 What would be your initial management?

This patient is showing signs of sepsis, I would assess her in an ABCDE fashion and initiate the sepsis 6 bundle. After ensuring she has IV fluids and antibiotics, I would take a focused history and examine the patient.

I would then like to read the operation note and previous ward round entries.

The operation note shows an uneventful laparoscopic ileo-caecectomy. The patient has been non-specifically well over the last 72 hours. You notice erythema at the extraction wound site.

Q. 14.2 What would be your next steps?

I would be concerned about a wound infection or an anastomotic leak. I would open the wound and organise for a CT scan.

Q. 14.3 You open the wound and you find purulent dark content, what is your diagnosis?

I would be concerned that the patient has developed an enterocutaneous fistula.

Q. 14.4 What is the management of this?

SNAP protocol
S: Treat the sepsis
N: Nutrition – if the output is above 500 mL in 24 hours, then start total parenteral nutrition (TPN)
A: Anatomy – after the sepsis has settled imaging is needed to delineate the anatomy of the fistula
P: Plan for surgery

Q 14.5 What are the common causes for enterocutaneous fistulae?

- Iatrogenic
- Secondary to Crohn's

The patient eventually settles and you plan to operate on this patient.

Q 14.6 What would be your approach?

As a day one consultant I would not undertake complex surgery like this on my own and I would involve a senior colleague. I would ensure that I have the availability of an all-day list and this would be the only case booked onto it. I would inform the theatre staff that the list may overrun as this is a complex procedure and may take many hours. I would ensure the patient has an intensive therapy units (ITU) bed available postoperative.

Q. 14.7 What are the main differences between Crohn's and UC?

	Crohn's	UC
Site	Anywhere in GI tract from mouth to anus	Start in rectum and spreads proximally towards caecum
Spread	Multiple skip lesions	Continuous
Inflammation	Transmural	Mucosal
Histology	Non caseating granulomas	Loss of goblet cells
Common complications	Fistulas/strictures	Toxic megacolon
Malignant potential	Very rare	Has malignant potential of 10% after 5 years

It can be very challenging to differentiate between Crohn's and UC. This can result in a diagnosis of indeterminate colitis and some patients have their initial diagnosis reconsidered in light of later clinical developments.

Further reading

Kumpf VJ, de Aguilar-Nascimento JE, Diaz-Pizarro Graf JI, et al. ASPEN-FELANPE clinical guidelines. JPEN J Parenter Enteral Nutr 2017; 41:104–112.

Lichtenstein GR, Loftus EV, Isaacs KL, et al. ACG clinical guideline: management of Crohn's disease in adults. Am J Gastroenterol 2018; 113:481–517.

Quinn M, Falconer S, Mckee RF. Management of enterocutaneous fistula: outcomes in 276 Patients. World J Surg 2007; 41:2502–2511.

Scenario 15

Appendiceal tumours

A 32-year-old woman presents with signs and symptoms of appendicitis. She is taken to theatre and undergoes a routine laparoscopic appendicectomy. The postoperative histology shows a 1 cm carcinoid tumour of the appendix at the tip.

Q. 15.1 What can you tell me about the histological classification if appendiceal carcinoid tumours and indication for further surgery?

Appendiceal carcinoid tumours are neuroendocrine tumours.

Appendicectomy alone is sufficient treatment in most cases with no follow-up required. Cases that require a formal right hemicolectomy are based on the following histological findings:

Size ≥2 cm
1–2 cm with any of the following adverse features:
- Located at base of appendix
- Evidence of extramural vascular invasion (EMVI)
- Evidence of lymphovascular invasion
- Involvement of appendix mesentery
- Involved surgical margins
- Ki67 index >2%

In a similar case on a different patient, the pathologist confirms that the histology reveals a low-grade appendiceal mucinous neoplasm (LAMN) with evidence of serosal involvement with mucinous epithelium.

Q. 15.2 What do you know of the classification of such lesions?

The classification of appendiceal mucinous neoplasms remains controversial. A consensus from the Peritoneal Surface Oncology Group International (PSOGI) agreed the following:
- Low-grade appendiceal neoplasm (reserved for lesions with no infiltrative invasion)
- High-grade appendiceal neoplasm (lesions with no infiltrative invasion but evidence of high-grade cytological atypia)
- Pseudomyxoma peritonei (PMP)
  – Low grade
  – High grade
  – High grade with signet cells

Q. 15.3 How would you manage a patient with LAMN?

There is no robust evidence base for the management of such lesions. I would therefore want to discuss this case at a tertiary pseudomyxoma MDT for further advice. In some cases, a right hemicolectomy may be advised.

Q. 15.4 What are the principles of management if the patient developed PMP?

Pseudomyxoma peritonei is a condition that requires specialist management at a recognised tertiary centre such as Basingstoke or the Christie Hospital.
The principles of treatment, provided the patient is fit, include:
- Cytoreductive surgery (CRS)
- Hyperthermic intraperitoneal chemotherapy (HIPEC)

Provided macroscopic control is achieved 5-year survival is favourable. Approximately one in four patients will develop a recurrence of disease, and in highly selected patients repeated CRS and HIPEC may be justified.

Further reading

Glasgow SC, Gaertner W, Stewart D, et al. The American Society of Colon and Rectal Surgeons, clinical practice guidelines for the management of appendiceal neoplasms. Dis Colon Rectum 2019; 62:1425–1438.

Guaglio M, Sinukumar S, Kusamura S, et al. Clinical surveillance after macroscopically complete surgery for low-grade appendiceal mucinous neoplasms (LAMN) with or without limited peritoneal spread: long-term results in a prospective series. Ann Surg Oncol 2018; 25:878–884.

Lord AC, Shihab O, Chandrakumaran K, et al. Recurrence and outcome after complete tumour removal and hyperthermic intraperitoneal chemotherapy in 512 patients with pseudomyxoma peritonei from perforated appendiceal mucinous tumours. Eur J Surg Oncol 2015; 41:396–399.

Misdraji J. Mucinous epithelial neoplasms of the appendix and pseudomyxoma peritonei. Mod Pathol 2015; 28:S67–79.

Moris D, Tsilimigras DI, Vagios S, et al. Neuroendocrine neoplasms of the appendix: a review of the literature. Anticancer Res 2018; 38:601–611.

Tiselius C, Kindler C, Shetye J, et al. Computed tomography follow-up assessment of patients with low-grade appendiceal mucinous neoplasms: evaluation of risk for pseudomyxoma peritonei. Ann Surg Oncol 2017; 24:1778–1782.

Scenario 16

Anal fissure

A 27-year-old female patient presents to the clinic complaining of a 6-week history of pain on defecation associated with fresh PR bleeding.

Q. 16.1 How would you proceed?

With the above history, my main concern would be that the patient has developed an acute anal fissure. I would take a focused history ensuring I rule out any 'red flag' symptoms. I would also ask a detailed bowel habit history including a history of constipation and straining. I would also ask about any change in bowel habits that may suggest an inflammatory aetiology for the fissure.

I would perform an inspection of the anal margin looking for areas of previous scarring and any obvious breaks in the skin. I would perform a gentle DRE with the patient's permission ensuring I stop if there is too much pain.

You diagnose an anal fissure.

Q. 16.2 What would your treatment be?

Initial treatment involves dietary modification including a high-fibre diet, good oral fluid intake, and stool softeners.

Specific treatment would be a topical GTN 0.2% ointment which is associated headaches or topical diltiazem 2% cream. My personal preference would be diltiazem due to its lower side effect profile.

Up to 70% of patients will be successfully treated with topical agents.

Q. 16.3 What is the pathophysiology of anal fissures?

Anal fissures are secondary to trauma, most commonly the passage of hard stools on defecation. The reason for nonhealing fissures is thought to be related to increased tone of the sphincter muscles. As the majority of chronic anal fissures are posterior, this is an area where the blood supply is relatively poor. Therefore, with increased sphincter tone this is further compromised leading to a relatively ischaemic area and thus poor wound healing.

The patient returns to your clinic in 6 weeks and is still symptomatic.

Q. 16.4 What would be your next management steps?

I would prescribe a further 6 weeks of topical treatment to the patient. I would also book the patient for an EUA under general anaesthetic and injection of Botox.

Q. 16.5 Describe what would you do intraoperatively

I would consent the patient for general risks of surgery including bleeding and infection. Specific to this operation I would consent for a risk of incontinence especially to flatus but also faces that would be temporary. I would also consent for recurrence of the fissure or failure of treatment.

After the WHO check, I would place the patient into the lithotomy position. I would then inspect the anal margin and anal canal using an Eisenhammer retractor. Then I would feel for the groove between the internal and external sphincters, injecting 20 units at two points (3 o' and 6 o'clock if the fissure was posterior). Other methods include injecting into the internal sphincter.

Your patient presents to your clinic after 6 weeks still symptomatic.

Q. 16.6 What is your next management step?

I would list the patient for further EUA and Botox injection.

Second-line Botox treatment has failed.

Q. 16.7 What is your next management step?

If Botox treatment has failed twice, the next option would be a lateral sphincterotomy. However, this carries a risk of permanent incontinence of up to 10% of cases. As this is a female patient, I would organise anorectal physiology testing to confirm high resting pressures are the cause of the fissure before consideration of performing a lateral sphincterotomy. If the patient had normal or low resting pressures, I would consider performing advancement flap surgery for the fissure rather than a lateral sphincterotomy.

Further reading

ACPGBI. https://www.acpgbi.org.uk//content/uploads/2017/08/Position-Statements-Management-of-Anal-Fissure-Management-of-Acute-Severe-Colitis.pdf [Accessed 1st April 2023]

Nelson RL, Thomas K, Morgan J, et al. Nonsurgical therapy for anal fissure. Cochrane Database Syst Rev 2012; 2012:Cd003431.

NICE. [online] Available from https://cks.nice.org.uk/topics/anal-fissure [Last accessed March, 2022].

Scenario 17

Endoscopy and polyp screening

A 65-year-old gentleman presents to your clinic as a 2- week wait referral with a change in bowel habit and altered per rectal bleeding. You decide to list him for an urgent colonoscopy.

Q. 17.1 Talk me through the technique you would use to perform this procedure.

In clinic I would ensure that I have taken a full history of the patient including all 'red flag' symptoms. I would also assess his past medical history and performance status to ensure he is fit for the investigation. I would examine the patient including a DRE and rigid sigmoidoscopy.

I would consent the patient in clinic, counselling him for the need for bowel preparation the day before endoscopy. I would also counsel the patient that he will be offered surgery and ensure he has someone who can be with him the night after the procedure otherwise he would need a hospital bed overnight. I ask if the patient is taking any anticoagulant medications and the reasons why, ensuring it is safe to stop them for the appropriate time prior to endoscopy. I would also counsel for the risks of bleeding and perforation.

On the day of the procedure, I would go through the consent process again and ensure the patient has taken the bowel preparation as described and that it has had the desired effect. I would ask if the patient would like sedation and also ensure he has someone available to pick him up and stay with him overnight.

After the patient has entered the room, I would ensure that the WHO checklist had been completed. I would then ensure the patient has a pulse oximeter attached and a flushing cannula. I would then inject the appropriate sedation and analgesia agents as per my trust guidelines. I would then ask the patient to assume the left lateral position raising their knees to their chest. I would then ensure the endoscope is functioning ensuring the insufflation and suction are correctly working. Then I would ask the patients permission to begin, firstly performing a DRE to check for any obvious masses. I would then place lubrication on the tip of the scope an insert in the anal canal past the dentate line. Then using a combination of torque steering and gentle movement

I would make my way to the caecum. During any difficult angulations I may change the position of the patient. If there is any evidence of looping, I may need to retract the scope with reverse torque, or use sigmoid pressure to aid in advancement. I would identify the caecum via visualising the appendix orifice, the ileocaecal valve and the triradiate fold. If any lesions are seen I would biopsy them as I slowly remove the scope back towards the rectum. Post-procedurally, I will write a full report and ensure any biopsies are correctly labelled.

Q. 17.2 What is the definition of a polyp and how can you classify them?

A polyp is defined as an abnormal growth of tissue projecting from a mucous membrane. Colonic polyps can be classified histologically and by their macroscopic appearance.

Histology

Adenoma
- Benign tumour of epithelial tissue of glandular origin
- Have malignant potential (associated dysplasia)

Serrated polyp
- Polyp has a saw-tooth appearance on histology
    - Hyperplastic
    - Sessile serrated
    - Serrated adenoma
    - Benign but malignant potential

Hamartoma
- Benign focal proliferation of cells typically found in the organ from which they arise
- The architecture of the cells is not maintained

Macroscopic appearance: Pedunculated (on a stalk) or sessile (flat)

Paris classification
- I pedunculated
- II flat (sessile)
- III depressed

Kudo pit pattern
- Broadly classified into types I to V
- Increasing irregularity of pit pattern implies – increasing risk of malignancy

Q. 17.3 What are the current British Society of Gastroenterology (BSG) guidelines for polyp surveillance?

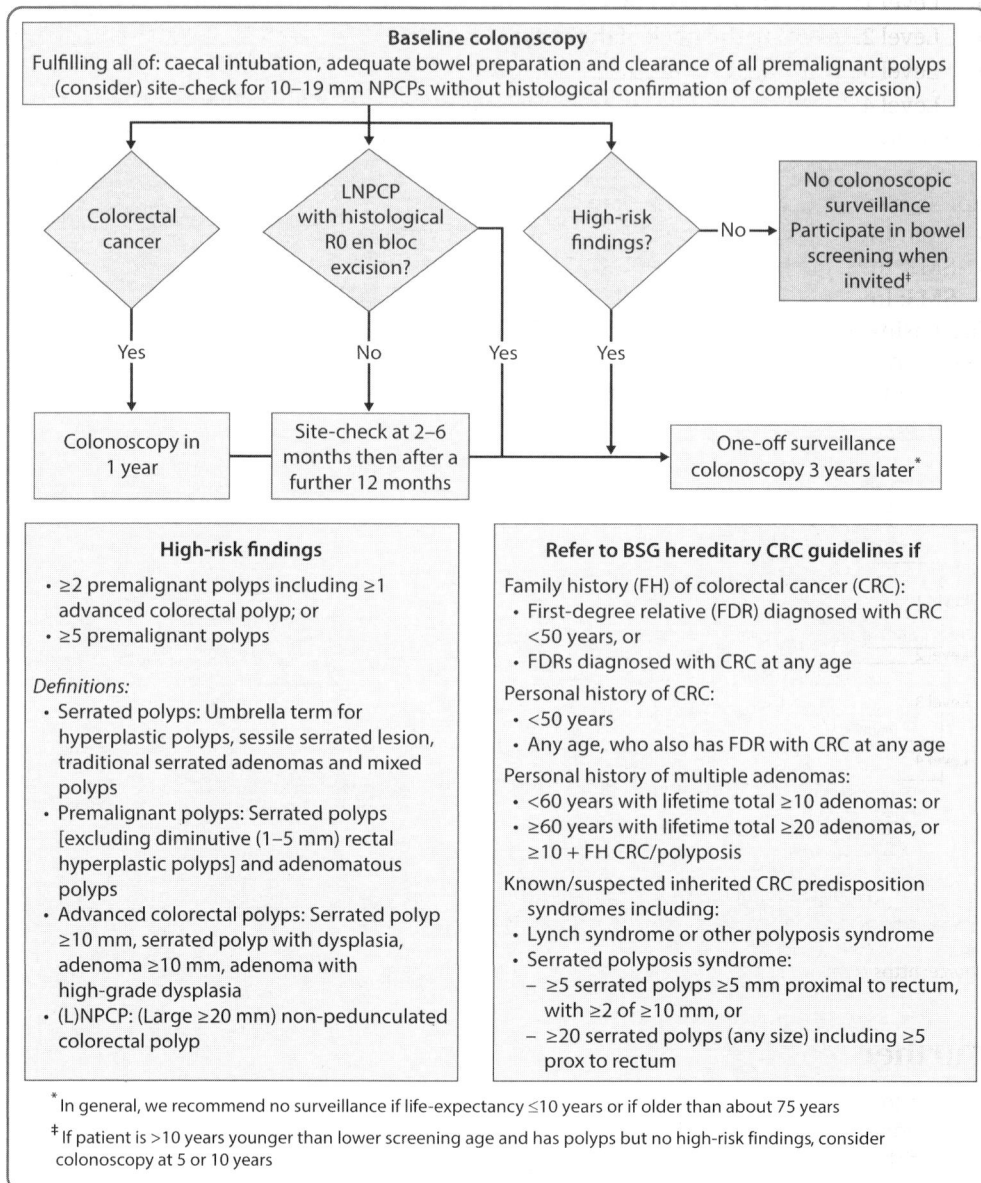

One of the polyps that you excised returns with histology showing a focal area of invasive carcinoma.

Q. 17.4 Do you know of any classification systems for polyp cancers?

There are two known classification systems based on if the polyp is sessile (flat) or pedunculated.

For pedunculated polyps, it is the Haggitt classification:
- Level 0: Non-invasive (severe dysplasia)
- Level 1: Through the muscularis mucosa but limited to the head of the polyp
- Level 2: Invading the neck of the polyp
- Level 3: Invading the stalk of the polyp
- Level 4: Invading into the submucosa below the stalk of the polyp

Increasing Haggitt level leads to increased risk of residual disease after excision.

For sessile polyps, it is the Kikuchi level:
- SM1: Invasion of the superficial 1/3 of the submucosa by neoplastic cells
- SM2: Invasion of the middle 1/3 of submucosa by neoplastic cells
- SM3: Invasion of the deepest 1/3 of submucosa by neoplastic cells

Increasing SM level relates to increased risk of nodal metastases (2, 8, and 23%, respectively)

Haggitt levels 0–3 are synonymous with SM1 of the Kikuchi level.

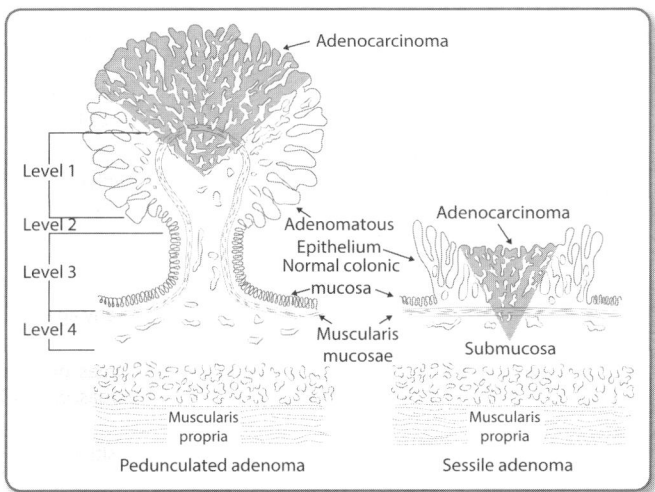

Source: https://onlinelibrary.wiley.com/doi/full/10.1111/codi.12262

Further reading

ACPGBI. [online] Available from https://www.acpgbi.org.uk/content/uploads/Management-of-the-Malignant-Colorectal-Polyp.pdf

The British Society of Gastroenterology. [online] Available from https://www.bsg.org.uk/clinical-resource/bsg-acpgbi-phe-post-polypectomy-and-post-colorectal-cancer-resection-surveillance-guidelines/ [Last accessed March, 2022].

Scenario 18

Bowel screening

You are running an endoscopy list and are about to consent your first patient, a 60-year-old gentleman who thinks he is here because of a 'test his GP did'.

Q. 18.1 What are the current guidelines for bowel screening in the UK?

As of 2019, the new NICE guidelines for bowel screening are for all patients between the ages of 60 and 74 years are offered a Faecal immunochemical test (FIT) every 2 years, except for Scotland where it is offered from 50 to 74 years.

Historically, in some areas of the UK, patients were offered a one-off flexible sigmoidoscopy at the age of 55 years. However, due to cost-effectiveness and the accuracy of FIT testing (the replacement for FOB tests), the one-off scope has largely been abandoned. Instead, the aim is to roll out the FIT test screening from 50 years old and the aim is to have this established by 2025 within the UK.

Q. 18.2 What are the current guidelines for a two-week wait (2WW) referral for suspected lower gastrointestinal (GI) cancer?

Any age with:
- Suspicious abdominal or rectal mass
- Unexplained anal mass or ulceration
- Positive FIT test

Consider referral in patients ≤50 years with rectal bleeding AND any of the following unexplained symptoms:
- Abdominal pain
- Change in bowel habit
- Weight loss
- Iron-deficiency anaemia

Consider referral in patients ≥50 years with any of the following:
- Unexplained rectal bleeding
- Unexplained weight loss
- Unexplained abdominal pain
- Unexplained change in bowel habit

Consider referral in patients ≥60 with unexplained anaemia even in the absence of iron deficiency.

Q. 18.3 What are the key performance indicators (KPI) for bowel screening?

Uptake:
- The proportion of men and women aged 60–74 years invited to take part in screening who adequately participate
- Acceptable level ≥52%
- Achievable level ≥60%

Bowel scope screening adenoma detection rate:
- Acceptable level ≥6.8%
- Achievable level ≥10%

The proportion of participants with an abnormal faecal occult blood test (FOBT) result who are offered a specialist appointment within 14 days of referral date (FIT test not included yet as KPI is based on previous years calculations).
- Acceptable level ≥95%
- Achievable level ≥98%

The proportion of patients given a diagnostic test date within 14 days of their specialist appointment:
- Acceptable level ≥90%
- Achievable level ≥95%

Pathology turnaround of 7 days from date received to date reported:
- Acceptable level ≥90%
- Achievable level ≥95%

Further reading

Atkin W, Wooldrage K, Parkin DM, et al. Long-term effects of once-only flexible sigmoidoscopy screening after 17 years of follow-up: the UK flexible sigmoidoscopy screening randomised controlled trial. Lancet 2017; 389:1299–1311.

https://www.gov.uk/government/publications/bowel-cancer-screening-programme-standards/bowel-cancer-screening-programme-standards-valid-for-data-collected-from-1-april-2018"\l "bcsp-s02-uptake

NICE. [online] Available from https://cks.nice.org.uk/topics/gastrointestinal-tract-lower-cancers-recognition-referral [Last accessed March, 2022].

Scenario 19

Hereditary colorectal cancer

A 25-year-old male patient presents to your clinic with symptoms of loose stools and PR bleeding. His father had colon cancer at the age of 30 years. He undergoes a colonoscopy.

Q. 19.1 What is the diagnosis?

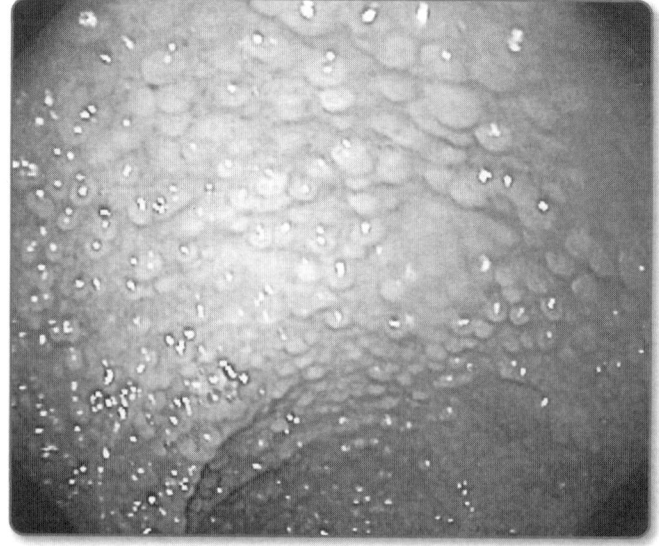

Source: https://en.wikipedia.org/wiki/Familial_adenomatous_polyposis.

The diagnosis is familial adenomatous polyposis (FAP).

Q. 19.2 What can you tell me about FAP?

- It is caused by a mutation on *APC* gene chromosome 5
- 85% of cases are familial
- Screening:
  - Initial colonoscopy at ages 13–15 years
  - Yearly flexible sigmoidoscopy thereafter until a clinical diagnosis made with a colonoscopy at 5-year intervals

- Annual colonoscopy after diagnosis has been made
- Should ideally have surgery by 30
- UGI:
  - 1–3 yearly OGD based on Spigelman score
  - Start at 25
  - Spigelman (size, number, histology and dysplasia)

Q. 19.3 When and what surgery would you offer?

I would offer surgery before the age of 30 years if possible. Ideally this could be performed during summer holiday periods during university time or before starting a new job. If it were a female patient, I would counsel the patient for risks of sexual dysfunction and infertility associated with surgery, and would delay surgery until family is completed if possible.

Surgery would be in the form of a panproctocolectomy.

Q. 19.4 What other hereditary colon cancer syndromes are you aware of?

Lynch syndrome
- Also known hereditary nonpolyposis colorectal cancer (HNPCC)
- Caused by a germline mutation of *MMR* gene [50–70% lifetime risk of colorectal cancer (CRC)]
- Associated with the microsatellite instability (MSI) pathway
- MLH1/MSH2/MSH6 are the most common genetic mutations
- CRC lifetime risk is 60%
- Endometrial CA lifetime risk is 60%
- Gastric and ovarian 10%
- Aspirin reduces risk of CRC (600 mg)
- Screening:
  - 1–2 yearly colonoscopies from the age of 25–75 years
- For extra-intestinal manifestations yearly:
  - TVUSS
  - CA125
- Amsterdam criteria (3-2-1 rule):
  - Three affected family members:
    - One must be 1st degree
    - FAP must be ruled out
  - Two successive generations
  - At least one below 50
  - Tells you how likely you are to have Lynch
- Right sided cancers more commonly. Surgical options include:
  - Subtotal colectomy and ileorectal anastomosis
  - Restorative proctocolectomy
  - Panproctocolectomy
- Commonly mucinous poorly differentiated signet ring

- Survival benefit years:
  - Screening 13.5 years
  - Subtotal colectomy 15.3 years
  - Proctocolectomy 15.6 years
  - Therefore, surgery does not offer much benefit over screening alone and patients must be counselled for this before undergoing any surgery

Peutz–Jeghers syndrome:
- It is autosomal dominant and associated with hamartomatous polyps
- Hyperpigmented macules on lips and oral mucosa
- Caused by the *STK11* gene mutation
- Screening:
  - Initial colonoscopy at age 8 years
    - Every 3 years if polyps found
    - If no polyps found screen only if symptomatic
  - If not symptomatic then screening at 18 years and 3 yearly after

MYH polyposis:
- Autosomal recessive polyposis syndrome
- Characterised by mutation in the *MYH* gene
- Similar to FAP, but much lower polyp burden and fewer extra GI manifestations
- Screening:
  - Same as FAP for colon (yearly from 25)
  - OGD 3–5 yearly from 30

Serrated polyposis syndrome
- WHO criteria any one of the following:
  - ≥5 serrated polyps proximal to sigmoid and ≥2 larger than 10 mm
  - Any number of serrated polyps proximal to sigmoid with 1st degree relative diagnosed
  - ≥20 serrated polyps of any size or distribution in colon
- Due to KRAS/BRAF mutations
- Annual colonoscopic surveillance:
  - 5 yearly screening for 1st degree relatives from 30

Further reading

BSG. [online] Available from https://www.bsg.org.uk/clinical-resource/bsg-acpgbi-guidelines-for-colorectal-cancer-screening-and-surveillance-in-moderate-and-high-risk-groups-update-from-2002/

Burn J, Gerdes AM, Macrae F, et al. Long-term effect of aspirin on cancer risk in carriers of hereditary colorectal cancer: an analysis from the CAPP2 randomised controlled trial. Lancet 2011; 378:2081–2087.

Bülow S, Christensen IJ, Højen H, et al. Duodenal surveillance improves the prognosis after duodenal cancer in familial adenomatous polyposis. Colorectal Dis 2012; 14:947–952.

Monahan KJ, Bradshaw N, Dolwani S, et al. Hereditary CRC guidelines eDelphi consensus group. Guidelines for the management of hereditary colorectal cancer from the British Society of Gastroenterology (BSG)/Association of Coloproctology of Great Britain and Ireland (ACPGBI)/United Kingdom Cancer Genetics Group (UKCGG). Gut 2020;69:411–444.

Scenario 20

Pouchitis

You see a 35-year-old female in whom you previously performed a restorative proctocolectomy on for UC. She is complaining of loose stools associated with blood per rectum and increased frequency.

Q. 20.1 What is the most likely diagnosis?
The most likely diagnosis is Pouchitis.

Q. 20.2 What is the treatment?
Initial treatment is with oral antibiotics for 2 weeks, either metronidazole or ciprofloxacin. If symptoms persist after 2 weeks you may switch to the other antibiotic or use combined therapy for a further 2 weeks. If symptoms still persist at this stage, then endoscopic assessment is needed.

Assessment may be carried out in one of two ways, either EUA +/− biopsies or pouchoscopy +/− biopsies. Often the two procedures are combined.

Q. 20.3 How would you define pouch failure?
Pouch failure is defined as either the need for a defunctioning stoma or formal pouch excision.

Q. 20.4 What would you do if symptoms persist?
The options include escalating medical therapy:
- 5-ASA
- Steroids

The final option is pouch excision:
- Either diversion stoma
- Formal pouch excision and end ileostomy

Q. 20.5 What scoring systems are you aware of for Pouchitis?

- St. Mark's triad
  - Diarrhoea
  - Endoscopic changes
  - Histological changes
- Pouchitis disease activity index (PDAI)
- Heidelberg pouchitis activity score

Further reading

Dalal RL, Shen B, Schwartz DA. Management of pouchitis and other common complications of the pouch. Inflamm Bowel Dis 2018; 24:989–996.

Segal JP, Ding NS, Worley G, et al. Systematic review with meta-analysis: the management of chronic refractory pouchitis with an evidence-based treatment algorithm. Aliment Pharmacol Ther 2017; 45:581–592.

Scenario 21

Radiation proctitis

You see a 65-year-old male in the clinic who has problems with loose stools and bleeding per rectum. He had a low anterior resection 10 years ago for a rectal tumour.

Q. 21.1 What further investigations would you organise?

I would organise:
- CT CAP (CT of the chest, abdomen, and pelvis)
- CEA
- Colonoscopy

Q. 21.2 On colonoscopy you see this, what is your diagnosis?

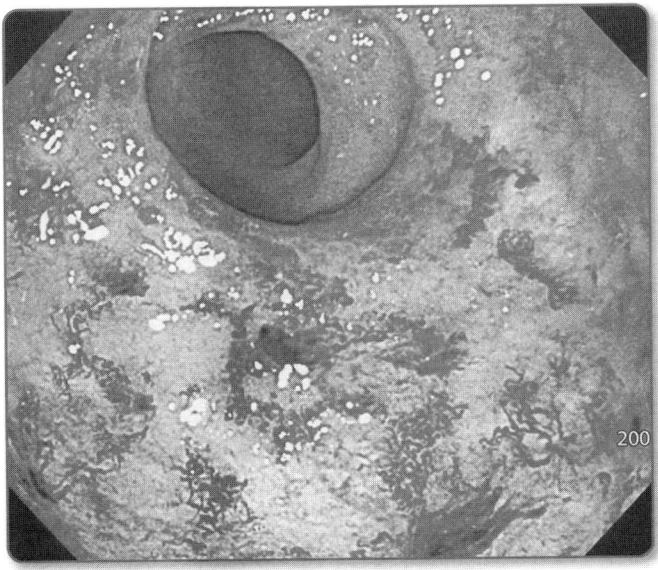

Source: https://www.nejm.org/doi/full/10.1056/NEJMicm0911437.

This is in keeping with radiation proctitis.

Q. 21.3 Would you biopsy this?

Biopsies can lead to complications such as nonhealing ulceration or fistula formation and thus should be avoided unless there is diagnostic uncertainty.

Q. 21.4 What are the risk factors?

The main risk factor is related to the dose of radiotherapy given. However, with more specific and targeted methods of delivering radiotherapy this is now seen less commonly.

Q. 21.5 What are the treatment options?

Conservative:
- Dietary modification including vitamin E supplements

Medical:
- Stool bulking agents
- Loperamide
- Sucralfate enemas (bleeding)
- Steroid enemas (inflammation)
- Vitamins A/E/C (poor evidence base)

Endoscopic:
- Argon plasma coagulation (APC)
- Topical formalin therapy
- Radiofrequency ablation (RFA)
- Cryotherapy

Surgical:
- Proctectomy +/− stoma
- This is a last resort

Further reading

BSG. [online] Available from https://www.bsg.org.uk/clinical-resource/practice-guidance-on-the-management-of-acute-and-chronic-gastrointestinal-problems-arising-as-a-result-of-treatment-for-cancer/ [Last accessed March, 2022].

Tabaja L, Sidani SM. Management of radiation proctitis. Dig Dis Sci 2018; 63:2180–2188.

Scenario 22

Obstructive defecation

You see a 60-year-old woman in the clinic who has problems opening her bowels over the past few months, with a need to digitate to help evacuate her bowels.

Q. 22.1 What would you do next?

I would like to take a detailed history including a full bowel history pertaining to stool consistency, urgency, the number of times needed to digitate per week, or any evidence of urgency or leakage. I would also need to elicit whether there are any 'red flag symptoms'.

I would take a past medical history including history of IBD, haemorrhoids, fissures, fistula-in-ano, or previous anal surgeries. I would like to take a detailed obstetric history including the number of births via SVD, if there was any instrumentation and any episiotomies or tears.

I would then perform a full physical examination, including an abdominal examination and DRE. On anal inspection I would look for evidence of any scarring, fistula openings, skin tags, or haemorrhoids. On DRE I would want to feel for any masses or rectoceles.

Q. 22.2 What is the definition of obstructive defecation?

This is a broad term used to describe defecatory dysfunction and constipation. Symptoms can include that of tenesmus. There are many causes including:
- Rectocele
- Enterocele
- Pelvic dyssynergy
- Rectal intussusception
- Pelvic prolapse

Q 22.3 What is the definition of constipation?

Constipation is defined as difficulty passing stools with an association of tenesmus and less than 3 motions per week.

The Rome criteria states:
- 3 months with 2 of the following in more than 25% of bowel motions
  - Straining
  - Lumpy or hard stools

- Tenesmus
- Manual manoeuvres (Self digitation)
- <3 motions per week
- Sensation of anorectal blockage
- No loose stools

Q 22.4 What scoring systems are you aware of for obstructed defecation syndrome (ODS)?

Wexner score

Symptom	Never	Rarely	Sometimes	Usually	Always
Flatus	0	1	2	3	4
Liquid	0	1	2	3	4
Solid	0	1	2	3	4
Pad	0	1	2	3	4
Urgency	0	1	2	3	4

Vaizey score

	Never	Rarely	Sometimes	Weekly	Daily
Solid stool	0	1	2	3	4
Liquid stool	0	1	2	3	4
Gas	0	1	2	3	4
Change in lifestyle	0	1	2	3	4
				No	Yes
Wear a pad/plug				0	2
Taking constipating agents				0	2
Inability to defer defecations for 15 minutes				0	4

Q. 22.5 What investigations would you do?

- Colonoscopy (To rule out any colonic lesions)
- Anorectal physiology:
    - Manometry
    - Rectal compliance
    - Colonic transit studies
    - Endoanal ultrasound
    - Defecating proctogram

Q. 22.6 What are the treatment options?

Treatment options for ODS are generally limited, and frank and honest conversations must be had with the patient that there will be no overall cure for their symptoms. Initially dietary modification and laxatives can help. If this fails biofeedback can be useful. Glycerine suppositories after defecation can also be given alongside rectal irrigation if needed.
Surgical options are a last resort.

The patients' proctogram shows evidence of a rectocele, what surgical options are you aware of?

After failure of medical treatment, there are several options depending on the approach:
- Perineal
- Transanal
- Transabdominal
- Transvaginal

Repair techniques include but not limited to:
- Stapled transanal rectal resection (STARR)
- Ventral mesh rectopexy

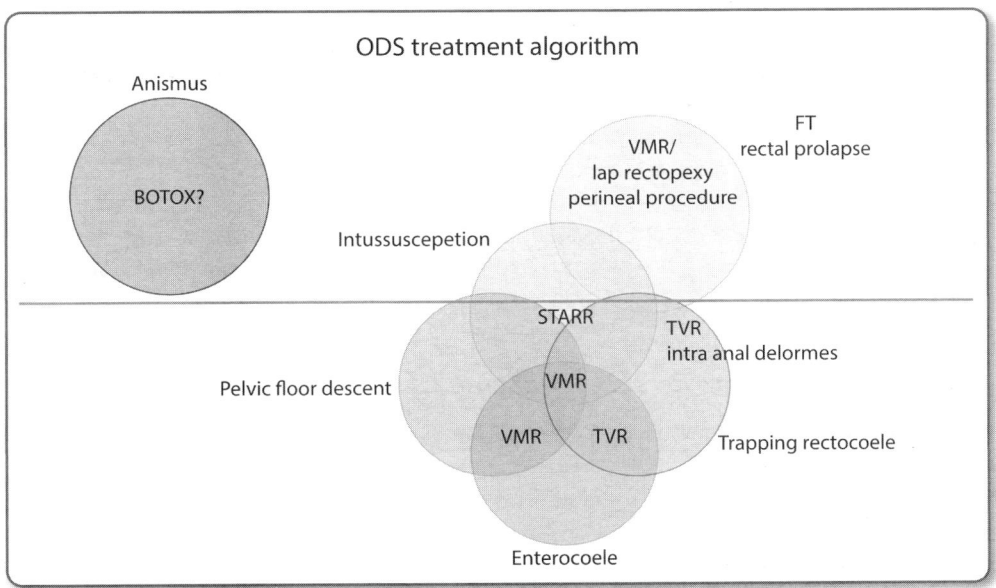

Further reading

Iacobellis F, Reginelli A, Berritto D, et al. Pelvic floor dysfunctions: how to image patients? Jpn J Radiol 2020; 38:47–63.

Van Geluwe B, Stuto A, Da Pozzo F, et al. 2014. Relief of obstructed defecation syndrome after stapled transanal rectal resection (STARR): A meta-analysis. Acta Chir Belg 2014; 114:189–197.

Thaha MA, Abukar AA, Thin NN, et al. Sacral nerve stimulation for faecal incontinence and constipation in adults. Cochrane Database Syst Rev 2015; Cd004464.

Scenario 23

Faecal incontinence

You see a 55-year-old woman in the clinic who has problems with passive incontinence and leakage of stools for 1 year.

Q. 23.1 What would you do next?

I would like to take a detailed history specifically what she is incontinent to whether it be gas, liquid, or faeces. I would like to take a full bowel history pertaining to stool consistency, urgency, the number of times needed to digitate per week, or any evidence of urgency or leakage. I would also need to elicit whether there are any 'red flag symptoms'.

I would take a past medical history including history of IBD, haemorrhoids, fissures, fistula-in-ano, or previous anal surgeries. I would like to take a detailed obstetric history including the number of births via SVD, if there was any instrumentation and any episiotomies or tears.

I would then perform a full physical examination, including an abdominal examination and DRE. On anal inspection I would look for evidence of any scarring, fistula openings, skin tags, or haemorrhoids. Specifically, I would like to check for any evidence of perineal decent by asking the patient to bear down, and make a rudimentary assessment of resting, and squeeze pressures by asking the patient to squeeze on my finger.

Q. 23.2 What investigations would you order?

- Colonoscopy (To rule out any colonic lesions)
- Anorectal physiology:
  - Manometry
  - Rectal compliance
  - Colonic transit studies
  - Endoanal ultrasound
  - Defecating proctogram

Q. 23.3 What are your treatment options?

Conservative
- Stool bulking agents such as Fybogel
- Biofeedback

Surgical options
- Sacral nerve stimulation
- Sphincter repairs
- Repair of any obvious cause (Such as a rectocele)

Further reading

Maeda Y, Lundby L, Buntzen S, et al. Outcome of sacral nerve stimulation for fecal incontinence at 5 years. Ann Surg 2014; 259:1126–1131.

Tan E, Ngo NT, Darzi A, et al. Meta-analysis: sacral nerve stimulation versus conservative therapy in the treatment of faecal incontinence. Int J Colorectal Dis 2011; 26:275–294.

Scenario 24

Pilonidal disease

You see a 25-year-old male in the accident and emergency department with a fluctuant swelling in the natal cleft. He has already been treated with oral antibiotics in the community.

Q. 24.1 How would you proceed?

The history is in keeping with the presence of a pilonidal abscess. I would take a focused history looking for previous episodes and/or any previous incision and drainages. I would pay attention to past medical history especially that of diabetes and would like to know the patient's occupation and if it involves long periods of being seated.

On examination I would like to confirm that it is indeed a pilonidal abscess, looking for any evidence of skin necrosis or spreading erythema. I would also like to assess for any anatomical relation to the anal verge. I would also look for signs of hirsutism in the natal cleft area.

Q. 24.2 What would be your management?

I would book the patient for a formal incision and drainage under general anaesthetic.

Q. 24.3 What is the recurrence rate of pilonidal disease following and incision and drainage?

50% of patients will suffer from recurrence.

Q. 24.4 What are the risk factors for the disease?

- Male gender
- Hirsute natal cleft
- Long periods of sitting
- Buttock friction
- Obesity
- Diabetes
- Sweating

Q. 24.5 What are the surgical options for a chronic pilonidal sinus?

- Lay open with curettage
- Karydakis procedure

- Rhomboid flap
- Sail flap

Q. 24.6 Can you describe one of these procedures?

For the exam you should be able to describe at least one of these procedures in detail. If you have not performed one before then watch videos, as it will be obvious to an examiner if you have just learnt from a textbook or have actually seen/performed the procedure.

Below we give a pictorial example of the Karydakis procedure:

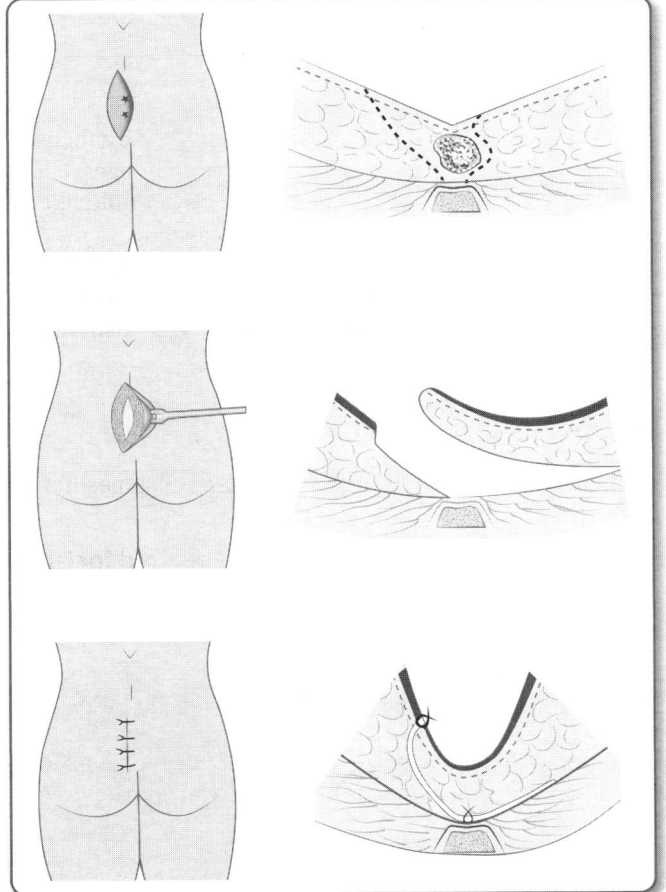

Source: https://www.aerzteblatt.de/int/archive/article/204214/The-management-of-pilonidal-sinus

Further reading

Al-Khamis A, Mccallum I, King PM, et al. Healing by primary versus secondary intention after surgical treatment for pilonidal sinus. Cochrane Database Syst Rev 2010; Cd006213.

Scenario 25

Perianal Crohn's disease

A 21-year-old man is referred to your colorectal clinic by the gastroenterologists with a discharging area next to his anus. He has a background of ileocaecal Crohn's disease for which he takes azathioprine.

Q. 25.1 What features in the clinical assessment are important?

I would start by taking a full clinical history, where I would look to address his luminal disease (bowel frequency, blood/mucus per rectum, abdominal pain/discomfort, partial obstruction) and his perianal symptoms (previous abscesses, abscess history, perianal pain, perianal discharge, and number of pads worn a day). I would also assess the patients for extra-intestinal manifestations of inflammatory bowel disease (eye/joint symptoms).

I would perform an examination where I would first look for other perianal manifestations of Crohn's (superficial fissuring, skin tags, and scars from previous surgeries), I would perform a careful digital rectal examination where I would attempt to identify the internal opening (this feels like a "grain of rice" and is particularly sore). Following this, I would attempt a proctoscopy looking for proctitis.

Q. 25.2 How would you manage him?

I would assess this gentleman's fistula by booking him for both an MRI scan and performing an examination under anaesthesia, as per the European Crohn's and Colitis Organisation (ECCO) guidelines.

I would discuss his case with the gastroenterologists. I am aware that perianal symptoms are a disease modifier in the Montreal Classification and indicate an aggressive step-up approach to medical management. Following the drainage of any sepsis, I think this gentleman should undergo a screen with the view to starting a biological therapy.

Q. 25.3 Having drained his sepsis by placing a seton and the patient having commenced infliximab the patient comes to see you to discuss his options?

First, in conjunction with the gastroenterologist his medications have been optimised, i.e. we have checked his drug levels (if these were low or he was symptomatic I would consider checking for antibodies with the view to switching biologic class).

Following this, I would assess my options in relation to the type of fistula the patient had. If the patient had a single, unbranched tract I would consider a ligation of intersphincteric tract (LIFT) procedure or an advancement flap; both of which I would consent the patient for an approximately 50% success rate. I would counsel them for signs of failure (i.e. abscess formation) and suggest they attend the AE as necessitated.

If the patient had a more complicated fistula, I would look to treat any undrained collections of secondary tracts using the video-assisted anal fistula treatment (VAAFT) scope and ensure the primary tract was draining well with a well-placed seton. I would assess the patient sequentially using MRI and once we had achieved a single, unbranched tract I would treat them as above.

Q. 25.4 Despite multiple attempts at repair the patient develops further external openings and a drastic decrease in his quality of life. He comes to your clinic and asks you what his options are?

This man has an aggressive perianal disease and the quality of life he has with his current medical/surgical therapy is poor. Prior to seeing him in the clinic, I would have discussed his case in the inflammatory bowel disease multi-disciplinary team (IBD-MDT) to ensure there were no other alternatives to consider (i.e. such as another class of biologic). I would offer this gentleman psychological support and I would consent him for a defunctioning colostomy, though I would be very clear that this could become a permanent ostomy. If despite his bowel being defunctioned, he was still symptomatic, I would be considering a proctectomy for him.

Further reading

European Crohn's and Colitis Organisation [ECCO], ECCO Guidelines on Therapeutics in Crohn's Disease: Surgical Treatment. J Crohn Colitis 2020; 14:155–168.

Geldof J, Iqbal N, LeBlanc JF, et al. Classifying perianal fistulising Crohn's disease: an expert consensus to guide decision-making in daily practice and clinical trials. Lancet Gastroenterol Hepatol 2022; 7:576–584.

Stellingwerf ME, van Praag EM, Tozer PJ, Bemelman WA, Buskens CJ. Systematic review and meta-analysis of endorectal advancement flap and ligation of the intersphincteric fistula tract for cryptoglandular and Crohn's high perianal fistulas. BJS Open 2019; 3:231–241.

Scenario 26

Robotic colorectal surgery

A 45-year-old male has a T3 caecal cancer confirmed on endoscopy and pre-operative work-up. Otherwise, he is fit and well, smokes 10/day with a 20-year pack history and no previous abdominal surgery or other medications/risk factors. The multidisciplinary team (MDT) have recommended surgical resection.

Q. 26.1 What are the potential arguments "for" proceeding with a robotic CME resection in this case?

Younger patient, potential for higher lymph node clearance owing to using the embryological planes and early evidence to suggest upstaging of "Staging" classification actually shows some improvement of outcomes in long-term survival.

Q. 26.2 And what additional risks would you consent your patent for during the work-up for a robotic CME?

For the increased risks associated with longer surgical time, increased bleeding risk-specifically the risk of injury to the superior mesenteric vein. (From excessive medial retraction on the vein from medial retraction at the hepatic flexure, and from the nature of high tie. Also potential for delayed gastric emptying.

Q. 26.3 Do you know of any guidelines referring to the use of CME?

There is a CME steering group committee consensus published in 2020 in surgical endoscopy and the German national guidelines recommending the CME approach to right-sided resections.

Q. 26.4 What is the difference between a D2 clearance of lymph nodes in a right hemicolectomy and a D3 clearance?

In a D2 clearance the D1 (paracolic lymph nodes) plus D2 (nodes along the blood supplying vessels) are removed. The minimum number required for accurate staging is 12.

In a D3 clearance the D1 and D2 nodes are taken but additionally, the nodes along the SMV and lateral to the SMA are taken. This is a technically more challenging procedure to perform than a D2 clearance.

Q. 26.5 What is stage migration in relation to CME surgery?

By taking additional nodes using the most radical CME technique with D3 lymphadenectomy there will be some stage 2 patients who, in fact, have more positive nodes therefore move up into the stage 3 disease class. However, the overall survival of both stages 2 and 3 is better. Stage 2: You have taken the highest risk ("sickest") patients and moved them into stage 3 but then these become the lowest risk patients in stage 3 and therefore improve outcomes in stage 3 also.

Q. 26.6 Can you describe the technical differences between a standard and CME for a right-sided colon cancer?

For the CME, you can approach the operation the same as for a medial to lateral standard right hemicolectomy. However, when isolating the ileocolic pedicle care must be taken to fully resect the fatty tissue around the origin before following up towards the middle colic artery and SMV. Set up is similar. Some units will use vascular software to identify any arterio-venous anatomical abnormalities almost like a sat-nav guide before embarking on the radical D3 lymphadenectomy in order to reduce the likelihood of injuring aberrant or replaced arteries and causing serious bleeding complications. The omentum must be taken with the corresponding transverse colon so the omentocolic vessels must also be safely ligated. ICG is a useful tool to use during the intracorporeal anastomosis to check vascularity. With the robot the anastomosis should be performed intracorporeally rather than extracorporeally in order to get the benefits of such.

Q. 26.7 When setting up for a CME right-sided resection what position would you set the table to as a standard?

15-degrees head down with some variable right-sided tilt up. This is more important if there is no smart operating table because the position cannot be altered without fully undocking the robot if there is no tilt table that talks to the robot.

Q. 26.8 What is your preference in port placement for a robotic CME on the abdomen and then also which instruments would you use in which port and why?

This is largely down to personal preference and how you have been trained. The newer robotic surgical systems are more forgiving with the port placements and ergonomics than earlier models; however, you need to have a standard set-up strategy in mind. Our preference is to set up with a port placement in a line 5-cm lateral to the midline oblique markings (placed from the right femoral head, through the umbilicus up towards the left mid-clavicular line). With approximate 6–8 cm between each port depending on patient abdominal size. This facilitates the instruments to be placed with the bipolar in R1, camera in R2 (move to R3 and enlarge later for the stapler device), scissors in R3 and "Cadiere" in R4. Be mindful of which port you will use for the stapler because this will need switching out for a 12-mm port or start with a 12-mm port and a reducer. Alternatives include a straight-line across the central abdomen or a curve across the central abdomen.

Q. 26.9 You have docked the robot but when you place the instrument in R4 it flashed orange and is not engaging. What do you do next?

Check the connections are correct; check that the drapes are placed properly and the robot has recognised them. Take the instrument back out and check that when it clicks in it fits properly into the port. If there is still a problem, then check the number of uses left on the instrument and that it has not expired. Once all of these checks have been done the instrument should dock properly. Further problems then you can check the port with a different instrument to differentiate between the connections and the instrument. Finally undocking, re-draping and re-starting the robot are all last measures to get the robot working.

Q. 26.10 Describe the potential advantages of robotic surgery.

- Lyapunov stability reducing tremor and improving accuracy
- Shortened learning curve of trainees in comparison to laparoscopic surgery
- Three-dimensional (3D) rather than two-dimensional (2D) images when compared with laparoscopic surgery
- Additional degrees of freedom when compared with laparoscopic surgery (facilitates narrow pelvic work)

Further reading

National Institute for Health and Care Excellence. (2020). Colorectal cancer (update) [C3] Optimal surgical technique for rectal cancer. NICE guideline NG151. [online] Available from https://www.nice.org.uk/guidance/ng151/evidence/c3-optimal-surgical-technique-for-rectal-cancer-pdf-7029391218 [Last accessed July, 2023].

Scenario 27

Complex diverticular disease

You review a 64-year-old patient in clinic who has had frequent episodes of diverticulitis, and multiple hospital admissions for IV antibiotics. They have tried altering their diet and still suffer with regular episodes of pain.

Q. 27.1 How does diverticulosis present as a chronic condition?

Chronicity could be due to recurrent episodes of simple diverticulitis. Over time this could lead to stricturing disease. More commonly an acute episode of diverticulitis with associated abscess or perforation, if managed conservatively, could lead to complex diverticular disease (stricturing or fistulating).

An example of complex diverticular disease would be fistula to the bladder. Colovesical fistula classically results in pneumaturia, suprapubic pain, sometimes (but not always) recurrent urine infections. There is often a palpable mass. Stricturing disease causes pain, there is sometimes palpable mass, and this can lead to a presentation of large bowel obstruction.

Q. 27.2 What are the possible underlying pathophysiologic mechanisms leading chronicity or complex diverticular disease?

Previous acute episodes managed conservatively, particularly if they were Hinchey 2–3 (with local perforation leading to pericolic abscess). Contributory factors could be smoking, obesity, and diabetes.

Q. 27.3 How would you manage complex diverticular disease?

It would depend very much on the patient, the severity of symptoms, effect on quality of life, and their general condition or frailty. A careful patient-focused clinical assessment, including history, examination, and imaging would be important.

Q. 27.4 How would you manage a patient presenting with large bowel obstruction secondary to a diverticular stricture?

My initial assessment would start with basic ABCDE and appropriate fluid and electrolyte replacement and adequate analgesia. History and examination to determine how acute, whether the patient was peritonitic (implying possible compromise of the caecum), general condition and frailty (Are they fit enough for major emergency surgery? Is major surgery even appropriate?). Imaging would be helpful, ideally CT scan.

It would be important to establish the cause of the obstruction and whether the stricture was benign (diverticular) or could it be ischaemic or underlying malignancy.

Q. 27.5 Why would this be important and how could you do this?

Depending on frailty, it would be very helpful and informative to know if we are dealing with benign or malignant disease. I could try and assess with flexible sigmoidoscopy and biopsy if possible. However, it is not always possible to determine in the acute setting. Generally, we can be guided by previous history and the CT findings. It is relevant to try and determine, as typically colonic stenting is not a viable option for benign strictures as there is a recognised increased risk of perforation in association with diverticula, it is also technically more challenging, and fibrotic strictures do not tend to open up with a stent. The Crest trial has also shown the limitations of colonic stenting in context of malignant large bowel obstruction, and we know that stenting is a temporary solution at best, so would not be suitable long term for a benign condition. So, if the obstruction was benign, the options would be a resection and Hartmann's procedure, or consider a defunctioning stoma if the patients were frail.

Q. 27.6 How would you manage a colovesical fistula?

A patient-focused assessment to determine the severity of symptoms, effect on quality of life, and their general condition or frailty. If the patient was fit enough, and this was having a significant impact on quality of life and health, then I would discuss options of resection.

Assessment would include a soluble contrast study such as enema, or cystogram. I would offer primary resection and anastomosis, ideally laparoscopically. Robotic surgery can be offered if available, this might enable a completely minimally invasive approach with robotic suturing to repair the bladder if necessary. I would use full bowel preparation, in case we decide to perform a defunctioning ileostomy. Most commonly a small Pfannenstiel incision can be used to assist, e.g. blunt dissection to pinch off the fistula, or dissect under direct vision from the bladder, enable repair of the bladder and be used as the extraction site. A small Alexis wound protector is an excellent device to enable to protect the wound, enable retraction and exposure, and re-establish pneumoperitoneum with the cap to facilitate intra-corporeal anastomosis. However, sometimes an anastomosis might be preferable under vision via the Pfannenstiel incision.

Q. 27.7 Would you take down the splenic flexure?

This is not always necessary, as the segment of involved bowel is sometimes quite short, and we do not need to be radical in resection. It should be considered, as the principles of anastomosis apply (no tension) however blood supply should be better as we do not need to be radical in taking IMA high, so this and the ascending left colic can be preserved ideally provided length and mobility are not an issue.

Q. 27.8 Are there any non-resectional options for colovesical fistula?

Yes, and these should be considered for frail patients. However, it might be that the symptoms are relatively minimal, and the cost of any intervention, e.g. defunctioning colostomy might have a more detrimental impact on quality of life than living with the fistula. It is also important to bear in mind that defunctioning might not fully resolve symptoms from the fistula, e.g. pneumaturia, dysuria, or urinary tract infections.

Further reading

Williams S, Bjarnason I, Hayee B, Haji A. Diverticular disease: update on pathophysiology, classification and management. Frontline Gastroenterology 2024; 15:50–58.

Diverticular disease: diagnosis and management (2019) NICE guideline NG147

Chapter 7

Endocrine surgery

Helen Elizabeth Doran, Ravi Acharya

Scenario 1

Incidentaloma and malignancy risk

Adrenals

A 60-year-old man with diverticulitis is successfully managed conservatively. A CT scan revealed an incidental 5 cm left adrenal mass.

Q. 1.1 How would you investigate this?

An incidentaloma is a clinically in-apparent adrenal mass discovered inadvertently in the course of diagnostic testing or treatment for other clinical conditions that are not related to suspicion of adrenal disease.

For example, if being investigated for headaches, palpitations, collapse and found to have an adrenal mass this is not an incidentaloma, whereas if being investigated for urinary incontinence and found to have an adrenal mass which proves to be a phaeochromocytoma, this is an incidentaloma.

Incidentalomas are very common, occurring in about 5% of all CT scans, with frequency increasing with age. Most should just be referred to an endocrinologist for routine investigation. It can be difficult to decide which requires urgent investigation particularly when found during staging for another malignancy. In general, all masses which are over 4 cm and/or look suspicious and/or have obvious clinical features of hormone excess should be referred urgently. This is to avoid operating on a patient with an undiagnosed phaeochromocytoma.

It is important to distinguish (i) whether the mass is producing hormones, as this will influence both the management decisions and perioperative care, and (ii) whether the patient has a current or prior history of malignancy; if they do the mass has a high likelihood of being a metastasis.

Q. 1.2 What are the hormones secreted by the adrenal gland and what are their actions?

The adrenal gland has two functional parts. The cortex secretes corticosteroids and mineralocorticoids, and is regulated by the hypothalamic pituitary adrenal (HPA) axis. The medulla (chromaffin tissue) secretes catecholamines and is under sympathetic control. Chromaffin tissue is derived from neuroectoderm that can occur anywhere from the adrenals down to the bladder, pelvis, and testes.

There are three histological zones in the cortex; the zona glomerulosa secretes aldosterone which is involved in blood pressure control, and salt and water balance, the zona fasciculata secretes cortisol which is involved in many nutritional and homeostatic functions, and the zona reticularis secretes sex hormones which influence sexual characteristics and behaviour. The medulla secretes the catecholamines, noradrenaline and adrenaline, which are inotropes and involved in the fight and flight response.

Q. 1.3 What is the proportion of adrenal masses that are secretory?

Pooled analysis from 26 international studies and several other series of adrenal masses showed about 10% of masses are functional.

Non-functional adenoma	71–82.4%
Subclinical Cushing's syndrome	5.3–7.9%
Phaeochromocytoma	5.1–5.7%
Aldosterone producing adenoma	1.0–1.2%
Malignant – Adrenocortical cancer	4.4–4.7%
Malignant – Metastasis	2.1–2.5%

Q. 1.4 How would you assess for adrenal function in patients with incidental adrenal lesions?

- All patients should be both clinically and biochemically assessed for adrenal hormone excess (see other scenarios)
- Catecholamines are measured by 24-hour urinary catecholamines or plasma metanephrines
- Glucocorticoids are assessed by serum cortisol, ideally at 9 AM, and if Cushing's is suspected, further testing by dexamethasone suppression tests with adrenocorticotrophic hormone (ACTH) measurement is required
- Aldosterone is measured by renin-to-aldosterone ratio (and serum K^+)
- Androgens, by serum dehydroepiandrosterone (DHEAS)

Scenario 2

Adrenocortical cancer

Q. 2.1 What is the risk of this incidentaloma being a malignancy, and specifically an adrenocortical cancer?

- Overall, 80% of incidentalomas are small, benign, non-functional adenomas
- Less than 5% are adrenocortical carcinoma (2/3 functional – multiple hormones are characteristic, 1/3 non-functional) and the risk of this is related to size
- 2.5% will be metastatic lesions and the remainder, ganglioneuroma, cyst, or myelolipomas
- The risk of an incidental adrenal nodule being a metastasis is dependent on a history of a primary cancer:
  - In patients with known current extra-adrenal primary malignancy, 50–75%
  - In patients without known extra-adrenal primary malignancy, 0.2–2%
  - In patients with only a prior (not current or suspected) malignancy, the risk is more variable and dependent on the primary lesions. Types of primary cancer most likely to metastasise to adrenals are lung, breast, stomach, kidney, lymphoma, and melanoma (+/– pancreas, oesophagus)

Q. 2.2 How can radiology help determine if the lesion is benign or malignant?

Cross-sectional imaging may show metastases or signs of local invasion, which would indicate that the lesion is malignant. About 70% of solitary lesions can be characterised on cross sectional imaging. Certain benign lesions are characteristic on CT, such as myelolipoma and cysts. Adenomas have low density and specific washouts on CT adrenal protocols. Malignancy is suspected if washout is delayed. Lesions that are indeterminate on CT washout may be characterised on magnetic resonance imaging (MRI), which gives detail on contrast enhancement and chemical shift. Radiologically, up to 30% of non-functional lesions will remain indeterminate and may be subsequently characterised as benign if stable on follow-up imaging.

PET avidity is increased in malignant lesions but also benign functional lesions.

The size of the lesion predicts the likelihood of malignancy (2% of lesions < 4 cm, 6% of lesions 4.1–6 cm, and 25% of lesions > 6 cm) and all lesions over 4 cm should be considered for resection unless clearly benign characteristics.

When reviewing previous imaging, rate of growth of differentials are:
- *Adrenocortical carcinoma (ACC):* Rapid growth and rarely <4 cm on detection. Absolute size increase of > 0.8 cm in 3–12 months is 71% sensitive and 81% specific at distinguishing benign vs. malignant adrenal masses
- *Metastasis:* Variable – may have very slow growth, fast growth, or reduction in size
- *Adenoma:* Up to 17% grow over the course of 2 years, by < 1 cm, 5% grow > 1 cm

With functional lesions, specialised imaging may show metastases, e.g. MIBG for malignant phaeochromocytoma. Phaeochromocytomas also have particular features of contrast enhancement on CT due to their vascularity.

Imaging gives information on the contralateral adrenal and anatomical relationships.

Q. 2.3 You are a colorectal surgeon working up a patient with a right-sided colon cancer for surgery and her staging CT shows this large left adrenal mass. The radiologist offers to biopsy it. What would you do?

Biopsy is rarely helpful except to differentiate a metastasis from a primary adrenal lesion as it cannot differentiate between adenoma and adenocarcinoma.

Biopsy of an adrenal lesion is indicated only if it is a suspected metastasis and if the result would alter the management of the patient (i.e. candidate for adrenalectomy or chemotherapy after discussion with an oncologist) after biochemically ruling out a phaeochromocytoma.

Presence of personal history of cancer increases the likelihood (50-75%) of malignant metastasis in the adrenals.

Q. 2.4 How are ACCs more likely to present and how are they treated?

Adrenocortical carcinoma (ACC) usually present, if large, with pressure effects (with pain or impaired venous return) or as incidentalomas. Multiple hormone secretion is characteristic of ACC. Most are sporadic but may be associated with rare genetic diseases – multiple endocrine neoplasia type 1 (MEN1), Beckwith–Wiedemann syndrome, and Li–Fraumeni syndrome.
- They are rare with an incidence of 2 per million and cause, 0.2% of cancer deaths
- Prognosis is poor with average survival of 18 months
- Often large and invade the renal vein or inferior vena cava
- On CT, ACC can be heterogeneous and, have signs of local invasion with lymphadenopathy
- ACC appears bright on T2-weighted MR, heterogeneous enhancement, delayed washout of contrast and do not show loss of signal on chemical shift imaging seen with lipid-rich adenoma. MRI is useful to detect vascular invasion or tumour thrombosis in suspected ACC
- 18FDG PET-CT is useful in detecting ACC and secondaries in the adrenal glands.
- Resection for tumour and amenable metastases increases survival
- Radiotherapy is of uncertain efficacy

Mitotane (DDT derivative) is given orally as an adjuvant therapy, has a 30% response and decreases risk of recurrence. As well as destroying cancer cells it blocks the production of hormones by the ACC, hence patients often need hydrocortisone replacement

Chemotherapy can be given in combination (cisplatin, doxorubicin, cisplatin).

Further reading

Barzon L, Sonino N, Fallo F, et al. Prevalence and natural history of adrenal incidentalomas. Eur J Endocrinol 2003; 149:273–285.

Fassnacht M, Arlt W, Bancos I, et al. Management of adrenal incidentalomas: European Society of Endocrinology Clinical Practice Guideline in collaboration with the European Network for the Study of Adrenal Tumors. Eur J Endocrinol 2016; 175:G1–G34.

Fassnacht M, Dekkers OM, Else T, et al. European Society of Endocrinology Clinical Practice Guidelines on the management of adrenocortical carcinoma in adults, in collaboration with the European Network for the Study of Adrenal Tumors. Eur J Endocrinol 2018; 179:G1–G46.

Hanna FWF, Issa BG, Sim J, et al. Management of incidental adrenal tumours. BMJ 2018; 360:j5674.

Harrison B. The indeterminate adrenal mass. Langenbecks Arch Surg 2012; 397:147–154.

Pantalone KM, Gopan T, Remer EM, et al. Change in adrenal mass size as a predictor of a malignant tumor. Endocr Pract 2010; 16:577–587.

Scenario 3

Phaeochromocytoma

A 29-year-old female with history of headache, palpitations and collapse has been found to have a left adrenal mass and is referred to your endocrine surgical clinic.

Q. 3.1 What is the most likely diagnosis and what would be your management?
Diagnosis
- The most likely diagnosis is a phaeochromocytoma. The classical presentation of phaeochromocytoma ("phaeo") is a history of headache, palpitations, and sweating. This may be associated with pallor, nausea, excess tiredness, anxiety, and collapse. This is due to the paroxysmal nature of catecholamine secretion
- The most common sign is hypertension (however, 10% are normotensive). Phaeochromocytoma can present as an emergency causing sudden death, myocardial infarction (MI), arrhythmia, heart failure, multiorgan failure, or a CVA. A phaeo crisis may be triggered by any surgical procedure, general anaesthesia or childbirth
- Usually, patients have some clinical symptoms but 5% of adrenal incidentalomas are phaeochromocytoma
- To confirm the diagnosis biochemically, blood samples should be sent for plasma-free metanephrines which have sensitivity and specificity of 96–100% and 80–100%
- Ideally these should be taken after 20 minutes of rest and be analysed immediately.
- Twenty-four hours or overnight urinary-free fractionated metanephrines have similar accuracy

Localisation (to confirm the site of the adrenaline excess) should be performed after securing a biochemical diagnosis.
- On CT, phaeos appear as homogenous lesions; 40–50 HU on non-contrast scans (lipid poor). Larger lesions may have necrosis, haemorrhage, calcification, or cyst
- On MR, lesions typically have high signal on T2-weighted scan; and can be useful to assess vascular structures

Functional localisation scans can detect multifocality, metastases and confirm the anatomical abnormality as the site of hypersecretion. Noradrenergic tissue can be anywhere from the base of the skull to the aortic bifurcation (organ of Zuckerkandl) and top of the bladder in pelvis. Imaging includes MIBG – methyl iodobenzyl guanidine with I^{123} or I^{131} which is taken up by chromaffin cells, 68-Gallium DOTATE PET (most sensitive and better resolution than MIBG), and 18FDG PET (more useful when scanning suspected de-differentiated malignant phaeos).

Pre-operative optimisation
- Phaeo patients need to be blocked pre-operatively to optimise intra-operative haemodynamic stability. This is initially with an alpha blocker (phenoxybenzamine) or selective alpha-1 blocking agent (doxazosin)
- The endpoint of block is postural hypotension and nasal stuffiness
- Reflex tachycardia is managed by addition of a beta blocker (propranolol)
- These patients should be reviewed pre-operatively by an anaesthetist experienced in the intraoperative management of this group due to the close invasive monitoring essential for safe surgery
- They need arterial and central lines, and use of agents like IV sodium nitroprusside, magnesium, hydralazine, phentolamine to control intra-operative hypertensive crisis

Post-adrenal vein ligation patients may need to be 'filled up' or noradrenaline administered to support blood pressure. Regular blood glucose monitoring is required to prevent hypoglycaemia.

Genetics
Majority of phaeochromocytoma are sporadic; 25–33% have genetic mutation. Phaeochromocytoma affects:
- 50% of MEN2 (50% symptomatic; 33% hypertensive)
- 10–20% of Von Hippel-Lindau (VHL) II (35% asymptomatic)
- 3–5% of neurofibromatosis 1

Genetic testing should be considered in the following patients:
- Paraganglioma
- Bilateral adrenal phaeochromocytoma
- Unilateral phaeochromocytoma + family history of phaeochromocytoma/ paraganglioma
- Phaeo in young age <45 years
- Clinical findings of syndromic disorder

Genes tested:
- This is evolving. Currently more than 17 genes are included in the genetic panel for phaeochromocytoma-paraganglioma syndromes
- MEN2 (RET), VHL, SDHB,~D,~A,~AF2,~C; FH (fumarate hydratase), TMEM127, MAX (mycosis associated factor X)

Relevance of genetics for planning surgery for phaeochromocytoma:
- Patients with bilateral phaeochromocytoma have either MEN2 or VHL with high penetrance for benign disease. Patients with SDHB and/or MAX mutation are at increased risk of malignancy
- Adrenal sparing surgery has been recommended for patients diagnosed with MEN2 or VHL when operating on both sides
- Complete removal of the phaeochromocytoma is recommended for succinate dehydrogenase subunit B (SDHB) and MYC-associated factor X (MAX) germline mutations

Routine assessment of patients' genotype after first operation can be crucial for adopting appropriate strategy for follow-up and future surgery.

Further reading

Gimenez-Roqueplo AP, Lehnert H, Mannelli M, et al. Phaeochromocytoma, new genes and screening strategies. Clin Endocrinol 2006; 65:699–705.

Grossman A, Pacak K, Sawka A, et al. Biochemical diagnosis and localization of pheochromocytoma: can we reach a consensus? Ann N Y Acad Sci 2006; 1073:332–347.

Rossitti HM, Söderkvist P, Gimm O. Extent of surgery for phaeochromocytomas in the genomic era. Br J Surg 2018; 105:e84–e98.

Scenario 4

Cushing's syndrome

A 60-year-old overweight man with diabetes and hypertension is referred by the endocrinologist with a 2.5 cm left adrenal mass. His cortisol levels are high.

Q. 4.1 What are the possible causes and how would you differentiate between them?

Most common cause of hypercortisolaemia is exogenous steroids.
Endogenous hypercortisolaemia can best classified into ACTH dependent: 80%
a. Pituitary adenoma (Cushing's disease) (70%)
b. Ectopic ACTH secretion (10%)
c. Ectopic corticotropin-releasing hormone (CRH) (very rare)

ACTH independent (adrenal): 20%
a. Adrenal adenoma
b. Adrenal cortical cancer
c. AIMAH and PPNAD
   (AIMAH, ACTH independent macronodular adrenal hyperplasia; PPNAD, primary pigmented nodular adrenal disease: associated with Carney's complex)

Diagnosis
Assess for clinical features of stigmata of cortisol excess:
- Abnormal body fat distribution – moon-like facies, facial plethora, acne
- Interscapular (Buffalo hump) supraclavicular pad of fat, truncal obesity
- Proximal myopathy
- Abdominal striae, bruising,
- Hirsutism – in ACTH dependent disease or ACC
- HTN, type 2 diabetes mellitus
- Kyphoscoliosis (due to osteoporosis)

Endocrine Society for Endocrinology recommends
Screening tests
1 mg overnight dexamethasone suppression test (ONDST) as screening test for hypercortisolaemia
- ≤50 nmol/L serum cortisol – suppressed (normal response)
- >138 nmol/L serum cortisol and no clinical signs of Cushing's autonomous cortisol secretion (instead of subclinical Cushing's)

- 51–138 nmol/L serum cortisol – 'possible autonomous cortisol secretion'

Other screening tests – 24-hour urinary free cortisol and midnight salivary cortisol

Confirmatory tests: Low-dose dexamethasone suppression (LDDST) test to confirm. (Steroid inhalers and excess alcohol – suppress the HPA axis and hence alter the screening tests. These should be stopped for 48–72 hours).

Pseudo Cushing's: This is a condition due to excess alcohol intake or endogenous depression which affects ONDST, LDDST and 24-hour FC. To differentiate it from Cushing's, LDDST followed by CRH is suggested.

Tests to differentiate aetiology

ACTH level: This will be suppressed in adrenal (ACTH independent) Cushing's; elevated significantly in ectopic ACTH and to a lesser extent in pituitary Cushing's disease.

To differentiate aetiologies of ACTH-dependent Cushing's syndrome; high-dose dexamethasone suppression test (HDDST) – helps differentiate pituitary Cushing's (where HPA axis is maintained) from ectopic ACTH syndrome (where there is no negative feedback control)

CRH; positive in pituitary Cushing's; negative in ectopic ACTH and adrenal Cushing's.

Pituitary MRI and inferior petrosal sinus sampling- to localise the lesion in pituitary Cushing's.

Q. 4.2 What are the treatment options, specifically for adrenal Cushing's?

This depends on the aetiology:
- ACTH dependent: Medical, neurosurgical, radiotherapy, bilateral adrenalectomy
- ACTH independent: Adrenalectomy

Adrenal surgery should be individualised for patients with autonomous cortisol secretion based on comorbidities related to cortisol excess (HTN, diabetes, osteoporosis), likelihood of malignancy, general health, age, and patient preference.

Perioperative optimisation
- Involves control of hypertension, diabetes, and weight management (including bariatric)
- Use of metyrapone (to suppress steroidogenesis) if diabetes is difficult to control and surgery likely to be delayed
- Physiotherapy: To improve mobility and respiratory muscle weakness
- Nutrition: To improve postoperative recovery
- Thromboembolism: To consider appropriate VTE prophylaxis

Q. 4.3 Can Cushing's adrenal nodules be malignant?

Aggressive/sudden onset of symptoms, presence of metastasis, and multiple raised steroids on biochemistry should raise concerns about the risk of malignancy.

Q. 4.4 What is the role of urinary steroid analysis?

Profiling urinary steroids by mass spectrometric analysis (metabolome) can help differentiate ACC from adenoma. Sensitivity and specificity is 88–90%.

Adrenocortical carcinomas produce multiple androgenic steroid precursors compared to adenoma which is mostly cortisol and very little androgens. Urinary analysis of 17-keto steroids is no longer used to assess Cushing's and congenital adrenal hyperplasia due to more specific tests.

Further reading

Arlt W, Biehl M, Taylor AE, et al. Urine steroid metabolomics as a biomarker tool for detecting malignancy in adrenal tumors. J Clin Endocrinol Metab 2011; 96:3775–3784.

Toniato A, Merante-Boschin I, Opocher G, et al. Surgical versus conservative management for subclinical Cushing syndrome in adrenal incidentalomas: a prospective randomized study. Ann Surg 2009; 249:388–391.

Scenario 5

Conn's syndrome

A 45-year-old man with hypertension that has been difficult to control for over 5 years is referred by the endocrinologist with hypokalaemia and a 2 cm adrenal nodule.

Q. 5.1 What is the most likely diagnosis and how would you manage him?

- Primary hyperaldosteronism (PA) also known as Conn's syndrome is the most likely diagnosis of this patient
- It is the most common endocrine cause of hypertension (> 10%) over the last decade since biochemical diagnosis has improved
- 25% of PA is due to unilateral adrenal adenoma (APA) which can be surgically managed; the other 75% of PA are chiefly due to bilateral adrenal hyperplasia and other rare genetic conditions like glucocorticoid remediable aldosteronism which are treated medically
- PA should be considered with a high index of suspicion in the following patients (as described by Endocrine Society Endocrinology)
- HTN with hypokalaemia
- Young < 30–35 years + HTN
- Difficult to control HTN requiring ≥ 3 drugs
- HTN + adrenal lesion (differential diagnosis phaeochromocytoma)

Symptoms are tiredness, muscle cramps, symptoms suggestive of cardio and renovascular end organ damage.

Diagnosis is confirmed in conjunction with an endocrinologist:
- This is by screening the suspected patient by ascertaining raised aldosterone-to-renin ratio (ARR) followed by confirmatory testing (saline infusion test, oral salt loading test, fludrocortisone test, and captopril challenge test)
- Medications which affect ARR-like angiotensin-converting enzyme (ACE) inhibitors (ramipril) and angiotensin receptor blockers (ARBs; candesartan), beta-blockers ideally have to be swapped to other anti-hypertensive medications to enable diagnosis. Patients also need to be normokalaemic as it affects renin level
- Once the biochemical diagnosis is secure, CT/MR is performed to image the adrenal lesion
- Selective adrenal vein sampling (AVS) is recommended to localise and lateralise the adrenal source of hyperaldosteronism only if the patient is a surgical candidate.
- This is required as beyond 40 years the incidence of incidental adrenal lesions on CT or MR increase

- AVS helps to avoid unnecessary surgery in some apparent unilateral adrenal lesions and helps to facilitate surgery in some apparent bilateral adrenal lesions on conventional CT or MR
- Appropriately selected PA patients undergoing adrenalectomy show resolution or significant improvement of HTN, thus improving long-term cardiovascular and renal morbidity
- Electrolyte imbalance and renal impairment can occur postoperatively, careful monitoring of urea and electrolytes (U&Es) and estimated glomerular filtration rate (eGFR) is required
- Surgically unfit patients and bilateral secretors (bilateral hyperplasia) are managed medically with aldosterone antagonists (spironolactone, eplerenone)

Q. 5.2 What operative approach would you use and what specific complications can occur?

Adrenalectomy can be done either via a transabdominal (i.e. through anterior abdominal wall) or retroperitoneal (i.e. through the back) approach. Either approach can be laparoscopic or open.

A laparoscopic approach is obviously less invasive, and can facilitate an improved view, but is less suitable for larger size lesions and where there is a high risk of bleeding. Neither of these two circumstances usually applies in Conns' patient so I would choose a laparoscopic approach.

The major benefit of the retroperitoneal approach is that it is not necessary to move any other organs out of the way (i.e. spleen, liver, pancreas, and colon) because the adrenal gland lies right against the ribcage in the back. Bleeding is reduced by the high-pressure insufflation, but if it does occur, the need to turn the patient supine for haemostasis can be an issue.

Around 3% will require conversion to an open approach. Reasons include bleeding, the tumour being stuck to surrounding structures, signs of malignancy (cancer), and tumours too large to be safely removed laparoscopically.

For very large and/or high lesions, cancers growing into other organs or where proximal and distal control of major vessels is required a thoracolumbar approach may be necessary.

Further reading

Beuschlein F, Mulatero P, Asbach E, et al. The SPARTACUS trial: controversies and unresolved issues. Horm Metab Res 2017; 49:936–942.

Dekkers T, Prejbisz A, Kool LJS, et al. Adrenal vein sampling versus CT scan to determine treatment in primary aldosteronism: an outcome-based randomised diagnostic trial. Lancet Diabetes Endocrinol 2016; 4:739–746.

Funder JW, Carey RM, Mantero F, et al. The management of primary aldosteronism: case detection, diagnosis, and treatment: an Endocrine Society Clinical Practice Guideline. J Clin Endocrinol Metab 2016; 101:1889–1916.

Hundemer GL, Vaidya A. Primary aldosteronism diagnosis and management: a clinical approach. Endocrinol Metab Clin North Am 2019; 48:681–700.

Williams TA, Reincke M. Management of endocrine disease: diagnosis and management of primary aldosteronism: the Endocrine Society guideline 2016 revisited. Eur J Endocrinol 2018; 179:R19–R29.

Young WF Jr. Diagnosis and treatment of primary aldosteronism: practical clinical perspectives. J Intern Med 2019; 285:126–148.

Scenario 6

Causes of hypercalcaemia, investigation, and medical management

Parathyroid

You are referred a 65-year-old patient with high calcium by a local GP who has undertaken preliminary blood tests including PTH, vitamin D levels, and myeloma screen.

Q. 6.1 Explain common causes of hypercalcaemia, and how you would differentiate between these?

Hypercalcaemia is a corrected calcium level above normal (usually 2.60 mmol/L). Causes are best classified as PTH and non-PTH-mediated.

PTH-mediated causes are primary hyperparathyroidism (HPT), renal hyperparathyroidism, and familial hypocalciuric hypercalcaemia (FHH). Non-PTH-mediated causes are mostly hypercalcaemia of malignancy, which includes metastatic osteoclastic bone activity, myeloma, paraneoplastic (PTH-rp), and rare PTH secreting tumours. Other non-PTH-mediated causes are immobilisation, endocrine (acromegaly, hyperthyroidism, phaeochromocytoma), and milk-alkali syndrome. In the general population primary hyperparathyroidism is the most common cause whereas hypercalcaemia of malignancy is the most common in hospital, and together they account for over 90% cases.

The diagnosis is entirely biochemical; there is no need for imaging other than to try and localise the source. It is very important to take a medication history as some drugs can affect calcium levels. To biochemically differentiate between causes the relationship between the serum calcium, PTH (and in some cases vitamin D levels), and urine calcium need to be interpreted.

Hyperparathyroidism occurs when excess parathormone is secreted by the parathyroid glands and disrupts the body's tightly controlled calcium homeostasis. Hypercalcaemia results from mobilisation from bone and reduced renal excretion. In non-PTH-mediated causes parathyroid hormone levels are suppressed.

In primary hyperparathyroidism, PTH may still be in normal range, but is inappropriately raised in the presence of the high serum calcium. The newer PTH assays (2nd and 3rd generation) which measure 'intact' PTH as opposed to fragments are much more sensitive and specific.

Vitamin D deficiency raises PTH and so should be treated and hyperparathyroidism confirmed after. Drug-induced hyperparathyroidism (thiazides which reduce calcium excretion, lithium which decrease parathyroid sensitivity to calcium) usually resolves on discontinuation.

24-hour urinary calcium or fractional excretion of calcium must be measured to exclude FHH. This is a rare autosomal dominant condition which mimics the serum biochemical picture of primary hyperparathyroidism. Mutations in the calcium sensing receptor (*CASR*) gene cause decreased receptor activity and increases the set point for calcium sensing. This makes the parathyroid glands less sensitive to calcium, thus a higher-than-normal serum calcium level is required to suppress PTH release. In the kidney, the higher set point leads to an increase in tubular calcium reabsorption resulting in hypercalcaemia (and hypocalciuria).

Q.6.2 Describe strategies for the medical management of hypercalcaemia.

Severe hypercalcaemia is typically a serum calcium above 3 mmol/L. Urgent treatment is required because of the risks of cardiac arrhythmia and coma.

Treatment principles are:
- Resuscitation with IV fluids (to keep UOP > 100 mL/h)
- Increase excretion of calcium: Give IV furosemide (once intravascularly replete)
- Reduce bone resorption: Bisphosphonates (concentrate in bone and reduce osteoclast function); calcimimetic – cinacalcet and others (calcitonin, gallium nitrate, plicamycin, glucocorticoids) which potentiate action of calcitonin, cause calciuresis, decrease intestinal absorption
- Treat the cause: Surgery for PHPT
- Dialysis

Further reading

Minisola S, Pepe J, Piemonte S, Cipriani C. The diagnosis and management of hypercalcaemia BMJ 2015; 350:h2723.

Scenario 7

Surgical role and strategies for hyperparathyroidism

You have confirmed the biochemical diagnosis of HPT. The patient has osteoporosis on a DEXA scan.

Q. 7.1 What would you advise?

Primary hyperparathyroidism has a spectrum of clinical manifestations with increasing severity dependent on time of onset and level of hypercalcaemia, but many patients are asymptomatic presenting as incidental findings on routine blood samples. The first key decision regarding intervention is at what point in the clinical spectrum it should occur; when end organ damage has occurred or earlier (effectively prophylactically). However, not all mild primary hyperparathyroidism will progress. Hence, fully informed consent of perceived benefits and available alternative therapies, including observation, are important.

The fourth international consensus in 2014 recommended surgical intervention where there is evidence of end organ damage (osteoporosis and renal stones) and/or severe hypercalcaemia, and in patients less than 50 years (due to the likelihood of eventual complications). As epidemiological studies increasingly suggested higher mortality from cardiovascular disease; the 2017 updated guidance focused on the asymptomatic/mild disease group and data from later epidemiological studies teasing out confounding factors, particularly for cardiovascular risk. Over time, the threshold for recommending surgery has greatly reduced, but with the caveat that although observational studies suggest mild HPT is associated with depression, decreased quality of life, and changes in cognition, the limited data from randomised controlled trials have not indicated consistent benefits after surgery. The recent 2019 NICE guidelines are consistent with this.

Patient expectation must be clear as many will, possibly incorrectly, assume intervention as better and/or will have been told they have a 'tumour'. Most asymptomatic patients will not experience any perceptible benefit after surgery. Risks of surgery include bleeding, voice change, failure to cure, and recurrence. If the main indication is osteoporosis, alternative management would be a bisphosphonate but there are limitations on length of treatment with this and gastrointestinal side effects.

If the patient opts for surgery increasingly this is undertaken as minimally invasive parathyroidectomy (MIP). I would explain the reason for imaging- to assess suitability for a minimally invasive approach, detect ectopic parathyroid tissue and identify concurrent thyroid pathology (which occurs in up to 30% of patients) and may influence the surgical approach. Types of imaging include USS, radionuclide imaging (sestamibi) and CT, increasingly 4D-CT. Each modality has its own sensitivity and specificity as well as tolerability.

There is confusion around exactly what both clinicians and patients mean by a minimally invasive approach. The principal of MIP is limited exploration based on radiological and sometimes biochemical information exploiting the fact that at least 85% of patients have a single parathyroid adenoma and therefore only one side of the neck will have hyperfunctioning parathyroid tissue.

The success of MIP is dependent on accurate imaging. Approaches are small incision, endoscopic, video-assisted and gas-less endoscopic parathyroidectomy. Intraoperative techniques used for MIP include image-guided (surgeon performed USS) and radio-guided (MIRP – injection of radiolabelled nucleotide). Intraoperative PTH can be very helpful in detecting the presence of multiple gland disease. A reduction in PTH levels on removal of the adenoma can exclude the need for further exploration.

Scenario 8

Parathyroidectomy

You are undertaking a targeted parathyroidectomy in a 36-year-old patient with primary hyperparathyroidism. You have found three normal parathyroid glands but cannot localise the left inferior gland.

Q. 8.1 What is your operative strategy?

I would review the biochemistry first to confirm the diagnosis and then the radiology.

My operative strategy would be along the following lines:
- Knowledge that most glands are within 2 cm radius of inferior thyroid artery
- Relate the search to embryology and rule of symmetry
  - Parathyroid embryology predicates their location, which can be variable and lie anywhere from the level of the submandibular glands to the mediastinum, particularly for the inferior glands which have a longer and more convoluted course of descent from 3rd pharyngeal pouch with thymus. Superior glands descend from the 4th pharyngeal pouch in a shorter and vertical course. About 80% of superiors are in typical location, above the intersection of the nerve and artery and 60% of inferiors below the thyroid lobe. The rest, however, can be undescended, along the track of descent or maldescended. Up to 1% can be in the chest, usually the inferiors, even around the heart or in the aorto-pulmonary window
- Look low for over-descended upper gland
- Check retro/parapharyngeal/oesophageal space for PLUG (posterior located upper gland)
- Look high (above the thyroid and up to submandibular gland) for non-descended lower gland
- Take down upper pole of thyroid and look behind
- Open carotid sheath, sloop great vessels, search from top to bottom
- Check thyrothymic ligament and consider cervical thymectomy (45% will have parathyroid tissue)

I would carefully consider whether to do any thyroidectomy, particularly if any scans had localised to one side. However, only 0.2% glands are in the thyroid and thyroidectomy potentially could make subsequent selective venous sampling more difficult to interpret.

Important to note carefully what I have found and obtain frozen sections:
- If available, I would ask for help
- Consider biopsy of normal glands
- Close neck

Further reading

Bilezikian JP, Brandi ML, Eastell R, et al. Guidelines for the management of asymptomatic primary hyperparathyroidism: summary statement from the fourth international workshop. J Clin Endocrinol Metab 2014; 99:3561–3569.

NICE. Hyperparathyroidism (primary): diagnosis, assessment and initial management; NICE guideline [NG132]. Published date: 23 May 2019.

Scenario 9

Persistent and recurrent hyperparathyroidism

You have undertaken parathyroid surgery on a 64-year-old male. He has biochemically confirmed hyperparathyroidism with negative localisation studies. You undertook a bilateral neck exploration and removed a large right superior parathyroid confirmed on frozen section. On 6 weeks postoperative visit, he has persistent hyperparathyroidism.

Q. 9.1 Explain difference between persistent and recurrent hyperparathyroidism. How would you manage this patient?

Persistent hyperparathyroidism is biochemical evidence of hyperparathyroidism within 6 months of parathyroid surgery. Recurrence is where the patient had a normal calcium post-op then recurrence of hyperparathyroidism more than 6 months after surgery.

I would have explained pre-operatively about possible failure. The British Association of Endocrine and Thyroid Surgeons (BAETS) audits up to 5% procedures – especially as the patient had not localised. Explaining this data may support the consultation.

First, I would confirm the biochemical diagnosis of persistent hyperparathyroidism, including evaluation of vitamin D status. I would then discuss the indications for revisional surgery (which must be very clear) and whether an alternative treatment (such as bisphosphonate) was more suitable. As both sides of the neck have been explored, I would try to avoid any revisional surgery for at least 6 months and so would need to manage the hypercalcaemia medically if significantly high.

This gentleman most likely has either a double adenoma or multiple gland disease. I would confirm the histology of the removed right superior which may be helpful.

The expected success rate and higher complication rate of revisional surgery need to be discussed. This is a situation requiring an experienced multidisciplinary team and maximal effort at localisation. Cure rate with and without localisation for recurrent disease are 95% and 60%, respectively (BAETS audit). Cross-sectional imaging can be supported by venous sampling, effectively a roadmap of PTH levels. This is a specialised interventional procedure, and risks include haematoma, anaphylaxis, contrast renal failure, stroke, and vessel injury.

The incidence of complications with revisional parathyroid surgery is much higher – 5-fold the risk of RLN injury in primary surgery. Nerve monitoring is recommended for these cases.

One cause of failure is surgical inexperience, although this is becoming less common as parathyroidectomy is now recognised as subspecialty practice. For trainees, the requirement of index procedures and tertiary experience is mandated. Currently, consultant annual case load is not specified in guidelines but there are recommendations. If necessary, I would consider referring the patient to a tertiary service.

Scenario 10

Renal hyperparathyroidism

A 65-year-old male with stage 5 chronic kidney disease (CKD) 5 and persistently raised PTH and hypercalcaemia.

Q. 10.1 How would you manage this patient?

Complex renal failure patients (irrespective of dialysis dependence) with bone mineral disease (BMD) are primarily managed medically by their renal physicians. Where there is evidence of mineral and bone disease and presence of osteoporosis or fragility fractures the treatment options (anti-resorptive therapies – bisphosphonates, etc.) should be individualised depending on the progression of CKD, BMD and may bone biopsy may be needed if it alters treatment options.

The majority of renal failure patients have secondary hyperparathyroidism due to constant stimulation of parathyroid glands due to vitamin D deficiency, hypocalcaemia, and hyperphosphatemia. This is managed medically with calcitriol/alfacalcidol, phosphate lowering agents, and dialysate.

Constant stimulation of parathyroid glands can cause somatic mutation in parathyroid glands leading to autonomous or tertiary hyperparathyroidism with resultant hypercalcaemia and bone disease. There is confusion in nomenclature about tertiary hyperparathyroidism; in many reports it does not just apply to transplant recipients. Some define 'tertiary' as persistent hyperparathyroidism despite reversal of the underlying cause and often occurs after transplantation.

As per Kidney Disease Improving Global Outcomes (KDIGO) Guidelines 2017. For patients with CKD on haemodialysis with persistently elevated/rising PTH requiring PTH lowering therapy, calcimimetics (cinacalcet), vitamin D analogues, and parathyroid surgery are all acceptable therapies. Individual treatment choices should be guided by consideration of concomitant therapies, calcium and phosphate levels, patient preference, and associated comorbidities and whether there is a possibility of future transplant.

The EVOLVE trial revealed cinacalcet substantially reduces (HR 0.31) the occurrence of severe unremitting HPT which is frequent in patients on haemodialysis. Cinacalcet decreased the risk of death and of major cardiovascular events in older, but not younger, patients with moderate-to-severe hyperparathyroidism who were receiving haemodialysis. Effect modification by age may be partly explained by differences in underlying cardiovascular risk and differential application of cointerventions (kidney transplant and parathyroidectomy) that reduce parathyroid hormone.

Patients on dialysis with persistently severely high PTH (suggested greater than nine times upper limit of normal as per KDIGO but with no clear consensus) and failure of medical and pharmacological management are suggested to have parathyroidectomy.

For patients with refractory hyperparathyroidism who are actively awaiting transplantation, decisions regarding parathyroidectomy should be jointly made with the transplant centre. Hyperparathyroidism often, but not always, resolves after kidney transplantation. Ideally if parathyroidectomy is indicated, this should occur before transplantation because of the risk of severe hypocalacaemia on graft function. Persistent refractory hyperparathyroidism in transplant patients can lead to increased mortality due to cardiovascular complications and allograft loss (ALERT trial). This is the rationale for offering parathyroid surgery. There have also been reports of reduction in eGFR after parathyroidectomy in these patients. However, it is not clear on whether this contributes significantly to allograft loss.

Q. 10.2 What are your surgical options/strategies?

The surgical options are subtotal parathyroidectomy (3 and ½ gland resection) or total parathyroidectomy (with or without autotransplantation). In patients with or likelihood of transplant there is a potential benefit of leaving some native parathyroid tissue, but this does increase the risk of recurrent hyperparathyroidism. Usually, the thymus is removed as this contains parathyroid rests. These patients do not need localisation studies unless primary hyperparathyroidism is suspected.

Further reading

Kidney Disease: Improving Global Outcomes (KDIGO) CKD-MBD Update Work Group. KDIGO 2017 clinical practice guideline update for the diagnosis, evaluation, prevention, and treatment of chronic kidney disease–mineral and bone disorder (CKD-MBD). Kidney Int Suppl 2017; 7:1–59.

Parfrey PS, Chertow GM, Block GA, et al. The clinical course of treated hyperparathyroidism among patients receiving hemodialysis and the effect of cinacalcet: the EVOLVE trial. J Clin Endocrinol Metab 2013; 98:4834–4844.

Parfrey PS, Drüeke TB, Block GA, et al. The effects of cinacalcet in older and younger patients on hemodialysis: the evaluation of cinacalcet HCl Therapy to Lower Cardiovascular Events (EVOLVE) Trial. Clin J Am Soc Nephrol 2015; 10:791–799.

Punch JD, Thompson NW, Merion RM. Subtotal parathyroidectomy in dialysis-dependent and post-renal transplant patients. A 25-year single-centre experience. Arch Surg 1995; 130:538–543.

Tominaga Y, Uchida K, Haba T, et al. More than 1,000 cases of total parathyroidectomy with forearm autograft for renal hyperparathyroidism. Am J Kidney Dis 2001; 38:S168–S171.

Scenario 11

Thyrotoxicosis

Thyroid

You are referred a 34-year-old lady with palpitations and a swelling in the neck who is 'concerned it's cancer and wants it out'. She has compressive symptoms and mild thyroid eye signs.

Q. 11.1 What are the steps in management?

First I would want to ascertain the cause of the palpitations and neck swelling as this would determine management options and whether surgery was appropriate. Her concern about possible malignancy also needs to be addressed. From the information given this is likely to be Graves' disease. To investigate this I would check her thyroid function tests and thyroid antibodies. Surgery may be the best treatment as she has compressive symptoms, but this may improve with treatment of hyperthyroidism.

Q. 11.2 These are her TFTs. What do they show? What are the causes and how would you manage this?

TSH	0.01	(0.27–4.2 nmol/L)
T4	32.1	(12–22 pmol/L)
T3	3.5	(3.1–6 pmol/L)

Thyrotoxicosis is confirmed by the elevated thyroxine and suppressed thyroid-stimulating hormone (TSH) concentrations. The most common cause is Graves' disease (80%), typically in young females aged 20–40 years, toxic multinodular goitre (10%) where patients are generally older with a marked goitre and solitary toxic nodule (10%). In this patient, as there are thyroid eye signs, the cause will be Graves and other potential extrathyroidal signs are pretibial myxoedema and thyroid acropachy.

Investigations I would consider include:
- Autoantibodies to thyroid peroxidase (TPO); present in 90% with autoimmune thyrotoxicosis and 10% of the general population. Very-high TPO and thyroglobulin (Tg) antibodies suggest Hashimoto thyroiditis. I would exclude thyroiditis [history, full blood count (FBC), and erythrocyte sedimentation rate (ESR)] before starting antithyroid treatment
- If TSH is suppressed and FT4 is normal, request FT3
- Thyroid receptor antibodies (TRAB) can help to predict response to medication
- Ultrasound of the thyroid is generally to investigate neck masses, not thyrotoxicosis

- Need CT neck if clinical retrosternal extension
- A thyrotropin-releasing hormone (TRH) test is unhelpful and not indicated

Treatment options for thyrotoxicosis include:
- Thionamides, i.e. anti-thyroid drugs (carbimazole and propylthiouracil)
- Radioactive iodine (RAI)
- Surgery

Beta-blockers may be considered for symptomatic relief in all patients with moderate or severe hyperthyroidism. Asthma is an absolute contraindication for their usage and heart failure a relative one. Beta-blockers may be the sole treatment required in thyrotoxicosis secondary to thyroiditis.

Initially, it is important to render the patient euthyroid. Side effects of carbimazole include neutropaenic sepsis and rarely agranulocytosis. Warn patients to stop the medication if they have a sore throat, rash or fever and report for medical advice. The complication usually occurs early after treatment but can occur up to several months later or even on a second course of thionamides. Agranulocytosis and other rare but serious side effects, including hepatitis and lupus-like syndromes, represent absolute contraindications to thionamide. Pruritus and rashes are common but often resolve with continued treatment. If these side effects necessitate a change in treatment, carbimazole can often be changed to propylthiouracil without recurrence.

Definitive treatment is surgery or radioactive iodine. As this patient is concerned about cancer surgery may be the preferred option. Other indications for surgery include large goitre, clinically suspicious nodule(s) in the gland, severe thyroid eye disease, patient preference (often due to having a young family or planning pregnancy), and Graves' disease in pregnancy if thionamides not tolerated (best in 2nd trimester).

Outcomes of surgery:
For both TMG and Graves:
- Total thyroidectomy is the standard procedure.
  - Previous accepted practice was to perform subtotal thyroidectomy as thought to reduce risk of injury to nerves and incidence of hypoparathyroidism. Now it has been shown that risk of surgical complications for endocrine-trained surgeons are no higher with total thyroidectomy and does not result in recurrent disease. Occasionally near total thyroidectomy is performed where a tiny remnant of thyroid is left near the entry point of the laryngeal inlet to safeguard the nerve. Hence all patients rendered hypothyroid permanently require lifelong thyroxine.
- Peri-surgical management:
  - Must be euthyroid prior to surgery
  - Beta-blockers and iodine have no routine role pre-operatively
  - Pre-operative vocal cord check may be offered (always for revisional surgery, cancer, changes to voice)
  - Check pre-operative calcium to detect coexisting primary hyperparathyroidism
- Complications:
  - Haemorrhage (<1%)
  - Wound infections (<0.5%)

- Recurrent laryngeal and external branch of the superior laryngeal nerve damage. Incidence of RLN nerve damage <2% and results in permanent change to voice. SLN damage has higher incidence but only rarely notable to patient
- Hypocalcaemia (transient in 20%, permanent in 2–5% depending on indication)
- Postoperative care:
  - Serum calcium should be checked
  - Anti-thyroid drugs should be stopped
  - Beta-blockers should be weaned
  - Length of stay is usually less than 48 hours postoperative
  - TFTs should be assessed 4 weeks postoperative, 3-monthly for 1 year, then yearly (GP)

Scenario 12

Thyroid swelling

A 28-year-old female patient with painless thyroid nodule has been referred to your clinic by her GP.

Q. 12.1 What could this be and how would you evaluate her?

Around 3–7% of adults have palpable thyroid nodule (s) and 30–70% on a neck ultrasound scan.

This is most likely to be a benign lesion: colloid nodule, dominant nodule in multinodular goitre, hyperplastic nodule, toxic adenoma, and cyst. It could be malignant, differentiated thyroid cancer (papillary thyroid cancer or follicular thyroid cancer), medullary thyroid cancer, anaplastic cancer, primary thyroid lymphoma, or thyroid metastases.

In her history, I would like to know:
- The duration – long standing or within a few weeks/months
- Any associated compressive symptoms – dysphagia, dyspnoea (positional), hoarseness of voice
- Any clinical features suggestive of hyper- or hypothyroidism
- Any history of radiation exposure, family history of thyroid cancer
- Any specific medications (lithium, amiodarone, anti-coagulants)

On examination, I would elicit answers to the following questions:
- Moves on swallowing. If central – ask patient to stick out the tongue
- Single or multiple nodules or diffuse enlargement; size, shape, consistency
- Can I get below it/retrosternal? Consider elevating arms to demonstrate superior vena cavalobstruction (Pemberton's sign)
- Trachea – central or deviated?
- Any lymphadenopathy
- Carotids palpable?
- Thyroid status examination: Palms, pulse, eye signs, skin

I would then check her thyroid function tests (TSH, T4, and T3) and review her ultrasound of the neck. Serum calcitonin is used selectively.

If not hyperfunctioning, and ≥1 cm and U3 or above as per BTA 2014 guidelines, I would arrange an USS-guided fine needle aspiration (FNA) biopsy.

If the nodule is <1 cm – ignore, unless extrathyroidal extension or suspicious lymph node(s) or high-risk clinical history.

Q. 12.2 What features are associated with increased risk of thyroid malignancy?

History: Age <20 or >60 years, dysphonia/hoarseness, rapid growth over weeks, history of neck irradiation, family history of thyroid cancer, Cowden's syndrome, or familial adenomatous polyposis.

On examination: Firm nodule with fixity to adjacent structures, regional lymphadenopathy.

On US thyroid: Solid nodules taller than wide with irregular margins, intranodular vascularity, microcalcifications are suspicious of malignancy.

Q. 12.3 On USS, it is 2.5 cm U3 nodule and the FNA is reported as Thy3. How would you manage her?

The risk of malignancy (ROM) for Thy3 category is 9.5–43%, the highest with suspicious ultrasound features.
  This could be Thy3a (atypia) or Thy3f (follicular lesion)
  Thy3a – denotes atypical features, unable to exclude papillary carcinoma or follicular neoplasm. These often need repeat US-guided FNA.
  Thy3f – denotes a follicular neoplasm suspected. This could be a hyperplastic nodule, follicular adenoma or follicular carcinoma, or possibly a follicular variant of papillary carcinoma or medullary carcinoma. This needs diagnostic hemithyroidectomy as histology is necessary to demonstrate capsular or vascular invasion.
  The ROM for Thy1 (inadequate/non-diagnostic) 0–10%; Thy2 0–2%; Thy3 10–40%; Thy4 60–75%; Thy5 98–99%.

Further reading

Chadwick D, Tani S. Management of the thyroid nodule. Surgery 2017; 35:563–568.
Perros P, Boelaert K, Colley S, et al. Guidelines for the management of thyroid cancer. Clin Endocrinol (Oxf) 2014; 81:1–122.

Scenario 13

Multinodular goitre

A GP has referred a 65-year-old lady with a long-standing lump in neck who has noticed a recent increase in size associated with some shortness of breath.

Q. 13.1 How would you assess her?

My concerns for this patient are multinodular goitre causing airway compression either due to increase in size or malignant transformation. The duration of symptoms is likely to give a guide to the cause: benign (gradual over few months), malignancy (few weeks), sudden (bleed into a cyst).
I would elicit a detailed history regarding progression of compressive symptoms:
- Dyspnoea – worse on lying down? Any stridor?
- Dysphagia/Pooling of secretions requiring frequent clearing of throat?
- Hoarseness of voice?
- Personal or family history of thyroid cancer; History to elicit thyroid function status
- Any history of neck irradiation

Physical examination would be to ascertain
If thyroid goitre: whether multinodular or smooth, any lymphadenopathy, any retrosternal extension (Pemberton's sign), tracheal position.

Thyroid status examination
I would arrange TFTs, US neck +/- biopsy if nodule U3 or above and CT neck and thorax, and respiratory flow volume loops if indicated.

Q. 13.2 How would you manage her and what are the options?

I would discuss this case with my radiologist ideally within an endocrine multidisciplinary team (MDT).
The key questions to be answered are:
- Is there any malignancy? This would need to be dealt with on its own merits
- Are the compressive symptoms attributable to goitre? Flow volume loops to elicit dynamic upper airway obstruction
- Radiological assessment is of paramount importance: Tracheal compression versus deviation?

- Extent of retrosternal goitre vis-à-vis aortic arch and the morphology of the goitre: pyramid and posteriorly situated vs. conical and in anterior mediastinum (retroclavicular)
- Any sign of toxicity?

The options are (1) Total thyroidectomy (2) Hemithyroidectomy (3) Reimage in 12 months to see if any progression in size in the absence of malignancy and asymptomatic.

Over 90% of retrosternal goitres can be resected transcervically. Other approaches are sternotomy or thoracotomy and video-assisted thoracoscopic surgery (VATS).

Patients at high risk of requiring sternotomy (Simo et al.) are those with goitre below the arch of aorta, recurrent goitres to the arch of aorta, iceberg or conical morphology, those involving multiple mediastinal compartments, extension to posterior pleura, and goitre with separate components.

Unplanned sternotomy is to be avoided.

Thyroidectomy for retrosternal goitre has increased risk of RLN injury (2–5%), bleeding and permanent hypoparathyroidism (2.1–3%), and 2–3% risk of tracheostomy due to bilateral RLN palsy.

Risk-minimisation strategies involve: Routine vocal cord check, intraoperative neural monitoring (IONM), hemithyroidectomy of the larger side, or staged total thyroidectomy.

Further reading

Dionigi G, Chiang FY, Dralle H, et al. Safety of neural monitoring in thyroid surgery. Int J Surg 2013; 11:S120–S126.

Gupta P, Lau KK, Rizvi I, et al. Video-assisted thoracoscopic thyroidectomy for retrosternal goitre. Ann R Coll Surg Engl 2014; 96:606–608.

Hardy RG, Bliss RD, Lennard TW, et al. Management of retrosternal goitres. Ann R Coll Surg Engl 2009; 91:8–11.

Landerholm K, Järhult J. Should asymptomatic retrosternal goitre be left untreated? A prospective single-centre study. Scand J Surg 2015; 104:92–95.

Simó R, Nixon IJ, Vander Poorten V, et al. Surgical management of intrathoracic goitres. Eur Arch Otorhinolaryngol 2019; 276:305–314.

Scenario 14

Thyroid surgery and complications

You review a 39-year-old lady who underwent total thyroidectomy for compressive symptoms on first postoperative day. Her voice is hoarse.

Q. 14.1 How would you assess her?

My main concerns are recurrent laryngeal nerve injury; temporary or permanent.
Other common cause is irritation of laryngopharynx due to endotracheal intubation.
After ascertaining her airway is secure and her vital signs are stable, I would review her operative notes. Was the RLN formally identified on both sides? Any suspicion of obvious malignancy? Was nerve monitoring used to confirm the integrity of the RLNs?
I would check if she has difficulty in projecting her voice and if she has bovine cough. I would also assess if can she swallow safely (SALT assessment).
I would examine her to check for any suggestion of an obvious haemoseroma in the neck.
I would arrange urgent flexible nasopharyngolaryngoscopy by an ENT colleague to directly visualise the vocal cords to check for palsy. Depending on the degree of injury, this patient may require early voice therapy/medialisation procedure/Teflon injection.
If swallow is unsafe, she would need fluid thickeners or in severe cases fine bore nasogastric feeding tube/percutaneous endoscopy gastrostomy (PEG) tube.

Q. 14.2 Describe the course of recurrent laryngeal nerves?

The right RLN arises from the right vagus in the thoracic inlet. It ascends from lateral to medial (more oblique than the left) in the paratracheal region.
The left RLN arises from the left vagus, travels anterior to the aortic arch, and runs in craniocaudal direction in the trachea-oesophageal groove.
As it ascends the next landmark is crossing of the inferior thyroid artery (ITA) followed by posterolateral nodular formation (tubercle of Zuckerkandl) at the thyroid mid-pole. Both these can be variable. Last relatively constant interaction of the nerve is with the ligament of Berry (condensation of true thyroid capsule) where it is usually dorsal or posterior to it. But rarely, it can traverse between anterior and posterior leaflets of Berry's ligament or even be anterior to it before it goes under the inferior most fibres of inferior constrictor of pharynx (the laryngeal entry point). Around 10% of patients have premature extra-laryngeal motor fibre branching below the laryngeal entry point and in over 90% this is distal to the ITA crossing point.

Q. 14.3 What is the incidence of RLN injury?

Permanent RLN injury ranges between 0.5% and 2% in expert hands. This risk is six times in revisional thyroid surgery.

Scandinavian Quality Register reports doubling of the rate of RLN injury identified when routine postoperative vocal cord check is performed.

Q. 14.4 Would you recommend pre-operative VC check via laryngoscopy?

The British Association of Endocrine & Thyroid Surgeons (BAETS), German Association of Endocrine Surgery & International Neural Monitoring Study Group recommend routine pre- and postoperative fibreoptic nasoendoscopy (FNE) to allow thyroid and parathyroid surgeons to know their personal nerve palsy rate, to avoid operating on patients with an undiagnosed pre-existing recurrent laryngeal nerve palsy and plan contralateral surgery.

Pre-operative laryngeal examination should be performed on all patients undergoing thyroid surgery who are at high risk for nerve injury (pre-operative voice abnormalities, history of cervical or upper chest surgery, thyroid cancer with known posterior extension, or extensive cervical node metastases) as per NCCN and American Thyroid Association and American Head & Neck Society Invasive Thyroid Cancer guidelines.

Q. 14.5 What does the current literature report regarding intraoperative neural monitoring (IONM) in thyroid/parathyroid surgery?

Dralle et al. (German multicentre non-RCT with 29,998 nerves at risk) revealed no statistical difference in permanent RLN injury between no routine RLN identification (0.93%), visual assessment only (0.89%), and IONM + VA (0.80%).

Barczyński et al. (2009) in an RCT with 1000 nerves at risk reported reduction in temporary RLN injury in the IONM group versus visual assessment alone; however, no difference in permanent RLN injury.

Pisanu et al. (2014) in a meta-analysis showed no statistical difference in rate of both transient and persistent vocal cord injury in thyroidectomy with and without nerve monitoring.

Further reading

Barczyński M, Konturek A, Cichoń S. Randomized clinical trial of visualization versus neuro-monitoring of recurrent laryngeal nerves during thyroidectomy. Br J Surg 2009; 96:240–246.

Dralle H, Sekulla C, Haerting J, et al. Risk factors of paralysis and functional outcome after recurrent laryngeal nerve monitoring in thyroid surgery. Surgery 2004; 136:1310–1322.

Pisanu A, Porceddu G, Podda M, et al. Systematic review with meta-analysis of studies comparing intraoperative neuromonitoring of recurrent laryngeal nerves versus visualization alone during thyroidectomy. J Surg Res 2014; 188:152–161.

Sinclair CF, Bumpous JM, Haugen BR, et al. Laryngeal examination in thyroid and parathyroid surgery: an American Head and Neck Society consensus statement: AHNS Consensus Statement. Head Neck 2016; 38:811–819.

Scenario 15

Thyroid cancer

A GP has referred a 44-year-old lady with gradually increasing, painless thyroid swelling noticed over last few months.

Q. 15.1 How would you assess her and investigate her?

My main concerns are regarding the nature of this thyroid swelling; benign or malignant.

History of increase in size over last few weeks, hoarseness of voice, dysphagia/dyspnoea, family history of thyroid cancer/FAP/Cowdens syndrome, exposure of neck to irradiation increases the risk of malignancy.

I would examine the patient to assess thyroid, neck lymph nodes, assess thyroid functional status, and request thyroid function test and arrange USS thyroid + FNA for nodules U3 or above and suspicious lymph nodes.

Q. 15.2 Ultrasound reveals 2 cm U4 lesion; on FNA thy 5; what would you do next?

Thy 5 lesion denotes a malignant lesion. I would discuss her case in thyroid MDT.

Thy 5 report should be able to differentiate between papillary, medullary or anaplastic carcinoma, metastasis or lymphoma.

I would review US neck to assess whether there are lymph nodes involved.

Q. 15.3 How would you manage her if she has papillary thyroid carcinoma (PTC)?

Surgical options are total or hemithyroidectomy.

She would need total thyroidectomy when:
- Tumour >4 cm
- Any size with high risk factors: Multifocal/Bilateral disease, gross extra-thyroidal spread, angioinvasion, clinical/radiologically involved lymph nodes (N1), familial thyroid cancer, and distant metastasis

Personalised decision making – hemi versus total thyroidectomy:
- Patients with 1–4 cm unifocal PTC without any of the above risk factors and previously <45 years but now 55 with TNM8
- Patients with history of radiation and 1–4 cm PTC and none of the above high-risk factors

For this patient – hemithyroidectomy would be advised for the above, if there are no high-risk features.

If any high-risk feature or if any compression symptoms are present – total thyroidectomy would be advised.

Therapeutic central compartment lymph node dissection (level 6 and 7) is indicated when lymph nodes are detected clinically/radiologically (cN1) or intra-operatively on frozen section.

If lateral lymph nodes (level 2–5) are involved, then selective lateral compartment dissection with central compartment lymph node dissection is performed.

There is no role for prophylactic central compartment node dissection when clinically/radiologically no nodes are involved with classical PTC, <55 years, unifocal <4 cm tumour and no extra thyroidal extension on USS, as the risk of lymph node metastasis is 2–4% when clinically/radiologically no nodes are involved (cN0).

Post-hemithyroidectomy: Histology revealed angioinvasion with multifocality and gross extrathyroidal extension, hence a completion thyroidectomy was performed.

Q. 15.4 What would you do next?

I would do a postoperative risk stratification for risk of recurrence of differentiated thyroid cancer to guide the intensity of follow-up and requirement for remnant radio iodine ablation therapy (RRA).

- High risk: (any of)
  Gross extra-thyroid extension (≥T3b), R2 resection (gross tumour left behind), and distant metastasis (M1)
- Intermediate risk: (any of)
  Microscopic invasion, lymph node METS(N1), aggressive histology [tall/columnar cell or diffuse sclerosing PTC, poorly differentiated features] or angioinvasion
- Low risk: (all need must be present)
  No local/distant metastases, R0/R1 resection (no gross tumour left behind); no local invasion (≤T2), no aggressive histology (as above).

She is likely to be in an intermediate-risk group and hence would need to be started on levothyroxine 2 µg/kg for TSH suppression and considered for RRA.

(Definite indications for RRA – T>4 cm, pT4 – gross extrathyroid extension, distant metastasis. No indication for RRA – T≤1 cm uni/multifocal classical PTC or follicular variant, or follicular minimally invasive with no angioinvasion and no invasion of thyroid capsule).

Around 9–12 months after total thyroidectomy (R0 resection) and RRA, dynamic risk stratification (DRS) is performed to check the response to therapy. DRS involves USS neck and, post-RRA stimulated thyroglobulin level. Excellent responders can have their TSH suppression relaxed (main a/e – osteoporosis and AF) and the follow up intensity can be reduced.

Q. 15.5 What would you do if you incidentally detect a 5 mm focus of medullary thyroid carcinoma (MTC) in a hemithyroidectomy specimen?

I would review this patient's histology, calcitonin, and *RET* gene analysis in thyroid MDT.

If RET negative, <5 mm incidental MTC, completion thyroidectomy is not essential.

As 20% of these may have lymph node metastases (>10 mm MTC have 40% lymph node metastases) postoperative calcitonin level would be helpful in deciding on completion thyroidectomy and central compartment lymph node dissection.

Further reading

Perros P, Boelaert K, Colley S, et al. Guidelines for the management of thyroid cancer. Clin Endocrinol (Oxf) 2014; 81:1–122.

Chapter 8

Transplant surgery

David van Dellen, Murali Somasundaram, Manikandan Kathirvel

Scenario 1

Renal transplantation

You are the consultant on-call receiving organ offers for renal transplantation. You review an electronic offering system (EOS) form for the following potential donor.

It is a named offer for one of your highly sensitized patients – a 34-year-old male, second transplant, unknown primary disease, currently on haemodialysis via a Tesio line who has been waiting for 8 years.

Q. 1.1 Please review the details and tell me your thoughts.

Donor type	Donor after cardiac death (DCD)
Sex	Male
Age	45 years
Occupation	Unemployed
Ethnic origin	White
Details	Out of hospital cardiac arrest (OOHCA) 3 days ago following head trauma due to altercation while drunk. Bystander cardiopulmonary resuscitation (CPR) for approximately 25 minutes. Paramedics continued CPR and achieve return of spontaneous circulation (ROSC) after approximately 45 minutes. CT brain-diffuse oedema and loss of grey/white differentiation. Intubated and ventilated at scene.
Body mass index (BMI)	19.3 kg/m^2

Urinalysis		
	Leucocytes	Small
	Ketones	Negative
	Blood	Haemolysed
	Glucose	+
	Nitrites	+

Virology		*Blood results*	
HBsAG	Negative	Hb g/dL	136
HBcAb	Negative	WCC × 10^9/L	17.6
Hepatitis C virus (HCV)	Positive	Plt × 10^9/L	205

Human immunodeficiency virus (HIV)	Negative	CRP mg/l	189
Cytomegalovirus (CMV)	Positive		
Epstein–Barr virus (EBV)	Awaited	ALP IU/L	99
Human T-lymphotropic virus (HTLV)	Negative	ALT IU/L	205
Toxo	Negative	Gamma GT IU/L	250
Syphilis	Negative	Bilirubin µmol/L	38
Hepatitis E virus (HEV)	Awaited		
Malaria	Not tested	Creatinine µmol/L	198
Trypanosoma cruzi	Not tested	Urea mmol/L	6
Coronavirus disease 2019 (COVID-19)	Negative	eGFR mL/min/1.73 m^2	34

Past medical history

History obtained from girl friend.	No other family
History of hypertension	No
History of cancer/malignancy	No
History of pulmonary disease	No
History of liver disease	Yes
History of diabetes	No
Family history diabetes	No
Units of alcohol per day	Very heavy > 9 U/day (1 bottle of cider per night)
History of drug use	Yes, previous IVDU, nil for > 10 years. Now regularly takes spice and smokes cannabis

To summarise, this is a 45-year-old male DCD donor. The aspects I would be concerned about are:
- The long cardiac arrest downtime
- The raised creatinine and reduced estimated glomerular filtration rate (eGFR)
- The positive hepatitis C virology
- The previous intravenous drug use (IVDU) history and the reliability of the current history giver
- The deranged liver function tests (LFTs) and the cause of this
- The patient also had an acute urinary tract infection

Q. 1.2 How would you proceed with this?

Firstly, I want more information. I would call the Hub to see if they could provide me with this, but the likelihood is I would need to speak to the specialist nurse for organ donation (SNOD). I would call the SNOD at the donor hospital. I specifically want to know the following:
- The reliability of the person giving the history – how long they have known the donor and the nature of their relationship with him

- Historical blood test results: I want to know what the historic LFTs and renal function are as well as the current urine output and whether he is on any renal replacement
- He is HCV positive, and I want to know any details about this – history, treatment/resistance, time of diagnosis, suspected mode of transmission. I would also specifically ask the retrieval team to check for any sign of hepatocellular carcinoma (HCC)
- Whether his liver function has been investigated previously, by whom and what the outcome of these investigations were
- Previous history of urinary tract infection

Q. 1.3 The person giving the history is a long-term partner, they have been in a relationship for > 10 years.

His liver function has been deranged for a number of years due to alcohol excess. He is under a gastroenterologist but has been uncompliant with treatment. He has been through various alcohol addiction programmes, but they have never been successful. His renal function from 4 months ago when he was last in hospital was normal with an eGFR of 88 mL/min/1.73 m². He is not currently on renal replacement and there is no previous history of urinary tract infection.

Regarding the HCV, this is the first time it has been noted. Would you accept this offer? Justify your reasoning.

There are recipient and donor factors to consider here.

Recipient factors:
- Highly sensitised patient who has been waiting for 8 years and will likely have a long-predicted wait time
- The patient is on HD via a Tesio line, which is high risk, especially in someone of his relatively young age
- This suggests a picture of someone who should be transplanted sooner rather than waiting for an ideal and low-risk donor

Donor factors:
- It seems that the history is reliable and from a source well known to the donor
- The history of high alcohol intake and deranged LFTs secondary to this are unrelated to the renal function
- The acute rise in creatinine is likely to be due to an acute kidney injury secondary to the prolonged downtime at cardiac arrest. I would expect that as the donor is young and otherwise has no history of renal disease this would recover, but the recipient would likely have delayed graft function (DGF) and is at slightly higher risk of primary non-function (PNF). This was the outcome of the paper by Boffa et al. (2017) investigating UK data. Dory Segev has also found the same outcomes using USRDS data

- Donor HCV is no longer a contraindication to donation or organ transplantation. It is now treatable and should not be an absolute reason for rejection of the donor

Weighing up these factors, I would accept the donor, but would want to speak to the patient about the above factors. They would need counselling about:
- Higher rate of DGF and potential of PNF
- Requirement for HCV prophylaxis post-transplantation
- The potential for excellent long-term graft function

Q. 1.4 What is hepatitis C?

Hepatitis C is a single-stranded RNA virus which is very common in Asia and Africa. It is transmissible by blood-to-blood contact. In the UK, it is commonly transmitted via intravenous drug use.

The acute infection is asymptomatic in approximately 85% of people. In the remainder, it can lead to generalised systemic symptoms which this donor may not have recognised or attributed to alcohol. 20% of patients will spontaneously clear the virus, leaving HCV antibodies detectable.

The chronic infection will develop in approximately 80% of patients. It can lead to cirrhosis or HCC.

Q. 1.5 What are the potential risks to the patient?

The concept of knowingly infecting a patient with an infectious disease poses important ethical issues which need to be addressed and discussed in detail with each patient. However, the very high likelihood of cure with direct acting anti-virals (95% with first-line treatment and 99–100% with second-line) mean that patients are extremely unlikely to have adverse effects from such intentional iatrogenic infection given that the cure will be obtained in months and complications typically take years or decades to develop. Transmission rates onwards from the infected patient can also be reduced to near zero with simple, non-onerous precautions.

However, in theory, if the patient is non-compliant or insensitive to direct acting anti-virals, HCV can develop, leading to cirrhosis and potentially HCC.

Q. 1.6 What treatment/monitoring regimen would you advise post-transplantation for this patient?

Our unit policy is adapted from the THINKER and EXPANDER trails which paved the way for the use of HCV positive donors in HCV-negative recipients. I would test the recipient for HCV polymerase chain reaction (PCR) on days 3–7 and then again on days 10–14. If they are HCV-PCR positive, then I would refer to hepatology for initiation of direct acting anti-viral therapy. This would last 12 weeks, following which we would expect a sustained viral response. If they continue to remain negative, further tests would be conducted at 1, 3, 6 and 12 months according to our unit policy.

In parallel, I would chase the genotype results from the donor hospital and convey these to our hepatologist to ensure the recipient is on the appropriate direct-acting antiviral (DAA) therapy.

Q. 1.7 What do you know about HEV? The results are still awaited, would this concern you?

Hepatitis E virus is a single-stranded RNA virus that is transmitted via the faeco-oral route. Infection via solid organ transplant is rare, as is chronic infection, unless the patient is immunocompromised, such as following transplantation. The SaBTO and BTS guidelines do not list the presence of HEV as a contraindication to transplantation and I am happy to transplant before the donor result is known. However, as the results are unknown I would counsel the patient accordingly and explain we would continue to chase the results following donation. If the donor was found to be positive, I would refer the recipient to hepatology who would likely screen the recipient for seroconversion. Potential treatment options include ribavirin therapy, but I would consult with my hepatology colleagues if this is the case.

Further reading

Boffa C, van de Leemkolk F, Curnow E, et al. Transplantation of Kidneys From Donors With Acute Kidney Injury: Friend or Foe? Am J Transplant 2017; 17:411–419.

Durand CM, Bowring MG, Brown DM, et al. Direct-Acting Antiviral Prophylaxis in Kidney Transplantation From Hepatitis C Virus- Infected Donors to Noninfected Recipients: An open-Label Nonrandomised trial. Ann Intern Med 2018;168:533–540.

Goldberg DS, Abt PL, Blumberg EA, et al. Trial of Transplantation of HCV-Infected Kidneys into Uninfected Recipients. N Engl J Med 2017; 376:2394–2395.

Scenario 2

Indications for pancreas transplantation

You are doing a transplant assessment clinic and 45-year-old female patient is on the list. She has end-stage renal disease secondary to type 1 diabetes mellitus and is currently pre-dialysis.

Q. 2.1 What are her transplant options?

This lady has ESRD secondary to T1DM and therefore, has multiple potential transplant options. She should be assessed and counselled for all of these. Her transplant options include:
- Kidney transplant alone (deceased or live donor)
- Kidney transplant combined with simultaneous β-cell replacement (or islets of pancreas)
- Kidney transplant followed by β-cell replacement (or islets of pancreas)

Q. 2.2 How would you go about tackling these issues and what specific information do you require to counsel the patient appropriately?

I would take a detailed, focused history and examination. The pertinent points to consider in this case in the history are:
- Diabetes treatment history-period for which she has suffered from diabetes, previous treatment regimens, current dose of insulin, whether the patient is on an/ or tried an insulin pump or any educational programmes to help to manage their diabetes (e.g. DAPHNE regimen)
- Complications related to diabetes [neuropathy, cardiovascular disease, peripheral vascular disease, history of cerebrovascular accident (CVA)/transient ischaemic attack (TIA), autonomic neuropathy, retinopathy, and hypoglycaemic unawareness]
- History of renal failure – whether she is currently on or pre-dialysis, fluid restriction, urine output, access for dialysis, how she is coping with renal replacement therapy (RRT)
- Her exercise tolerance and current quality of life
- In addition, I would want to know whether she has any potential live donors and what (if any) of her renal failure or her diabetes is the greatest burden on her life? These, together with the history, will help me to evaluate what her preferred transplant options should be
- Once I have taken my history, I would like to do an examination of the cardiovascular and peripheral vascular systems, respiratory system and perform an abdominal examination

Q. 2.3 What is hypoglycaemic unawareness?

This is defined as two or more episodes of hypoglycaemia requiring third party assistance over the last 2 years. It is an objective method used to identify patients eligible for islet only transplant or those at very high risk of mortality.

Q. 2.4 She is on hospital HD via a fistula, currently on an insulin regimen as advised by her general practitioner (GP) and suffers with retinopathy, peripheral neuropathy and suffered from a myocardial infarction 3 years ago. She does not have any live donors.

With the absence of a live donor, she would ideally be better served with a simultaneous pancreas and kidney transplant as long as there were no contraindications to a pancreas transplant. Given that she is not under the care of a diabetologist I would also refer her to one of my colleagues for optimisation of her diabetes care.

Q. 2.5 What contraindications are there specific to pancreas transplantation as opposed to islet transplant?

- Cardiovascular fitness
- Anatomical considerations, preventing safe pancreas implantation

Q. 2.6 What are the indications for whole organ pancreas transplantation?

There are three categories of whole organ pancreas transplantation:
1. Simultaneous pancreas and kidney transplantation: The indication is insulin dependent diabetes mellitus with end-stage renal failure (ESRF), and with an eGFR < 20 mL/min
2. Pancreas transplantation alone: The indication is insulin-dependent diabetes mellitus either resulting in end-organ failure or labile blood sugars (± hypoglycaemic unawareness). Renal function should be an eGFR at least > 40 mL/min
3. Pancreas after kidney transplantation: The indication is insulin-dependent diabetes mellitus with ESRF which has been corrected with a previous renal transplantation. Renal function should be an eGFR at least > 40 mL/min

Q. 2.7 What are the potential complications of pancreas transplantation?

Complications of pancreas transplantation can be defined under the following headings:
- Immediate surgical complications:
  - Bleeding requiring a return to theatre (5%)
  - Pancreas thrombosis (8%)
  - Peri-pancreatic collections
  - Intra-abdominal sepsis
  - Graft pancreatitis

- Relaparotomy (30%)
- Anastomotic leak (5%)
- Medium/Long-term surgical complications
  - Pseudoaneurysm
  - Wound infection
- Complications of major surgery
  - Infection (urinary and respiratory)
  - Hernia
  - Damage to surrounding structures
  - Cardiac complications
  - Pulmonary embolism (PE)/deep vein thrombosis (DVT)
- General complications of immunosuppression/transplantation
  - Opportunistic infection
  - Cancer [skin cancer, post-transplant lymphoproliferative disorder (PTLD), Kaposi's sarcoma]
  - Post-transplant diabetes [PTD, previously known as new-onset diabetes after transplant (NODAT)]
  - Transmission of virus or tumour from the donor

Q. 2.8 What are the graft and patient survivals after pancreas transplantation?

These vary slightly between the various categories of solid organ pancreas transplantation.

For simultaneous pancreas and kidney transplantation, 1-year patient survival is 95% in the UK. Pancreas and kidney graft survival are 85–90% and 95% respectively.

For pancreas alone transplant (PTA and PAK) 1-year survival approaches 100% in the UK, but graft survival is slightly worse than simultaneous pancreas-kidney (SPK) at about 80–85%.

Further reading

https://bts.org.uk/wp-content/uploads/2019/09/FINAL-Pancreas-guidelines-FINAL-version-following-consultation.-Sept-2019.pdf [Accessed 1st April 2023]

Scenario 3

Immunosuppression for transplant surgery

A 23-year-old man presents for his first kidney transplantation from a deceased donor. His primary disease is IgA nephropathy. It is ABO compatible and a 1:1:1 mismatch.

Q. 3.1 What immunosuppressive regimen would you use?

Immunosuppressive regimens are divided into induction, maintenance and treatment for rejection.

In my unit, for standard immunological risk recipients (such as this one) we use galiximab induction with intraoperative methylprednisolone, followed by dual maintenance immunosuppression with tacrolimus and mycophenolate mofetil (MMF). Post-operatively, steroids are used in a rapidly weaning regimen for 5 days, unless otherwise indicated (*please note, your local policies regarding induction and maintenance immunosuppression will suffice, if you can justify them).

Q. 3.2 Tell me about basiliximab.

Basiliximab is a non-depleting antibody. It is a chimeric monoclonal antibody (the variable region is mouse-derived). It targets the alpha-subunit on CD-25 of the interleukin (IL)-2 receptor and is therefore, classified as an IL-2 receptor antagonist. It provides this blockade for approximately 1–1.5 months. IL-2 stimulates the cell-cycle via a number of intracellular signalling proteins, including mTOR.

Q. 3.3 How is it administered?

Basiliximab is given as 2, 20 mg IV doses, the first given at time of induction and the second on day 4 post-transplantation.

Q. 3.4 Tell me about induction therapy.

Induction agents are used in the acute phase; peri-operatively to prevent rejection during this phase, when the risk is often highest. Induction agents can be steroids at higher doses, but are often antibodies, which are either T-cell depleting or non-depleting agents. The T-cell depleting agents can further be classified into mono-clonal or polyclonal agents, depending on the number of binding sites they act upon on the T-cell.

Q. 3.5 In the perioperative period the patient makes a good recovery from a surgical perspective, but on day 6 his creatinine spikes from a baseline of 120 to 200. What is your differential diagnosis and how would you investigate this?

Within a week following renal transplantation my differential diagnoses would be:
- Dehydration – either as a result of poor fluid intake or increased output, either due to polyuria or diarrhoea
- Infective complication – urinary tract infection, gastroenteritis, pneumonia, infection transmitted from the donor leading to systemic symptoms
- Vascular complication – in the absence of any sign of acute bleeding, my concerns would be either renal vein or artery thrombosis
- Rejection
- Ureteric stenosis
- Overdose/Intolerance to immunosuppression

My first-line investigations would be blood tests including full blood count (FBC), urea and electrolytes (U and E), LFTs, trough tacrolimus levels, donor-specific antibodies (DSA), coagulation screen, group and save and virology screen (to include CMV, EBV, BK and JC). I would crossmatch blood if there was any suggestion of bleeding. I would also want to send a stool culture if there was any evidence of diarrhoea. I would request an urgent USS duplex of the kidney to exclude a vascular complication and hydronephrosis.

Q. 3.6 The patient has diarrhoea and nausea, but is otherwise well. Prior to transplantation, he had no gastrointestinal symptoms. Your registrar has instituted IV fluids which helps to improve his creatinine. His stool culture is negative. It is now day 8 post-transplantation, and the patient wants to go home. What do you do?

Given that all the investigations are negative, and IV fluids have improved his renal function, but his symptoms persist, this is likely to be due to dehydration secondary to an intolerance to MMF leading to gastrointestinal disturbance, one of the most common complications of MMF. I would therefore, split his dose from our standard 1 g BD to 500 mg QDS and reassess his symptoms after 24–48 hours. If this did not relieve his symptoms, the overall dose could be reduced to 500 mg BD. I would not be happy to send him home until we are confident that, there are no other issues to contend with.

Q. 3.7 You do this, but it has no impact on his symptoms. He has now been discharged, but he sees you in clinic with persistent diarrhoea and nausea. What do you do?

The options now are to switch from MMF to either Myfortic or to azathioprine. Enteric-coated mycophenolic acid (Myfortic) has a better side-effect profile than the generic MMF and may be a suitable alternative. If this was not an option or fails, my second-line choice would be to switch to azathioprine. Prior to doing this, however, I would want to counsel the patient appropriately and check thiopurine methyltransferase (TPMT) levels to ensure adequate metabolisation of azathioprine is possible and therefore prevent overdose.

Common maintenance immunosuppressive agents

Medication	Dosage	Mechanism of action	Common/Serious side effects
Tacrolimus	0.1–0.2 mg/kg/day (divided into two equal doses)	Tacrolimus binds to immunophilin to form the FK-506 binding protein. This complex inhibits calcineurin leading to an inhibition of its phosphatase reaction, required in the activation of NFAT. Inhibition of this causes an inhibition of IL-2 dependent gene transcription	Neurotoxicity, nephrotoxicity, anaemia, insomnia, diabetes, anxiety, tremors, gastrointestinal disturbances, alopecia, headaches, electrolyte abnormalities, posterior reversible encephalopathy syndrome (PRES)
Mycophenolate mofetil (MMF)	1 g twice daily	MMF is also known as an anti-proliferative. It is a pro-drug of mycophenolic acid (MPA) which inhibits inosine monophosphate dehydrogenase, an enzyme required for production of guanine nucleotides (a purine) for DNA synthesis and therefore, prevents B and T lymphocyte activation	Gastrointestinal disturbance, myelosuppression, alopecia, depression **Congenital malformations and spontaneous abortions**
Cyclosporin	5–10 mg/kg/day (divided into two equal doses)	Very similar to tacrolimus. It is also a calcineurin inhibitor that inhibits the phosphatase reaction of NFAT, therefore, inhibiting IL-2 dependent gene transcription	Hyperlipidaemia, hypertension, hirsutism, gingival hyperplasia, nephrotoxicity (diabetes and neurotoxicity, but less likely than tacrolimus)
Azathioprine	1–3 mg/kg daily in one dose	Another anti-proliferative agent that also inhibits purine synthesis required for B and T lymphocyte proliferation in the cell cycle	Gastrointestinal disturbance, myelosuppression **Not associated with congenital malformations and abortions, therefore, an alternative to MMF**

Continues overleaf

Continued

Medication	Dosage	Mechanism of action	Common/Serious side effects
Prednisolone	5–20 mg once daily	• Blockade of T-cell- and APC-derived cytokine expression • It also has anti-inflammatory properties	Sodium and fluid retention, hypertension, hyperglycaemia, weight gain, increased appetite, indigestion/heartburn, insomnia, changes in mood/behaviour, osteoporosis, thinning of the skin, bruising, cushingoid appearance
Sirolimus	2 mg once daily	mTOR (mammalian target of rapamycin) inhibitor: It also binds to immunophilin to form the FK-506 binding protein, but this complex inhibits mTOR which is required in IL-2 stimulated T-cell proliferation	Fever, cold-sores, gastrointestinal symptoms, hypercholesterolaemia, hypertension, acne, poor wound healing

Common induction immunosuppressive agents

Medication	Dosage	Mechanism of action	Common/Serious side effects
Basiliximab	20 mg IV, 1st at induction and then 4 days post-transplantation	Basiliximab is a non-depleting monoclonal antibody, which targets the IL-2, CD-25 receptor, leading to inhibition of T-cell proliferation	Generally, very well tolerated with side effects rarely reported
*Alemtuzumab	30 mg SC (one or two doses, 24 hours apart)	Humanised T-cell depleting monoclonal antibody, anti-CD52 Ag on the surface of B and T lymphocytes, macrophages, NK cells and monocytes	Bone marrow suppression (specifically leucopenia) – effects can be profound and last up to 6 months, increased risk of cancers, including PTLD Rarely, it can lead to anaphylaxis, therefore, often given with antihistamine and methylprednisolone
Rabbit anti-thymocyte globulin (rATG)	1.5 mg/kg IV, daily for 4–7 days	Polyclonal IgG leading to T-cell depletion	Gastrointestinal disturbance, fevers, rigors, chills, tachycardia, and bone marrow suppression

*Used off-license in transplantation.

Further reading

https://www.nice.org.uk/guidance/ta481 [Accessed 1st April 2023]

Scenario 4

Graft dysfunction

You are in transplant outpatient clinic and see a 62-year-old female patient at 36 months after her first renal transplant. Her primary disease is IgA nephropathy. You notice the creatinine has gone from a baseline of 180 to 250 over the last 9 months. The history and examination were unremarkable.

Q. 4.1 What would you do next?

Assuming the history and examination did not reveal anything of concern, I would want to check the operation note, donor history and day 0 biopsy, if available. I want to know the patient's blood pressure, compliance with medication and trend of renal function and trough tacrolimus levels.

I would organise some investigations. I would like an FBC, U/Es, LFTs, clotting profile, group and save, DSA, virology (CMV, BK, and EBV) and trough tacrolimus levels. I will send the urine off for urinary PCR and microscopy, sensitivities and culture. I would also organise a USS duplex of the kidney to exclude a vascular complication and check for hydronephrosis. Depending on the outcomes of these results I would request a renal transplant biopsy. I would also like to know the outcome and function of the paired kidney.

Q. 4.2 You do all the above and you note the creatinine has been worsening progressively for the last 9 months. There was no day 0 biopsy, virology is negative, but the donor history reveals a history of type 2 diabetes mellitus and hypertension, controlled on three agents. Tacrolimus trough levels have ranged between 8 and 12 ng/ml. All else is normal. What do you do?

The possibilities here are:
- Donor-related vascular disease
- Calcineurin inhibitor (CNI) nephrotoxicity
- Rejection (unlikely)
- Interstitial fibrosis and tubular atrophy

The next step would be to perform a renal biopsy. I would request for this to be done.

Q. 4.3 The kidney biopsy shows interstitial fibrosis and tubular atrophy (IFTA). What does this mean and what would you do now?

The IFTA is interstitial fibrosis and tubular atrophy. It describes specific chronic histologic changes often due to multiple non-specific insults.

In a patient with this history, it is likely to be due to pre-existing donor vascular disease, chronic rejection and calcineurin toxicity. The creeping creatinine study, although based on ciclosporin, would suggest withdrawal (or minimisation) of the CNI with maintenance of the MMF (± prednisolone if required). This is likely to prolong graft longevity. I would therefore initially aim for trough tacrolimus levels of 4–6 ng/mL, maintain MMF at 1 g BD and avoid prednisolone due to the long-term complications of steroids in this cohort of patients. This gives me scope to minimise the tacrolimus further and add prednisolone, if required.

Q. 4.4 How do you withdraw tacrolimus?

This patient is suitable for tacrolimus withdrawal as she has been transplanted 3 years ago, has had no recent episodes of rejection and has a biopsy showing no evidence of rejection.

I would ensure she is on a stable, therapeutic dose of MMF and reduce the tacrolimus dose by 50% every 2–3 weeks until it was stable between 4 and 6 ng/ml.

Q. 4.5 What would you do if the kidney biopsy suggested chronic T-cell-mediated rejection? The DSAs are positive.

This is something that would often be dealt with by the transplant nephrologists as part of the transplant multidisciplinary team (MDT) because there are multiple treatment options. Patients with positive DSA are at higher risk of graft loss when compared to patients with absent DSA. I would therefore discuss the case with one of our nephrologists, the parent consultant and the patient.

My preferred option would be to give a steroid pulse to the patient and then optimise the immunosuppression. I would, therefore, admit the patient for 3 days of 1 g IV hydrocortisone and monitor the renal function. I would then start 20 mg prednisolone orally, daily with the aim of weaning down to 5 mg OD over 3–4 weeks. I would re-check the DSA as per departmental protocol.

Q. 4.6 In general terms, what is the Banff criteria for diagnosing rejection?

The Banff classification of renal transplant biopsies is an international consensus on histological grading of renal transplant biopsies, that first came into inception in 1991 and are now updated every 2 years.

Biopsies are classified into six grades, but within each grade there are multiple further sub-classifications:

1. Normal
2. Antibody mediated changes – either acute or chronic rejection
3. Borderline for T-cell-mediated rejection
4. T-cell-mediated rejection
5. Interstitial fibrosis and tubular atrophy
6. Other changes, inconsistent with acute or chronic rejection

Q. 4.7 If CMV log was raised (log3.2), how would this change your management?

This would suggest that she is over immunosuppressed and her immunosuppression needs modifying. I would again aim for lower trough tacrolimus levels of 6–8 ng/mL and I would also minimise her MMF dosage. At our unit, for immunologically uncomplicated patients over the age of 60 years our standard MMF dose is 750 mg BD so I would change her to this dose.

Finally, I would start her on oral valganciclovir, dosed according to her renal function. I would continue to treat her until she had two consecutive, negative CMV logs spaced 1 week apart before reducing her down to prophylactic dose for a further 2–4 weeks. I would want to check her CMV logs initially once weekly, and then fortnightly until her treatment was complete.

Further reading

Dudley C, Pohanka E, Riad H, et al. Mycophenolate Mofetil Substitution for Cyclosporine a in Renal Transplant Recipients With Chronic Progressive Allograft Dysfunction: The "Creeping Creatinine" Study. Transplantation 2005; 79:466–475.

Lefaucheur C, Loupy A, Hill GS, et al. Preexisting Donor-Specific HLA Antibodies Predict Outcome in Kidney Transplantation. J Am Soc Nephrol 2010; 21:1389–1406.

Roufosse C, Simmonds N, Clahsen-van Groningen M, et al. A 2018 Reference Guide to the Banff Classification of Renal Allograft Pathology. Transplantation 2018; 102:1795–1814.

Scenario 5

Organ retrieval

You are performing retrieval surgery for a donor. The coordinator has given you the following details:
- Departure in 2 hours' time with 2-hour travel time
- Donation after brain death (DBD) retrieval of liver and kidneys with cardiothoracic team attending for heart retrieval
- A 49-year-old donor with history of subarachnoid haemorrhage

When you arrive at the donor hospital and meet the SNOD, they offer to handover but say they are very new to the role.

Q. 5.1 Explain how you would proceed?

I would introduce all members of my team to the SNOD and the relevant hospital staff including theatre and anaesthetic team. I would conduct myself professionally at all times in accordance with NHS Blood and Transplant (NHSBT) retrieval standards guidelines. I would review the relevant donor details and documentation including certification of brainstem death, medical history, body mapping data, virology, blood group and biochemistry results. I would request to see any relevant imaging such as a CT scan if the patient has had one to assess for any aberrant anatomy. I would confirm the relevant organ support the patient is on and their current clinical state. I would seek any relevant medical history that may affect the retrieval such as previous thoracoabdominal surgery. I would confirm the theatre has adequate facilities with a minimum of two suction systems and a local member of staff to act as a runner. I would confirm with the SNOD if there are any special requests from the transplanting centres such as additional photographs or information.

Q. 5.2 You take some rest in the coffee room while the cardiothoracic team are completing their preliminary assessments. After a period, the SNOD attends and informs you the cardiothoracic team are keen to start operating in your absence and begin the thoracic dissection phase. How do you respond and why?

I would not support this and suggest we commence simultaneously. It is possible for massive exsanguination on entering the thoracic cavity and I would like to have performed a laparotomy and slung the aorta for an emergency cannulation if necessary to prevent losing the abdominal organs.

Q. 5.3 Explain how you would proceed with the warm phase dissection abdominal part of the retrieval.

I am aware of numerous different approaches but mine is as follows. I would perform a generous midline laparotomy incision in continuity with the open thorax. Initially, I would perform a laparotomy to assess for any undiagnosed disease such as malignancy. I would initiate warm phase dissection by a limited medial visceral rotation to enable access to the aorta. I would apply vessel slings to the abdominal aorta just above the bifurcation to enable cannulation later. I would then identify the left renal vein as it crosses the aorta and dissect superiorly to the origin of the superior mesenteric artery (SMA) which I would encircle with a vessel sling. I would then inspect and assess the liver in detail, assessing the edges, the level of steatosis and size. I would look and palpate for any aberrant anatomy, particularly an accessory left hepatic artery from left gastric and accessory right hepatic artery from the SMA.

I would then turn my attention to the hepatic hilum and identify the origins of the common hepatic, gastroduodenal and splenic arteries. I would dissect out the extra-hepatic portal vein as it passes supero-posteriorly to the pancreas and encircle it with a vessel sling. Finally, I would dissect out the common bile duct distally, ligate and divide it, before opening the gallbladder and flushing it with saline until the duct is clear of bile.

I would discuss with the cardiothoracic team to establish where aortic cross clamping should occur and venting of the vena cava. This would complete the warm phase dissection.

Q. 5.4 Your training registrar feels that the dissection is incomplete. They suggest slinging all the vessels at the hilum, furthering the Kocherisation and starting dissection of the kidneys as this will enable better identification of anatomy. What is the rationale against this?

Extensive warm phase dissection is not favourable, particularly of arteries as it may promote spasm. It is also not preferable to completely dissect vessels for the transplanting centre as the risk of injury may be greater. There is a balance to be struck however, as some structures may be difficult to identify in the cold phase of dissection based on the surgeon's experience.

Q. 5.5 The cardiothoracic team advise you they are ready for cross clamping. Explain what the 'cold phase' is and what how you would proceed?

The 'cold phase' commences once cold perfusion starts and cross clamping of the aorta takes place. After ensuring the patient has received IV heparin, I would select an appropriately sized aortic cannula and choose an appropriate perfusion solution [University of Wisconsin (UW) Solution], then ensure that the circuit runs free of air and is flushed. I would ligate the aorta just superior to the bifurcation and occlude it several centimetres above manually. I would then make an incision and cannulate the aorta and secure the cannula. Once the perfusion has started, I would ensure the supracoeliac aorta has been successfully cross clamped indicating the start of the cold ischaemic time (CIT) period. Venting of venous blood would ideally take place in the chest.

Q. 5.6 What is a DCD? How would the described scenario be different if the donor was to be classified as a DCD?

The crucial difference when attending for a DCD retrieval is that the donor has not, at the time of planning donation, died. This is in contrast to a DBD case where brainstem death is established. In DCD retrieval, patients are identified as suitable donors based on characteristics and anticipated to die once support is withdrawn. Death may not occur in an appropriate time frame following withdrawal and retrieval may not therefore, proceed. Following withdrawal of support, the donor may arrest, and death is declared by the anaesthetist who has withdrawn support. There follows a 'no touch' period of 5 minutes before the retrieval can take place. The goal is then to begin cold perfusion as soon as possible. This is achieved by purposeful and rapid thoracotomy and laparotomy to cannulate the aorta and cross clamp as soon as possible. The entire retrieval then takes place in a cold phase dissection state.

Q. 5.7 What do you understand by the terms 'agonal phase' and 'warm ischaemic time' in the context of DCD organ retrieval? What is the significance of these in transplantation?

The agonal phase commences at the start of withdrawal of treatment and ends at the time of circulatory arrest. During the phase, patients experience a period of hypoxia and hypotension which may vary in severity and duration. The definition of 'warm ischaemic time' is not universally accepted and may correspond to time from withdrawal, significant hypotension or circulatory arrest until the start of cold perfusion. It corresponds to the time that organs are subjected to ischaemic injury at body temperature.

Certain organs are not suitable for DCD transplantation such as the heart and small intestine. DCD organs have been used in lung, kidney, liver and pancreas transplantation. The duration of the agonal phase is important and if greater than 60 minutes, organs are likely to be declined for the lung, liver and pancreas. The kidney is more resistant to ischaemic injury and the current NHSBT guidelines recommend a minimum of 3 hours wait of agonal phase before declaring that the retrieval should not proceed. Organs may be declined if the agonal phase is shorter than 1 hour, but the perceived 'warm ischaemic time' is unacceptable, for example, if the patient had a sustained period of severe hypotension after withdrawal of treatment and a long period before actual circulatory arrest.

Q. 5.8 You complete the retrieval described in the scenario and remove the liver. While perfusing the liver and assessing it on the bench, you leave your registrar to retrieve the kidneys with an assistant as you have seen them do this before and they have adequate experience. Later, on your bench assessment of the right kidney, you feel the artery does not have an adequate patch and the ureter has been significantly stripped. How would you deal with this situation?

I would carefully inspect the organ and record the damage according to the Human Tissue Authority (HTA) guidelines as per the NHSBT protocols. I would arrange to speak with a representative from the receiving transplanting centre (either surgeon or coordinator) to explain the damage in detail because if they were considering the organ for a marginal recipient, they may not wish to receive it with the damage sustained. Finally, I would review the case with the registrar in a structured method for feedback and training.

Q. 5.9 What do you know about 1-year survival rates after liver, pancreas and kidney transplantation? Are DCD donors commonly used for transplantation of these organs?

Outcomes after renal transplantation are the most favourable with 1-year survival for DBD quoted variably at around 90–95%. In more recent years, DCD outcomes have been stated as equivalent increasing the utilisation of DCD kidney donors. 1-year survival after DBD liver transplantation is quoted at 90% with DCD organs achieving less favourable outcomes though these have improved in recent years. Survival rates after 1 year for either simultaneous kidney pancreas (SKP) or isolated pancreas transplants approach 95%. DCD pancreas grafts are not routinely utilised.

Further reading

Summers DM, Watson CJ, Pettigrew GJ, et al. Kidney donation after circulatory death (DCD): state of the art. Kidney Int 2015; 88:241–249.

Zalewska K, Ploeg R. National Standards for Organ Retrieval from Deceased Donors. NHSBT 2018; MPD1043/8.

Scenario 6

Organ preservation

You are the on-call transplant surgeon due to receive a kidney for implantation, the offer was accepted by your colleague, the donor details are as follows:
- 68-year-old male
- Cause of death: Traumatic brain injury with haemorrhage following a fall. Lower limb fracture also sustained
- No known past medical history, however the NOK believes the patient has been using IV drugs recently
- Renal function indicates an AKI (stage 1) but a blood test by the GP 3 months ago revealed normal kidney function

You assess the recipient, who is a 27-year-old male who contracted ESRF and dialysis dependency following a UTI and severe sepsis 2 years ago. He has been discussed in the MDT. He arrives with his partner, who wishes to be a donor for him if possible.

Q. 6.1 How would you proceed?

I would be initially concerned about using this organ for this recipient as there is information indicating a possible marginal graft. Firstly, I would like to know more information about the donor, particularly the results of the virology and if there were any concerning features during the retrieval. I would like to know the body mass index (BMI), urinalysis results and specifically whether diabetes and hypertension have been excluded. Finally, I would like to know the human leukocyte antigens (HLAs) mismatch for the proposed recipient.

If the proposed recipient wants to explore a living donor option, the NHSBT guidelines are that these should be explored. I would review the MDT and consultation outcomes to confirm that these options have been discussed. Finally, if a new option was available and he wanted to explore this, I would discuss the case in detail with the patient his nephrologist to ascertain what would be in his best interests. It may be better to defer if this particular donor does not seem optimal for him.

Q. 6.2 What is meant by the term 'marginal kidney graft'?

This refers to an organ for transplant that is a higher risk for transplantation based on donor characteristics. In renal transplant, such donors are also referred to as 'extended criteria donors' (ECD). According to NHSBT guidelines, this refers to any renal grafts in which the donor was ≥ 60 years at the time of death or is aged 50–59 years with at least two of three characteristics (hypertension/creatinine > 130 μmol/L/death due to intracranial haemorrhage).

Q. 6.3 You decide against using this organ for the proposed recipient and request the coordinator to call a closer age matched recipient for transplant. While this is being done, the (left) kidney arrives and you perform the bench preparation with the assistance of a medical student. The kidney arrives in UW solution. What is UW solution?

University of Wisconsin (Viaspan) solution is an organ preserving solution used for cold perfusion and storage of transplant organs. It was developed in the 1980s and mimics intracellular electrolyte composition (high potassium and low sodium). It utilises a phosphate buffer system and osmotic membrane-impermeable agents to counteract transmembrane water shifts and prevent cellular oedema. It has allowed organs to be preserved for longer periods thus expanding the limits of transplantation.

Q. 6.4 What other preservation solutions do you know of?

- Marshall's hypertonic citrate (Soltran)
  - Contains potassium and sodium citrate, mannitol and magnesium sulphate. Used for kidney perfusion only in the UK.

University of Wisconsin (UW) and Marshall's are the primary perfusion fluids used in the UK in abdominal visceral transplantation. I am also aware of:
- Histidine-tryptophan-ketoglutarate (HTK) (Custodial)
  - Has an intracellular sodium concentration (15 mmol/L) and slightly elevated extracellular potassium concentration (10 mmol/L). Initially designed as a cardiac preservation solution, it is now widely used for liver preservation.
- Euro-Collins
  - Derived from Collins solution it has similar attributes to UW with an intracellular electrolyte composition to prevent transmembranous fluid and electrolyte shifts. The later development of UW and HTK has largely superseded its wide use.

Q. 6.5 Explain how you would bench prepare the kidney for transplantation?

The kidney should be kept cool and in solution as far as possible but not in direct contact with ice. I first identify the ureter inferiorly and place an artery clip at the very tip for orientation. I then examine to assess if the anatomy and described features in the donor documents correspond to what I can identify. I place Prolene stay sutures on the vein and dissect it from distal to proximal reaching the hilum. By dissecting directly superior to the vessel in the midline, no significant branches are typically encountered. I ligate the adrenal vein and any other small branches to give good mobility on the vein. I then examine the arterial patch and remove excess tissue as a large patch of aorta is typically provided. I dissect the artery in a similar fashion as the vein to the hilum. Finally, I dissect the fat of Gerota's fascia off the kidney, taking care not to injure the capsule from superiorly to inferiorly. As I reach the inferior border, I take care to leave adequate fat on the ureter and avoid stripping it as the blood supply originates partially from the peri-ureteric fat. I finally perfuse the kidney again with solution to ensure clear arteriovenous flow, identify any leaks that may need ligation and flush out any remaining blood.

Q. 6.6 An alternative recipient was selected for the donor. Unfortunately, their COVID swab was positive, and an alternative has to be called. There will be a significant delay before the organ can be implanted. What methods are you aware of to preserve the organ prior to transplantation? Are you aware of any other preservation methods for abdominal organs?

The simplest and most cost-effective organ preservation method is static cold storage which is most widely used in the UK within transplantation. NHSBT guidelines stipulate that UW should be used when retrieving the liver or pancreas and therefore, Soltran is used for kidney only perfusion and storage.

Organs may also be machine perfused at different temperatures and using different systems. In the UK, some renal transplant centres utilise hypothermic machine perfusion and the LifePort system which involves bench preparing the kidney and cannulating the artery to enable pulsatile perfusion using a designated solution. The kidney can be transported while on the machine. This has been shown in an international randomised clinical trial to reduce the risk of DGF and improve survival in the first year after transplantation. There are a number of considerations to its use and typically it is used for DCD kidneys in the UK.

Other perfusion methods include the use of normothermic temperatures and in the UK, this is now used for liver transplant organs [normothermic machine perfusion (NMP)]. The machine licensed is the OrganOx metra which utilises oxygenated blood perfusion of the liver graft by a centrifugal pump with a recycling reservoir. This has been shown in clinical trial to increase utilisation of DCD liver grafts for transplantation.

I am aware that there are numerous other machine perfusion devices available and in development with different indications for use, but the important point is that they must demonstrate improvement in clinical outcomes to justify use. Minimising CITs still remains the most important factor in improving outcomes in almost all cases.

Q. 6.7 What is normothermic regional perfusion (NRP) and what do you know about its application for abdominal transplantation?

Used in DCD retrievals, the method involves re-establishing flow of oxygenated blood into donors following circulatory arrest. This aims to prevent the effects of warm ischaemic injury and uses similar principles to cardiopulmonary bypass and ECMO. Venous cannulation can be achieved from the inferior vena cava (IVC), or femoral vein and the siphoned blood is then passed through a heat exchanger and membrane oxygenator before returning to the donor by an arterial cannula, typically via the femoral artery.

In addition to enabling recovery from warm ischaemia and replenishing adenosine triphosphate (ATP) stores, NRP can permit assessment of organ function and allow for a less hasty retrieval process. It is associated with reduced incidence of cholangiopathy after DCD liver transplant at 1 year.

Q. 6.8 What is a Maastricht category 4 donor? What is the relevance to the classification in the UK?

A patient who is declared brainstem dead but then undergoes circulatory arrest is classified as a Maastricht category 4 donor. This is in contrast to a category 3 donor who endures withdrawal of organ support and then arrests – the typical DCD in the UK.

Maastricht category 3 and 4 donors are known as 'controlled' donors and are utilised in the UK. Category 1 and 2 donors are 'uncontrolled' and involve those who are dead on arrival to hospital and those who undergo unsuccessful resuscitation respectively. Such donors are not utilised for transplantation in the UK but may be in some other European countries such as Spain.

Further reading

Moers C, Smits JM, Maathuis MH, et al. Machine Perfusion or Cold Storage in Deceased-Donor Kidney Transplantation. N Engl J Med 2009; 360:7–19.

Nasralla D, Coussios CC, Mergental H, et al. A randomized trial of normothermic preservation in liver transplantation. Nature 2018; 557:50–56.

Watson CJE, Hunt F, Messer S, et al. In situ normothermic perfusion of livers in controlled circulatory death donation may prevent ischemic cholangiopathy and improve graft survival. Am J Transplant 2019; 19:1745–1758.

Scenario 7

Brainstem death, ethics and incompatible transplants

You are covering the on-call for renal transplant, general surgery and trauma. A 27-year-old male attends as a trauma call after sustaining a blow to the head. He suffered a skull fracture and cerebral haemorrhage and is pronounced brainstem dead shortly after admission.

Q. 7.1 What is brainstem death?

Brainstem death is the irreversible loss of all functions of the brain, including those of the brainstem. It consists of a state of coma, absence of brainstem reflexes and ultimately apnoea. The diagnosis can only be made on patients under mechanical ventilation.

Q. 7.2 How is brainstem death diagnosed?

The patient must first be identified to be in a coma (prolonged state of unconsciousness) with clinical evidence supportive of a cause (such as head injury). After ascertaining this, certain clinical scenarios need to be excluded including:
- Hypothermia
- Intoxication
- Sedative drugs
- Neuromuscular blocking agents
- Severe electrolyte, acid-base or endocrine abnormalities as a cause

The patient must be found to have absent brainstem reflexes, absent motor response and apnoea when $PaCO_2$ is > 6.5 KPa.

Q. 7.3 You are informed by the ITU team that the patient has been pronounced brainstem dead. He was on the organ donor register and the family support donation. They meet you and thank you for trying to save his life but are not sure about his death. They ask you to confirm it for them. How would you proceed?

Brainstem death can only be certified under certain conditions. The tests must be performed twice at an interval that is not specified. The time of death is that of the first certification. The test must be performed by two doctors, one of which is consultant level and the other must have been qualified for 5 years minimum. Members of the transplant team should not be involved in certification. I would sensitively explain this to the family and that I could not be involved in the certification. I would ensure that they receive adequate support from the SNOD involved in the donation.

Q. 7.4 The patient is planned for DBD retrieval in your hospital. The family are in agreement and support donation of heart, lungs, liver, pancreas and kidneys. There are multiple delays in allocation of organs by the national network, but a retrieval is ultimately planned, and teams are due to be mobilised, 20 hours after the process starts. At this stage, the family have decided that they withdraw their consent and ask the SNOD to stop the entire process. Do the family have the right to prevent donation by law?

If the patient has given their consent and is on the organ donor register then the donation can legally proceed, irrespective of the family's wishes. Practically speaking though, donation is unlikely to go ahead if the family object.

Q. 7.5 You turn your attention to other clinical commitments in a combined medical and surgical renal transplant assessment clinic. Mr X, a 50-year-old man with ESRF, attends with a friend who he says lives with him. The friend claims that he wants to donate a kidney to Mr X. What is this kind of donation called and what procedure should be followed?

This donation would be classed as 'live unrelated directed' donation. Although all live donation relies on altruism, typically the term 'altruistic donor' is used when the donation is not directed to one individual.

I would assess the donor in accordance with the national guidelines described by the British Transplant Society (BTS). This assessment is typically performed by an independent nephrologist. It involves taking a full history and examination. Important points to consider are the presence of any significant comorbidities such as hypertension, diabetes mellitus, obesity, cardiovascular disease and any history of malignancy. The examination should assess suitability for surgery and include urinalysis to identify any proteinuria or microscopic haematuria. If the patient is medically suitable then imaging should be performed to assess for any anatomical abnormalities such as multiple renal arteries which would be relevant in the nephrectomy. The reasons for donation should be explored and the donor should understand the process and the long-term implications and risks of donation.

Q. 7.6 The friend of Mr X appears to understand the procedure, risks and potential long-term consequences. It transpires on further questioning that he has made an agreement with Mr X to donate so that he can remain living with him, rent free indefinitely. Both parties are still keen to proceed with the process. Is there any relevant legislation to guide your decision whether to offer the surgery?

Yes – the Human Tissue Act (HTA) of 2004 (updated in November 2021) governs the process of organ donation in the UK and stipulates that reward should not be a motivating factor in donation. The described situation would contravene this and therefore, the donation should not take place.

Q. 7.7 You see another patient, Mr Y in the clinic with ESRF who attends with his wife as a potential donor for transplant. A full assessment of Mr Y has been completed and he fulfils criteria for renal transplantation. His wife is physically fit with no comorbidities and appears to be a suitable donor. What are the essential aspects of assessing their immunological compatibility?

This essentially involves screening for clinically important antibodies, the presence or absence of them in the donor/recipient and the mismatches between them. The ABO antibody system used in assessing compatibility for blood transfusion will form part of this to ascertain if the wife can donate to Mr Y based on blood group. The HLA system also has great clinical relevance and the number of mismatches between the important HLA antigens will typically be used to determine immunological risk of transplantation.

Q. 7.8 What HLA antibodies listed in a quoted 'HLA match' such as '2-1-2'? Are there any other important HLA antibodies?

This is actually the number of mismatches between the important antibodies HLA-A, HLA-B and HLA-DR. This is determined from the number of donor HLA specificities from each locus that are absent in the recipient, where '0-0-0' has no incompatibilities and '2-2-2' is a fully mismatched combination. Other important HLA antibodies are HLA-C, HLA-DQ and HLA-DP.

Q. 7.9 It transpires that Mr Y and his wife are not blood group compatible and the HLA match is not favourable either. What would you advise them to do?

According to BTS guidelines, they should be offered to enter into the UK Living Kidney Sharing Scheme (UKLKSS). This would enable a possible paired donation, where another living donor (perhaps even altruistic) is a better match for Mr Y and his wife could go on and donate to another patient for whom she is a better match. In this way, a domino donation could also be arranged nationwide where multiple kidneys are donated simultaneously.

Q. 7.10 The final patient in your clinic approaches you with a potential live donor option and full assessment has been completed. The main concern is lack of ABO compatibility. The pair are unable to enter into the UKLKSS. Can the transplant proceed?

Yes, ABO incompatible transplant is possible. This should only be undertaken once entry into the UKLKSS has been fully explored as an option.

Q. 7.11 How does the process of ABO incompatible transplantation differ from routine living donor transplant?

Patients should be fully informed of the alternatives to ABO incompatible transplantation (e.g. paired donation). A thorough risk assessment should take place to assess risk of accelerated acute rejection, antibody mediated rejection and death. Extracorporeal therapies (e.g. plasmapheresis) should be used prior to transplantation to remove relevant ABO antibodies from the recipient to reduce the risk of antibody-mediated rejection at the time of transplantation. Patients should receive pre-transplant conditioning to reduce immune response, typically using intravenous immunoglobulin (IVIG), rituximab and mycophenolate.

The surgery can take place routinely but following the transplant, more aggressive monitoring of patients should take place, particularly in the first 2 weeks post-operatively (when the risk of rejection is highest). Samples should be taken daily to assess antibody levels and supplemental immunosuppression medications may be required such as monoclonal antibodies (e.g. alemtuzumab).

Further reading

Kumar L. Brain death and care of the organ donor. J Anaesthesiol Clin Pharmacol 2016; 32:146–152.

Scenario 8

Peritoneal dialysis and intestinal transplant

You assess a 45-year-old male patient in clinic who has a background of type 1 diabetes mellitus. He has been referred for insertion of a peritoneal dialysis (PD) catheter.

Q. 8.1 What is PD?

Peritoneal dialysis is a form of dialysis used to treat ESRF. It utilises the peritoneal cavity as a partially permeable membrane. Dialysate which contains a solution of electrolytes (e.g. sodium, calcium, and chloride) and other compounds (e.g. glucose and lactate) is infused into the peritoneum by a catheter. As the peritoneum is highly vascular, dialysis then takes place by a combination of diffusion, osmosis and ultrafiltration, leading to removal of waste products from the blood stream and into the dialysate. The dialysate is then discarded via the catheter.

Q. 8.2 What types of PD do you know of? How does it compare to HD?

Peritoneal dialysis can either be continuous ambulatory PD (CAPD) or automated PD. CAPD involves allowing dialysate to drain into the peritoneal cavity manually by gravity, allowing a 'dwell' time in which dialysis takes place and then allowing the fluid to drain out by gravity. Automated PD involves use of a machine to cycle the dialysate into the peritoneal cavity by a pump and also remove it. There are different ways this can be performed (cycling/intermittent) but the patient will usually be connected to the machine overnight.

The obvious differences between HD and PD are the access routes and some patients may be more suitable for fistula formation rather than PD catheter insertion and vice versa. The efficacy of HD is greater than that of PD, but this must be offset against the cardiovascular disadvantages. HD is performed over shorter periods of hours and then patients may be treatment free for 2 days, whereas PD may require several exchanges in a single day. Traditionally, one drawback of HD was the need to attend hospital, but home HD is now possible with adequate training. It still requires the machinery, and this may be limiting for patients travelling. Choice of dialysis modality for a patient is, therefore, a combination of medical and patient choice factors.

Q. 8.3 How will you assess the patient for surgery for a PD catheter?

I would take a full history, focusing particularly on the renal disease, duration, renal function and expected date of need for dialysis. I would need to take a detailed surgical history, particularly focusing on any previous abdominal surgery which may preclude PD catheter insertion (e.g. inflammatory bowel disease, adhesions, and hernias). Co-morbidities (e.g. obesity and COPD) may be relevant to both completion of surgery and the ability to comfortably and safely perform exchanges. I would assess if the patient was capable of performing exchanges and managing their dialysis at home and also their wishes and understanding of the process.

Examining the patient, I would assess the shape of their abdomen, look for the presence of any previous scars, hernias and assess their general health. I would arrange routine blood tests in preparation for surgery and if necessary, arrange imaging to assess the abdominal anatomy further.

Q. 8.4 You deem the patient a suitable candidate for PD after discussion with their nephrologist. Explain how you would perform the procedure?

I am aware of different methods for insertion of PD catheter, but I would choose an open surgical procedure. I would arrange for the patient to be seen and marked pre-operatively by a PD nurse for the best exit site for the catheter – typically lateral border of rectus, midpoint between the anterior superior iliac spine on the left side. In a fully anaesthetised patient, under antibiotic prophylaxis cover I would perform a mini laparotomy 3 cm inferior to the umbilicus in the midline. Upon entering the peritoneal cavity by standard direct vision technique, I would select a curled Tenckhoff catheter and introduce this into the pelvis using a long straight instrument such as a sponge holding forceps. The catheter should pass easily and rest within the pelvis without recoiling. I would instil some saline via the catheter and aspirate to check free flow. I would line up the inner Dacron cuff with the abdominal wall sheath and secure it temporarily. I would then make a small opening at the exit site and tunnel the catheter subcutaneously from the incision to the exit site and deliver it there. I would perform a final instillation of saline via the catheter to check adequate drainage. I would then secure the inner Dacron cuff to the sheath using a Vicryl suture and the outer cuff to the skin using Monocryl. I would then close the midline incision and recover the patient routinely. Postoperatively, I would obtain an abdominal X-ray to assess catheter position was adequate. PD can commence after 14 days.

Q. 8.5 The patient is discharged following the procedure with no concerns. You review them in your follow-up clinic 2 weeks later and ascertain all is well and dialysis is ongoing without concern. 6 weeks later you are called as the patient attends the emergency department with severe abdominal pain and a temperature of 38°C. Explain how you would assess this patient and what would you be concerned about?

The patient should be assessed routinely with an ABC approach – oxygen administered, IV access obtained and 'sepsis 6 bundle' completed with blood cultures, lactate levels and a blood gas taken, as well as checking blood glucose and ketones. Any PD fluid within the abdominal cavity should be emptied and sent for culture and microscopy. They should receive broad spectrum antibiotics and a modest fluid challenge in view of ESRF. After administration of analgesia, I would perform a full clinical assessment including history and examination. I would be concerned about PD peritonitis. If there was any doubt regarding the diagnosis, I would arrange a CT scan of the abdomen and pelvis.

If the diagnosis of PD peritonitis is made, I would prescribe vancomycin to be administered via the PD catheter as treatment and ciprofloxacin orally. If the patient was well, they could be managed as an outpatient and may not require admission. If they do not respond to this regimen they should be admitted for treatment and if necessary, the PD catheter removed. If this was the case, a temporarily dialysis line should be placed for HD.

Q. 8.6 **The patient recovers from the acute episode and continues PD without event. Over the course of the next few years, the patient is advised to consider other management of their ESRF but is resistant and wants to remain on PD. They present 5 years later with intestinal obstruction to their local hospital who contact you directly – what would be your main concern?**

Intestinal obstruction in the presence of a long history of PD would raise the concern of encapsulating peritoneal sclerosis (EPS) as a diagnosis.

Q. 8.7 **What is EPS?**

This is sometimes also referred to as sclerosing peritonitis and is a rare complication of PD that results in fibrosis and scarring of the peritoneum which results in an encapsulating fibrous cocoon that causes bowel obstruction. It is thought to be due to chronic peritoneal injury though the precise pathogenesis is unknown. It occurs in patients who have been on PD for long durations and may be precipitated by episodes of PD peritonitis or acute cessation of dialysis.

Q. 8.8 **The patient receives initial resuscitation with nasogastric tube, bowel rest and IV fluid. They are transferred to your unit in London without consultation. On assessment, you find the patient to be critically unwell with a peritonitic abdomen. What is the ideal management within the UK setup and what would be your concern?**

Encapsulating peritoneal sclerosis remains very rare and treatment is difficult, complex and requires an MDT approach. As outcomes in UK were historically poor, services have been centralised to either Manchester or Cambridge. The patient should ideally be managed at one of these centres. If the patient is critically unwell, I would be concerned that they may need emergency treatment and may not be fit for transfer.

Q. 8.9 **You proceed to laparotomy with another consultant. It is extremely difficult and a number of enterotomies are made, and a significant bowel resection is undertaken. A segment of intestine appears compromised, so**

you perform laparostomy and return for a re-look after 48 hours. At second look, the segment of intestine is non-viable and is resected. The patient is left with 40 cm of small intestine from the duodenal-jejunal (DJ) flexure and commences on total parenteral nutrition (TPN).

What is intestinal failure (IF)?

Intestinal failure is the inability of the intestine to absorb nutrients (macro and micro), electrolytes and water sufficiently to sustain life and therefore, requires intravenous supplementation or replacement. It can be classified into three types, based on duration of onset. Type I IF is acquired and lasts <28 days. It is usually self-limiting and can include postoperative issues such as ileus. Type II is also classified as acute and its duration may be from weeks to months and patients remain unstable in their intestinal function. Patients may progress from type II to type III which signifies a chronic state which may be reversible or irreversible.

Intestinal failure can also be classified based on nutritional support required (e.g. kcal/kg/day) or by aetiology; short bowel syndrome (SBS), fistulae, dysmotility, mechanical obstruction or small bowel mucosal disease.

Q. 8.10 Does this patient qualify for an intestinal transplant? What are the indications?

No. Intestinal transplantation is indicated in patients who have irreversible intestinal failure and life-threatening complications of parenteral nutrition such as intestinal failure associated liver disease (IFALD), multiple episodes of line sepsis and loss of venous access. There are other relative indications, but this is the main one. The procedure has considerable morbidity and as outcomes on long-term TPN are good with modern treatment, the number of patients suitable for transplant is low.

Further reading

Kaufman SS, Avitzur Y, Beath SV, et al. New Insights Into the Indications for Intestinal Transplantation: Consensus in the Year 2019. Transplantation 2020; 104:937–946.

Scenario 9

Liver transplantation

You are on-call for liver transplantation and are contacted by an ITU consultant within the hospital regarding a patient with fulminant hepatic failure who is deteriorating. They feel that the patient should undergo a liver transplant.

Q. 9.1 What are the indications for liver transplant?

Liver transplantation in adults can be indicated for patients with acute liver failure (liver failure within 8 weeks of onset of symptoms and no prior history of dysfunction), chronic liver disease (e.g. primary biliary cirrhosis and hepatitis), liver tumours (e.g. HCC) and variant syndromes (e.g. polycystic liver disease and hepatopulmonary syndrome). Patients who develop acute liver failure on background of chronic liver failure (ACLF) may also be suitable if specific criteria are met.

Patients should be referred early for assessment by a transplant centre and evaluated in an MDT. Specific diseases have criteria, for example, patients with chronic disease must have a projected 1-year mortality without transplantation of >9% and a UKELD score of ≥ 49. Those with tumours such as HCC have specific criteria to meet such as Milan criteria.

Q. 9.2 How would you assess this patient?

I would assess the patient by an ABC approach on the ITU, paying attention to their oxygen and ventilation requirements, the presence of any haemodynamic support (e.g. inotropes) or renal failure requiring haemofiltration. I would examine the patient, particularly the abdomen to plan potential surgery. Crucially, I would be looking for signs of hepatic decompensation (ascites, encephalopathy, jaundice, and variceal haemorrhage) and any evidence of multiorgan failure.

I would carefully review the history to ascertain if there was any history of previous liver disease or alcohol abuse. A collateral history may be very useful in this case. I would review the full past medical, surgical, drug and social history to assess for any contraindications to transplantation (e.g. active malignancy). I would review all her recent investigations including LFTs, clotting profile and review her arterial anatomy by CT scan if not already performed. Finally, I would discuss the case with a hepatologist and arrange for an MDT to list the patient if appropriate.

Q. 9.3 The patient is listed for a super urgent liver transplant. You are approached by the patient's mother in the corridor who wants to 'donate her liver' for the patient. Would this be possible?

Liver donation would not be suitable in this case as the patient is in fulminant hepatic failure and the time needed to work up the mother as a donor would take too long. Liver donation has limited application in the UK due to the presence of a strong national deceased donor programme. It is used more in other countries without such a network such as Japan or India.

Q. 9.4 You accept an offer for a liver for this patient from a 45-year-old DBD liver. The donor died from a head injury and had no co-morbidities. The liver has been retrieved with normal anatomy reported and no injuries. It will arrive in 4 hours. The anaesthetist asks about starting a pre-emptive recipient hepatectomy – what would the benefit of this be?

By starting pre-emptively, the recipient could undergo the dissection for hepatectomy and then, once the liver arrives it could be transplanted after the bench preparation is complete. This would likely reduce the CIT, even if two teams were working simultaneously on the bench preparation of the liver and hepatectomy of the recipient. This would be especially useful if the recipient hepatectomy was anticipated to be difficult (e.g. large polycystic liver). Reducing CIT has consistently shown to improve patient outcomes, and this is of great importance.

Q. 9.5 You begin the hepatectomy for the recipient. There is significant portal hypertension and patient is bleeding profusely on dissection. What is portal hypertension? What strategies could you use to circumvent this?

Portal hypertension occurs when the portal pressure rises above the normal value of 1–5 mmHg but clinically significant portal hypertension occurs when pressure rises above 12 mmHg. This may be caused by intrinsic liver disease or obstruction to flow but is typically seen in cirrhosis as the liver fibrosis increases resistance to flow. Patients may develop varices in the classical locations due to the formation of portosystemic anastomoses (e.g. oesophagus, paraumbilical area, bare area of liver, and retroperitoneum) and resultant haemorrhage.

It is therefore, frequently seen in liver transplant recipients and at the time of surgery may result in massive bleeding. Strategies to approach this include use of additional cell saver system, aggressive correction of any coagulopathy and meticulous technique. Bleeding may still be profuse and veno-venous bypass or a porto-caval shunt could be used.

Q. 9.6 You are ready to complete the recipient hepatectomy and implant the donor liver. Explain the key steps in performing a liver transplantation.

In order to implant the liver, the donor liver has to be fully bench-prepared and ready. The recipient's native liver can be removed once all the major structures are dissected

Scenario 9 Liver transplantation

free and encircled with vessel slings (bile duct, portal vein, and hepatic arteries). The liver needs to be mobilised and access to the vena cava possible.

The major hilar structures are clamped and divided high in the hilum preserving length. The donor liver can be implanted either by caval replacement technique or piggyback. Depending on the technique the cava is either side clamped or fully cross clamped infra- and supra-hepatically. The recipient liver can then be removed. A caval anastomosis is then performed, either side-by-side in the case of piggyback or infra- and supra-hepatic end-to-end for caval replacement. The portal vein is than anastomosed end-to-end after which the liver can be re-perfused. The arterial anastomosis site can vary but will usually involve the confluence of the gastroduodenal artery (GDA) and common hepatic artery (CHA) in the recipient native vessels to a similar location on the graft. Finally, the bile duct is anastomosed end-to-end.

Q. 9.7 The operation is completed without event. The patient is started on aspirin and low-molecular weight heparin to prevent graft thrombosis. After 24 hours, your registrar asks if you can review the patient as they are concerned about bleeding. They report that one of the drain bags that was placed has filled with blood. Explain the key points in your assessment of this patient and how you might manage them.

I would assess the patient by an ABC approach. If the patient is still on ITU, I would want to know if the patient is intubated, the FiO_2 and if oxygen requirements are increasing. I would ascertain if the patient requires inotropic support to maintain blood pressure and examine the patient carefully including the cardiovascular parameters. Specifically, I would assess for any abdominal distension or haematoma, the nature of the drain output and volumes and requirement for any blood products.

If bleeding was significant, I would first stop any anticoagulation, ensure the patient has adequate volume filling with transfusion of packed red cells and correction of any coagulopathy by transfusion of products (e.g. platelets, cryoprecipitate, etc.). If the patient is stabilised initially and it was safe, I would arrange a CT angiogram to identify the source of bleeding and target management more clearly. The exception to this would be if the patient was exsanguinating profusely and transfusion was unable to keep up with the bleeding – in this case I would arrange for the patient to go to theatre immediately.

Q. 9.8 You find evidence of a low-grade bleed but feel it is better to manage the patient conservatively with stopping anticoagulation and giving supportive treatment. The patient makes a good recovery and is transferred to the ward from ITU. On day 5, blood tests indicate an abrupt rise in bilirubin, aspartate aminotransferase (AST) and alanine aminotransferase (ALT). A tacrolimus level is measured at 3 ng/ml. What would you be worried about? How would you manage the patient?

The findings of raised transaminases on day 5 of post-transplantation and a sub-therapeutic tacrolimus level would concern me for acute rejection. I would be worried about this patient but would first want to exclude an acute surgical problem.

I would arrange an urgent US Doppler of the liver to assess for any arterial thrombosis and establish that flow was adequate. If this demonstrated normal vascular flow, I would arrange an urgent transjugular (TJ) liver biopsy to assess for rejection. In the meantime, I would increase the tacrolimus dose to achieve therapeutic levels (circa 8–12 ng/mL depending on local protocols).

Q. 9.9 A biopsy demonstrates acute cellular rejection. How would you treat this?

I would prescribe IV methylprednisolone as treatment based on local protocols, which usually involves a dose of 1 g IV initially. I would ensure that tacrolimus levels were in range, although this may take more than a couple of days to optimise.

Q. 9.10 The patient makes a good recovery and is discharged. Six months later, they re-attend with a raised bilirubin, ALP and gamma-glutamyl transferase (GT). Transaminases are mildly raised. The patient has been diligent with their immunosuppression and tacrolimus levels are within range. What would be your main concern? How would you manage the patient?

I would be worried about a post-transplant biliary stricture given the time of presentation and the cholestatic picture of the blood results. I would arrange full assessment of the patient and admission, if necessary. I would review the history and examine the patient. I would arrange repeat blood tests to assess the trend and organise an MRCP to assess for the presence of any biliary stricture and intrahepatic duct dilatation. If no mechanical problem was demonstrated with the transplanted liver, I would arrange an urgent TJ liver biopsy to assess further.

Q. 9.11 A diagnosis of biliary stricture is made, what is the management?

Treatment should initially be by ERCP and balloon dilatation. Plastic stents can also be placed across the stricture to improve flow. More recently, fully covered self-expanding metal stents (FC-SEMS) have been used in treatment, in particular the Kaffes stent. Strictures can also be accessed by percutaneous transhepatic cholangiography (PTC) route, but this is second line as risks are greater. This may be the only option if the patient had a hepatico-jejunostomy at the time of surgery. Strictures that are refractory to dilatation and stenting should be treated surgically by revision with excision of duct-to-duct anastomosis and formation of hepatico-jejunostomy.

Further reading

Millson C, Considine A, Cramp ME, et al. Adult liver transplantation: A UK clinical guideline - part 1: pre-operation. Frontline Gastroenterol 2020; 11:375–384.

Millson C, Considine A, Cramp ME, et al. Adult liver transplantation: UK clinical guideline - part 2: surgery and post-operation. Frontline Gastroenterol. 2020; 11:385–396.

Scenario 10

Arteriovenous fistula

A 45-year-old female patient with ESRF and eGFR of 18 mL/min, pre-dialysis, is referred to vascular access clinic to consider arteriovenous fistula (AVF) creation.

Q. 10.1 How will you proceed?

- *Detailed history*: Cause for renal failure, previous history of fluid overload, previous history of RRT, chronic medical problems such as heart disease and diabetes
- *Smoking history*: Prolonged smoking/long-standing diabetes increase the risk of peripheral arterial disease and risk of AVF thrombosis
- *Medication history*: Antiplatelets and oral anticoagulants. Oral anticoagulants need to be stopped prior to the surgery. Prophylactic and postoperative aspirin is indicated in patients with a previous history of fistula failures and patients with a high risk of atherosclerosis
- *Hand dominance*: Arteriovenous fistula creation is always preferred in the non-dominant hand whenever possible
- *Clinical examination*: Both limbs need assessment. Prominent veins on the inspection are very much favoured. Palpate arterial pulsations from distal to proximal (radial–ulnar–brachial–axillary–subclavian artery)
- *Perform modified Allen's test*: A test used to assess the patency of the palmar arterial arch. Patency of both radial and ulnar arteries is mandatory before planning a wrist fistula because of the risk of arterial occlusion
- *Tourniquet test*: Apply tourniquet snug to the arm. The patient is asked to clench and unclench their fist. If the veins are clinically felt and palpable, perform a tap/thrill to look for vein patency
- *Duplex ultrasound*: Measures the vein diameter and assesses the patency by compressing the vein

Q. 10.2 What is an ideal AVF?

- The AV fistula must be accessible with the patient in a comfortable sitting position
- In the forearm, the AV fistula should be on the volar surface
- The AV fistula should be on the anterior or lateral surface in the upper arm
- The AV fistula must be able to be reliably cannulated repeatedly
- The AV fistula should be within 5–6 mm of the skin surface. Hence, cephalic vein is more preferred than the basilic vein
- A relatively straight segment 8–10 cm long needs to be available for cannulation

- Blood flow must be adequate to support the dialysis prescription, generally at least 500–700 cc/min

Q. 10.3 What is the vein diameter ideal to construct AV fistula?

Vein diameter (measured by ultrasound) of at least 2–2.5 mm under tourniquet in a warm room is generally considered the minimum diameter to create a fistula reliably.

Q. 10.4 What is fistula maturation, and what is the time taken for a wrist fistula to mature?

Fistula maturation is defined as a fistula that can be used clinically for dialysis vascular access (usable vein diameter with adequate flow). The minimum time for AV fistula maturation is 1 month. Successful maturation rates for wrist fistulae are 50%, and elbow fistulae is 80%.

Q.10.5 Which artery and vein are commonly used in AVF creation in the lower extremity?

The superficial femoral artery and the saphenous or femoral/popliteal vein in the thigh.

Q. 10.6 Why are distal fistula creations preferred over proximal fistulae?

Its use as the first access preserves the most proximal arm vessels for later access attempts. It is generally a more comfortable means of dialysis that requires less frequent superficialisation. It also dilates the most proximal veins to enable easier fistula creation in the future.

Q. 10.7 What do you know about the brachiobasilic fistula?

Brachiobasilic fistulae are created when the wrist options and brachiocephalic fistula options are unavailable. The basilic vein has a deeper course than the cephalic vein in the arm. Hence, brachiobasilic fistula creation needs fistula creation followed by superficialisation of the basilic vein from the deeper planes to the subcutaneous plane for easy access (basilic vein transposition). Hence, it is a more extensive operation and is usually performed under GA or regional block. It can be created as a one-stage procedure or in two stages.

Q. 10.8 What is the advantage of having an elbow fistula over the wrist?

The flow rates are better than the wrist fistula, and the maturation time is quicker than the wrist fistula. The arm's cephalic vein is larger and easier to cannulate than the forearm cephalic vein.

The disadvantages are shortened accessible vein length, less long-term patency, more arm swelling and high risk of steal syndrome.

Q. 10.9 What is Steal syndrome?

Steal syndrome is a collection of ischaemic symptoms due to preferential arterial blood flow through the fistula and decreased distal flow. They are rare with a wrist fistula. They tend to be more common for brachial artery-based fistulae. Usually, the symptoms occur during dialysis or when the patient uses the arm for work. The presence of rest pain or ischaemic changes in the palm is an indication to ligate the fistula to prevent further ischaemia or banding of the fistula if AVF needs preservation.

Q. 10.10 What are the risk factors of Steal syndrome?

End-stage renal failure with long-term diabetes, old age, female sex, and use of polytetrafluoroethylene (PTFE) grafts.

Q. 10.11 What are the complications of AV fistula creation?

Predominantly local complications – bleeding, venous hypertension, limb swelling, aneurysm/pseudoaneurysm formation, infection, primary failure, failure to mature and steal syndrome. Other problems include neuropathy and heart failure.

Q. 10.12 What is the common reason for limb swelling after AV fistula creation?

Slight limb swelling is expected after AV fistula creation. Central venous occlusion should be suspected if there is abnormal limb swelling. Clinically, the patient might have prominent veins on the chest wall, and these patients have issues with blood flow during dialysis and a high risk of fistula failure.

Q. 10.13 What is primary AV fistula failure? What are the risk factors for this?

Arteriovenous fistula that is never usable or fails within the first 3 months of its use. Risk factors include:
- Obesity
- Older age
- Female sex
- Cardiovascular disease
- Diabetes
- Thrombophilia

Q. 10.14 How do you assess for AV fistula stenosis and what are the possible interventions?

A duplex ultrasound and/or venography are commonly used to assess the anatomy of stenosis. Angioplasty/stenting/surgical revision are the options to correct the stenosis. It depends upon the location and the length of the stenosis.

Further reading

Percutaneous endovascular forearm arteriovenous fistula creation for haemodialysis access (2021) NICE guideline IPG710

Scenario 11

Paediatric kidney transplantation

A 6-year-old boy with stage 5 chronic kidney disease (CKD), pre-dialysis, is referred for kidney transplant assessment

Q. 11.1 What is the threshold at which referral to a kidney transplant service is done?

As the eGFR declines to <30 mL/min/1.73 m^2 (CKD stage 4), preparations for RRT are initiated. Although RRT is not needed until eGFR is <15 mL/min, patients are usually referred to plan AVFs, initiate the assessment for kidney transplant and to identify and prepare live donors if the family opts for live donor kidney transplant.

Q. 11.2 What are the options for RRT in children?

- Pre-emptive kidney transplantation
- Peritoneal dialysis
- Haemodialysis

Q. 11.3 How do you classify CKD based on GFR?

KDIGO classification: Kidney Disease Improving Global Outcomes
- *G1*: Normal or high GFR (≥90 mL/min/1.73 m^2)
- *G2*: Mildly decreased GFR between 60 and 89 mL/min/1.73 m^2
- *G3a*: Mildly to moderately decreased GFR between 45 and 59 mL/min/1.73 m^2
- *G3b*: Moderately to severely decreased GFR between 30 and 44 mL/min/1.73 m^2
- *G4*: Severely decreased GFR between 15 and 29 mL/min/1.73 m^2
- *G5*: Kidney failure GFR of <15 mL/min/1.73 m^2 ESRD

Q. 11.4 What is the most common cause of paediatric end-stage kidney disease (ESKD)?

Congenital anomalies of the kidney and urinary tract (CAKUT): CAKUT accounts for 60% of paediatric CKD. These disorders include kidney aplasia/hypoplasia/dysplasia, reflux nephropathy, obstructive uropathy anomalies (e.g. posterior urethral valves) and polycystic kidney disease.

Glomerular causes account for 10–20% of children with CKD [e.g. focal segmental glomerulosclerosis (FSGS – most common), haemolytic uraemic syndrome, secondary glomerular disease, and systemic lupus nephritis].

Other disorders:
- Genetic disorders such as cystinosis, oxalosis, and hereditary nephritis (also referred to as Alport syndrome)
- Interstitial nephritis
- Unidentified or unknown primary underlying aetiology

Q. 11.5 What are the indications for emergency HD?

Fluid overload, uraemic symptoms, and uncontrolled metabolic abnormalities (e.g. hyperkalaemia, hyperphosphataemia).

Q. 11.6 What are the advantages of pre-emptive kidney transplantation over other forms of RRT?

- Better health-related quality-of-life measures, growth, and development than either PD or HD
- Mortality is higher in patients undergoing chronic dialysis compared to those with pre-emptive transplantation
- Graft survival is better for children who received a pre-emptive transplant as initial RRT versus dialysis
- Dialysis is more disruptive to family lifestyle, schooling and social interactions
- Avoidance of dialysis preserves vascular and peritoneal access sites for future use (i.e. lifetime for a child) if the transplant should fail
- Less dietary and fluid restrictions are needed in the post-transplant setting than on dialysis
- Dialysis is associated with an increased risk of cardiovascular disease (e.g. ischaemic heart disease, cerebrovascular disease, heart failure, cardiac arrest/arrhythmias, and cardiomyopathy) and vascular calcification, which occur at a proportionately earlier age

Q. 11.7 What are the contraindications of pre-emptive transplants?

- Need for pre-transplant nephrectomies (e.g. malignant renovascular hypertension, chronic pyelonephritis)
- ESKD from autoimmune disease with persistently high titres of autoantibody (e.g. anti-glomerular basement membrane disease)
- Ongoing active infections
- Underlying active kidney disease and associated rapidly progressive disease (e.g. haemolytic uraemic syndrome or crescentic glomerulonephritis)
- If the patient or his/her caregivers are not yet able to cope with the regimented care necessary for the transplant recipient as exhibited by non-adherence to his/her CKD care

Q. 11.8 What are the contraindications for paediatric kidney transplant?

- Uncontrolled extrarenal malignancies

- Systemic sepsis
- Severe irreversible multi organ system failure not correctable by organ transplant
- Severe cardiac or pulmonary dysfunction in a patient who is not a candidate for multiorgan transplantation
- Life-threatening disorder of extrarenal origin that is not correctable by organ transplant
- Elevated levels of circulating anti-glomerular basement membrane antibodies

Q. 11.9 What are the advantages of having a living donor kidney over a deceased donor?

- The incidence of delayed allograft function is lower
- Long-term allograft survival is higher
- Dialysis can be avoided, or the period on dialysis can be shortened because the time of transplantation is decided in advance. This may limit dialysis-related complications, such as growth impairment

Q. 11.10 What are the goals of pre-transplant evaluation of the paediatric transplant recipient?

- Detection of anti-HLA antibodies to the donor (detection of sensitisation)
- Correction of any significant urinary tract abnormality
- Detection and treatment of any infection prior to transplantation
- Completion of routine childhood immunisations
- Review of whether nephrectomy would be beneficial long-term

Q. 11.11 What is DGF?

Kidney failure persisting after transplantation is called DGF. The definition of DGF varies in different studies, but generally refers to oliguria or the requirement for dialysis within the first week of post-transplantation.

Q. 11.12 What are the causes of DGF?

- Post-ischaemic acute kidney injury is the most common cause of DGF
- Thrombosis or embolization of the renal artery or vein
- Accelerated rejection superimposed on ischaemic acute tubular necrosis (ATN)
- Urologic abnormalities (e.g. urinary leak or haematoma)
- Hyperacute rejection (generally preventable)
- Factors related to the donor (e.g. cardiovascular instability, older donor age, kidney function based on serum/plasma creatinine)

Q. 11.13 What are the common causes of early graft insufficiency (1–12 weeks after transplantation)?
- Acute allograft rejection
- CNI toxicity
- Urinary obstruction
- Infection
- Hypovolaemia
- Recurrent disease

Q. 11.14 What are the common causes of disease recurrence in the graft kidney?
- Membranoproliferative glomerulonephritis
- Haemolytic uraemic syndrome
- Primary hyperoxaluria

Further reading

https://www.clinicalguidelines.scot.nhs.uk/nhsggc-guidelines/nhsggc-guidelines/kidney-diseases/renal-transplantation-paediatric-management-of/

Scenario 12

Living donor renal transplantation assessment

A 35-year-old male patient with ESRF presents to the transplant clinic with his wife as a potential live donor.

Q. 12.1 How would you proceed with the assessment of the donor?

I would first confirm the donor's relationship with the recipient and their reason for donation. Following this, I would explore their understanding of the process of donation, that they were aware of what it involves, the aims and the potential risks. Providing their understanding was appropriate, I would obtain verbal consent from the donor candidate for further evaluation.

I would assess the donor as per NHSBT and BTS guidelines. The donor should be assessed by a nephrologist independent of the recipient's nephrologist. Patients who attend the surgical clinic have usually been deemed suitable for donation by a nephrologist, but I would confirm appropriate details. The medical assessment involves standard history and examination initially. Important points of note in the history are any known important diseases, such as hypertension, gout, cardiac disease, nephrolithiasis and diabetes mellitus. Family history is important and should be sought to assess for any history of kidney disease and diabetes. Present and past use of tobacco products should be obtained. The examination and investigations are extensive so I will briefly describe some important points. It includes estimation of GFR, measurement of albumin-to-creatinine ratio, testing for microscopic haematuria and fasting blood glucose and/or glycated haemoglobin (HbA1c) measurement. Screening for important conditions should be performed (e.g. HIV, hepatitis B/C, CMV). The donor should be assessed for compatibility with the recipient by determination of ABO blood type and HLA compatibility.

Presuming the medical assessment is appropriate I would review the surgical history, particularly for any previous urological or abdominal surgery which may affect completion of laparoscopic nephrectomy. The donor BMI is important both from the medical and surgical perspective and should ideally be within the normal range. Patients should be highly motivated to permit a smooth postoperative course. Imaging of the kidneys to assess anatomy is important in selection of the kidney for donation (preferably left).

By completing the above, the donor can be provided with individualised estimates of short- and long-term risks to their health and the challenges that the recipient may face with transplantation. I would inform incompatible donors about exchange programmes and incompatible living donor transplantation options.

Q. 12.2 What is the advantage of living over deceased donation?

Live donation is associated with both improved graft and patient survival. There are a series of factors that this can be attributed to. The opportunity to proceed to planned elective surgery with minimal delay permits pre-emptive, or early transplantation and the avoidance of dialysis reduces overall morbidity in a patient's lifetime. The ability to co-ordinate the donor operation and transplant well allows a decrease in cold ischaemia time which is associated with improved outcomes in all forms of transplantation.

Q. 12.3 What type of kidney transplants are you aware of based on donation schemes?

- *Directed donation* – a healthy person donates an organ or part of an organ to a specific recipient
- *Paired or pool donation* – a healthy person from one donor-recipient pair (pair 'A') donates an organ to a recipient in another pair (pair 'B'). The donor in pair 'B' then donates to the recipient in pair 'A' in a reciprocal arrangement. The donors are not genetically related or known to their respective recipients. 'Paired donations' involve two pairs in an exchange and 'pooled donations' include a series of paired donations, each of which is linked to another in the same series
- *Non-directed altruistic donation* – an organ or part of an organ is donated by a healthy person to an unknown recipient
- *Directed altruistic donation* – an organ or part of an organ is donated by a healthy person and contact between the donor and recipient has been made because the recipient requires a transplantation

Q. 12.4 In which situations are split kidney functions assessed?

Differential kidney function, determined by 99mTc DMSA scanning, is recommended where there is > 10% variation in kidney size, significant renal anatomical abnormality or difference in size of 2 cm or more between the kidneys.

Q. 12.5 What is the risk of acquiring ESRD in a living kidney donor?

This can be quoted as <1% risk and therefore, extremely low. It is important that donors understand that there is a risk, however, and if illness is contracted in the future which confers a risk of renal complications, they should inform the relevant medical teams involved so they are aware of the solitary kidney.

Q. 12.6 What is the threshold of live donor blood pressure before deciding on proceeding with organ donation?

Blood pressure must be assessed on at least two separate occasions. Blood pressure < 140/90 mmHg is considered safe to proceed in the donor. Patients whose blood pressure are controlled to <140/90 mmHg with medications without evidence of end-organ damage can be considered for donation. Where these parameters are not met, live donation is contraindicated due to the hypertension.

Q. 12.7 Which kidney will be considered for donation if one kidney has a stone with no other metabolic abnormality identified?

In appropriate donors with unilateral kidney stone(s), the stone-bearing kidney can be considered for donation (if vascular anatomy and split kidney function permit) in order to leave the donor with a stone-free kidney after donation.

Q. 12.8 How would you proceed with organ donation if the donor had angiomyolipoma in the kidneys?

Bilateral angiomyolipoma and angiomyolipoma > 4 cm generally preclude living kidney donation. Unilateral large (> 4 cm) angiomyolipoma can be used if ex vivo excision of the angiomyolipoma is feasible. Kidneys containing a single angiomyolipoma between 1 and 4 cm can be considered for donation depending on position, consideration of whether ex vivo excision is feasible, and if when left in situ in the recipient, it can be followed with serial ultrasound imaging.

Q. 12.9 Which kidney is preferred for laparoscopic donor nephrectomy?

The left kidney is usually preferred, assuming both kidneys have equal numbers of arteries, due to the greater length of the left renal vein.

Further reading

https://bts.org.uk/wp-content/uploads/2018/07/FINAL_LDKT-guidelines_June-2018.pdf [Accessed 1st April 2023]

Scenario 13

Liver transplantation assessment

A 45-year-old male patient is being considered for liver transplantation for alcohol-related chronic liver disease.

Q. 13.1 How would you assess him and work him up for liver transplantation?

The work-up should be completed as part of a multidisciplinary team approach and ideally this involves a hepatologist, dietician, anaesthetist, psychologist and radiologist in addition to the surgeon. I would ensure that this is done in accordance with BTS guidelines. Each relevant team member's assessment should form the basis of discussion for suitability for listing.

From the surgical perspective, I would take a detailed history of the patient's liver failure; in this particular case the duration and nature of alcohol abuse, confirmed abstinence and how the patient has and will cope in the future. A history of the liver failure should include details of any episodes of decompensation with ascites, jaundice, encephalopathy, portal venous thrombosis and variceal bleeding. I would obtain details of the patients past medical and surgical history, particularly any previous operations which may affect the liver explantation approach. Social history is very important, and the patient needs to be highly motivated with an adequate support network and understanding of what liver transplantation involves. My examination of the patient would involve assessment of BMI, examination for any hernias and signs of portal hypertension which may affect surgery.

Investigations are extensive including full biochemical liver screen, ABO-Rh blood typing, tumour markers (serum alpha-fetoprotein), serology (e.g. CMV, EBV, HIV, etc.), blood alcohol levels, urinalysis and drug screen. Specific anaesthetic assessments may include cardiac stress testing and contrast-enhanced echocardiography in addition to standard ECG, pulse oximetry, arterial blood gas and CXR. Contrast-enhanced abdominal CT scan or MRI should assess vascular anatomy and the presence of any portal venous thrombosis or HCC.

I would combine the information from my assessment with the other care professionals at the MDT and contribute to the decision as to whether to list the patient for transplantation.

Q. 13.2 What differentiates acute from chronic liver failure?

The duration of symptoms: Liver failure symptoms lasting > 6 months is considered as chronic liver failure.

Q. 13.3 What are the causes of acute liver failure?

[As with all approaches to this kind of question, at this stage you should list important causes grouped appropriately. For example, mention infective (e.g. hepatitis A/B/C), drug related (e.g. alcohol, paracetamol), genetic (e.g. Wilson's disease) and so forth. Avoid reeling off rare causes robotically and boring the examiners. The A–I mnemonic below can help to refresh your memory if you get stuck.]

- A: *A*cetaminophen, hepatitis *A*, *A*utoimmune hepatitis, *A*denovirus
- B: Hepatitis *B*, *B*udd–Chiari syndrome
- C: *C*ryptogenic, hepatitis *C*, *C*MV
- D: Hepatitis *D*, *D*rugs and toxins
- E: Hepatitis *E*, *E*BV
- F: *F*atty infiltration
- G: *G*enetic – Wilson's disease
- H: *H*ypoperfusion (ischaemic hepatitis, sepsis), *H*ELLP syndrome, *H*SV, *H*epatectomy
- I: *I*nfiltration by tumour

Q. 13.4 What is King's College Criteria for transplantation for liver failure?

The King's College Criteria form a predictive tool and are used to assess patients in fulminant hepatic failure and their suitability for liver transplantation. Originally described in the 1980s, the scoring system has been validated in a number of different publications and has predictive accuracies of 85–95%. The criteria used in patients follow acetaminophen ingestion include:

- Arterial pH < 7.3
- INR > 6.5
- Creatinine > 300 µmol/L
- Presence of encephalopathy (of grade III or IV)

Different weighting is given to the parameters (e.g. arterial pH alone <7.3 in acetaminophen overdose is more significant than INR > 6.5).

Where liver failure is due to another cause, additional criteria include serum bilirubin, aetiology, patient's age and interval duration of jaundice-encephalopathy.

Q. 13.5 What are the indications in a cirrhotic patient to recommend liver transplantation?

Decompensated liver disease manifesting as either variceal haemorrhage, ascites, encephalopathy or hepatorenal syndrome. HCC is also a common indication in the cirrhotic patient.

Q. 13.6 What scoring systems do you know of to assess patients for liver transplantation? What are the principles behind these scoring systems?

Various scoring systems are available. They are typically used to predict survival in patients with chronic liver disease and therefore, the risk of death without transplantation. These data can then be used to advise which patients are likely to benefit from transplantation based on the risks of the procedure itself.

I am most familiar with the United Kingdom Model for End-stage Liver Disease (UKELD) which has been modelled specifically to detect the risks in the population of the UK. The model applies to death from liver failure and does not apply to many cases, such as cancer, hepatopulmonary syndrome, etc. It uses laboratory measurements and application of a formula to generate a score. A UKELD score of > 49 is considered as the threshold for referral for liver transplantation.

I am also familiar with the Model for End-stage Liver Disease (MELD) score, Na-MELD and Child's Pugh scoring systems. Each has different advantages, disadvantages and appropriate applications. Any scoring system should be used with common sense, understanding its strengths and limitations.

Q. 13.7 What are the survival rates for liver transplantation in the UK?

1-year survival rate is typically quoted at 90% although there may be some variation between centres. 5-year survival rate is quoted at 70–75%.

Q. 13.8 What are MELD exception points?

The MELD score accurately predicts 3-month mortality for most patients with cirrhosis but underestimates risks of mortality and waiting list dropout for patients with HCC. Since 2002 patients were given extra 'exception points' to balance their risk and make allocation fairer when compared to non-HCC patients. Studies since have indicated that such points have often given advantage to HCC patients leading to adjustment of allocation of exception points. Conditions which allow for exception points include HCC, hepatopulmonary syndrome and cholangiocarcinoma.

Q. 13.9 What are the Milan criteria for liver transplantation?

These criteria are used to assess patients with HCC for suitability for liver transplantation. They include:
- One lesion smaller than 5 cm; alternatively, up to three lesions, each smaller than 3 cm
- No extrahepatic manifestations
- No evidence of gross vascular invasion

Another similar scoring system for patients with HCC is the UCSF criteria which includes:
- A single tumour up to 6.5 cm
- Or, up to three lesions each <4.5 cm with cumulative tumour burden of ≤8 cm
- No extrahepatic manifestations
- No evidence of gross vascular invasion

Q. 13.10 What are the contraindications for liver transplantation?

Some contraindications include cardiopulmonary disease that cannot be corrected and is a prohibitive risk for surgery, acquired immunodeficiency syndrome (AIDS), malignancy outside of the liver not meeting oncologic criteria for cure, uncontrolled sepsis and persistent non-adherence to medical care.

'Geographical differences in donor availability' means that some conditions (usually those controversial indications like colorectal liver metastases) could be treated in some countries due to organ availability whereas in others, such cases could not be listed. As advances in care of diseases improve, other conditions may provoke further debate as to whether contraindication is appropriate (e.g. cholangiocarcinoma).

Further reading

https://bts.org.uk/wp-content/uploads/2016/09/03_BTS_LivingDonorLiver-1.pdf [Accessed 1st April 2023]

Scenario 14

Post-transplantation lymphoproliferative disorder

A 46-year-old patient who is a recipient of a DBD liver transplant 6 years previously presents with abdominal pain and fevers. On assessment, the patient has complained of feeling generally unwell with fevers and fatigue for the last 3 weeks. Clinical examination reveals a tender abdomen with localized peritonism on the right. Tacrolimus levels were raised.

Q. 14.1 What would you be concerned about?

Given the background history of transplantation and long-term immunosuppression my first differential diagnosis is PTLD.

Q. 14.2 What is PTLD?

PTLD means post-transplant lymphoproliferative disorder. These are lymphoid and/or plasmacytic proliferations that occur as a result of immunosuppression in the setting of solid organ or allogeneic haematopoietic cell transplantation. Clinically, this manifests similarly to a lymphoma.

Q. 14.3 What is the pathogenesis of PTLD?

In most affected patients (70%), PTLD is an EBV-positive B cell proliferation occurring in the setting of immunosuppression and decreased T-cell immune surveillance. Normally, EBV infection leads to a polyclonal expansion of B cells harbouring the virus. In immunocompetent individuals, cytotoxic T-cell response eliminates the vast majority of the infected B cells. When T-cell immunity is suppressed as seen in transplant recipients, these B cells proliferate and give rise to lymphoproliferative disorders such as PTLD.

Q. 14.4 What are the risk factors for acquiring PTLD post-liver transplantation?

- Degree and duration of T-cell immunosuppression (CNI and induction agents like monoclonal and polyclonal antibodies)
- EBV negative recipient receiving organ from an EBV positive donor
- History of pre-transplantation malignancy
- Fewer HLA matches

Q. 14.5 What are the signs and symptoms of PTLD?
- Non-specific constitutional symptoms such as fever, weight loss, and fatigue
- Lymphadenopathy
- Extranodal mass
- Dysfunction of involved organs (typically gastrointestinal tract, lungs, skin, liver, and central nervous system)
- Symptoms related to compression of surrounding structures
- Involvement of the allograft can lead to allograft dysfunction, including renal failure, heart failure, and respiratory dysfunction

Q. 14.6 What are the biochemical abnormalities in a patient with PTLD?
- Unexplained anaemia, thrombocytopaenia, or leucopaenia
- Elevated level of serum lactate dehydrogenase (LDH)
- Hypercalcaemia
- Hyperuricaemia
- Monoclonal protein in the serum or urine

Q. 14.7 What types of PTLD do you know?
- Early lesion (plasmacytic hyperplasia and infectious mononucleosis-like PTLD)
- Polymorphic PTLD
- Monomorphic PTLD
- Classic Hodgkin lymphoma-like PTLD

Q. 14.8 You suspect PTLD in this patient, how would you manage the patient and confirm the diagnosis?

Post-transplantation lymphoproliferative disorder has significant morbidity and may be fatal so I would be concerned about this patient. I would complete an ABC approach style resuscitation of this patient using the CCRISP protocol. I would ensure that the sepsis six bundle has been completed as patients can often develop superimposed infections. I would carefully review the patient's transplant history to check their pre-transplant EBV status and that of the donor and any history of malignancy or additional immunosuppressive treatments for rejection in the past.

I would make sure that the patient's current immunosuppressants are reduced as this is the main initial treatment strategy. Serology should be sent routinely with particular attention to EBV result. The patient should have initial imaging with a contrast CT of the chest, abdomen and pelvis to assess for the presence of any localised lesions and any lymphadenopathy. Radiological findings may be highly suggestive and if any doubt is present a PET scan could be used to support the diagnosis. Ultimately, a biopsy will confirm the diagnosis and should be sought if feasible, safe and indicated.

Q. 14.9 What is the treatment for PTLD?

The initial management is reduction of immunosuppression. For early diagnosed lesions with mild manifestation, this may be all that is required. Some patients may not tolerate reduction of immunosuppression well and require additional treatment with immunotherapy with the CD20 monoclonal antibody, rituximab. Additional treatments can include chemotherapy, radiation therapy, localised surgery or a combination of these.

A key factor in guiding treatment is whether the lesion(s) express CD20 based on biopsy results. Tumours which do not express CD20 are not candidates for rituximab therapy and are treated with combination chemotherapy plus reduction of immunosuppression predominantly.

Further reading

Shah N, Eyre TA, Tucker D, et al. Front-line management of post-transplantation lymphoproliferative disorder in adult solid organ recipient patients – A British Society for Haematology Guideline. Br J Haematol 2021; 193:727–740.

Chapter 9

Hepatopancreatobiliary surgery

Aali J Sheen, Saurabh Jamdar, Ajith K Siriwardena

Scenario 1

Obstructive jaundice

A 33-year-old lady presents with epigastric pain and is noted to be mildly jaundiced in the outpatient clinic.

Q. 1.1 How would you investigate this patient and manage her condition?

This patient should be managed with the initial approach used for all patients; a careful history and examination. Below are outlined the particular steps that are required in terms of the salient points which must be raised for the purposes of the examination. If a patient is jaundiced in your outpatient clinic, it is best to add that hospital admission is almost certainly required to investigate further.

Plan of care

- History:
    - *Symptoms of obstructive jaundice*: Dark urine and pale stools.
    - Presence or absence of pain
    - Duration of jaundice
    - Associated pruritus
    - Weight loss
    - History of rigors or fever
- Examination:
    - General:
        - *Inspection*: Jaundice (inspect in normal light); scratch marks.
        - *Eyes*: Scleral jaundice, Kayser–Fleischer rings (dark ring around iris)
        - *Hands*: Clubbing, evidence of weight loss (thenar wasting)
    - Abdominal examination:
        - *Inspection*: Distension, caput medusa (anterior abdominal wall varices)
        - *Palpation*: Hepatosplenomegaly. Palpable gallbladder, Courvoisier's sign (palpable gallbladder in the presence of obstructive jaundice is typically due to distal bile duct obstruction).
        - *Ascites*
    - Urinalysis
- *Admit* the patient
- Serum investigations:
    - Full blood count and clotting profile
    - Urea and electrolytes
    - Enzymatic liver function tests
    - Serum amylase (or lipase)
- Trans-abdominal ultrasound

The key here is to diagnose gallstones as this will be the most common diagnosis in a patient of this age.

If gallstones are diagnosed, the presence of jaundice also indicates likely bile duct obstruction.

Q. 1.2 What are the options in management after an ultrasound identifies gallstones and a dilated bile duct?

Options include:
- Magnetic resonance cholangiopancreatography (MRCP) (for further non-invasive delineation of biliary anatomy)
- Laparoscopic cholecystectomy with intraoperative cholangiogram and extraction of stone with laparoscopic bile duct exploration
- Endoscopic retrograde cholangiopancreatography (ERCP) followed by laparoscopic cholecystectomy
- Laparoscopic cholecystectomy followed by ERCP

The question must be answered according to your skill set and training. MRCP is invaluable in providing imaging of biliary anatomy. Diagnostic ERCP is no longer recommended.

If you are a specialist in the field of laparoscopic surgery, then laparoscopic cholecystectomy with laparoscopic bile duct exploration is a suitable option. Evidence favours this approach in a younger patient with a bile duct of at least 1 cm in diameter or more. Alternatively, ERCP and duct clearance can be undertaken, followed by surgery.

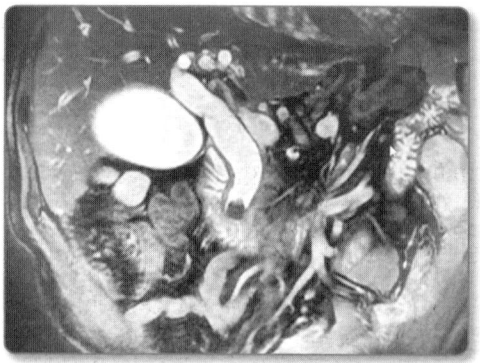

MR scan (coronal view) depicting a solitary stone in the distal end of a dilated common/main bile duct.

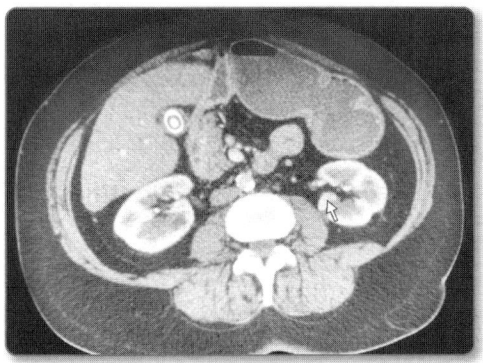

CT scan showing a gallbladder with a large and calcified gallstone.

Further reading

British Society of Gastroenterology. Updated guidelines on the management of common bile duct stones 2023. [online] Available from https://www.bsg.org.uk/resource/Updated-guideline-on-the-management-of-common-bile-duct-stones-(CBDS).html [Last accessed Feb., 2023].

European Association for the Study of the Liver (EASL). EASL Clinical Practice Guidelines on the prevention, diagnosis and treatment of gallstones. J Hepatol 2016; 65:146–181.

National Institute for Health and care Excellence. Gallstone disease: diagnosis and management 2014. [online] Available from https://www.nice.org.uk/guidance/cg188/chapter/1-Recommendations#managing-gallbladder-stones [Last accessed Feb., 2023].

Scenario 2

Acute cholecystitis

A 48-year-old man presents with epigastric pain and is Murphy's positive on examination.

Q. 2.1 How would you investigate this patient and manage his condition?

This scenario addresses the basic issues of management of acute abdominal pain.

The importance of the basic steps in assessment cannot be over-emphasised.

You would take a detailed history and confirm the examination findings of right upper quadrant tenderness with a positive Murphy's sign (A Murphy's sign is a "catch" in the breath elicited by gently pressing on the right upper quadrant and asking the patient to take a deep breath and is due to pressure on a distended, inflamed gallbladder).

The following serum and other tests will be required: Full blood count (FBC), urea and electrolytes (U&Es), coagulation profile, liver function tests (LFTs), C-reactive protein (CRP) and amylase, and also an urgent ultrasound is required.
Ultrasound findings are:
- Thick-walled gallbladder
- Pericholecystic fluid

A CT scan was undertaken, of which an image is shown below.

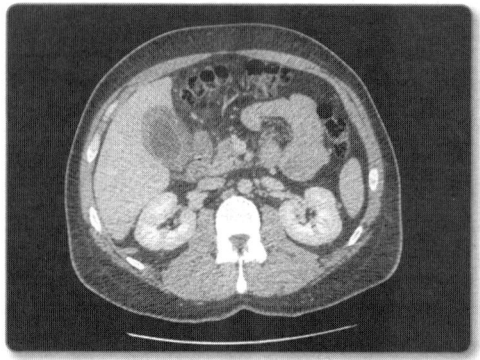

CT image showing a thick-walled gallbladder with a small amount of pericholecystic fluid.

Q. 2.2 Once a diagnosis of acute cholecystitis is made how would you manage the patient?

This answer relies on you stating that all measures to stabilise the emergency admission have been taken with the standard ABC assessment.
Treatment includes:
- Mandatory admission to hospital
- Intravenous antibiotics
- Analgesia
- Emergency laparoscopic ± open cholecystectomy
- Cholecystostomy in patients who are acutely ill but are too unwell for surgery

Key tips
- Admission to hospital is essential for confirmation of diagnosis and regular monitoring of the patient
- Transabdominal ultrasonography for diagnosis is the first-line test and should be performed within 24 hours of admission to hospital
- Intravenous fluids and intravenous antibiotics are baseline care
- Cholecystectomy is the treatment of choice, and the patient should be assessed and prepared for this operation

The main risks of acute laparoscopic cholecystectomy include:
- General complications of surgery such as deep vein thrombosis (DVT), pulmonary embolism (PE), and wound complications
- Bile duct injury <0.3% or bile leak
- Risk of conversion to open up to 4%
- Reoperation
- Bowel and/or other visceral injury

Q. 2.3 if you are presented with the CT scan images below – what is the diagnosis and how will you manage this patient?

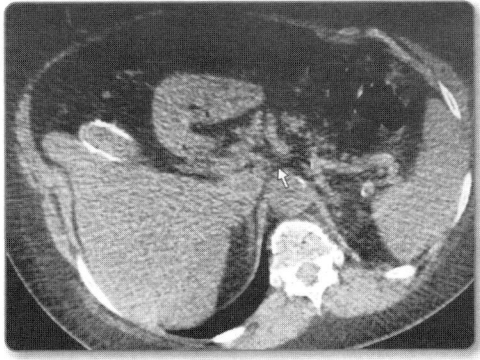

This is an image of a *porcelain* gallbladder and is recognised as a "gallbladder" wall which is heavily calcified. This is usually associated with a large number of gallstones as well as a diagnosis of chronic cholecystitis. There is an association with gallbladder cancer, but this association has neither been confirmed nor proven. Surgery to remove the gallbladder is generally offered to most patients if they are fit enough.

Further reading

Ansaloni L, Pisano M, Coccolini F, et al. 2016 WSES guidelines on acute calculous cholecystitis. World J Emerg Surg 2016; 11:25.

Association of Upper Gastrointestinal Surgeons of Great Britain and Ireland. Pathway for the management of acute gallstone diseases. 2015.

DesJardins H, Duy L, Scheirey C, Schnelldorfer T. Porcelain Gallbladder: Is Observation a Safe Option in Select Populations? J Am Coll Surg 2018; 226:1064–1069.

https://cks.nice.org.uk/cholecystitis-acute#!scenario [Accessed 1st April 2023]

Schnelldorfer T. Porcelain Gallbladder: A Benign Process or Concern for Malignancy?. J Gastrointest Surg 2013; 17:1161–1168.

Stephen AE, Berger DL. Carcinoma in the porcelain gallbladder: A relationship revisited. Surgery 2001; 129:699–703.

Scenario 3

Bile leak

A 23-year-old woman is admitted with acute abdominal pain 2 days after a laparoscopic cholecystectomy.

Q. 3.1 How would you manage this patient?

When managing such a patient or anyone that presents so soon to hospital after surgery the initial answer must always begin with the "*A*irway, *B*reathing, and *C*irculation" (ABC) of resuscitation followed by a careful history and examination. In this scenario, you must add that you will ensure that you look at the patient's recent operative records paying particular attention to the operation and whether it was difficult, if there was any excessive bleeding and also whether clear anatomy was documented when dissecting Calot's triangle. *A phone call to the consultant who undertook the operation will also be helpful.* This patient requires serum investigations as well as intravenous antibiotics as indicated, oxygen and analgesia as well as blood cultures. Imaging is best served with an urgent ultrasound, but if the patient is exhibiting systemic inflammatory response syndrome (SIRS), it is also worth considering an urgent CT scan as well as a return to theatre with a laparoscopy. Possible differential diagnosis includes:

- Bile leak from "cystic duct" stump
- Bleed from the "cystic" artery stump or "gallbladder" fossa
- Bile duct injury
- Suspected other visceral injury
- Hepatic abscess

Q. 3.2 How would you manage the patient if the CT scan shows fluid only in the abdomen and intact biliary anatomy?

The fluid will need to be drained and is most likely to be bile. Bile can leak from the cystic duct stump as a result of a surgical clip coming loose, but generally is related to an increase in the pressure in the bile duct due to a distal obstruction. The distal obstruction can be due to a stricture of the bile duct or more likely a stone.

In this scenario, a percutaneous drain is recommended which is preferably placed under ultrasound guidance. This is followed by ERCP. The ERCP will delineate biliary anatomy, identify the leak and allow a stent to be placed in the bile duct which will help to dry up the leak by creating a path of least resistance for the passage of bile through the main duct rather than the leak. If a stent is not possible, a sphincterotomy usually is enough to divert the bile away from the leak. If there is a tear or damage to the bile duct noted, then a stent is always preferable.

In rare cases if the leakage does not settle, a larger stent may be required. This management is adequate for most patients.

Key points:
- Resuscitate the patient
- Identify the presence of bile in the abdomen
- Drain the bile
- Control the leak with an ERCP

Please see below Strasberg's classification of biliary injury post-cholecystectomy, which is pertinent to the specialist trainee.

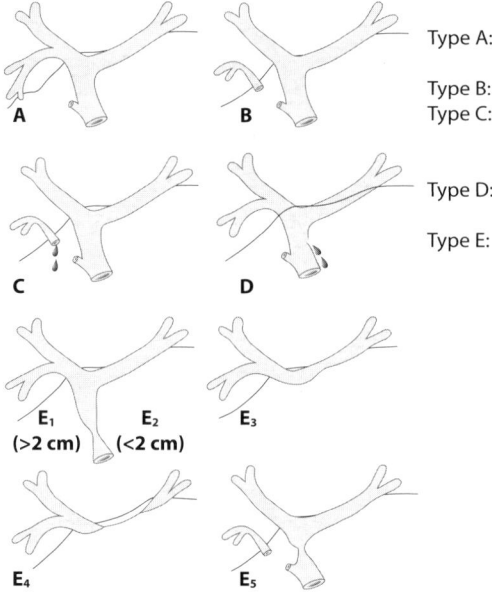

Type A: Bile leak from cystic duct stump or gallbladder fossa (duct of Luschka)
Type B: Damage to an aberrant posterior sectoral duct
Type C: Bile leak from an aberrant right hepatic duct that is not communicating with the main duct
Type D: Lateral injury to the main duct with no loss of continuity
Type E: 1–5 as per Bismuth's classification—circumferential injury of the main duct (transection)
- \>2 cm from confluence
- <2 cm from confluence
- Injury at the confluence
- Separation of major ducts at the confluence
- Complete occlusion of all bile ducts

Further reading

de'Angelis N, Catena F, Memeo R, et al. 2020 WSES guidelines for the detection and management of bile duct injury during cholecystectomy. World J Emerg Surg 2021; 16:30.

Scenario 4

Acute pancreatitis

A 68-year-old woman is admitted with a diagnosis of acute gallstone pancreatitis.

Q. 4.1 How would you determine the diagnosis and manage this condition?

The diagnosis of acute pancreatitis requires two of the following three features:
1. Abdominal pain consistent with acute pancreatitis (acute onset of a persistent, severe, and epigastric pain often radiating to the back)
2. Serum lipase activity (or amylase activity) at least three times greater than the upper limit of normal
3. Characteristic findings of acute pancreatitis on contrast-enhanced computed tomography (CECT) and less commonly magnetic resonance imaging (MRI) or transabdominal ultrasonography

If abdominal pain suggests strongly that acute pancreatitis is present, but the serum amylase and/or lipase activity is less than three times the upper limit of normal, as may be the case with delayed presentation, imaging will be required to confirm the diagnosis. If the diagnosis of acute pancreatitis is established by abdominal pain and by increases in the serum pancreatic enzyme activities, a CT is not usually required for diagnosis in the emergency room or on admission to the hospital.

Further management of a patient with acute pancreatitis will include:
- Confirmation of diagnosis
- Stratifying the severity of the disease
- Monitoring for complications of pancreatitis
- Treating the complications

Patients require analgesia, supplemental oxygen, serum investigations including full blood count (FBC), urea and electrolytes (U&Es), clotting, arterial blood gases, CRP, calcium (bone profile), liver function tests, amylase and lipase.

An ultrasound is the first-line imaging investigation, as gallstones need to be ruled out as they are the most common cause of pancreatitis.

Patients are usually dehydrated and in extreme pain when they come to hospital, so adequate analgesia as well as oxygen is required with IV fluids. In some cases when the patient is scoring high on modified early warning score (MEWS) or SIRS, further monitoring with a urinary catheter to measure adequate urine output is also highly recommended.

Q. 4.2 What are the common causes of pancreatitis?

Common causes of pancreatitis should be listed as follows:
- Gallstones

- Alcohol-induced
- Post-ERCP
- Traumatic pancreatitis
- Hyperlipidaemia
- Hypercalcaemia
- Drug-induced
- Idiopathic

Q. 4.3 How would you stratify the severity of the disease?

- APACHE (*A*cute *P*hysiologic *A*ssessment and *C*hronic *H*ealth *E*valuation) scoring system
- Ranson's or Glasgow criteria
- BISAP (Bedside Index of Severe Acute Pancreatitis)
- PANC-3 (three variables in 24 hours; high haematocrit, high BMI and presence of pleural effusion on chest X-ray)
- HAPS (Harmless Acute Pancreatitis Score)
- Japanese Severity score

Most scoring systems require the score to be calculated over 48 hours. The APACHE scoring is immediate but has a greater positive predictive value after 48 hours – it should be used in conjunction with the serum CRP and if more than 8 with a CRP of more than 150 then the patient can be diagnosed with severe acute pancreatitis with care and further management of the patient suggested to be with critical care physician involvement or on the high dependency unit.

Key point: Whichever scoring system you choose to use please ensure that you know the variables involved in the scoring system.

Q. 4.4 How would you distinguish between mild and severe acute pancreatitis?

"An acute inflammatory process of the pancreas with variable involvement of other regional tissues or remote organ systems"
- *Mild acute pancreatitis* is self-limiting and resolves in 48 hours with little or no involvement of other organs
- *Severe acute pancreatitis* involves more than one organ failure and/or local complication such as pancreatic necrosis, pseudocyst or abscess

Be prepared to discuss systemic inflammatory response syndrome (SIRS).
SIRS:
- Temperature <36°C or >38°C
- Heart rate >90 beats/min
- Respiratory rate >20 breaths/min or $Paco_2$ <32 mmHg
- White blood cell count >12,000 or <4,000 cells/mm^3

An early CT scan is justified in scenarios where the diagnosis is uncertain in order to rule out another possible cause of an acute abdomen such as a perforated viscous, small/large bowel ischaemia, abdominal aortic aneurysm and acute pyelonephritis.

This is an important differential as the initial management of acute pancreatitis is nonoperative whereas intestinal infarction requires surgery.

Further reading

Bradley EL 3rd. A clinically based classification system for acute pancreatitis. Summary of the International Symposium on Acute Pancreatitis, Atlanta, Ga, September 11 through 13, 1992. Arch Surg 1993; 128:586–590.

Scenario 5

Severe acute pancreatitis

A patient presents with severe acute pancreatitis.

Q. 5.1 How would you manage their condition?
- If there is diagnostic doubt, then CT should be considered
- The diagnosis can be made by a combination of history, examination and serum diagnostic tests
- Ideally, patients should be nursed in a critical care setting with careful attention to analgesia, intravenous fluid replacement, supplemental oxygen and organ system monitoring
- Urine output, oxygen saturation, blood pressure should be monitored
- There is no role for antibiotics in the early management of severe acute pancreatitis. Early, inappropriate use simply encourages the emergence of multiple resistant microbes at a later stage
- Attention should be paid to nutrition and current evidence indicates that patients should be allowed oral calorie intake as tolerated. The concept of "pancreas rest" is obsolete
- Early surgical treatment is not indicated in severe acute pancreatitis
- Fluid collections are part of the pathophysiology of the disease and do not require drainage

Q. 5.2 What features would you look for on a CT scan in patients with a diagnosis of severe acute pancreatitis?
Once a diagnosis is made, the following features can be seen in pancreatitis.
- Pancreatic necrosis – poor parenchymal necrosis of the pancreas (**Figure a** showing acute interstitial oedematous pancreatitis)
- Pseudocyst of the pancreas – although this is typically a late finding (**Figure b**)
- Walled off necrosis (**Figure c**)
- Infected pancreatic necrosis (**Figure d**)
- Acute necrotic collections (**Figure e**)

Please see the images of examples of the relevant CT scan findings described above which can be seen in patients with severe acute pancreatitis.

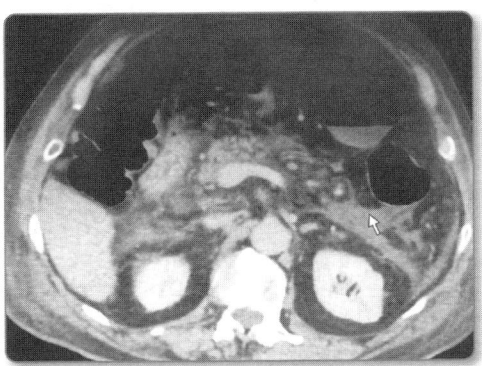

Figure a CT scan image showing acute interstitial oedematous pancreatitis – this is seen in the very early stages of acute pancreatitis – note the local swelling and small degree of collection below the head and tail of the pancreas.

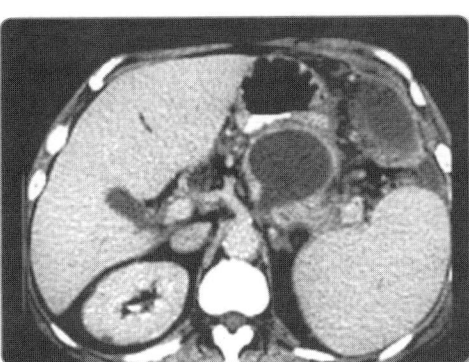

Figure b CT scan image depicting a pancreatic pseudocyst – note the thick white outer wall of the cyst filled cavity below the air-filled stomach.

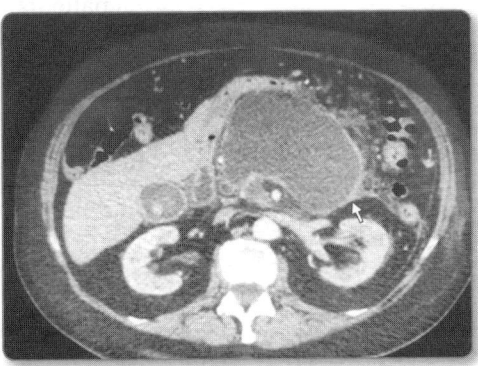

Figure c Computed tomography (CT) scan image showing "walled-off necrosis," which can be managed using endoscopic ultrasound (EUS) and placement of an AXIOS stent – all interventions are carried out depending upon local expertise.

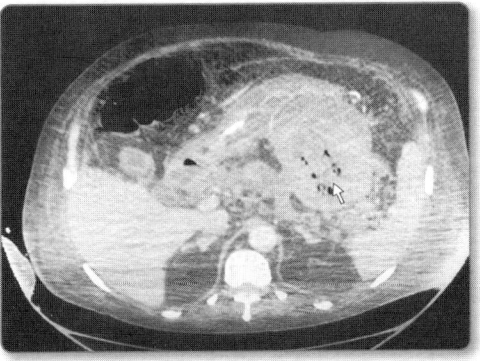

Figure d CT scan image with arrow indicating infected pancreatic necrosis with a large peri-pancreatic collection containing gas. The tip of the nasogastric tube can be seen in the distal stomach.

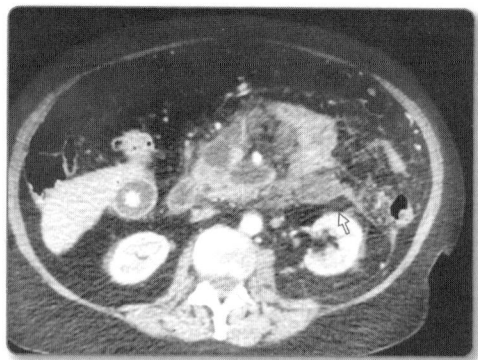

Figure e CT scan image showing acute necrotic collection with a large gallstone also evident in the gallbladder – a case of severe acute gallstone pancreatitis.

Q. 5.3 What management options are available for patients with severe acute pancreatitis and walled off necrosis?

Such patients should have the basic essential care of high-dependency unit (HDU), close monitoring and ideally delayed treatment with the following interventions being possible:
- Endoscopic drainage of the area of necrosis using endoscopic ultrasound techniques
- Percutaneous radiological drainage of the area of necrosis – this may give the patient a sustained pancreatic fistula
- Laparoscopic or open necrosectomy – requires surgery and the relevant expertise available in the department
- Minimal access necrosectomy

Q. 5.4 How would you manage a bleeding complication in a patient with severe acute pancreatitis (they may present with haematemesis, melaena or sudden collapse with hypovolaemia)?

In such a question the initial answer must be the basic management of a patient who is haemodynamically unstable. This is the ABC and resuscitation. In addition, this patient will require urgent CT scan with angiography followed by possible mesenteric angiography and embolisation of the bleeding vessel.

CT angiography consists of a non-contrast phase followed by an early arterial phase CT scan. Selective mesenteric angiography is an invasive technique which requires selective catheterisation of the hepatic artery and superior mesenteric artery.

False aneurysms in patients with severe acute pancreatitis can arise from any of the following:
- Superior mesenteric artery
- Inferior pancreaticoduodenal artery
- Superior pancreaticoduodenal artery
- Gastroduodenal artery
- Splenic artery

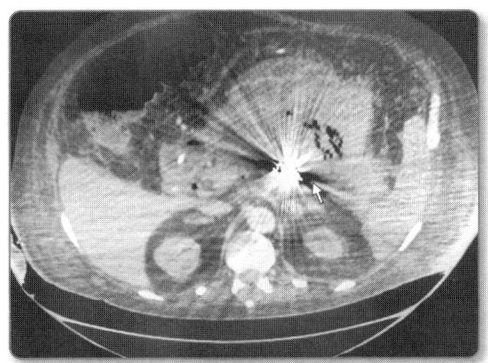

CT scan image with an arrow indicating embolisation coils in a false aneurysm of the splenic artery used to control bleeding.

Further reading

Baron TH. American Gastroenterological Association Clinical Practice Update: Management of Pancreatic Necrosis. Gastroenterology 2019; pii:S0016-5085(19)41293-6.

Goodchild G, Chouhan M, Johnson GJ. Practical guide to the management of acute pancreatitis Frontline Gastroenterol 2019; 10:292–299.

Isaji S, Takada T, Kawarada Y, et al. JPN Guidelines for the management of acute pancreatitis: surgical management. J Hepatobiliary Pancreat Surg 2006; 13:48–55.

Leppäniemi A, Tolonen M, Tarasconi A, et al. 2019 WSES guidelines for the management of severe acute pancreatitis. World J Emerg Surg 2019; 14:27.

National Institute for Health and Care Excellence. (2023). Pancreatitis: All NICE products on pancreatitis. Includes any guidance and advice. [online] Available from https://www.nice.org.uk/guidance/conditions-and-diseases/digestive-tract-conditions/pancreatitis [Last accessed Feb., 2023].

Working Party of the British Society of Gastroenterology; Association of Surgeons of Great Britain and Ireland; Pancreatic Society of Great Britain and Ireland; Association of Upper GI Surgeons of Great Britain and Ireland. UK guidelines for the management of acute pancreatitis. Gut 2005; 54:iii1–iii9.

Scenario 6

Jaundice

A 74-year-old man presents with weight loss and jaundice, pale stools and dark urine for about 2–3 weeks.

Q. 6.1 How would you diagnose and manage his condition?

Once a diagnosis of jaundice is made is it important to know how to classify jaundice into prehepatic, hepatic or post-hepatic. For the large majority of scenarios in the Fellow of the Royal College of Surgeons (FRCS) exit examination, you will invariably be presented with an example of post-hepatic jaundice or obstructive jaundice.

Jaundice classification:

Prehepatic	Hepatic	Post-hepatic
• Gilbert's (5%)	• Viral hepatitis	• CHD stones
• Crigler–Najjar (Neonates)	• Alcoholic	• Periampullary tumours
• Dubin–Johnson	• PBC	• Benign CBD (↓ stricture excretion)
• Bilirubin	• PSC	• Pancreatitis
	• Haemochromatosis	• Pseudocyst
	• Wilson's	• Cholangiocarcinoma
	• Pregnancy	

Investigations required include serum tests including full blood count (FBC), urea and electrolytes (U&E), liver enzymes, clotting profile and C-reactive protein (CRP). Further tests are carried out if required to determine whether the patient has unconjugated or conjugated hyperbilirubinaemia as set out in the table below.

Test	Prehepatic	Hepatic	Post-hepatic
Total bilirubin	Normal/Increased	Increased	Increased
Conjugated bilirubin	Normal	Increased	Increased
Unconjugated (Conj) bilirubin	Normal/Increased	Increased	Normal
Urobilinogen (UB)	Normal/Increased	Decreased	Decreased/None
Urine colour	Normal	Dark (UB + Conj)	Dark (Conj)
Stool colour	Normal	Normal/Pale	Pale
Conjugated bilirubin in urine	Not present	Present	Present

Further investigations will centre on determining the cause of obstructive jaundice and then the relief of jaundice.
- Ultrasound of the abdomen
- CT scan ± MRI including a magnetic resonance cholangiopancreatography (MRCP)
- Endoscopic retrograde cholangiopancreatography (ERCP) for any distal bile duct stricture or occlusion together with biopsy and/or brush cytology for a tissue diagnosis
- Percutaneous transhepatic biliary drainage (PTBD) with cholangiogram (PTC) for occlusion either more proximally in the biliary tree or not accessible by ERCP

Q. 6.2 What does this MRCP image show and how will you manage this patient with obstructive jaundice?

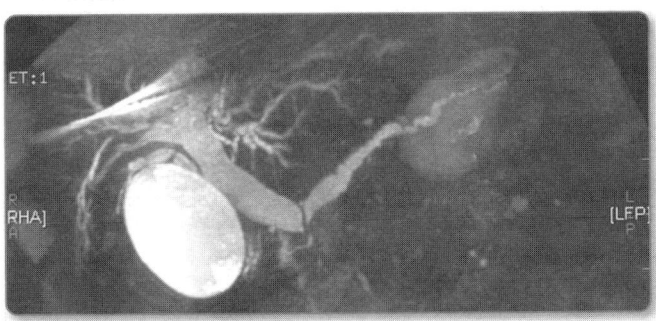

Image shows a "***double duct sign***" (dilatation of both the bile and main pancreatic ducts) this can be due to:
- Ampullary tumour
- Head of pancreas carcinoma
- Duodenal carcinoma
- Distal bile duct carcinoma

Treatment will be to achieve biliary decompression with an endobiliary stent placed by ERCP in the first instance and then PTBD if this fails.

Historically, plastic endobiliary stents were used. These are narrow in calibre (7-Fr) and are prone to occlude and may not provide satisfactory biliary drainage. In modern practice, self-expanding metallic stents are used. A covered metal stent can be removed either endoscopically or at surgery and thus should be used in patients who may be candidates for surgical resection. Uncovered and self-expanding metal stents can be used if there are no plans for subsequent removal.

CT scan images are then required of the abdomen, chest and pelvis to ensure that there is no metastatic disease.

Current NICE guidance in the UK is that an ^{18}fluorodeoxyglucose (FDG)-positron emission tomography (PET)/CT scan aids detection of distant metastases.

Important features to exclude in imaging in order to decide on operability are:
- Presence of liver, peritoneal or lung metastases
- Presence of nodal metastases

- Size of the primary tumour:
  - If the tumour is <3 cm in size it may not abut the portal/superior mesenteric vein.
  - If there is abutment of 180° of the circumference of the superior mesenteric vein and no contact with the superior mesenteric artery, this is regarded as borderline resectable.
  - Encasement of the portal vein/SMV or abutment of 180° of the SMA is regarded as inoperable disease.

Other tests that may be needed include:
- MRI of the liver – specifically for the presence of metastases
- Diagnostic laparoscopy for small volume of peritoneal disease
- Endoscopic ultrasound and nodal biopsy for tissue

Any decision is based on both disease staging and the patient's performance score (PS) and made by a multidisciplinary team (MDT) for either:
- Surgery with adjuvant chemotherapy
- Neoadjuvant chemotherapy for borderline resectable tumours
- Palliative chemotherapy
- Best supportive care

Eastern Co-operative Oncology Group (ECOG) Performance core	Criteria
0	Fully active, able to carry on all pre-disease (activities)? without restriction
1	Restricted in physically strenuous activity but ambulatory and able to carry out work of a light or sedentary nature, e.g. light housework, office work
2	Ambulatory and capable of all self-care but unable to carry out any work activities. Up and about >50% of waking hours
3	Capable of only limited self-care, confined to bed or chair >50% of waking hours
4	Completely disabled, cannot self-care, totally confined to bed or chair
5	Dead

All patients should have access to a hepato-pancreato-biliary (HPB) specialist nurse, Macmillan support in the community as well as dietetic advice, as poor nutrition in patients with periampullary cancers is commonly seen.

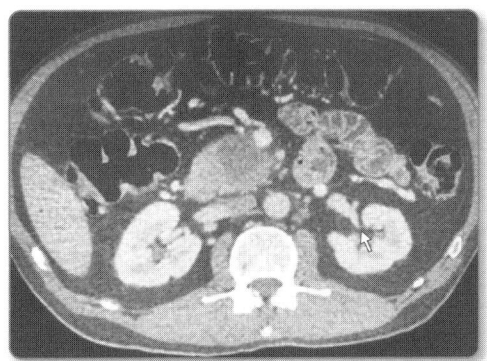

CT scan image of a patient with a head of pancreas mass as depicted with the hypodense lesion – note that there is abutment of 180° of the superior mesenteric vein at the level of origin of the middle colic vein. This patient's disease would be regarded as borderline resectable and may therefore be offered neoadjuvant chemotherapy.

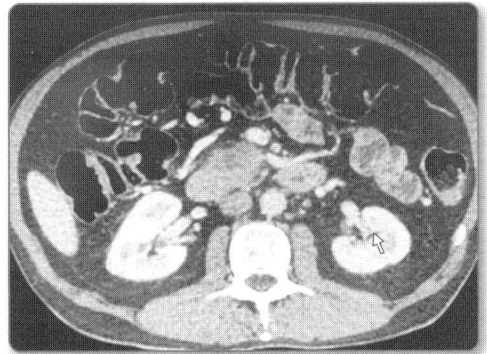

CT scan image showing the superior mesenteric vein (SMV) with a margin away from the tumour mass and the first jejunal branch of the SMV, the superior mesenteric artery (SMA) is clear from the tumour and this lesion is potentially operable.

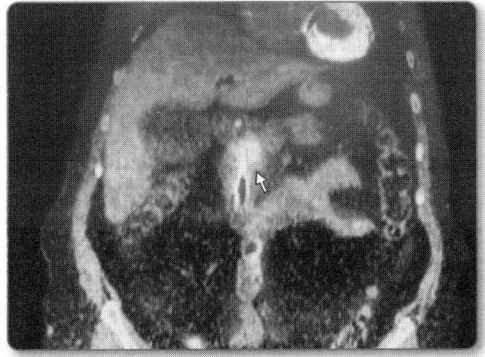

Fluorodeoxyglucose (FDG)-positron emission tomography (PET)-CT showing the endobiliary stent next to a small tumour in the head of the pancreas with no other signs of metastases.

Q. 6.3 If a patient has an operable tumour in the head of the pancreas and is deemed surgically fit for a Whipple pancreaticoduodenectomy, how will you obtain consent from the patient?

Obtaining consent involves a detailed discussion in terms of what the operation involves as well as the risks and benefits.
- General risks of any operation. These can be described in a systematic fashion
- Cardiac
- Respiratory
- Thrombotic [deep vein thrombosis (DVT)/pulmonary embolism (PE)]
- Metabolic (hypokalaemia and hyponatraemia) such as DVT and PE as well as wound infection and dehiscence
- Complications specific to pancreatectomy:
  - Finding unsuspected metastases at surgery
  - Unsuspected unresectability of the tumour
  - Haemorrhage (either during or after surgery)
  - Biliary anastomotic leak (2%)
  - Pancreatic anastomotic leak (up to 30%)
  - Gastric stasis
  - Chyle leak
  - Deep-seated collection
  - Wound infection, breakdown, late incisional hernia
  - Respiratory complications including acute lung injury and chest infection
  - Reoperation
  - Overall procedure-related risk of death of 3–5%
  - Postoperative diabetes mellitus
  - Postoperative exocrine insufficiency

Key points: Most serious complications are rare and inpatient stay can be anything from 10 days to 3 weeks and in some cases longer. Most pancreatic leaks are subclinical and drain fluid is now routinely checked for amylase level at day 3 and the drain removed if normal. A high-volume amylase rich leak requires the drain to stay in longer and in some cases the patients are sent home with the drains in and removed at a later date in clinic.

Further reading

https://www.nccn.org/patients/guidelines/pancreatic/ [Accessed 1st April 2023]

Marchegiani G, Todaro V, Boninsegna E, et al. Surgery after FOLFIRINOX treatment for locally advanced and borderline resectable pancreatic cancer: increase in tumour attenuation on CT correlates with R0 resection. Eur Radiol 2018; 28:4265–4273.

O'Reilly D, Fou L, Hasler E, et al. Diagnosis and management of pancreatic cancer in adults: A summary of guidelines from the UK National Institute for Health and Care Excellence. Pancreatology 2018; 18:962–970.

Tempero MA. NCCN Guidelines Updates: Pancreatic Cancer. J Natl Compr Canc Netw 2019; 17:603–605.

Wagner M, Antunes C, Pietrasz D, et al. CT evaluation after neoadjuvant FOLFIRINOX chemotherapy for borderline and locally advanced pancreatic adenocarcinoma. Eur Radiol 2017; 27:3104–3116.

Scenario 7

Alcoholic liver disease

A patient who has recently been diagnosed with alcoholic liver disease presents with severe jaundice and weight loss as well as abdominal distension.

Q. 7.1 How would you manage his jaundice and investigate his possible diagnosis?

A careful history is required for this patient with an emphasis placed on their relevant past medical history particularly for risk factors associated with the development of liver cirrhosis. A history of travel abroad with any injections received while abroad particularly immunisations, blood transfusions and intravenous drug abuse become pertinent. Patients of South-East Asian origin may be hepatitis B surface antigen carriers and this is relevant so such patients will require a mandatory hepatitis screen. In the history provided above, the alcohol consumption is the likely cause for liver damage, so it is worth knowing the degree and duration of alcohol consumption that the patient has taken over the years (national UK advice for men is ≤ 20 IU and women ≤ 14 IU/week).

Further investigations will centre around determining the cause of jaundice and then relief of jaundice.
- Ultrasound of the abdomen
- CT scan ± MRI including a magnetic resonance cholangiopancreatography (MRCP)
- Endoscopic retrograde cholangiopancreatography (ERCP) for any distal bile duct stricture/occlusion with biopsy and/or brush cytology for a tissue diagnosis
- Percutaneous transhepatic biliary drainage (PTBD) with cholangiogram (PTC) for occlusion either higher up in the biliary tree or not accessible by ERCP

Q. 7.2 What scoring system do you know to help to determine the severity of alcoholic liver disease?

The scoring system used for classifying the degree of liver cirrhosis is called the Child–Pugh classification – below is a table commonly used to determine the score – surgery is only contemplated in patients with a score of A. Points of 1–3 is given for each variable.

Measure	1 point	2 points	3 points
Total serum bilirubin (µmol/L)	<34	34–50	>50
Serum albumin 9 g/dL	>3.5	2.8–3.5	<2.8
Prothrombin time (s)	<4.0	4.0–6.0	>6.0
INR	<1.7	1.7–2.3	>2.3
Ascites	None	Mild	Moderate-to-severe
Hepatic encephalopathy	None	Grade I–II	Grade III–IV

Below is a guide to the interpretation of these results:

Class A
- 5–6 points
- 1–5 years survival rate: 95%

Class B
- 7–9 points
- Moderately severe liver disease
- 1–5 years survival rate: 75%

Class C
- 10–15 points
- Most severe liver disease
- 1–5 years survival rate: 50%

Q. 7.3 In the absence of jaundice what are the treatment options for a patient with a hepatoma?

The treatment algorithm outlined by the Barcelona liver clinic is the most widely used. This combines disease stage with optimal treatment and is seen below.

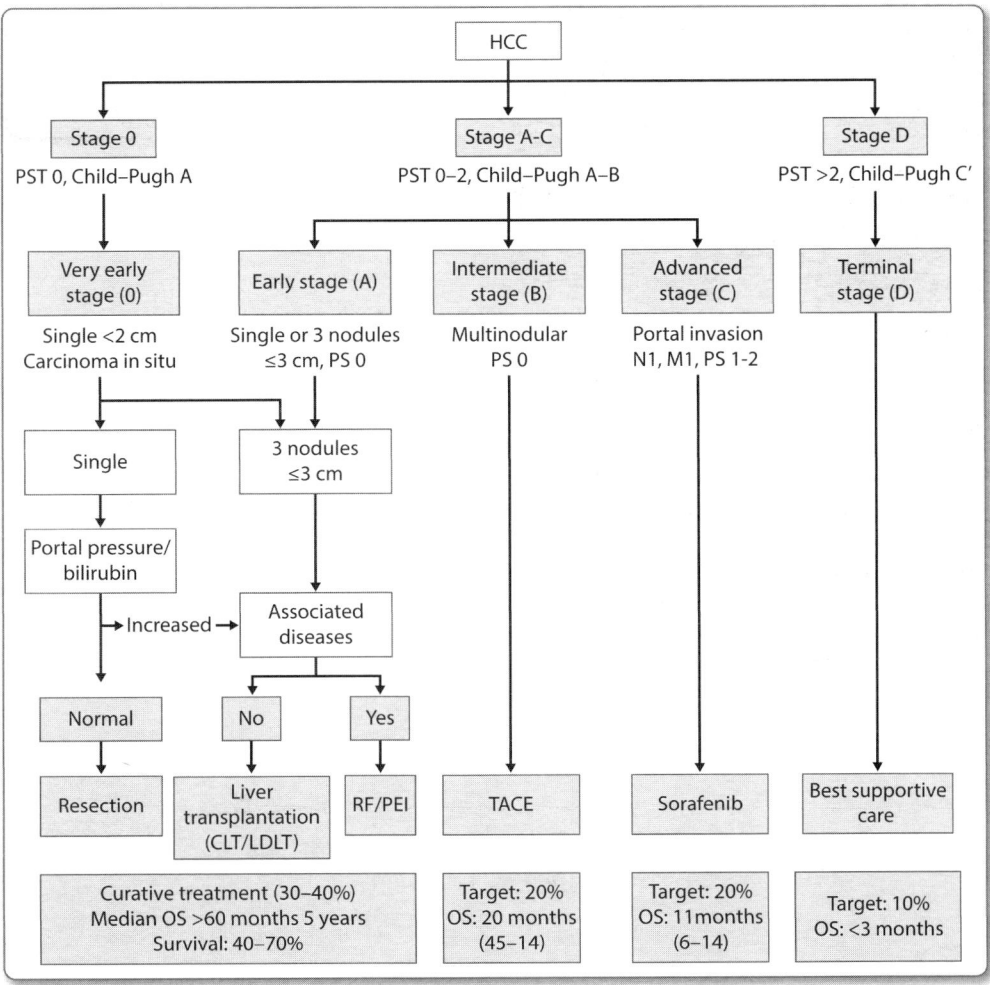

(CLT, cadaveric liver transplant; HCC, hepatocellular carcinoma; LDLT, living donor liver transplant; PEI, percutaneous ethanol injection; RF, radiofrequency; TACE, transarterial chemoembolisation)

Milan criteria: Transplantation considered for decompensated liver disease and hepatocellular carcinoma (HCC) if one lesion not larger than 5 cm, or up to 3 lesions each 3 cm or smaller.

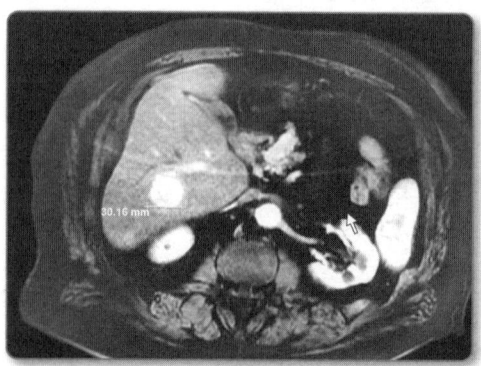

MR image showing a 3-cm hepatoma in the right lobe of the liver.

Further reading

Galanakis N, Kehagias E, Matthaiou N, Samonakis D, Tsetis D. Transcatheter arterial chemoembolization combined with radiofrequency or microwave ablation for hepatocellular carcinoma: a review. Hepat Oncol 2018; 5:HEP07.

Jindal A, Thadi A, Shailubhai K. Hepatocellular Carcinoma: Etiology and Current and Future Drugs. J Clin Experiment Hepatol 2019; 9:221–232.

Raza A, Sood GK. Hepatocellular carcinoma review: current treatment, and evidence-based medicine. World J Gastroenterol 2014; 20:4115–4127.

Scenario 8

Liver metastases

A patient with a known diagnosis of bowel cancer has now been referred with a diagnosis of a liver metastasis which has been picked up on a surveillance computed tomography (CT) scan.

Q. 8.1 What are the basic principles in managing a patient with colorectal liver metastases?

At the first opportunity, this case will be discussed at the regional hepato-pancreato-biliary (HPB) MDT followed by assessment of the patient's fitness for surgery. The MDT will fully stage the tumour burden in the liver by mapping out which lobes/segments/hemi-liver the tumours are located in as well as their proximity to the inflow and outflow blood vessels and whether there will be enough residual tumour volume in order for the liver to function adequately once the affected tumours are removed surgically. An understanding of the liver architecture is also important to try and determine any serious liver parenchymal disease such as an abnormal increase in steatosis (which can arise from chemotherapy) and cirrhosis. A poor liver parenchymal function and reserve will be a contraindication to liver surgery.

Key steps include:
- All patients should have full staging with CT chest and PET-CT as well as liver-specific MR (Primovist). Physical examination as well as serum markers of disease with a carcinoembryonic antigen (CEA) is indicated
- Identification of the tumours in the liver and their exact anatomical location
- If resection of all the tumours will leave sufficient functioning liver volume (>30%)
- Exclusion of extrahepatic disease, and if present, if treatable, such as lung metastases
- Adequate patient medical fitness for surgery ideally tested for by cardiopulmonary exercise testing
- Surgery can take the form of:
  - Classical pathway – bowel first followed by liver surgery
  - Synchronous surgery with both liver and bowel operations undertaken at the same time
  - Liver first surgery with bowel second
  - Downstaging of liver disease followed by restaging and possible liver surgery
- Continued surveillance of follow-up of patients is advised with regular 3–6 monthly CT imaging and serum CEA

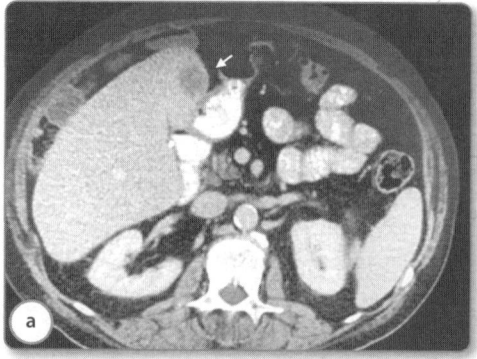
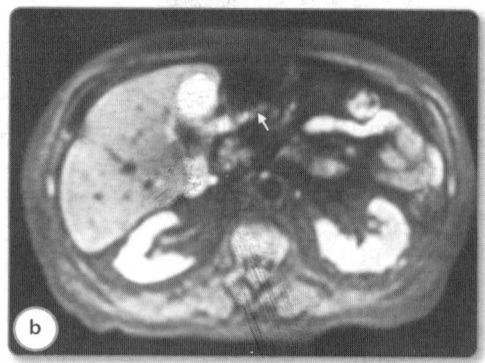
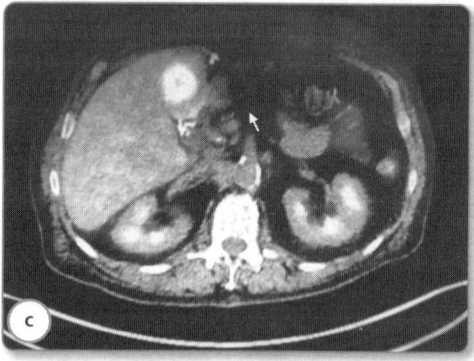

Figures a to c (a) Computed axial tomography (CT) scan image with a hypodense lesion on portal-venous phase, white arrow pointing to lesion in segment IVB; (b) Diffusion-weighted image (DWI) on liver specific MR scan depicting lesion/deposit as hyperintense and (c) PET-CT showing the corresponding colorectal liver metastases deposit.

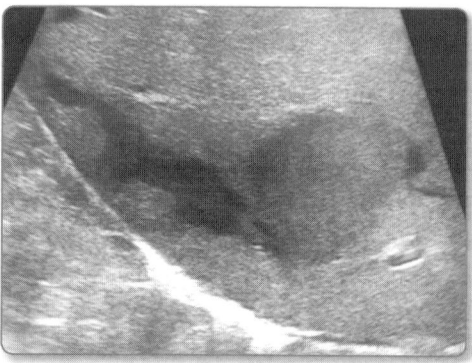

Figure d Intraoperative ultrasound image of the liver during surgery, showing a large metastatic deposit close to the right hepatic vein (for this scenario a right hepatectomy is required).

Q. 8.2 What do you understand by the term down-staging chemotherapy and how to assess patients for potential surgery with advanced metastatic colorectal cancer?

Down-staging chemotherapy is based on the premise that preoperative chemotherapy can potentially reduce the tumour load to allow previously unresectable metastases in the liver to undergo resection. In 2001, Adam et al. showed a 13.5% increase in resectability of patients previously deemed to have unresectable metastases (5-FU, folinic acid and oxaliplatin). Although the overall numbers of patients that can undergo resection remains small, it does provide a benefit to the selected patient with improved overall survival.

When assessing metastatic colorectal cancer, the European Society for Medical Oncology (ESMO) 2014 guidelines have categorised patients into the four groups outlined below:
- Group 0: Upfront resectable disease of the liver and or lung
- Group 1: Potentially, resectable disease – may need preoperative chemotherapy, e.g. FOLFIRI but also KRAS status of patients is important (WT – cetuximab)
- Group 2: Disseminated disease or technically "never" or unlikely resectable – ablative therapies can be used – intermediate intensive treatment
- Group 3: Never-resectable metastatic disease – nonintensive sequential treatment

Other factors such as the biology of the disease should also be considered:
- Synchronous versus metachronous
- Aggressiveness of the tumour
- Progression time (from bowel disease)

Seventy five percent of patients suffer from relapse of disease of which the majority occurs in the liver remnant. The aim of any treatment is for R0 resection where possible as well as the use of systemic chemotherapy to control the disease process at a cellular level.

Q. 8.3 If surgery is not possible what other treatment modalities are you aware of?

As discussed above there are various other measures that you should be aware of in any discussion when presented with a case of advanced metastatic colorectal cancer.
- The use of ablative measures such as radiofrequency and/or microwave ablation
- Ablative measures in conjunction with surgery for liver metastases
- Neoadjuvant chemotherapy for unresectable disease followed by postoperative FOLFOX if resected
- Systemic chemotherapy alone or palliative chemotherapy

Further reading

Adam R, Avisar E, Ariche A, et al. Five-year survival following hepatic resection after neoadjuvant therapy for nonresectable colorectal. Ann Surg Oncol 2001; 8:347–353.

Adam R, Hoti E, Bredt LC. Evolution of neoadjuvant therapy for extended hepatic metastases – have we reached our (non-resectable) limit? J Surg Oncol 2010; 102:922–931.

Albiin N. MRI of Focal Liver Lesions. Curr Med Imaging Rev 2012; 8:107–116.

Imai K, Adam R, Baba H. How to increase the resectability of initially unresectable colorectal liver metastases: A surgical perspective. Ann Gastroenterol Surg 2019; 3:476–486.

Morine Y, Ikemoto T, Iwahashi S, et al. Clinical Impact of FOLFOXIRI Aiming for Conversion Surgery in Unresectable Multiple Colorectal Liver Metastasis. Anticancer Res 2019; 39:5089–5096.

Van Cutsem E, Cervantes A, Nordlinger B, Arnold D, on behalf of the ESMO Guidelines Working Group. Metastatic colorectal cancer: ESMO Clinical Practice Guidelines for diagnosis, treatment and follow-up. Ann Oncol 2014; 25:iii1–iii9.

Scenario 9

Hilar mass

A deeply jaundiced 68-year-old man with weight loss and severe itching attends your clinic.

Q. 9.1 What will your initial management involve and how will you relieve his jaundice?

Please see *Scenario 6* for the initial part of the answer to this question including jaundice graph and table for jaundice.

Resultant serum investigations identify a picture of obstructive jaundice with a high bilirubin, alkaline phosphatase and an ultrasound have shown dilated intrahepatic biliary tree but a collapsed extrahepatic bile duct and gallbladder.

Please see below an image taken from the CT scan of this patient.

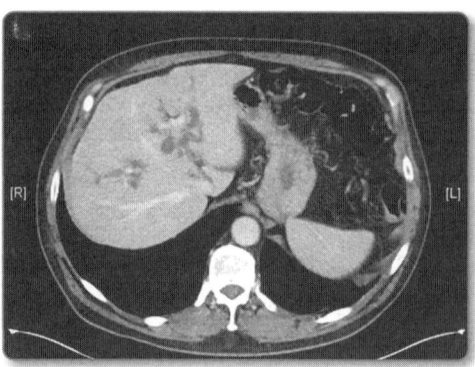

The CT scan depicts intrahepatic duct dilatation with atrophy of the left lobe.

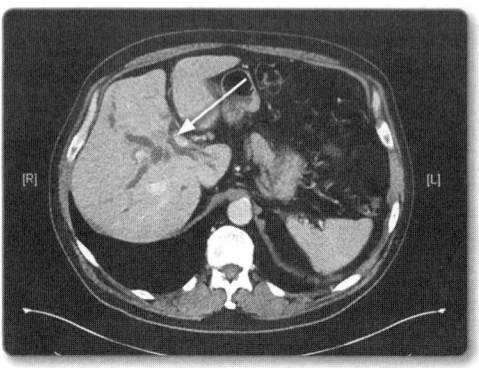

CT image showing the "Hilar" mass with a suspected type IV cholangiocarcinoma (white arrow).

Important aspects to determine resectability:
- Location and staging of tumour – CT scan of the thorax
- Distant and local spread – confirming no small metastatic deposits in the liver is key
- Relationship of arterial and portal inflow of planned remnant lobe
- Volume of size of remnant lobe of liver
- Liver volumetry is also advised to ensure that the future liver remnant is sufficient (>25%)
- If liver volume is not sufficient then one can consider portal vein embolisation
- Adequate biliary drainage of an obstructed system and especially of future remnant lobe – bilirubin that does not come down well, may compromise patient outcome as well as prognosis
- Further imaging recommended includes MR liver with contrast as well as fluorodeoxyglucose (FDG)-positron emission tomography (PET) imaging

Classification of hilar cholangiocarcinoma

Bismuth–Corlette classification of perihilar cholangiocarcinoma (PH-CCA).

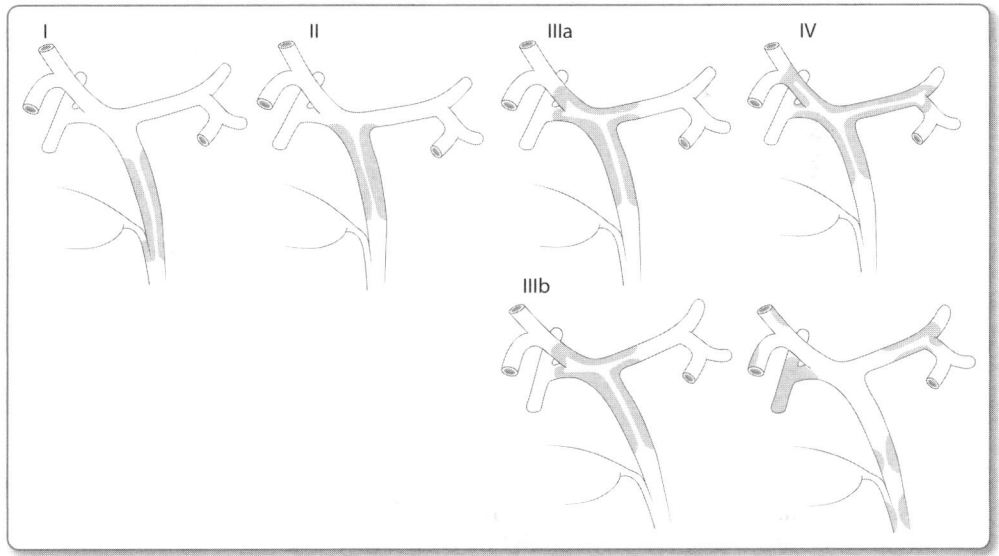

If a tumour is operable then the flowing considerations in planning for surgery should be considered:
- Percutaneous drainage of future remnant first
- Second-step drainage of resection side if bilirubin does not fall
- Also consider drainage of future resection side if portal vein embolisation planned

Resection will involve careful dissection of hilar nodes and vessels with preservation of the vasculature of the remnant liver. In addition, the caudate lobe is resected with the extrahepatic biliary tree excised and reconstruction of the remnant lobe biliary tree with a hepaticojejunostomy. Please see diagram below which details the hilar nodes and harvest, which should be undertaken, particularly stations 8 and 12 for adequate histological staging.

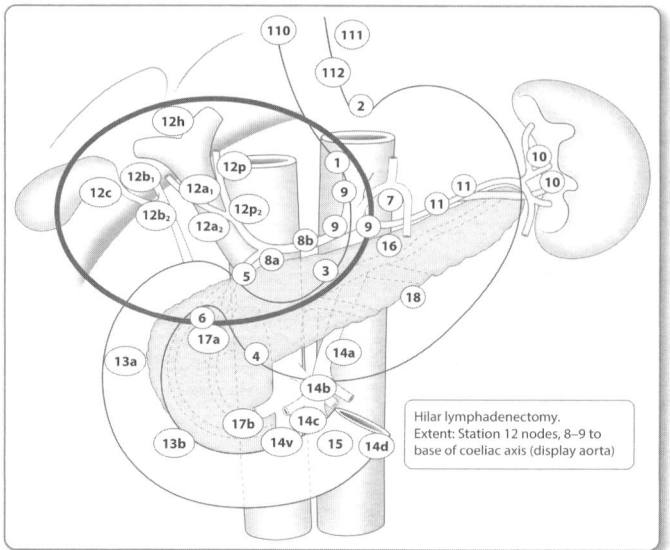

Hilar lymphadenectomy.
Extent: Station 12 nodes, 8–9 to base of coeliac axis (display aorta)

If unresectable, then the plan will involve good biliary drainage and palliation of symptoms with a tissue diagnosis possible from biopsy of any mass and/or brush cytology from percutaneous transhepatic biliary drainage (PTBD).

Postoperatively, at present adjuvant capecitabine is proposed based on the evidence from the BILCAP study results for resected biliary tract cancers over observation alone. Briefly, the study showed an increase in disease-free survival in the capecitabine group from 17.4 to 25.9 months.

In summary:
- Perihilar cholangiocarcinoma (PH-CCA) is a rare tumour
- The majority are not resectable by surgery and so palliation of jaundice with PTBD and stent as well as supportive care is the mainstay of treatment
- About 10% of patients have disease that can be removed
- Surgery requires near faultless preoperative preparation
- Hepatectomy with en bloc caudate resection plus excision of the extrahepatic biliary tree and radical hilar lymphadenectomy followed by Roux hepaticojejunostomy is the most complex non-transplant adult hepatobiliary operation

Further reading

Adeva J, Sangro B, Salati M, et al. Medical treatment for cholangiocarcinoma. Liver Int 2019; 39:123–142.
Bismuth H, Corlette MB. Intrahepatic cholangioenteric anastomosis in carcinoma of the hilus of the liver. Surg Gynecol Obstet 1975; 140:170–178.
Primrose JN, Fox RP, Palmer DH, et al. Capecitabine compared with observation in resected biliary tract cancer (BILCAP): a randomised, controlled, multicentre, phase 3 study. Lancet Oncol 2019; 20:663–673.

Scenario 10

Cystic neoplasm of the pancreas

A patient complained of abdominal pain for weeks and underwent a computed axial tomography (CT) scan which identified a cystic neoplasm of the pancreas.

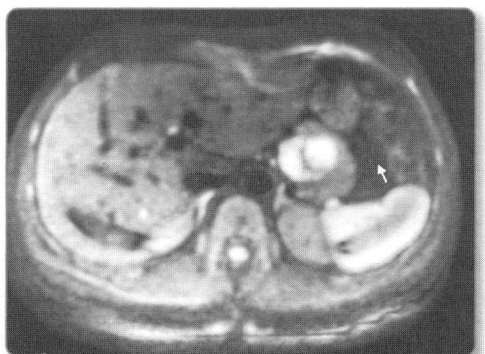
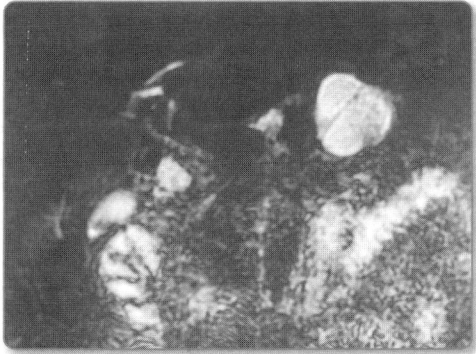

MR image above showing a large cystic neoplasm of the tail of the pancreas, which is closely related to the hilum of the spleen and compressing the stomach above – note the septations in the cyst on the sequences shown.

Q. 10.1 How would you classify cystic neoplasms of the pancreas?

Cystic neoplasms of the pancreas as per the European Study Group on cystic tumours of the pancreas are divided into 'epithelial neoplastic' and 'epithelial non-neoplastic' tumours.
Commone epithelial neoplasms include:
- Intraductal papillary mucinous neoplasm (IPMN) of all types
- Mucinous cystic neoplasm
- Serous cystic neoplasm

Commone epithelial non-neoplastic include:
- Mucinous non-neoplastic cyst
- Enterogenous cyst
- Periampullary duodenal wall cyst

MRI/MRCP is the preferred imaging modality for any cysts considered for surgical resection, followed which an endoscopic ultrasound (EUS) + fine-needle aspiration cytology (FNAC) is recommended. FNAC can help to distinguish between mucinous and nonmucinous cysts. Cyst fluid evaluation for carcinoembryonic antigen

(CEA) (≥192 ng/mL), amylase (indicative of an inflammatory cyst) and cytology is recommended. CEA value of 192 or greater will help to differentiate between mucin producing and non mucin producing cysts. However, as with all cysts a combination of MR findings, mucin content, CEA level and cytology is required to distinguish between benign mucinous cysts and cysts with high-grade dysplasia or an associated invasive carcinoma – so no test should be used in isolation as the diagnostic accuracy of a single test is not sufficient.

Below are the findings on imaging and cytology that raise the suspicion of malignant transformation of a pancreatic cyst/intraductal papillary mucinous neoplasm (IPMN).
- Main pancreatic duct dilatation of between 5 and 9.9 mm or ≥10 mm
- Communication with, or arising from the main pancreatic duct
- Cyst growth rate of ≥5 mm/year
- Increased serum CA-19.9 level (>37 U/mL)
- Enhancing mural nodules (<5 mm) or solid component
- Cyst diameter ≥40 mm

Follow-up of cysts for 3–5 years is recommended. In patients with signs of weight loss, jaundice related to the cyst, new-onset diabetes, pancreatitis and abdominal pain, closer surveillance as well as reassessment and staging of the cyst is required.

Side-branch IPMN is observed for the above factors and surgery considered in cases where there are changes in size, positive cytology for high-grade dysplasia or cancer, mural nodules or solid component. Mixed type IPMN is managed as per main duct IPMN due to a higher risk of malignant transformation.

Q. 10.2 This patient has a 3.5-cm mucinous cystic neoplasm of the pancreas – how would you confirm the diagnosis and what are the treatment options?

In the first instance, this case is discussed at the HPB MDT with details of a careful history including any weight loss, jaundice, new-onset diabetes and pancreatitis. A contrast-enhanced MR pancreas with MRCP is advised to identify any features that suggest surgery is possibly required. This is followed by an EUS + FNAC. 3.5 cm is a large cyst and if EUS confirms that there is mucin then this cyst should be considered for resection. Depending on the location in the pancreas, the cyst will undergo most likely a distal pancreatectomy. If the cyst is closely related to the hilum of the spleen, then a splenectomy will most likely need to be undertaken, otherwise there is no clear evidence to suggest that in all mucinous cystic neoplasms of the pancreas without any proven cancer on cytology, a splenectomy is advised. If frozen section of the transected margin is undertaken then only if there is high-grade dysplasia or cancer, up to a total pancreatectomy may be undertaken (careful counselling required as the patient will become diabetic and require preoperative vaccination as well as antibiotics for life due to loss of spleen).

Absolute and relative indications for surgery in intraductal papillary mucinous neoplasm (IPMN).

Absolute indications	Relative indications
Positive cytology for malignancy/HGD	Growth rate ≥ 5 mm/year
Solid mass	Increased serum levels of CA-19.9 (>37 U/mL)
Jaundice (tumour related)	MPD dilatation between 5 and 9.9 mm
Enhancing mural nodules (≥5 mm)	Cyst diameter of ≥40 mm
MPD dilatation ≥10 mm	New onset diabetes
	Acute pancreatitis (caused by IPMN)
	Enhancing mural nodule (<5 mm)

(HGD, high-grade dysplasia; IPMN, intra-ductal papillary mucinous neoplasm; MPD, main pancreatic duct)

Q. 10.3 What are the risks associated when performing a laparoscopic distal pancreatectomy?

Distal pancreatectomy is an operation largely undertaken by laparoscopic or minimally invasive techniques. Prior to surgery the following steps are required:
- Vaccinations to pre-empt loss of spleen at least 2 weeks before surgery:
  - *Haemophilus influenzae*
  - *Streptococcus pneumoniae*
  - *Neisseria meningitidis*
- Medical fitness for operation
- In terms of consent:
  - Loss of spleen
  - Pancreatic leak/fistula
  - New onset diabetes or worsening of glycaemic control
  - Damage to splenic flexure of colon/greater curvature of stomach
  - Generalised complications of surgery as well as overwhelming sepsis secondary to loss of spleen

Further reading

European Study Group on Cystic Tumours of the Pancreas. European evidence-based guidelines on pancreatic cystic neoplasms. Gut 2018; 67:789–804.

Scholten L, van Huijgevoort NCM, van Hooft JE, Besselink MG, Del Chiaro M. Pancreatic Cystic Neoplasms: Different Types, Different Management, New Guidelines. Visc Med 2018; 34:173–177.

Nilsson LN, Keane MG, Shamali A, et al. Nature and management of pancreatic mucinous cystic neoplasm (MCN): A systematic review of the literature. Pancreatology 2016; 16:1028–1036.

Scenario 11

Choledochal cyst

A young lady presents with vague abdominal pain and an ultrasound scan shows large bile duct with a diameter of 4 cm. There are no stones within the gallbladder or bile duct.

Q. 11.1 What is the differential diagnosis and how will you investigate this further?

In the absence of jaundice one must always start any answer as per before by describing that a full history and clinical examination will take place followed by serum investigations including liver enzymes and CA-19.9, as well as cross-sectional imaging with either a contrast-enhanced computed axial tomography (CT) scan or preferably an MR scan with magnetic resonance cholangiopancreatography (MRCP).

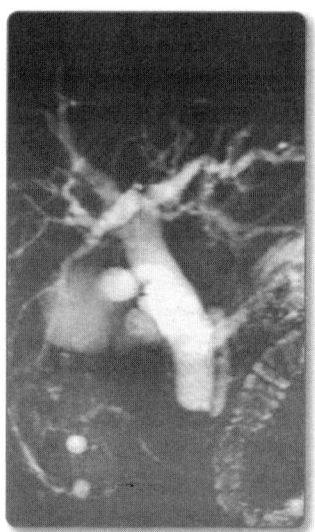

Magnetic resonance cholangiopancreatography image showing a grossly dilated extrahepatic bile duct – the intrahepatic ducts are normal – Type I choledochal cyst.

The differential diagnosis will include:
- Non-obstructing distal bile duct stone
- Distal bile duct cholangiocarcinoma
- Small periampullary tumour

- Head of pancreas tumour
- Choledochal cyst

Choledochal cysts are congenital abnormalities of the bile duct. They present mainly in childhood, but about 20% present in adulthood. It is identified as a disproportionate dilation of the biliary system which can affect both the intra- or extra hepatic biliary tree, or both. They occur predominantly in women and present with vague abdominal complaints.

First classified by Alonso-Lej in 1959 and revised by Totani in 1977 into five subtypes (I–V).

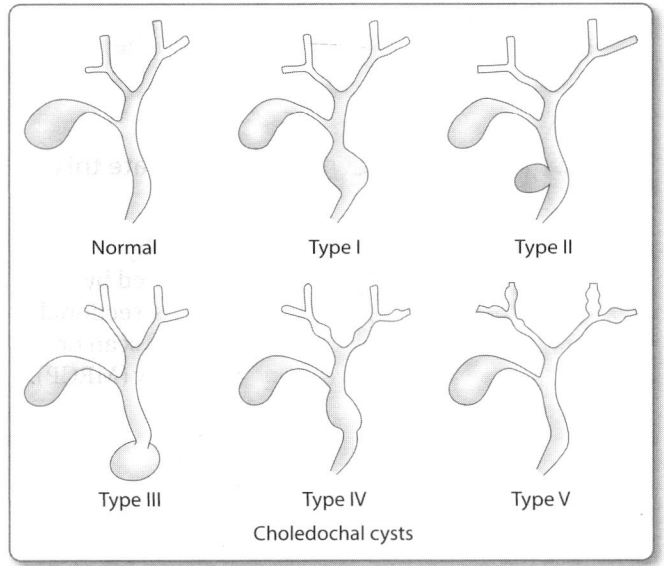

Choledochal cysts

- Type I: Fusiform dilatation of the extrahepatic biliary tree only (IA, Cystic; IB, Focal; and IC, Fusiform)
- Type II: Diverticulum of the common duct (CD)
- Type III: Cystic dilatation of the intramural portion of the CD, also described as a choledochocoele
- Type IV: Dilatation of the intra- and extrahepatic ducts (IVA) both intra- and extrahepatic ducts, (IVB) multiple cysts of extrahepatic ducts only
- Type V: Caroli's disease – dilatation of the intra-hepatic ducts only

Can present with pain, jaundice, cholangitis, malignant stricture and pancreatitis as well as weight loss.

Q. 11.2 What surgical option is available and how would you undertake the operation?

If malignancy is present, then prognosis is poor and survival is low as they are often diagnosed late. Once imaging is carried out treatment ideally rests with surgical resection, with types I–III locally resectable with reconstruction involving hepaticojejunostomy. Treatment for types IV–V can involve partial hepatectomy and relief of obstruction if present, but management here is neither straightforward nor conventional. Surgery for type I–III can be undertaken by minimal access techniques, but largely open surgery is undertaken especially if partial hepatectomy is considered.

Further reading

Khandelwal C, Anand U, Kumar B, Priyadarshi RN. Diagnosis and management of choledochal cysts. Indian J Surg 2012; 74:29–34.

Ulas M, Polat E, Karaman K, et al. Management of choledochal cysts in adults: a retrospective analysis of 23 patients. Hepatogastroenterology 2012; 59:1155–1159.

Scenario 12

Liver trauma

After a major road traffic accident, a patient is in extreme abdominal pain and has a suspected liver injury.

Q. 12.1 What are your initial management steps for a patient with liver trauma?

For this question always answer with the initial assessment of a patient in a trauma or emergency situation. ABC of resuscitation with establishment of the patients' airway, ensure breathing has been assessed, intravenous resuscitation with at least ×2 wide bore cannulae and fluid replacement (Hartmann's solution or colloids for a haemodynamically unstable patient). A patient with suspected intra-abdominal trauma, particularly a liver injury, the history of the accident is of importance – especially high impact collisions. The patient may also describe intense abdominal pain as well as other injuries and you must make the examiner aware that you will assess the patient for any other serious injuries – initially if the patient is stable a CT scan of the C-spine, thorax, abdomen and pelvis is important and mandatory with intravenous contrast.

Rules for fluid resuscitation include:
- Limit crystalloids
- Resuscitate with blood products:
  - 1:1:1 packed red blood cells (PRBCs): fresh frozen plasma (FFP): Platelets
- Consider tranexamic acid:
  - Antifibrinolytic agent that prevents clot breakdown
  - ≤3 hours: 1 g bolus, followed by 1 g over 8 hours
- CRASH-2 trial:
  - 1.5% all-cause mortality reduction
  - 0.8% haemorrhage mortality reduction

With all such patients in resuscitation, it is important to continuously monitor the patient with close liaison with the trauma team as well as the anaesthetic staff – the physiological signs below are important to be aware of:
- >4–5 litres of suspected blood loss
- pH ≤ 7.25
- Core temperature < 36°C
- Diffuse bleeding

In patients with suspected liver trauma, the points below help to ascertain a suspected liver injury. In the UK, blunt trauma (60%) is the most common cause of liver injury with penetrating trauma more often seen in the USA/South Africa (65/85%).
- *Blunt trauma*: Look for signs of bruising on the abdomen and on back
- *Crush injury*: Direct blow to the abdomen
  - Central portion of liver is affected – IV, V and VIII

- Fractures of ribs are also a sign of possible liver injury.
- Decelerating injury: RTA, attachments to the diaphragm and falciform ligament can be sheared.
- Parenchymal fractures in right lobe – VI/VII and V/VIII

The mainstay of treatment for any liver injury is conservative for most patients – the degree of injury is classified as per the *American Association for the Surgery of Trauma* (AAST) classification of liver trauma (I–V). Even grade IV and sometimes V can be managed with conservative measures.

Any haemodynamic instability is firstly treated with resuscitation and arteriography with embolisation. This treatment is almost certainly regarded as first choice. Quick and decisive action in this regard improves outcomes for patients with liver trauma and can save lives without the need for a laparotomy.

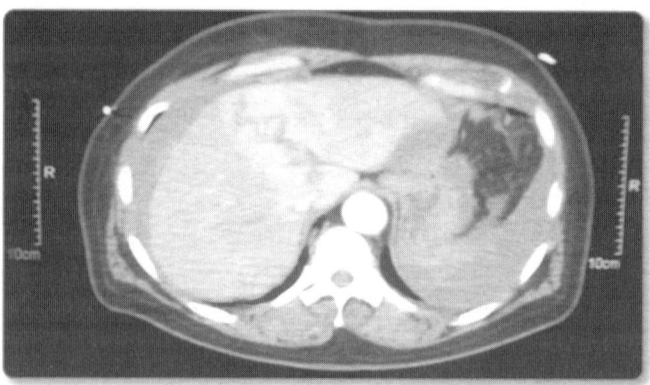

Computed axial tomography (CT) scan image showing a fracture of the liver with fluid in the abdominal cavity consistent with haemorrhage/bile.

AAST classification of liver trauma

Grade	Haematoma	Laceration/Vascular
I	Subcapsular, <10% surface area (SA)	Capsular tear, <1 cm parenchymal depth
II	Subcapsular, 10–50% SA Intraparenchymal <10 cm diameter	Capsular tear 1–3 cm parenchymal depth, <10 cm length
III	Subcapsular, >50% surface area of ruptured subcapsular or parenchymal haematoma intraparenchymal > 10 cm	Capsular tear >3 cm parenchymal depth vascular injury – with active bleeding contained within liver parenchyma
IV		Parenchymal disruption involving 25–75% hepatic lobe or involves 1–3 Couinaud segments
		Vascular injury with active bleeding breaching the liver parenchyma into the peritoneum
V		Parenchymal disruption involving >75% of hepatic lobe
		Vascular: Juxtahepatic venous injuries (retrohepatic vena cava/central major hepatic veins)

Q. 12.2 What are the basic principles that govern whether an operation is required or not?

The following are recognised as reasons for an urgent laparotomy.
- Multiple injuries with suspected bowel perforation and patients with peritonitis
- Failure to maintain haemodynamic stability with IV fluid resuscitation alone
- Continued bleeding of patient after embolisation – decreasing haemoglobin even after blood transfusions and sustained hypovolaemic shock after continued IV resuscitation

Surgery is rarely undertaken with most liver trauma. >80% is managed with conservative measures and interventional radiology. Any surgery undertaken is designed to control haemorrhage from the damaged liver and the liver itself does not require any repair, and rarely resection – patients in such a condition are grossly fluid depleted, exhibit a profound inflammatory response and may well have a clotting abnormality.

Patients require full intubation and general anaesthetic with both arterial and venous monitoring as well as a urinary catheter.

A midline laparotomy is undertaken and with clearance of any blood, and packing of the peritoneal cavity with large swabs. The liver should be packed around it to close the "injury" often seen as a large fracture in the capsule and parenchyma. To control bleeding, a pringle clamp (clamp applied to the porta hepatis) can be applied and in extreme circumstances (e.g. if the patient remains unstable despite packing and attempting the Pringle manoeuvre), a caval or hepatic vein injury is more likely. In this scenario, total vascular exclusion can be applied but the prognosis is poor in such circumstances with survival which is not always possible.

If the patient remains stable after packing and there are no other injuries, the abdomen is closed with the packs remaining in situ – the patient should be kept on the intensive care unit with close monitoring:
- Warm the patient
- Correct any coagulopathy
- Correct any acid-base disturbance
- Re-image the patient if necessary necessary, with IV contrast CT
- Further arteriography and embolisation may be required

Re-laparotomy is considered at least after 48–72 hours and when the patient is stable. Indications for stability include corrected coagulopathy and no further decrease in haemoglobin. Removal of packs usually is all that is required and again a completion hepatectomy is rarely undertaken. Sometimes a small drain can be inserted in case the patient develops a bile leak as a result of the parenchymal damage. Any resultant high-volume bile leak is managed conservatively with ERCP and stent indicated on occasion.

Complications of liver trauma include:
- Bile leak (Nagano classification)
- Liver abscess formation
- Liver failure
- Jaundice and coagulopathy

Nagano classification of bile leak into four types:
1. Type A: Minor leaks from small bile radicles on the surface of the liver which are usually self-limiting

2. Type B: Leaks from inadequate closure of the major bile duct branches on the liver's surface
3. Type C: Injury to the main duct commonly near the hilum
4. Type D: Leakage due to a transected duct disconnected from the main duct

Treatment of types A to D

- Type A leaks usually close spontaneously with external drainage although sometimes ERCP and sphincterotomy may be required
- Types B and C:
  - These can be managed by ERCP and stenting combined with drainage of the bile collection.
- Type D leaks:
  - Require surgery and bilioenteric anastomosis or, if the draining segment is small, fibrin glue occlusion or acetic acid ablation.
  - Sometimes operative excision of the excluded segment may be required.

Overall outcome of liver trauma can be quoted as per below:
- Blunt trauma mortality: 10–30%
- Penetrating mortality: 0–10%
- Overall mortality is 10–12%
  - Grade I: 11%
  - Grade II: 10%
  - Grade III/IV: 13%
  - Grade V: 33%

Further reading

Binz S, McCollester J, Thomas S, et al. CRASH-2 Study of Tranexamic Acid to Treat Bleeding in Trauma Patients: A Controversy Fueled by Science and Social Media. J Blood Transfus 2015; 2015:874920.

Como JJ, Bokhari F, Chiu WC, et al. Practice management guidelines for selective nonoperative management of penetrating abdominal trauma. J Trauma 2010; 68:721–733.

Di Saverio S, Catena F, Filicori F, et al. Predictive factors of morbidity and mortality in grade IV and V liver trauma undergoing perihepatic packing: single institution 14 years experience at European trauma centre. Injury 2012; 43:1347–1354.

Lin BC, Fang JF, Chen RJ, Wong YC, Hsu YP. Surgical management and outcome of blunt major liver injuries: experience of damage control laparotomy with perihepatic packing in one trauma centre. Injury 2014; 45:122–127.

Nagano Y, Togo S, Tanaka K, et al. Risk factors and management of bile leakage after hepatic resection. World J Surg 2003; 27:695–698.

Schweizer W, Tanner S, Baer HU, et al. Management of traumatic liver injuries. Br J Surg 1993; 80:86–88.

Srinivasan T, Wig JD, Gupta R, et al. Complex Hepatic Injuries: an Audit from a Tertiary Center. Eur J Trauma Emerg Surg 2007; 34:287–293.

Scenario 13

Non-alcoholic fatty liver disease

A 58-year-old man with a BMI of 41 attends your clinic. He has been referred to your clinic with deranged LFTs and an ultrasound scan revealing non-alcoholic fatty liver disease.

Q. 13.1 How many morbidly obese patients do you think would have co-existing non-alcoholic fatty liver disease (NAFLD)?

Nearly 94% of obese patients with body mass index (BMI) > 30 have NAFLD. Patients classed as being overweight (BMI > 25) would have NAFLD in 67% of cases. Furthermore, nearly 25% of people with normal BMI can have NAFLD.

Q. 13.2 Can you define NAFLD and is it included in NICE guideline for Bariatric Surgery?

It is a wide spectrum of liver damage caused by the presence of fat in >5% of the hepatocytes, in the population consuming less 70 g/week for women and less 140 g/week for men of alcohol consumption.

On its own, NAFLD is not included in the NICE guidelines for bariatric operations; however, it is a part of metabolic syndrome in obese patients and hence eligible as part of other obesity related co-morbidities like diabetes and hypertension.

Q. 13.3 What would be your expectation of resolution of NAFLD after bariatric operations?

Meta-analysis of bariatric surgery results in an improvement of histopathological features of NAFLD in the majority of simple fatty liver disease. However, once non-alcoholic steatohepatitis (NASH) settles in, improvement happens to a lesser degree. In cases that have already progressed to fibrosis or cirrhosis, resolution is fairly poor.

Q. 13.4 Can you enumerate some bariatric operations that you are aware of?

Nearly all bariatric procedures are now performed laparoscopically and will increasingly be robotic. Such bariatric operations include:
- Roux-en-Y gastric bypass
- Sleeve gastrectomy (most common worldwide)

- Gastric band (much less used currently)
- Duodenal switch
- Biliopancreatic diversion

Further reading

Non-alcoholic fatty liver disease (NAFLD): assessment and management (2016) NICE guideline NG49.

Cusi K, I Scott, B Diana, et al. American Association of Clinical Endocrinology clinical practice guideline for the diagnosis and management of nonalcoholic fatty liver disease in primary care and endocrinology clinical settings: Co-sponsored by the American Association for the Study of Liver Diseases (AASLD). Endocr Pract 2022; 28:528-562.

Chapter 10

Oesophagogastric surgery

Pranav H Patel, Nima Abbassi-Ghadi, Sacheen Kumar

Scenario 1

Gastric cancer

A 54-year-old lady is referred to your tertiary oesophago-gastric cancer service on the 2-week-wait pathway. The referral states she has a 'T2 lesser curve adenocarcinoma'.

Q. 1.1 How would you manage this patient?

Completion of initial assessment

Complete a full history and clinical examination with initial assessment of airway patency, and with a respiratory and cardiac examination.

Abdominal examination would encompass peripheral stigmata of malignancy including scleral icterus and lymphadenopathy (including supraclavicular fossae).

Proceed to clinically stage the gastric cancer with a CT chest, abdomen and pelvis; staging laparoscopy; endoscopic ultrasound (EUS) and a CT whole body positron emission tomography (PET) if suspected to have metastatic disease.

Note: Endoscopic ultrasound is not part of the standard staging protocol in all institutions; however, it can provide information regarding resectability for early lesions (T1 tumours suitable for endoscopic resection) or advanced lesions suggesting invasion into local structures such as pancreas (T4a or T4b).

The findings will be discussed within a specialist UGI cancer multi-disciplinary team in order to determine a management plan. All staging investigations must be completed prior to final agreed treatment plan.

Q. 1.2 What is the staging criteria?

The staging of gastric cancer is based on the 8th edition of the American Joint Committee on Cancer (AJCC) staging of stomach cancers (see **Table** below). There are separate classifications for clinical (cTNM), pathologic (pTNM), and postneoadjuvant (ypTNM) stage groups.

The American Joint Committee on Cancer (AJCC) staging criteria for stomach cancer (8th Edition).

T stage	
Tx	Unable to histologically assess primary tumour
T0	No evidence of primary tumour
Tis	Carcinoma in situ: intraepithelial tumour without invasion of lamina propria, high-grade dysplasia
T1	Tumour invades the lamina propria, muscularis mucosae, or sub-mucosa
T1a	Tumour invades the lamina propria or muscularis mucosae
T1b	Tumour invades the sub-mucosa
T2	Tumour invades the muscularis propria
T3	Tumour penetrates the sub-serosal connective tissue without invasion of the visceral peritoneum or adjacent structures
T4	Tumour invades the serosa
T4a	Tumour invades the serosa (visceral peritoneum)
T4b	Tumour invades through serosa into adjacent structures/organs
N category	
Nx	Regional lymph nodes cannot be assessed
N0	No regional lymph nodes not metastases
N1	Metastasis in 1–2 regional lymph nodes
N2	Metastasis in 3–6 regional lymph nodes
N3	Metastasis in 7 or more regional lymph nodes
N3a	Metastasis in 7–15 regional lymph nodes
N3b	Metastasis in 16 or more regional lymph nodes
M category	
M0	No distant metastases
M1	Distant (visceral) or solid-organ metastases

Q. 1.3 What histological sub-types may this patient have?

Gastric adenocarcinoma is defined by the Laurén classification as intestinal-type or diffuse-type with the additional variability of a mixed-type.

Intestinal-type cancers are more common in men over 60 years of age, more common in Eastern countries (such as Japan and South Korea) and typically located in the antrum. Diffuse-type cancers are more common in younger women, have equal incidence in the East and West and are predominantly in the proximal body of the stomach.

Q. 1.4 The staging of this patient has confirmed the tumour to be at 44 cm extending along the lesser curve, how would you treat this patient?

Once staging has confirmed the absence of metastatic (M1) disease, MDT ratification for treatment on a potentially curative pathway will require neoadjuvant chemotherapy and surgical resection of the tumour. This is a predominantly western treatment paradigm with the use of neoadjuvant chemotherapy followed by surgery showing a significantly increased survival benefit in the seminal MAGIC trial with perioperative *E*pirubicin, *C*isplatin, and *F*luorouracil (ECF) followed by surgery. The FLOT4 randomised control trial identified a significantly increased median survival of 50 months versus 35 months between fluorouracil plus leucovorin, oxaliplatin and docetaxel (FLOT) and ECF. This has now become the standard regimen for perioperative systemic chemotherapy for gastric and gastro-oesophageal junction adenocarcinomas.

Additional trials are being conducted on perioperative management with systemic chemotherapy with addition of immunotherapy agents. These are phase 2 trials and are in the recruitment phase awaiting presentation of initial results.

In Eastern centres, particularly Japan and South Korea, clinicians favour a primary surgery with adjuvant chemotherapy model, rather than the neo-adjuvant model utilised in the west. This is in part due to the identification of patients with earlier stage disease. The adoption of national screening programmes in the East has identified a high volume of patients with earlier disease. This has enabled the development of minimally invasive and advanced endoscopic techniques in the East, which are now utilised internationally. Early surgical resection has been shown to be curative in these patients.

Q. 1.5 How would you pre-operatively assess the patient?

A fitness assessment for major surgery should be conducted in conjunction with a multi-disciplinary team with an enhanced recovery protocol in practice. It is important to include a comprehensive assessment of functional capacity. Determining a patient's physical activity and past medical history will aid in the subjective investigations of their fitness. Cardiac or respiratory assessment tools may be utilised, such as the Revised Cardiac Risk Index (RCRI) by the American College of Cardiology (ACC).

Cardiac

- *ECG:* The most basic cardiac assessment to identify electrical conductional abnormalities
- *Transthoracic echocardiography (TTE)*: Assessment of structural abnormalities associated with underlying cardiac disease and limited functional assessment
- *Stress echocardiogram*: Assessment of baseline cardiac function and abnormalities as well as cardiac function and signs of dysrhythmia when undergoing increased stress and cardiac load

Functional assessment

Cardio-pulmonary exercise testing (CPEX): The 2014 ACC guidelines on perioperative cardiovascular assessment indicate the use of CPEX testing for patients undergoing high-risk surgery when functional capacity is unknown. The discriminatory ability for CPEX to predict increased morbidity and mortality after surgery suggests an anaerobic threshold of approximately 10 mL O_2/kg/min as an optimal level.

Q. 1.6 This patient has a lesser curve tumour. What are the surgical options?

Radical surgery depends on the location of the tumour and the type of gastrectomy performed depends on sufficient clearance of tumour margins. A 5-cm longitudinal margin is traditionally recommended with some guidelines (Japanese Gastric Cancer Association) suggesting an 8-cm margin for diffuse-type tumours. The surgical options given below.

Total gastrectomy

This involves the excision of the whole stomach including the cardia (oesophago-gastric junction) and the pylorus. It is indicated for tumour arising and invading the proximal stomach.

Distal (subtotal) gastrectomy

This involves the removal of the stomach including the pylorus but preserving the cardia. Two-thirds or more of the stomach is usually removed for gastric cancer.

Proximal (pylorus preserving) gastrectomy

This is typically only performed for early gastric cancers in Eastern centres and involves the removal of the stomach, including the cardia, but preserving the pylorus. It is indicated in proximal tumours, where more than half of the distal stomach can be preserved.

Lymphadenectomy

Lymph node (LN) metastasis is the most common mode of spread for gastric adenocarcinomas. Histological assessment has shown in T4a/T4b tumours, there is an 80% probability of lymph node metastasis; even T1 tumours have a 10% probability (T1a 3% and T1b 18%).

The distribution of lymph nodes is classified by the Japanese Classification of Gastric Carcinomas (JCGC) with the current (3rd English edition) grouping lymph node stations by a 'D' criterion.

The anatomical locations of each LN station and chain of nodes are as follows (see **Box** below):

I. Right paracardial LNs
II. Left paracardial LNs
III. Lesser curve LNs (IIIa: Left gastric branch LNs; IIIb: Distal lesser curve along right gastric artery)
IV. Greater curve LNs [IVsa: Along short gastrics; IVsb: Left greater curvature along left gastroepiploic artery (GEA); IVd: Right greater curvature along right GEA]

Continues opposite

Continued

> V. Suprapyloric LNs, along first branch and proximal to the right gastric artery
> VI. Infrapyloric LNs, along first branch and proximal to the right GEA down to the confluence if the right gastroepiploic vein (GEV)
> VII. Along the trunk of the left gastric artery down to its trunk
> VIII. Common hepatic artery (VIIIa: Anterosuperior LNs; VIIIb: Posterior LNs)
> IX. Coeliac artery LNs
> X. Splenic hilum LNs
> XI. Splenic artery LNs (XIp: Proximal splenic artery LNs; XId: distal splenic artery LNs)
> XII. Hepatoduodenal ligament LNs (XIIa: Proper hepatic artery LNs; XIIb: Bile duct LNs up to the confluence of the hepatic ducts and upper border of the pancreas; XIIp: LNs along the portal vein)

The JCGC criteria describe a lymphadenectomy as D1, D1+ and D2 categories (see Table below).

Lymphadenectomy station dissection and excision as recommended by JCGC.

Lymphadenectomy	Total gastrectomy	Distal (subtotal gastrectomy)
D1	Stations I–VII	Stations I, III, IVsb, IVd, V, VI, VII
D1+	Stations I–VII, VIIIa, IX	Stations I, III, IVsb, IVd, V, VI, VII, VIIIa, IX
D2	Stations I–VII, VIIIa, IX, XIp, XIIa	Stations I, III, IVsb, IVd, V, VI, VII, VIIIa, IX, XIp, and XIIa

In Japan, the benefits of D2 versus a less extensive dissection have never been tested in a randomised study. In the West, two large and randomised trials have been conducted testing D0/D1 as standard lymphadenectomy with D2 lymphadenectomy ('Dutch trial' and 'MRC trial'). These trials concluded no significant survival benefit with D2 compared to D1 lymphadenectomy; however, a higher morbidity and mortality rate were reported. They were both performed in a 'western' centre with a patient cohort consisting of a majority of stage II or III cancers.

Q. 1.7 Can you describe the surgical procedures?

Open subtotal/distal gastrectomy + D2 lymphadenectomy

A roof-top incision is performed, and a laparotomy performed with intra-operative staging to assess for tumour location, presence of macroscopic peritoneal or liver metastases.

The omentum (± bursectomy – although limited evidence to suggest improved outcome) is removed from the right side of the transverse colon and followed along the transverse colon up to the lower pole of the spleen. If omentectomy is performed without full bursectomy, it should be incised at least 3 cm away from the right gastroepiploic (RGE) arcade in order that station IV lymph nodes are excised entirely.

Mobilisation of the duodenum enables safe visualisation of arterial and venous anatomy and subsequent infra-pyloric lymphadenectomy. The peritoneum close to the duodenum should be incised and extended along D2 (Kocherisation manoeuvre), the duodenum can then be 'rolled' upwards to identify and ligate the superior pancreaticoduodenal veins to aid safe ligation of postpyloric D1.

The left gastroepiploic (LGE) vessels are divided from the lower pole of the spleen by identifying their origin from the splenic artery. For tumours of the greater curve, lymph node metastasis may occur in the splenic hilum LNs (Station X) and these should be sampled. On the greater curve of the stomach, there is an avascular space between the LGE artery and the short gastrics vessels, and this will be the upper limit of dissection for a subtotal gastrectomy.

The infra-pyloric (Station VI) lymphadenectomy is performed by identification of the 'gastrocolic trunk vessels'. This is achieved by dissection of the middle colic branches from the transverse colon mesentery to the SMV, this enables the safe mobilisation of the gastric antrum. As the antrum is 'pulled upwards' the gastroduodenal artery (GDA) is identified between the duodenum and the pancreas. The GDA is exposed distally as far as the origin of the RGE artery; the infra-pyloric artery arises near the origin of the RGE artery – both are ligated. The GDA should be pursued proximally to its origin form the common hepatic artery (CHA) where station VIII lymphadenectomy is performed from its surface. Using this technique station V as well as VIII clearance is achieved in entirety.

Further supra-pyloric dissection and lymphadenectomy can be achieved by drawing down the pylorus to reveal the right gastric artery (RGA) and the superior duodenal arteries (SDAs). The tissue between the vessels is divided and their origins are traced to the proper hepatic artery (PHA). The origin of the right gastric vein (RGV) is the portal vein, therefore once the RGA and RGV are identified, they can be safely ligated and excised with station V LNs. The anterior peritoneum of the hepatoduodenal ligament is removed to fully expose the PHA for subsequent station XIIa lymphadenectomy. The postpyloric D1 is then excised by linear stapler or incision and primary sutured closure.

The inferior retraction of the stomach enables dissection of pars flaccida up to the upper end of the lesser omentum and peritoneum covering the right diaphragmatic crus. The crus is exposed towards the coeliac artery, which aids further dissection of the coeliac axis LNs (Station IX).

The core of the D2 lymphadenectomy is performed by dissection of the upper border of the pancreas. The stomach is elevated, and the pancreas retracted downwards to expose the coeliac trunk vessels. The CHA origin is identified and any further tissue remaining on station VIII is excised. The lymphadenectomy is then completed by identifying the origin of the LGA and splenic artery (SA). The origin of the LGA and left gastric vein (LGV), which originates from the PV or splenic vein (SV), is identified and ligated with station VII LNs. The surface of the diaphragmatic crus is also encountered here and station IX, which was previously dissected can be completed here.

The lymphadenopathy is then completed by dissection along the SA from its origin up to the splenic hilum with excision of all tissues from the arterial surface (station XIp).

The LNs along the lesser curve (Station I and III) are most frequently involved with tumours of the gastric body, therefore complete excision is essential. The stomach is retracted inferiorly towards the cardia and the anterior branch of the vagus nerve is cut to enable dissection of the left cardiac LNs (Station I). The posterior vagal trunk is then cut, and the stomach reflected to complete stations I and III dissection by excision of the LNs from the posterior aspect of the cardia.

The line of gastrectomy is then determined, typically two-thirds of the stomach with a remnant consisting of a quarter to a third of the total stomach volume. Reconstruction is completed by a Roux-en-Y (R-Y) reconstruction as explained below with a gastro-jejunal anastomosis either anteriorly or posteriorly placed.

An abdominal drain is typically placed adjacent to the anastomosis.

Total gastrectomy + D2 lymphadenectomy

Most aspects of D2 lymphadenectomy in total gastrectomy are common to sub-total gastrectomy. The additional dissection involves the completion of the proximal gastrectomy and dissection of the upper greater curve LNs. Following division of the LGE artery at its origin, the gastro-splenic ligament is divided, and the short gastric vessels ligated towards the superior pole of the spleen up to the left diaphragmatic crus, adjacent to the gastric cardia. Station II and IV lymphadenectomy is completed following this dissection, with care taken to avoid injury to the sub-phrenic vessels which is close proximity to this dissection.

The abdominal oesophagus is then divided with a linear stapler or incised prior to reconstruction with a stapled or handsewn oesophago-jejunal anastomosis and Roux-en-Y reconstruction as described below.

In cases where the tumour is a Siewert Type III, with the tumour epicentre being 2 cm below the GOJ with extension into the oesophagus, an extended total gastrectomy with hiatal extension may be utilised. Surgeon preference may dictate the use of a left thoracoabdominal approach to enable extension of the dissection and anastomosis above the hiatus.

Q. 1.8 What are the possible reconstruction options?

While Roux-en-Y (R-Y) and Billroth II (B-II) reconstructions are widely used, Billroth I gastroduodenostomy (B-I) is also frequently employed in Eastern Asia.

Roux-en-Y reconstruction after subtotal gastrectomy

The advantages of the R-Y over Billroth 1 reconstructions are the absence of duodenal (biliary) reflux, safe anastomosis with a very low leak rate and a low risk of obstruction by gastric bed recurrence. The disadvantages include the loss of endoscopic access to the duodenal papilla.

Procedure

The duodenum is transected using a linear-type stapler and many surgeons add covering seromuscular stitches. The jejunum 20–30 cm distal to the Treitz ligament is divided and the jejunal limb is pulled up either via the ante- or retrocolic route. In T4a/T4b tumours that have a significant risk of local recurrence involving the mesocolon, the antecolic route is preferred. Gastrojejunostomy is achieved either by stapler or hand-sewing; a differing 'lie' of the anastomosis is selected accordingly. The Jejunojejunostomy is made 40 cm distal to the gastrojejunostomy. The mesentery holes are closed to prevent internal hernia.

When the retrocolic route is selected, the gastrojejunostomy site should be pulled down below the mesocolon and be fixed to it to prevent torsion or obstruction of the jejunal limb in the narrow space above the mesocolon.

Billroth I reconstruction for subtotal gastrectomy

The advantages of B-I over R-Y are physiological food passage, simple anastomosis without jejunal manipulation, and preserved endoscopic access to the duodenal papilla. B-I is useful for distal tumours at an early stage for which a relatively large proximal stomach can be preserved, and recurrence is not thought likely. The disadvantages of B-I are duodenal (biliary) reflux, anastomotic leak and possible obstruction at recurrence.

Thus, B-I should be avoided in cases with high operative risks, small remnant stomach, preoperative presence of oesophageal reflux or locally advanced disease.

Gastroduodenostomy is made either by hand-sewing or using a circular stapler. When the anastomotic tension is high, Kocher's mobilisation of the duodenum is required to relieve it.

R-Y reconstruction after a total gastrectomy

The jejunum is transected 20–30 cm from the Treitz ligament. Either the ante- or retrocolic route is selected according to the criteria mentioned in the section on distal gastrectomy. The retrocolic pathway provides the shortest route and the least tension on the limb mesentery, especially in obese patients with a large omental residue.

Jejunal vessels are carefully prepared so that the mesentery tension is reduced, preserving the blood supply to the anastomotic site.

Oesophagojejunostomy is undertaken using a circular stapler. A 25-mm anvil is applicable in most cases. A larger size can be selected in patients with large oesophagus and jejunum.

Jejunojejunostomy is performed 40–50 cm below the oesophageal anastomosis. A shorter limb may cause reflux and a longer one may be disadvantageous from a nutritional viewpoint. In the double tract method, Jejunojejunostomy is made 20 cm distal to the duodenojejunostomy.

Jejunal interposition after total gastrectomy

This method is employed to maintain the physiological food passage to the duodenum. However, there is no solid evidence that this reconstruction has long-term nutritional advantage over standard R-Y. The length of the interposed jejunum can be shorter (20–30 cm) than the jejunal limb in R-Y, probably because the jejunal juice can flow down the natural route without reflux.

Q. 1.9 What is the postoperative management and what are the early postoperative complications?

Postoperative patients are managed in critical care by experienced intensivists. The patient will have central access [central venous catheter (CVC)], arterial line for BP monitoring, spinal or epidural analgesic catheters and a nasogastric tube (NG) tube. Monitoring of vital signs and serum haematology and biochemistry results will be conducted daily with recovery to a soft diet determined by adherence to an enhanced recovery protocol.

The recognised postoperative complications include:
- *Anastomotic leak*: Most anastomotic leaks after gastrectomy occur at the oesophagojejunostomy. Possible causes are tissue ischaemia or tension on the anastomotic line. These should be avoided by careful preparation of the jejunal loop.
  Early anastomotic leak occurring within 72 hours would be life-threatening without proper management. It may present as septic episodes or contaminated drain discharge. A CT with oral contrast (Gastrografin) should be performed whenever a leak is suspected. Drainage is crucial to treat anastomotic leakage. The management of a delayed leak is controversial. Usually, drains have already been removed and meals are started. When a contrast study reveals only a minor leak, fasting and adequate nutrition will be sufficient. A naso-jejunal tube placed beyond the jejunojejunostomy may be useful for enteral feeding. If the patient is septic, a drain must be placed.
- *Duodenal stump leak*: A properly stapled duodenal stump rarely leaks. However, stump leak occurs when the duodenal tissue is damaged or becomes ischaemic. There is no evidence that covering stiches reduce leak, but some surgeons use them. A prophylactic drain that is placed near the stump gives good information. If its discharge contains bile, it is an indication for immediate re-operation. Re-closure of the stump is usually very difficult due to tissue inflammation. If there is a major defect, a Foley-type catheter can be placed in the duodenum with a plan to form a controlled fistula.
- *Pancreatic fistula*: After D2 lymphadenectomy, pancreatic leak may occur even without pancreatectomy. It is more common when the pancreatic capsule has been removed as a part of bursectomy or the pancreas has been mobilised for splenectomy. Increased amylase content in the drain fluid on the first or second postoperative day is a useful marker to predict later development of pancreatic fistula.
  When pancreatic leak occurs, the management should concentrate on prevention of infection and abscess control. Adequate drainage is essential and radiological intervention should be considered.
- *Haemorrhage*: Haemorrhage within the first few hours of surgery should be treated by early re-laparotomy. It must be remembered that drains can occlude with blood clot and the clinical suspicion of bleeding in a haemodynamically unstable patient is a sufficient indication to operate.

Secondary haemorrhage caused by intra-abdominal infection following anastomotic leak and/or pancreatic fistula is truly life-threatening. A poorly drained abscess causes pseudo-aneurysm of a major artery (most frequently the splenic artery) and then causes massive haemorrhage. Once massive bleeding occurs, immediate angiography again should first be considered because it is able to identify and embolise the bleeding point.

Further reading

Al-Batran S. Phase II Study of Atezolizumab + FLOT vs. FLOT Alone in Patients With Gastric Cancer and GEJ - NCT03421288. Clin Trial 2018.

Al-Batran SE, Homann N, Pauligk C, et al. Perioperative chemotherapy with fluorouracil plus leucovorin, oxaliplatin, and docetaxel versus fluorouracil or capecitabine plus cisplatin and epirubicin for locally advanced, resectable gastric or gastro-oesophageal junction adenocarcinoma (FLOT4): a randomised, phase 2/3 trial. The Lancet 2019; 393:1948–1957.

Amin MB, Edge S, Greene F, et al. AJCC Cancer Staging Manual, 8th edition. New York, NY: Springer, 2017.

Bonenkamp JS, Hermans J, Sasako M, et al. Randomised comparison of morbidity after D1 and D2 dissection for gastric cancer in 996 Dutch patients. Lancet 1995; 25:745–758.

Cunningham D, Allum WH, Stenning SP, et al. Perioperative Chemotherapy versus Surgery Alone for Resectable Gastroesophageal Cancer. N Engl J Med 2006; 355:11–20.

Cuschieri AFP, Fielding J, Craven J, et al. Postoperative morbidity and mortality after D1 and D2 resections for gastric cancer- preliminary results of the MRC randomised controlled surgical trial. The Surgical Cooperative Group. Lancet 1996; 13:995–999.

Fleisher LA, Fleischmann KE, Auerbach AD, et al. 2014 ACC/AHA guideline on perioperative cardiovascular evaluation and management of patients undergoing noncardiac surgery: a report of the American College of Cardiology/American Heart Association Task Force on practice guidelines. J Am Coll Cardiol 2014; 64:e77–e137.

Hamashima C, Shibuya D, Yamazaki H, et al. The Japanese guidelines for gastric cancer screening. Jpn J Clin Oncol 2008; 38:259–267.

Japanese Gastric Cancer. Japanese gastric cancer treatment guidelines 2018 (5th edition). Gastric Cancer 2020.

Jiménez Fonseca P, Carmona-Bayonas A, Hernández R, et al. Lauren subtypes of advanced gastric cancer influence survival and response to chemotherapy: real-world data from the AGAMENON National Cancer Registry. Br J Cancer 2017; 117:775–782.

Mansukhani S, Davidson M, Gillbanks A, et al. ICONIC Study – Peri-operative Immuno-Chemotherapy in Operable Oesophageal and Gastric Cancer. J Clin Oncol 2018; 36:Suppl.

Mortensen K, Nilsson M, Slim K, et al. Consensus guidelines for enhanced recovery after gastrectomy: Enhanced Recovery After Surgery (ERAS(R)) Society recommendations. Br J Surg 2014; 101:1209–1229.

Sano T, Aiko T. New Japanese classifications and treatment guidelines for gastric cancer: revision concepts and major revised points. Gastric Cancer 2011; 14:97–100.

Scenario 2

Oesophageal cancer

A 76-year-old man presents to primary care with a 6-month history of intractable gastro-oesophageal reflux, despite long term proton pump inhibitor (PPI) use. He has lost 7 kg of weight over the last 2 months.

Q. 2.1 How would you assess this patient?

Completion of initial assessment

Complete a full history including family history of malignancy, and clinical examination with initial assessment of airway patency with a respiratory and cardiac examination.

Abdominal examination would encompass peripheral stigmata of malignancy including clubbing, scleral icterus and lymphadenopathy (including supraclavicular fossae).

Initial investigation would be a diagnostic oesophagogastro duodenoscopy (OGD) and CT of chest, abdomen and pelvis to investigate the upper gastrointestinal (GI) symptoms and weight loss.

Q. 2.2 The OGD shows macroscopic appearance of a distal oesophageal tumour, how might you proceed?

The appearance of a suspected tumour on OGD would require tissue confirmation, a minimum of 6–8 biopsies should be sampled in a 4-quadrant fashion from the tumour as per the Japanese Esophageal Society guidelines. The location of the tumour should be well defined with a measure of distance from the GOJ, known as Siewert grading, and total length of the tumour in order to determine the final surgical strategy. The OGD should be completed by full assessment of the stomach, pylorus and duodenum up to D2 (duodenal papilla). Retroflexed views of the GOJ should be attained to determine if there is gastric extension of a GOJ tumour.

Histological confirmation of carcinoma would require completion of clinical staging by CT of chest, abdomen and pelvis; whole-body PET; staging laparoscopy ± peritoneal cytology and endoscopic ultrasound.

Following completion of the staging investigations, the results will be discussed in a specialist UGI cancer MDT for management plan ratification. The stage is assigned by the TNM (8th edition).

TNM classification for oesophageal and GOJ adenocarcinoma.

T stage	
Tx	Unable to histologically assess tumour
T0	No evidence of primary tumour
Tis	High-grade dysplasia, defines as malignant cells confined to basement membrane
T1	Tumour invades the lamina propria, muscularis mucosae, or sub-mucosa
T1a	Tumour invades the lamina propria or muscularis mucosae
T1b	Tumour invades the sub-mucosa
T2	Tumour invades the muscularis propria
T3	Tumour invades the adventitia
T4	Tumour invades the adjacent structures
T4a	Tumour invades the pleura, pericardium, azygos vein, diaphragm or peritoneum
T4b	Tumour invades wider adjacent structures, such as the aorta, vertebral body or trachea
N category	
Nx	Regional lymph nodes cannot be assessed
N0	No regional lymph nodes not metastases
N1	Metastasis in 1–2 regional lymph nodes
N2	Metastasis in 3–6 regional lymph nodes
N3	Metastasis in 7 or more regional lymph nodes
N3a	Metastasis in 7–15 regional lymph nodes
N3b	Metastasis in 16 or more regional lymph nodes
M category	
M0	No distant metastases
M1	Distant (visceral) or solid-organ metastases

Staging considerations

Laparoscopy

Staging laparoscopy is advised for GOJ (Siewert Types II and III) tumours to assess for peritoneal metastasis and perform abdominal fluid cytology. De Graaf et al. concluded that staging laparoscopy was most useful in distal oesophageal, GOJ and gastric cancers; and not indicated in tumours of the upper two-thirds of the oesophagus. Furthermore, the EORTC guidelines have suggested only GOJ Siewert Types II, III and gastric cancers benefit from staging with laparoscopy, with <5% of cases of distal and Siewert Type I cancers have peritoneal metastases.

Endoscopic ultrasound

All ultrasonographic investigations, the results are operator-dependent. Endoscopic ultrasonography (EUS) and EUS-guided fine-needle aspiration (EUS-FNA) are the most accurate techniques for locoregional staging of oesophageal cancer. Puli et al. concluded that EUS should be strongly considered for staging oesophageal cancer, in particular for those staged at T1 and T4, with particular importance for T1 lesions which may be amenable for endoscopic mucosal resection (EMR).

Q. 2.3 What are the risk factors for oesophageal cancer?

Gastro-oesophageal reflux disease (GORD) is now the most common symptomatic presentation of all conditions affecting the upper gastrointestinal tract. Estimates suggest that 4–9% of all adults experience daily heartburn and up to 20% experience symptoms on a weekly basis. Of these, 60% have no endoscopic abnormality, 30% have oesophagitis and 10% have Barrett's columnar lined oesophagus. Many patients are self-treated and do not attend for further investigation, yet 80% with Barrett's are asymptomatic.

Disease associations with oesophageal cancer.

Tissue type	Disease association
Oesophageal squamous cell carcinoma	Corrosive ingestion, achalasia, tylosis palmarum, family history
Oesophageal adenocarcinoma	GORD: Barrett's metaplasia, obesity, *Helicobacter pylori – protective*

Q. 2.4 How would you treat this patient?

The principles of management are common across upper GI adenocarcinomas and include neoadjuvant chemotherapy with resectional surgery on a potentially curative pathway. The evidence for this has already been discussed in the gastric adenocarcinoma vignette.

There is some international variation to this practice with certain countries and treatment centres preferring neo-adjuvant chemoradiotherapy (CRT) and subsequent resectional surgery. CRT with follow-up surgery was shown to show a benefit to surgery alone in the seminal CROSS trial, this method of neo-adjuvant CRT remains the established treatment standard in the Netherlands. However, subsequent studies have suggested that neo-adjuvant CRT provides no long-term survival benefit over neoadjuvant chemotherapy with increased morbidity from the radiotherapy component of the peri-operative treatment.

Definitive CRT without surgery has been shown to have local recurrence rates of 40–75% are recognised following definitive CRT. Indeed, it is generally recognised that local failure is more common after chemoradiation than with surgery.

For SCC, definitive CRT treatment has reported good overall survival figures, rivalling those of surgery, stage for stage. Many squamous cancers are in the mid and upper oesophagus and their pattern of lymph node spread is less predictable. These areas can be safely treated with CRT. In the FFCD 9102 French study, SCC patients were assessed after induction CRT using 5-FU and cisplatin. If they had achieved an objective response they were randomised (295 out of 455 patients) to carry on with CRT or go to surgery. There was no significant difference between the 2-year survival rates for patients who had surgery (33.6%) and those who had CRT alone (39.8%). There were more early deaths in the surgery arm, but CRT required more dilatations and stents.

Q. 2.5 What are the surgical options for this patient?

The choice of approach in oesophageal cancer is dependent on tumour location, the extent of spread, and the fitness, age and build of the individual patient. Traditionally, oesophagectomy was performed by open surgery but there has been an increase in totally minimally invasive oesophagectomy (MIO) and hybrid surgery during the last 10 years.

Tumour location primarily dictates the access (incision) by dictating the position of anastomosis and therefore the reconstruction. Approaches for GOJ tumours may be abdominal (Transhiatal), thoracic (Two stage/Ivor Lewis) or if lesions are more proximal a thoracic and cervical approach (three stage) may be required.

Two-phase (Ivor Lewis oesophagectomy)

The first phase is abdominal mobilisation of the stomach through an upper midline or rooftop incision (or laparoscopically). The second phase is mediastinal dissection and oesophageal resection through a right thoracotomy. The stomach is delivered into the chest and an anastomosis fashioned at the thoracic inlet.

Abdominal phase

The procedure begins with a laparotomy to assess the primary tumour and exclude the presence of distant metastases. The stomach is mobilised on the right gastroepiploic and right gastric arcades, which remains critical to the blood supply of the gastric conduit. Care must be taken when performing medial dissection in order not to injure the right GEA insertion on the gastroduodenal artery. It is important that all posterior attachments of the stomach and the duodenocolic ligament are divided to allow full mobility of the stomach. Preservation of a significant flap of omentum along the greater curve allows the formation of an omentoplasty around the anastomosis and conduit in the chest.

During hiatal dissection it is important to take an envelope of tissue around the tumour and to ensure adequate room for passage of the gastric conduit. For lower oesophageal and oesophagogastric junction tumours it is routine to take a cuff of hiatal muscle and, anteriorly, all tissue posterior to the pericardium. The left and right pleura are entered and resected en bloc with the specimen. On the left (para-aortic) hiatal dissection, it is important to be vigilant to ligate the small lymphatic branches traversing over the abdominal to thoracic aorta.

The lymphadenectomy begins at the origin of the right gastric artery, skeletonising the common hepatic artery, the root of the left gastric artery and the splenic artery to the level of the posterior gastric artery. This is best performed using either diathermy scissors or forceps with formal ligation of larger lymphatic channels to prevent postoperative lymph leak. The left gastric vein should be ligated with care just above the upper border of the pancreas gland.

A feeding jejunostomy is routinely placed for postoperative nutrition.

Thoracic phase

The patient is placed in the left lateral decubitus position. The operating table is broken to widen the intercostal space. The mediastinal phase is performed via a right posterolateral thoracotomy through the fifth intercostal space with the proximal extent of the incision following the medial border of the scapula. It is important to count the ribs by palpation to avoid too low an incision.

Division or resection of the arch of the azygos vein is required for exposure. The pleural incision is deepened along the line of the azygos vein to expose the adventitia on the descending aorta. The thoracic duct is identified at the level of the azygos vein and dissected off the aorta. It is then ligated with the tissue between aorta, oesophagus and azygos, just above the hiatus. The para-aortic lymph nodes and thoracic duct are mobilised en bloc, ligating aortic branches to the oesophagus. The anterior plane of dissection is along the pericardium to the inferior pulmonary vein, allowing the oesophagus to be slung. Dissection continues caudally to the right pulmonary hilum and the right bronchial, subcarinal and left bronchial nodes are dissected. Care must be taken with monopolar diathermy in this region to prevent injury to the membranous parts of the tracheobronchial tree.

In high tumours, such as middle-third squamous lesions, a supra-azygous dissection is performed, with the mediastinal pleura incised along the course of the right vagus nerve towards the brachiocephalic and subclavian arteries. The right recurrent laryngeal nerve is preserved and the lymph node chain alongside it meticulously dissected. The pleura is incised along the border of the superior vena cava and the right paratracheal lymph nodes, located between the trachea and cava, are dissected.

The stomach is delivered into the chest and the specimen removed after sleeve resection of the lesser curvature to form the gastric conduit. This is usually performed with a linear stapler by elevation at the fundus and resection of the specimen to leave a conduit of 5 cm diameter. The oesophagus is transected once sufficient gastric conduit length is confirmed. The oesophagogastric anastomosis is fashioned at the supra-azygous level in the upper thorax. In addition to ensuring an adequate resection margin, it is important that the gastric conduit is aligned correctly, without a twist, for good drainage and a good functional outcome. If a lower anastomosis is fashioned, differences in abdominal and mediastinal pressure promote reflux and inhibit gastric emptying, resulting in troublesome symptoms and reduced quality of life. Once the anastomosis and the gastrotomy line closure are completed, the omentum is passed posterior to the conduit and forms a 'wrap' around both the anastomosis and the staple line. It provides a further barrier between the conduit and the membranous trachea.

Left thoracoabdominal oesophagectomy

The left thoracoabdominal approach provides excellent exposure of the hiatus and is still appropriate for selected patients with tumours that have significant involvement of the cardia, and for those requiring extended total gastrectomy. It is important to use a circumferential incision to divide the diaphragm rather than a radial incision that denervates part of the left diaphragm. The Japanese Clinical Oncology Group trial has shown that, for proximal gastric cancer, the left thoracoabdominal approach has a higher complication rate and no survival benefit compared to the alternative trans-hiatal approach to gastrectomy.

Three-phase oesophagectomy

Exposing the oesophagus in the left neck provides good access for anastomosis. Although it does not allow resection of much more oesophagus than a two-phase approach, it should be considered for tumours of the upper middle third of the oesophagus when there is concern about involvement of the proximal margin. It does allow for a formal nodal dissection in the neck in patients with high nodal disease in the mediastinum. It was originally thought that leakage of a cervical anastomosis is less catastrophic than a thoracic leak. This is not always the case and must be balanced against the potential increased risk of gastric tip necrosis and anastomotic stricture with cervical anastomosis.

When a preoperative decision is made then the first phase should mirror the thoracic dissection described in the preceding section with additional mobilisation of the oesophagus to the root of the neck. It is useful here to secure a tape around the cervical oesophagus to aid the cervical dissection. The second phase of the operation is routine gastric mobilisation with the patient supine. This can be performed synchronously with a left-sided cervical dissection (third phase). The oesophagus is divided in the neck, and the oesophagus and stomach delivered on a tape to the abdomen, allowing the gastric tube to be formed with resection of the specimen. The gastric tube is then delivered to the neck, often within a laparoscopic camera bag, for anastomosis. When an intra-operative decision is made to convert to a three-stage procedure then the gastric tube is created during the thoracic phase and delivered into the neck during the third (cervical) phase.

Transhiatal oesophagectomy

Controversy exists about the role of oesophagectomy without thoracotomy for oesophageal cancer. Proponents of the technique argue that outcome is dependent on disease stage rather than the operative technique employed. Opponents claim improvements in survival for some undergoing oesophagectomy with two-field lymphadenectomy, which is not performed with a transhiatal approach. The approach is akin to the abdominal phase in a two-stage ILO with dissection of the supra-hiatal/distal oesophagus under direct vision from the abdomen.

For early (T1a/T1b/T2 without nodal disease) oesophageal adenocarcinoma, there are endoscopic resection techniques available, which enable local resection of the tumour.

Endoscopic resection

Endoscopic mucosal resection

The principle of EMR is the removal of a mucosal lesion by resecting it from its deeper layers using a snare instrument. This method does not allow for lesions larger than 2 cm to be removed en bloc. Larger lesions can be removed by EMR, but only in a piecemeal fashion. The technique is fundamentally different from ESD, where the submucosal layer is carefully dissected in a stepwise manner. Using EMR, early neoplasia is often lifted from the proper muscle layer before resection using different solutions of saline for submucosal injection. This method is mostly used in early Barrett's cancer but is also applicable in the cardia and antrum of the stomach.

Endoscopic submucosal dissection

Endoscopic submucosal dissection (ESD) was originally developed in Japan for the local treatment of superficial oesophageal lesions limited to the mucosal layer or with minimal invasion of the submucosal layer. The main goal of submucosal dissection is to retrieve the lesion en bloc for histopathological staging and to minimise the chance for local recurrence. ESD is performed in several steps. First, the lesion is delineated by placing circumferential dots using electrocautery around the lesion with a few millimetres of free margin. The lesion is then lifted from the proper muscle layer by submucosal injection in the same fashion as in EMR.

Q. 2.6 Is a radical lymphadenectomy required for an oesophagectomy?

As for many solid-organ tumours, controversy persists as to the value of lymphadenectomy in oesophageal cancer. Some authors believe that lymph node metastases are simply markers of systemic disease, while others believe that cure can be obtained in many patients with positive nodes by a radical lymphadenectomy with clear resection margins.

- *Radical lymphadenectomy:*
  - One-field lymphadenectomy describes an upper abdominal lymphadenectomy including removal of diaphragmatic, right and left paracardial, lesser curvature, left gastric, coeliac, common hepatic and splenic artery nodes
  - Two-field lymphadenectomy describes removal of the first field along with removal of paraoesophageal nodes, para-aortic nodes (together with the thoracic duct), right and left pulmonary hilar, subcarinal and right paratracheal nodes
  - Three-field lymphadenectomy describes removal of the first and second fields along with a neck dissection clearing the brachiocephalic, deep lateral and external cervical nodes, as well as right and left recurrent nerve lymphatic chains (deep anterior cervical nodes)
- Non-radical lymphadenectomy – in which only the nodes in direct proximity to the tumour, the oesophagus and upper stomach are removed

Q. 2.7 What are the complications following a two-phase oesophagectomy?

The complications from an oesophagectomy can be divided into immediate, delayed and long-term.

Anastomotic leakage and gastric conduit necrosis

Anastomotic leak is defined as a full-thickness defect involving oesophagus, anastomosis, staple line, or conduit irrespective of presentation or method of identification. The tables below present the International Consensus on the classification of anastomotic leak and conduit necrosis.

Classification of anastomotic leak and conduit necrosis.

Anastomotic leak	Classification
Type I	Local defect requiring no therapy or treated medically/with dietary modification
Type II	Local defect requiring interventional but not surgical therapy (e.g. interventional radiology drain, stent or bedside opening of wound)
Type III	Local defect requiring surgical therapy
Conduit necrosis	
Type I	Focal conduit necrosis identified at endoscopy. Treatment – additional monitoring or non-surgical therapy
Type II	Focal conduit necrosis identified at endoscopy and not associated with free leakage. Treatment – surgical therapy not involving oesophageal diversion
Type III	Extensive conduit necrosis. Treatment – conduit resection with diversion

While there is no role for a routine postoperative contrast swallow following oesophagectomy, patients with clinical suspicion of a leak or failure to progress should be actively investigated. The preferred diagnostic tests for investigation of anastomotic leaks are endoscopic assessment (OGD) and computed tomography (CT) with intravenous and oral contrast. The former typically being the investigation of choice due to greater sensitivity and the additional advantage of assessment of defect size, gastric conduit necrosis and endoscopic salvage options to promote resolution.

Early anastomotic disruption (within 48–72 hours) is rare and is the result of technical error. The patient should be re-explored for correction of the technical fault. Total gastric necrosis can, rarely, occur with catastrophic consequences. This must be diagnosed early by endoscopy, the patient can then be resuscitated and immediately returned to theatre for the formation of a cervical oesophagostomy and closure of the viable component of the gastric remnant. At a later date, a retrosternal colonic interposition is used to restore intestinal continuity.

Chylothorax

Damage to the thoracic duct during oesophagectomy can be minimised by formal identification during dissection and carefully ligating the duct low in the mediastinum between the oesophagus, azygos and aorta. An incidence of 2–3% during open resection is commonly reported and is more common with squamous cell carcinoma. High-volume chyle leaks, of over a litre per day, are usually apparent during the first few days after surgery when jejunostomy feed is commenced. Early re-exploration is recommended for these leaks, as the damaged thoracic duct or side branch is usually identified at the time of re-exploration. If left untreated the chyle leak results in malnutrition and significant immune suppression. Leaks of <500 mL/day often resolve with enteral feeding using medium-chain triglycerides.

Diaphragmatic herniation

The widened hiatus, through which the gastric conduit has passed, is a potential site of herniation in the early and late postoperative period. The reported incidence is approximately 15% at 1 year follow-up. Ganeshan D, et al. reported, in a series of 440 patients, a variation in incidence for patients by type of surgery with 17% for a transhiatal approach, 12% for an ILO, and 10% for MIO.

The gastrocolic omentum or transverse colon is usually the lead point, but other intra-abdominal contents including small bowel can be involved. In the acute setting, it is crucial to recognise this complication on a postoperative chest radiograph as, once confirmed by a CT scan, urgent re-operation is indicated if there is significant obstruction, or the patient is toxic.

Delayed gastric emptying

The incidence of delayed gastric emptying is minimised by the routine use of pyloroplasty or pyloromyotomy. Emptying problems are also reduced with good alignment of the pylorus with the base of the conduit. Pyloric procedures and endoscopic pneumatic dilatation may contribute to dumping syndrome; however, this typically resolves in the first year after resection and can be avoided by limiting carbohydrate load.

Medical management with regular prokinetics, such as metoclopramide, can also aid conduit emptying.

Benign anastomotic strictures

Strictures are relatively common following stapled intrathoracic anastomosis and usually respond to endoscopic dilatation (median 1–3). Refractory strictures, although rare, are more common with cervical anastomosis.

Further reading

Bedenne L, Michel P, Bouché O, et al. Chemoradiation followed by surgery compared with chemoradiation alone in squamous cancer of the esophagus: FFCD 9102. J Clin Oncol 2007; 25:1160–1168.

de Graaf GW, Ayantunde AA, Parsons SL, Duffy JP, Welch NT. The role of staging laparoscopy in oesophagogastric cancers. Eur J Surg Oncol 2007; 33:988–992.

Ell CMA, Gossner L, Pech O, et al. Endoscopic Mucosal Resection of Early Cancer and High-Grade Dysplasia in Barrett's Esophagus. Gastroenterology 2000; 118:670–677.

Ganeshan DM, Correa AM, Bhosale P, et al. Diaphragmatic hernia after esophagectomy in 440 patients with long-term follow-up. Ann Thorac Surg 2013; 96:1138–1145.

Japan Esophageal Society. Japanese Classification of Esophageal Cancer, 11th Edition: Part I. Esophagus 2017; 14:1–36.

Japan Esophageal Society. Japanese Classification of Esophageal Cancer, 11th Edition: Parts II and III. Esophagus 2017; 14:37–65.

Low DE, Alderson D, Cecconello I, et al. International Consensus on Standardization of Data Collection for Complications Associated With Esophagectomy: Esophagectomy Complications Consensus Group (ECCG). Ann Surg 2015; 262:286–294.

Lutz MP, Zalcberg JR, Ducreux M, et al. Highlights of the EORTC St. Gallen International Expert Consensus on the primary therapy of gastric, gastroesophageal and oesophageal cancer - differential treatment strategies for subtypes of early gastroesophageal cancer. Eur J Cancer 2012; 48:2941–2953.

Messager M, Warlaumont M, Renaud F, et al. Recent improvements in the management of esophageal anastomotic leak after surgery for cancer. Eur J Surg Oncol 2017; 43:258–269.

Miao L, Zhang Y, Hu H, et al. Incidence and management of chylothorax after esophagectomy. Thorac Cancer 2015; 6:354–358.

Oyama TTA, Hotta K, Morita S, et al. Endoscopic Submucosal Dissection of Early Esophageal Cancer. Clin Gastroenterol Hepatol 2005; 3:67–70.

Park JY, Song HY, Kim JH, et al. Benign anastomotic strictures after esophagectomy: long-term effectiveness of balloon dilation and factors affecting recurrence in 155 patients. AJR Am J Roentgenol 2012; 198:1208–1213.

Peyre CG, Hagen JA, DeMeester SR, et al. Predicting systemic disease in patients with esophageal cancer after esophagectomy: a multinational study on the significance of the number of involved lymph nodes. Ann Surg 2008; 248:979–985.

Pimentel-Nunes P, Libânio D, Bastiaansen BAJ, et al. Endoscopic submucosal dissection: European Society of Gastrointestinal Endoscopy (ESGE) Guideline. Endoscopy 2015; 47:829–854.

Puli SR, Reddy JB, Bechtold ML, et al. Staging accuracy of esophageal cancer by endoscopic ultrasound: a meta-analysis and systematic review. World J Gastroenterol 2008; 14:1479–1490.

Rice TW, Patil DT, Blackstone EH. AJCC/UICC staging of cancers of the esophagus and esophagogastric junction: application to clinical practice, 8th edition. Ann Cardiothorac Surg 2017; 6:119–130.

Sasako M, Sano T, Yamamoto S, et al. Left thoracoabdominal approach versus abdominal-transhiatal approach for gastric cancer of the cardia or subcardia: a randomised controlled trial. The Lancet Oncol 2006; 7:644–651.

van Hagen PH, van Lanschot JJB, Steyerberg EW, et al. Preoperative Chemoradiotherapy for Esophageal or Junctional Cancer. N Engl J Med 2012; 366:2074–2084.

von Döbeln GA, Klevebro F, Jacobsen AB, et al. Neoadjuvant chemotherapy versus neoadjuvant chemoradiotherapy for cancer of the esophagus or gastroesophageal junction: long-term results of a randomized clinical trial. Dis Esophagus 2019; 32.

Scenario 3

Gastrointestinal stromal tumours

A 67-year-old male patient a long-standing history of gastro-oesophageal reflux disease (GORD) on medical management presents with an episode of haematemesis. An urgent oesophagogastroduodenoscopy (OGD) is performed and reveals a submucosal lesion in the gastric fundus. Biopsies come back as 'inflamed gastric mucosa'.

Q. 3.1 What are your differentials?

- Gastrointestinal stromal tumour (GIST) of the stomach
- Leiomyoma – benign sarcomatous lesion
- Leiomyosarcoma – malignant sarcomatous lesion
- Gastric lymphoma
- Gastric carcinoid

Q. 3.2 How would you differentiate a gastric gastrointestinal stromal tumour (GIST) from the other diagnoses?

Gastrointestinal stromal tumours are soft-tissue sarcomas of mesenchymal origin arising in the gastrointestinal (GI) tract. They are rare, accounting for 0.1–3% of all gut tumours and 5% of all soft tissue sarcomas. The sub-categorisation between benign (leiomyoma) and malignant (leiomyosarcoma) sarcomas of the GI tract with GISTs being stromal tumours with smooth muscle, neural or undifferentiated features.

Diagnosis is made by histological confirmation, and tissue diagnosis is secured by endoscopic ultrasound-guided fine-needle biopsy (FNB) for solid lesions or fine-needle aspiration (FNA) for cystic-solid lesions. GISTs are of the stomach and are from the intestinal cells of Cajal and express the receptor tyrosine kinase *KIT*. Therefore, tissue shows CD-117 positivity, DOG-1 positive and desmin negative. Approximately 85% of GISTs have active mutations in the *KIT* gene.

Q. 3.3 Are gastrointestinal stromal tumours (GISTs) malignant?

The size of the tumour, the symptoms at diagnosis, the organ of origin (small bowel GISTs have the worst prognosis) and mitotic count are the critical when assessing prognosis. Miettinen M et al. reviewed the long-term follow-up of 1,765 gastric GISTs showed that tumours < 10 cm diameter or with a mitotic count < 5/50 high power fields (HPFs) had a 2–3% risk of having metastasised whereas those >10 cm diameter or mitotic count > 5/50 HPFs had an 86% risk of metastatic spread.

Modified Miettinen score specifying the risk of gastrointestinal stromal tumour (GIST) recurrence by histological grading.

Tumour parameters		Risk of progressive disease			
Mitotic index	Size	Stomach	Duodenum	Jejunum or ileum	Rectum
<5 per 50 HPF	<2 cm	none	None	None	None
	>2 < 5 cm	Very low (1.9%)	Low (8.3%)	Low (4.3%)	Low (8.5%)
	>5 < 10 cm	Low (3.6%)	Insufficient data	Moderate (24%)	Insufficient data
	>10 cm	Moderate (10%)	High (34%)	High (52%)	High (57%)
>5 per 50 HPF	<2 cm	None	Insufficient data	High (51%)	High (54%)
	>2 < 5 cm	Moderate (16%)	High (50%)	High (73%)	High (52%)
	>5 < 10 cm	High (55%)	Insufficient data	High (85%)	Insufficient data
	>10 cm	High (86%)	High (86%)	Very high (90%)	High (71%)

Presentation is typically incidental with small GISTs (<3 cm) being asymptomatic. The most common symptom at presentation is GI bleeding and abdominal pain, which may be reported in up to 50% of patients at presentation. Most duodenal GISTs are in the second part of the duodenum and can cause gastric outlet obstruction or infiltrate the pancreas.

Q. 3.4 What are the best imaging modalities?

Endoscopic ultrasound

Although EUS is an invasive diagnostic investigation, it is able to identify the classical features of a hypoechoic mass contiguous with the muscularis propria or muscularis mucosae layers of the normal gut wall. EUS + FNA has been reported to have a diagnostic accuracy of between 91 and 97%.

Computed tomography

Gastrointestinal stromal tumours imaging by CT scanning typically shows an extraluminal mass, often with central necrosis, arising from the digestive tract wall. Small tumours typically appear as sharply margined, smooth-walled, homogeneous, soft-tissue masses with moderate contrast enhancement. Large tumours tend to have mucosal ulceration, central necrosis and cavitation, and heterogeneous enhancement following IV contrast. A CT of chest, abdomen and pelvis is advised to fully stage a

GIST prior to further treatment or surgical intervention. CT imaging can also be used for response to neoadjuvant therapy.

Magnetic resonance imaging

Magnetic resonance imaging (MRI) offers no additional information regarding the intralesional tissue characterisation of primary GISTs. However, MRI provides excellent soft-tissue contrast resolution and can help to delineate the relationships of the tumour and adjacent organs.

Positron emission tomography

Positron emission tomography (PET) scanning using a standard fluorodeoxyglucose (FDG)-PET technique has proven extremely useful in the prediction of tumour response to the tyrosine kinase inhibitor imatinib, now used in the treatment of unresectable and metastatic malignant GISTs. PET imaging can be utilised to distinguish between tumour progression and increase in volume due to intra-tumour bleeding.

Q. 3.5 What is the role of systemic chemotherapy?

Systemic chemotherapeutic drugs do not play a role in GIST management, however, there is a specific indication for the tyrosine kinase inhibitor's imatinib and sunitinib. These drugs are generally well tolerated although most patients experience some mild or moderate adverse events. Serious adverse events occur in around 20% of patients, the most serious of which is life-threatening tumour haemorrhage in approximately 5%.

Unresectable, metastatic or recurrent disease

Imatinib has been shown to have response rates of 80–90% in metastatic disease. Over 50% of patients with metastatic or unresectable GISTs will survive >5 years if treated with imatinib.

Q. 3.6 What are the surgical principles of GIST surgery?

Loco-regional disease

The principles of surgery for loco-regional resectable disease are:
- A wide local resection with macroscopic and microscopic removal of the entire tumour is recommended (R0)
- Extended lymphadenectomy is normally not required
- Tumours of the gastric fundus, body and greater curve (diameter < 5 cm) may be excised with a local resection as long as a 2-cm margin is preserved. This may be performed laparoscopically
- Where adjacent organs are involved, en bloc resection is recommended whenever possible – input from other specialist surgeons should be considered prior to embarking on a resection
- Endoscopic resection is not recommended

Unresectable and/or metastatic disease:
- Mutational analysis to assess sensitivity to imatinib is mandatory prior to starting treatment

- Imatinib should be used as treatment for unresectable and/or metastatic GISTs
- Unresectable GISTs may be rendered resectable after 6–12 months of imatinib

Surgery for GISTs at anatomical locations where a 2-cm margin is not possible (proximity to major vasculature, pylorus, etc.) a formal gastric resection may be required. For distal lesions, this would be a subtotal gastrectomy; large lesions of the cardia or lesser curve may require a total gastrectomy. Alternatively, a proximal gastric resection may be reconstructed by the Merendino procedure or transgastric GIST excision, which is a combined endoscopic-laparoscopic excision.

Further reading

Akahoshi KSY, Matsui N, Oya M, et al. Preoperative diagnosis of gastrointestinal stromal tumor by endoscopic ultrasound-guided fine needle aspiration. World J Gastroenterol 2007; 13:2077–2082.

Ando N, Goto H, Niwa Y, et al. The diagnosis of GI stromal tumors with EUS-guided fine needle aspiration with immunohistochemical analysis. Gastrointest Endosc 2002; 55:37–43.

Gronchi A, Fiore M, Miselli F, et al. Surgery of residual disease following molecular-targeted therapy with imatinib mesylate in advanced/metastatic GIST. Ann Surg 2007; 245:341–346.

Hong XCH, Loyer EM, Benjamin RS, Trent JC, Charnsangavej C. Gastrointestinal Stromal Tumor – Role of CT in Diagnosis and in Response Evaluation and Surveillance after Treatment with Imatinib. RadioGraphics 2006; 26:481–495.

Kochhar R, Manoharan P, Leahy M, Taylor MB. Imaging in gastrointestinal stromal tumours: current status and future directions. Clin Radiol 2010; 65:584–592.

Miettinen M, Sobin LH, Lasota J. Gastrointestinal Stromal Tumors of the Stomach A Clinicopathologic, Immunohistochemical, and Molecular Genetic Study of 1765 Cases With Long-term Follow-up. Am J Surg Pathol 2005; 29:52–68.

Mughal TI, Schrieber A. Principal long-term adverse effects of imatinib in patients with chronic myeloid leukemia in chronic phase. Biologics 2010; 4:315–323.

Novelli M, Rossi S, Rodriguez-Justo M, et al. DOG1 and CD117 are the antibodies of choice in the diagnosis of gastrointestinal stromal tumours. Histopathology 2010; 57:259–270.

Søreide K, Sandvik OM, Søreide JA, et al. Global epidemiology of gastrointestinal stromal tumours (GIST): A systematic review of population-based cohort studies. Cancer Epidemiol 2016; 40:39–46.

Scenario 4

Syllabus theme A: Gastro-oesophageal reflux disease

A 40-year-old male patient who smokes and drinks an average of 30 units/week presents to the surgical outpatients clinic with persistent dyspepsia and a hoarse voice in the morning. His symptoms have not improved following commencement of a proton pump inhibitor (PPI) by the GP.

Q. 4.1 What is the diagnosis?

This patient is experiencing signs and symptoms of gastro-oesophageal reflux disease (GORD), the symptoms may vary considerably and may occasionally be absent. Mucosal damage can be associated with a spectrum of motility, endoscopic and physiological abnormalities. A persistence in GORD can result in and increased incidence of Barrett's oesophagus and metaplasia, progressing to oesophageal adenocarcinoma.

The classification of GORD is adapted from the Montreal classification (see **Flowchart** below). The adult incidence GORD is particularly high in the West at 5 per 1,000 person years in the UK.

The modified Montreal classification of gastro-oesophageal reflux disease (GORD) and its associated syndromes.

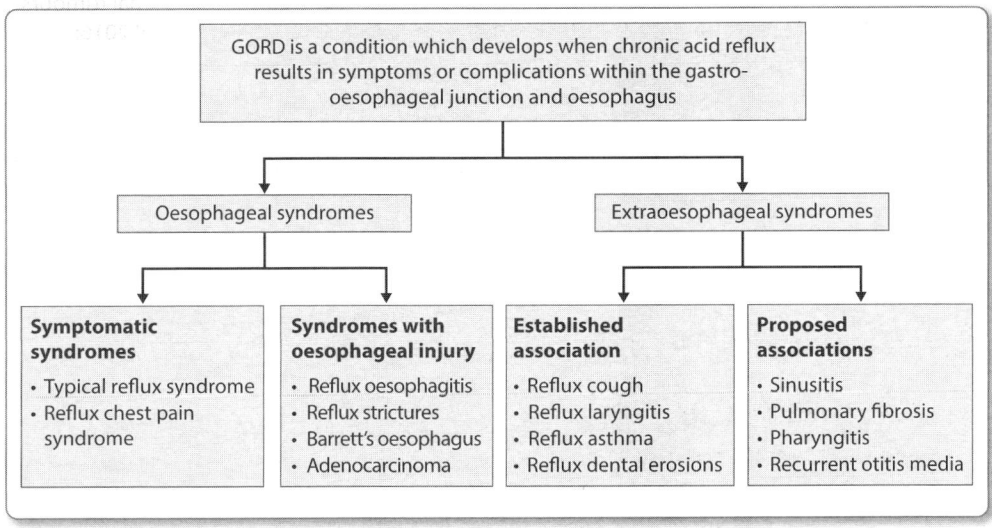

Q. 4.2 What are the risk factors for GORD, how are they classified?

There are a number of modifiable and non-modifiable risk factors, which have a significant impact on the development and exacerbation of GORD to oesophageal disease.
- *Modifiable risk factors*: Obesity, alcohol intake, tobacco smoking, hiatal hernia, Helicobacter pylori infection or recurrent infections, pregnancy and type 1 diabetes mellitus and type 2 diabetes mellitus
- *Non-modifiable risk factors*: Genetic prevalence of Barrett's oesophagus or family history of upper GI malignancy, connective tissue disorders such as limited scleroderma and Zollinger–Ellison syndrome

Q. 4.3 What is normal oesophageal anatomy?

The oesophagus is approximately 25 cm long, running from the pharynx to the stomach. It is sub-divided into three anatomical segments: (1) cervical, (2) thoracic and (3) abdominal.
(1). The cervical oesophagus (5 cm) is a direct continuation of the hypopharynx, between cricopharyngeal muscle and the thoracic inlet (first thoracic vertebra).
(2). The thoracic oesophagus (18 cm) ends at the 10th thoracic vertebra at the oesophageal hiatus.
(3). The abdominal oesophagus (1–2 cm) ends at the oesophagogastric junction (OGJ).

The muscle configuration of the oesophagus is unique with both smooth and striated muscle present within the oesophageal wall. Striated muscle is exclusively at the proximal end (including the cricopharyngeal muscle), mixing progressively with smooth muscle over the proximal and middle thirds; the lower third is entirely smooth. Blood supply is predominantly from the inferior thyroid arteries (cervical oesophagus), direct aortic branches (thoracic) and left gastric artery (abdominal). Parasympathetic innervation of the smooth muscle is provided directly from the vagus nerves with some indirect contribution proximally from the recurrent laryngeal nerves. Sympathetic innervation of the striated muscle is from the middle cervical ganglion proximally, and upper four thoracic ganglia distally.

The oesophagus has two sphincters: upper (UOS) and lower (LOS). The UOS is the cricopharyngeal muscle, the LOS is less discrete and is a complex of structures.

Q. 4.4 What are the anti-reflux mechanisms in the oesophagus?

A 10-mmHg positive-pressure gradient spans the stomach and oesophagus; the stomach and abdominal oesophagus lying within 5 mmHg of positive intra-abdominal pressure, and the thoracic oesophagus exposed to about 5 mmHg negative pressure.

Lower oesophageal sphincter

The lower oesophageal sphincter (LOS) is the primary anti-reflux mechanism. Although not an anatomically discrete sphincter, it is a dynamic high-pressure zone (HPZ) in the distal oesophagus, which relaxes to allow swallowing, belching and vomiting, and constricts to prevent reflux. It is composed of specialised smooth muscle, arranged in either clasp or sling formation, running in the distal 2–4 cm of the oesophagus and cardia.

Diaphragmatic sphincter

The slings of the right crus constitute a 'pinchcock' mechanism. In the absence of a hiatus hernia, it is difficult to separate the relative contributions of the diaphragmatic sphincter (DS) and LOS to the HPZ. DS relaxation and distensibility are controlled both central via diaphragmatic vagal efferent fibres and local via neuromuscular stretch receptors.

Distal oesophageal compression

The phreno-oesophageal ligament originates from the abdominal surface of the diaphragm and anchors the oesophagus. This anchor maintains the abdominal oesophagus within the LOS and preserves its function within the HPZ. Disruption predisposes to sliding hiatus hernias which can result in GORD.

Q. 4.5 How do you investigate the symptoms of GORD described by this patient?

The National Institute of Clinical Excellence (NICE) guidelines for GORD and dyspepsia in adults recommend that the presumptive diagnosis can be made in the presence of typical symptoms (heartburn and regurgitation) with the commencement of empirical therapy with PPIs. It is important to rule out cardiac and biliary causes of symptoms described by the patient as part of the investigations undertaken. Further investigations include:

Endoscopy

The National Institute of Clinical Excellence guidelines recommend an oesophagogastro duodenoscopy (OGD) on an immediate basis with significant bleeding; an urgent basis (within 2 weeks) for patients presenting with dysphagia or aged over 55 years with reflux/dyspeptic symptoms and weight loss; and on a non-urgent basis for patients aged over 55 years with refractory symptoms, or associated with anaemia, raised platelets or nausea and vomiting. OGDs are used more widely in comparison to the NICE guidelines. Exclusion of Barrett's disease or oesophageal adenocarcinoma and the investigation of oesophageal motility disorders are common indication for the use of an OGD.

Contrast radiology

The widespread availability of endoscopy has made contrast studies less frequent; however, they retain a complementary role when used selectively. They are particularly indicated for oesophageal dysmotility syndromes, where they may be diagnostic, for example, achalasia or diffuse oesophageal spasm (corkscrew/nutcracker oesophagus).

pH studies

Ambulatory pH studies and impedance monitoring remain the only tests that can objectively measure reflux and compare it with symptoms. Patients use a button to mark symptoms, which can then be correlated with reflux episodes (using acid as a surrogate). In most patients, testing off acid suppression therapy is recommended, however, testing on therapy may be useful for those with refractory symptoms.

Positioning of the pH probe 5 cm above the top of the LOS is crucial. As distance from nose to LOS is variable, manometry is routinely used to place the pH probe. When the probe registers a pH < 4, it records a reflux episode lasting usually until the pH rises above 5. 24-hour studies remain standard. Parameters generated include the number of reflux episodes and the total reflux time. Normal physiological reflux is typically defined as: <5% of total time with oesophageal pH < 4; less than 8% of upright time of pH < 4; < 3% of supine time pH < 4; and < 3 episodes of pH < 4 lasting 5 minutes. These parameters can then be used to generate composite scores with reference to controls, the most popular being the DeMeester score.

Oesophageal impedance monitoring

Multi-channel intra-luminal impedance involves placement of paired electrodes in the oesophageal lumen to enable detection and differentiation of gas versus liquid reflux (irrespective of pH). This study is most effective in assessment of volume or food bolus reflux.

Oesophageal manometry

Oesophageal manometry is the gold standard assessment for motor function. It is typically combined with pH studies and is recommended prior to anti-reflux surgery in order to exclude a primary dysmotility disorder such as achalasia for which surgery is contraindicated.

High-resolution manometry (HRM) uses a larger number of more closely spaced ports to generate a three-dimensional representation, combining time, position and amplitude with increased spatial resolution.

This has three advantages for the assessment of GORD:
1. The definition of the associated oesophageal dysmotility
2. Acid clearance can be better predicted
3. Better assessment of LOS function

Q. 4.6 What are the management options for this patient?

The management for this patient's symptoms is focussed on a multi-factorial risk reduction, which will include life-style measures, medical and surgical management.

Life-style measures

Avoidance of precipitating substances including smoking, excess alcohol, late night meals, spicy or excessively fatty meals, reduction in weight in particular truncal obesity.

Medical management

Pharmacological intervention is focussed on PPIs of H2 antagonists, PPIs should be commenced immediately in primary care to assess the efficacy while further investigations are undertaken.

Surgical

Referral to specialist upper gastrointestinal surgery unit for clinical assessment and investigation for potential anti-reflux surgery.

Further reading

Bredenoord AJ, Weusten BL, Smout AJ. Symptom association analysis in ambulatory gastro-oesophageal reflux monitoring. Gut 2005; 54:1810–1817.

Gyawali CP, Kahrilas PJ, Savarino E, et al. Modern diagnosis of GERD: the Lyon Consensus. Gut 2018; 67:1351–1362.

Pandolfino JE, Fox MR, Bredenoord AJ, Kahrilas PJ. High-resolution manometry in clinical practice: utilizing pressure topography to classify oesophageal motility abnormalities. Neurogastroenterol Motil 2009; 21:796–806.

Portale G, Peters J, Hsieh CC, et al. When are reflux episodes symptomatic? Dis Esophagus 2007; 20:47–52.

The National Institute of Clinical Excellence (NICE). Gastro-oesophageal reflux disease and dyspepsia in adults – investigation and management. London: National Institute for Health and Care Excellence (NICE), 2014.

Tutuian RV, Shay MF, Castell SS. Multichannel Intraluminal Impedance in Esophageal Function Testing and Gastroesophageal Reflux Monitoring. J Clin Gastroenterol 2003; 37:206–215.

Scenario 5

Anti-reflux surgery

A 46-year-old male patient returns to you surgical outpatient clinic with persistent symptoms of GORD including retrosternal pain and episode volume reflux. He denies dysphagia but reports some unintentional weight loss. He has used a PPI regularly for 6 months with some improvement in symptoms.

Q. 5.1 How would you manage this patient?

Completion of initial assessment

History and examination including inspection for peripheral stigmata of malignancy including clubbing, scleral icterus and lymphadenopathy. Abdominal inspection and palpation to identify previous surgical scars or evidence of ventral, umbilical or paraumbilical hernias which may impact on further surgical access (open or laparoscopic).

Medical therapy

The initial assessment for this case should include a clinical review of symptoms while on anti-acid therapy (PPI and H2-receptor antagonists) and on its cessation. Symptom control by addition of alternative pharmacology must be considered.

In this case vignette, it is important to discuss initial medical management to include a repeat OGD to ensure that there is no evidence of malignancy or *H. pylori* (endoscopic CLO test).

Q. 5.2 What are the selection criteria for surgery?

Those patients selected to undergo anti-reflux surgery should have objective evidence of reflux. This may be the demonstration of erosive oesophagitis on endoscopy or an abnormal amount of acid reflux demonstrated by 24-hour pH monitoring. Neither of these tests is sufficiently reliable to base all preoperative decisions on their outcome, as a number of patients with troublesome reflux will have either a normal 24-hour pH study or no evidence of oesophagitis at endoscopy. Therefore, all tests must be interpreted in conjunction with the patient's clinical presentation and response to medical therapy. A final recommendation for surgery should be based on all available clinical and objective information.

Patients selected for surgery fall into two general groups:
1. Patients who have failed to respond (or have responded only partially) to medical therapy
2. Patients whose symptoms are fully controlled by medications, but who have developed side-effects or do not wish to continue medications throughout their lives

The first group represent the large majority of patients presenting for surgery. The second group are less common but are typically younger patients who face decades of acid suppression to alleviate their symptoms.

In the first group, the response to surgery is usually more certain if the patient has had a good response to acid suppression in the past, or at least has had some symptom relief from medication. In patients who have had no response to PPIs, particularly those presenting with atypical symptoms, their symptoms are often due to something other than reflux, despite concurrent objective evidence of reflux (which can be asymptomatic). Such patients will usually not benefit from anti-reflux surgery.

Q. 5.3 Are there any other groups that would benefit from anti-reflux surgery?

Reflux with stricture formation

The treatment of peptic oesophageal strictures has been greatly altered since PPIs became available, and thus the role for surgery has declined. It is now unusual to see patients with refractory strictures. Strictures in young and fit patients are usually best treated by anti-reflux surgery and dilatation. However, many patients who develop strictures are elderly or infirm and the use of PPIs with dilatation is usually effective in this group.

Reflux with respiratory complications

When gastro-oesophageal regurgitation results in aspiration and chronic airway diseases such as recurrent pneumonia, asthma or bronchiectasis. There is also an establishing role for anti-reflux surgery in patients with chronic lung disease requiring transplantation with a significant reduction in decline of lung function seen post-anti-reflux surgery.

Reflux with Barrett's disease

Despite numerous publications on the role of anti-reflux surgery in Barrett's oesophagus, there are few randomised controlled trials. Parilla et al. compared the results of H2-receptor antagonists and PPIs versus open Nissen fundoplication with the primary outcome being preventing Barrett's oesophagus progression to dysplasia and adenocarcinoma. A median follow-up of 5 years was adopted, and the authors have no significant difference between the two groups in terms of progression to dysplasia or malignancy. This trial concluded that surgery cannot be advocated as the treatment of choice in patients with Barrett's oesophagus.

Q. 5.4 What is the evidence for surgical verses medical treatment?

There have been a number of trials to determine the primary efficacy of either medical or surgical management for GORD. To date, six randomised controlled trials comparing medical with surgical intervention for GORD, follow-up ranges for these studies were from 1–10.6 years. A summary of these studies is as follows:

- *Spechler SJ et al. (2001)*: Long-term outcome of medical and surgical therapies for gastro-oesophageal reflux disease: follow-up of a randomised controlled trial. 239 participants with median follow-up of 10.6 years. The authors concluded that this study suggests that anti-reflux surgery should not be advised with the expectation that patients with GORD will no longer need to take anti-acid medications or that the procedure will prevent oesophageal cancer among those with GORD and Barrett oesophagus
- *Spechler SJ et al. (2019)*: Randomised control trial for medical therapy versus surgery for refractory heartburn. The trial enrolled an initial 306 patients, but subsequently identified 99 patients in the cohort with functional reflux. The assigned groups were surgical treatment [laparoscopic Nissen fundoplication (LNF)], active medical treatment (omeprazole plus baclofen), or control medical treatment (omeprazole plus placebo). The authors concluded that for this highly selected group of patients with refractory heartburn, surgery was more successful for symptom control
- *Mahon D et al (2005)*: Randomised clinical trial of LNF compared with proton-pump inhibitors for treatment of chronic gastro-oesophageal reflux. A total of 340 patients with a history of GORD for at least 6 months were investigated by endoscopy, 24-hours pH monitoring and manometry. The authors concluded that LNF leads to significantly less acid exposure of the lower oesophagus at 3 months and significantly greater improvements in both gastrointestinal and general well-being after 12 months compared with PPI treatment
- *Mehta S et al. (2006)*: Prospective trial of LNF versus proton pump inhibitor therapy for gastro-oesophageal reflux disease: 7-year follow-up. 183 included in randomised controlled trial comparing LNF and PPI therapy for the treatment of GORD. The authors concluded that both optimal PPI therapy and laparoscopic Nissen fundoplication are effective treatments for GERD. However, surgery offers additional benefit for those who have only partial symptomatic relief while on PPIs
- *Grant A et al. (2008); UK REFLUX TRIAL*: The effectiveness and cost-effectiveness of minimal access surgery among people with gastro-oesophageal reflux disease – a UK collaborative study. There were 810 patients – 357 patients were recruited to the randomised arm of the trial (178 patients were allocated to surgical and 179 patients were allocated to medical management). A further 453 patients were included in parallel non-randomised preference arm (261 patients chose surgical, 192 patients chose medical management).

    Among patients requiring long-term medication to control symptoms of GORD, surgical management significantly increases general and reflux-specific health-related quality of life measures, at least up to 12 months after surgery
- *Attwood SE et al. (2008)*: Medical or surgical management of GERD patients with Barrett's oesophagus: the LOTUS trial 3-year experience. A total of 554 patients

with gastro-oesophageal reflux disease, 60 patients had Barrett's oesophagus-28 randomised to esomeprazole and 32 to LNF. Four patients crossed over secondary to treatment failure. The authors suggest that the success of LNF is similar in patients with or without BE and matches optimised medical therapy
- *Galmiche JP et al. (2011), LOTUS randomised clinical trial*: This publication presented the 5-year follow-up of the randomised trial, which enrolled 554 patients with well-established chronic GORD who initially responded to acid suppression. The authors demonstrated that with contemporary anti-reflux surgery for GORD, either by drug-induced acid suppression with esomeprazole or by LNF, most patients achieve and remain in remission at 5 years
- *Anvari M et al. (2011)*: A randomised controlled trial of LNF versus PPIs for treatment of patients with chronic gastroesophageal reflux disease – 1-year comparison of optimised medical therapy using PPI (n = 52) LNF (n = 52). Patients were monitored for 1 year. The primary endpoint was frequency of gastro-oesophageal reflux disease symptoms. Surgical patients had improved symptoms, pH control, and overall quality of life health index after surgery at 1 year compared with the medical group

Q. 5.5 Describe the surgical technique?

Anti-reflux surgery technique

The choice of technique for anti-reflux surgery has traditionally been based on anatomic considerations and the surgeon's preference and expertise, this approach results in a lack of standardisation making outcome comparisons difficult. Attwood et al. attempted to standardise surgical practice by identifying a consensus opinion on surgical technique in their randomised trial designed to compare medical and surgical therapy.

Based on a consensus of 40 experienced upper GI surgeons, the following standardised approach to Nissen fundoplication was followed:
- Opening the phreno-oesophageal ligament in a left to right fashion
- Preservation of the hepatic branch of the anterior vagus nerve
- Dissection of both crura
- Transhiatal mobilisation to allow approximately 3 cm of intra-abdominal oesophagus
- Short gastric vessel division to ensure a tension-free wrap
- Crural closure posteriorly with non-absorbable sutures
- Creation of a 1.5–2 cm wrap with the most distal suture incorporating the anterior muscular wall of the oesophagus
- Bougie placement at the time of wrap construction

This standardisation led to excellent postoperative outcomes comparable with medical treatment and included a 2% conversion rate, 3% postoperative complication rate, and a median postoperative length of stay of 2 days.

Nissen fundoplication

Nissen originally described a procedure that entailed mobilisation of the oesophagus from the diaphragmatic hiatus, reduction of any hiatus hernia into the abdominal cavity, preservation of the vagus nerves and mobilisation of the posterior gastric fundus around behind the oesophagus, without dividing the short gastric vessels, and suturing of the posterior fundus to the anterior wall of the fundus using non-absorbable sutures, achieving a fundoplication of 5 cm in length.

Posterior fundoplication

A variety of fundoplication operations have been described in which the fundus is wrapped partially round the back of the oesophagus with the aim of reduction of the possible side effects of total fundoplication due to over competence of the cardia, i.e. dysphagia and gas-related problems. Toupet described a posterior partial fundoplication in which the fundus is passed behind the oesophagus and sutured to the left lateral and right lateral walls of the oesophagus, as well as to the right diaphragmatic pillar, creating a 270° posterior fundoplication.

Anterior partial fundoplication

Several anterior wraps have been described, the most commonly used in European practice is the 'Dor' fundoplication, in which the distal oesophagus is mobilised, the fundus is sutured to the left and right sides of the oesophagus (with or without suturing to diaphragm).

The 'Dor' procedure is commonly used in combination with an abdominal cardiomyotomy for achalasia as it is unlikely to cause dysphagia, and it may reduce the risk of gastro-oesophageal reflux following cardiomyotomy.

Collis procedure

The Collis procedure is useful for patients whose oesophagogastric junction cannot be reduced below the diaphragm (short oesophagus). This is less common in clinical practice, especially with laparoscopic mobilisation and reduction of a paraoesophageal hernia sac. The Collis procedure entails the construction of a tube of gastric lesser curve to recreate an abdominal length of oesophagus, around which a fundoplication can then be constructed to help with oesophageal shortening.

Partial versus total fundoplication

There are 10 recent randomised controlled trials and two meta-analyses which have investigated the differences between partial and total fundoplication.

No significant differences between the two types of procedures were noted in the incidence of oesophagitis, heartburn, persisting acid reflux, in the proportion of patients experiencing a good or excellent long-term outcome.

Note: Evidence suggests that the outcomes of patients with oesophageal dysmotility are not affected by the type of fundoplication.

Anterior versus Nissen fundoplication

Four randomised controlled trials reporting on 457 patients with a follow-up ranging from 6 months to 10 years have been published and have compared laparoscopic anterior fundoplication with the LNF. Based on the findings of these trials, the anterior fundoplication was associated with significantly less postoperative dysphagia according to at least one of the evaluated dysphagia parameters compared with the LNF even during long-term follow-up (up to 10 years). However, the anterior fundoplication was found to be less effective for reflux control (based on patient symptoms and objective tests) as more patients required re-operations for reflux control. Patient satisfaction ratings were similar between the groups in all studies up to 10 years after surgery.

Toupet versus Nissen fundoplication

Six recent randomised controlled trials (including both open and laparoscopic techniques) with follow-up of 1–5 years have compared the Toupet fundoplication with the Nissen. The majority of published studies have demonstrated lower dysphagia rates after a Toupet fundoplication and no difference in heartburn control between the two procedures at follow-up.

Postoperative complications

There are several complications associated with a fundoplication procedure, these are generally divided into short- and long-term results. In general, a laparoscopic fundoplication is a safe and effective procedure and confers a good 10-year outcome on the control of GORD. The effects of postoperative dysphagia are not long lasting in a number of studies the effect of acid reflux results in a greater degree of dysphagia pre-operatively compared to 12 months postoperatively.

Further reading

Abbassi-Ghadi N, Kumar S, Cheung B, et al. Anti-reflux surgery for lung transplant recipients in the presence of impedance-detected duodenogastroesophageal reflux and bronchiolitis obliterans syndrome: a study of efficacy and safety. J Heart Lung Transplant 2013; 32:588–595.
Anvari M, Allen C, Marshall J, et al. A Randomized Controlled Trial of Laparoscopic Nissen Fundoplication Versus Proton Pump Inhibitors for Treatment of Patients With Chronic Gastroesophageal Reflux Disease- One-Year Follow-Up. Gastroenterology 2011; 5:885.
Attwood SE, Lundell L, Hatlebakk JG, et al. Medical or surgical management of GERD patients with Barrett's esophagus: the LOTUS trial 3-year experience. J Gastrointest Surg 2008; 12:1646–1654.
Baigrie RJ, Cullis SN, Ndhluni AJ, Cariem A. Randomized double-blind trial of laparoscopic Nissen fundoplication versus anterior partial fundoplication. Br J Surg 2005; 92:819–823.
Cai W, Watson DI, Lally CJ, et al. Ten-year clinical outcome of a prospective randomized clinical trial of laparoscopic Nissen versus anterior 180 (degrees) partial fundoplication. Br J Surg 2008; 95:1501–1505.
Catarci M, Gentileschi P, Papi C, et al. Evidence-based appraisal of antireflux fundoplication. Ann Surg 2004; 239:325–337.
Chrysos E, Tsiaoussis J, Zoras OJ, et al. Laparoscopic surgery for gastroesophageal reflux disease patients with impaired esophageal peristalsis: total or partial fundoplication? J Am Coll Surg 2003; 197:8–15.
Dor J, Humbert P, Paoli JM, Miorclerc M, Aubert J. Treatment of reflux by the so-called modified Heller-Nissen technic. Presse Med 1967; 75:2563–2565.
Fibbe C, Layer P, Keller J, et al. Esophageal motility in reflux disease before and after fundoplication: a prospective, randomized, clinical, and manometric study. Gastroenterology 2001; 121:5–14.
Galmiche JP, Hatlebakk J, Attwood S, et al. Laparoscopic antireflux surgery vs esomeprazole treatment for chronic GERD: the LOTUS randomized clinical trial. JAMA 2011; 305:1969–1977.

Grant AWS, Ramsay C, Bojke L, et al. The effectiveness and cost-effectiveness of minimal access surgery amongst people with gastro-oesophageal reflux disease – a UK collaborative study. The REFLUX Trial. Health Technol Assess 2008; 12:1–181.

Hagedorn C, Lönroth H, Rydberg L, Ruth M, Lundell L. Long-term efficacy of total (Nissen-Rossetti) and posterior partial (Toupet) fundoplication: results of a randomized clinical trial. J Gastrointest Surg 2002; 6:540–555.

Jobe BA, Horvath KD, Swanstrom LL. Postoperative Function Following Laparoscopic Collis Gastroplasty for Shortened Esophagus. Arch Surg 1998; 133:867–874.

Lundell L, Abrahamsson H, Ruth M, et al. Long-term results of a prospective randomized comparison of total fundic wrap (Nissen-Rossetti) or semifundoplication (Toupet) for gastro-oesophageal reflux. Br J Surg 1996; 83:830–835.

Mahon D, Rhodes M, Decadt B, et al. Randomized clinical trial of laparoscopic Nissen fundoplication compared with proton-pump inhibitors for treatment of chronic gastro-oesophageal reflux. Br J Surg 2005; 92:695–699.

Mehta S, Bennett J, Mahon D, Rhodes M. Prospective trial of laparoscopic nissen fundoplication versus proton pump inhibitor therapy for gastroesophageal reflux disease: Seven-year follow-up. J Gastrointest Surg 2006; 10:1312–1316.

Nissen R. A simple operation for control of reflux esophagitis. Schweiz Med Wochenschr 1956; 18:590–592.

Parrilla P, Martínez de Haro LF, Ortiz A, et al. Long-Term Results of a Randomized Prospective Study Comparing Medical and Surgical Treatment of Barrett's Esophagus. Ann Surg 2003; 237:291–298.

Salminen PT, Hiekkanen HI, Rantala AP, Ovaska JT. Comparison of long-term outcome of laparoscopic and conventional nissen fundoplication: a prospective randomized study with an 11-year follow-up. Ann Surg 2007; 246:201–206.

Spechler SJ, Hunter JG, Jones KM, et al. Randomized Trial of Medical versus Surgical Treatment for Refractory Heartburn. N Engl J Med 2019; 381:1513–1523.

Spechler SLE, Ahnen D, Goyal RK, et al. Long-term outcome of medical and surgical therapies for gastroesophageal reflux disease: follow-up of a randomized controlled trial. JAMA 2001; 18:2331–2338.

Spence GM, Watson DI, Jamiesion GG, Lally CJ, Devitt PG. Multicenter, prospective, double-blind, randomized trial of laparoscopic nissen vs anterior 90 degrees partial fundoplication. J Gastrointest Surg 2006; 10:698–705.

Strate U, Emmermann A, Fibbe C, Layer P, Zornig C. Laparoscopic fundoplication: Nissen versus Toupet two-year outcome of a prospective randomized study of 200 patients regarding preoperative esophageal motility. Surg Endosc 2008; 22:21–30.

Toupet A. Technique d'oesophago-gastroplastie avec phrenogastropexie appliquée dans la cure radicale des hernies hiatales et comme complement de l'operation de Heller dans les cardiospasmes. Med Acad Chir 1963; 89:374–379.

Varin O, Velstra B, De Sutter S, Ceelen W. Total vs Partial Fundoplication in the Treatment of Gastroesophageal Reflux Disease: A meta-analysis. Arch Surg 2009; 144:273–278.

Watson DI, Jamieson GG, Lally C, et al. Multicenter, prospective, double-blind, randomized trial of laparoscopic nissen vs anterior 90 degrees partial fundoplication. Arch Surg 2004; 139:1160–1167.

Zornig C, Strate U, Fibbe C, Emmermann A, Layer P. Nissen vs Toupet laparoscopic fundoplication. Surg Endosc 2002; 16:758–766.

Scenario 6

Barrett's oesophagus

A 47-year-old male patient with Barrett's oesophagus presents for his surveillance endoscopy and the endoscopist reports a 'long segment of Barrett's disease extending from the GOJ at 40 cm with an associated hiatal hernia'. A nodular lesion is biopsied and sent for histology.

Q. 6.1 The endoscopist sends the patient to you for a surgical opinion, what would you do?

Initially perform a complete history and examination including review of risk factors and pharmacology.

The primary investigation would be a repeat OGD which enables assessment of the pharynx and epiglottis for reflux pharyngitis. Passage of the endoscope distally enables assessment of the length of the Barrett's and classify the extent of the disease by the Prague classification criteria to determine if there is progression of disease. Four quadrant mucosal biopsies can also be taken following endoscopic assessment using the Seattle protocol methodology.

Q. 6.2 You determine that this patient has a long-term history of GORD and Barrett's oesophagus. He has been on PPI therapy since his mid-twenties. He has adopted the lifestyle changes as advised but still suffers with daily reflux related symptoms. Provide a definition of Barrett's disease of the oesophagus?

Definition of Barrett's oesophagus

Barrett's oesophagus is the metaplastic replacement of stratified squamous epithelium of the oesophagus by columnar epithelium.

Internationally, there is no universally accepted definition, however, the presence of specialised intestinal metaplasia (SIM), characterised by the presence of goblet cells is typical. SIM is associated with an increased risk of progression to low grade dysplasia (LGD), high-grade dysplasia (HGD) and adenocarcinoma.

Q. 6.3 How does the OGD report correlate with this patient's clinical presentation?

This patient is failing with the medical management of his Barrett's oesophagus, he has a long segment of disease as per the Prague classification and has persistent acid-related symptoms, which would require further assessment by pH and manometry studies. The Hiatal hernia may be contributing to his symptoms and the nodule may suggest dysplastic changes to the distal oesophagus which would require endoscopic excision or surgical resection if confirmed histopathologically.

Q. 6.4 What is the Prague classification?

At endoscopy, Barrett's epithelium (BE) has a salmon pink colour with a velvet-like texture compared to the pale, glossy appearance of squamous epithelium. The key anatomical landmark is the oesophagogastric junction (OGJ), which is usually identified as the proximal extent of the upper gastric folds. The squamo-columnar junction (Z line) is the point at which squamous mucosa of the oesophagus meets columnar mucosa of the stomach. In the absence of SIM, the Z line and OGJ coincide.

The Prague classification enables the assessment and monitoring of Barrett's oesophagus in patients during their surveillance endoscopies (see **Figure** below). The criteria define the assessment of the circumferential (C) and maximum (M) extent of the endoscopically visualised Barrett's oesophagus segment as well as endoscopic landmarks such as the OGJ and pathology such as hiatal hernias. The classification conferred an overall reliability co-efficient above 0.9.

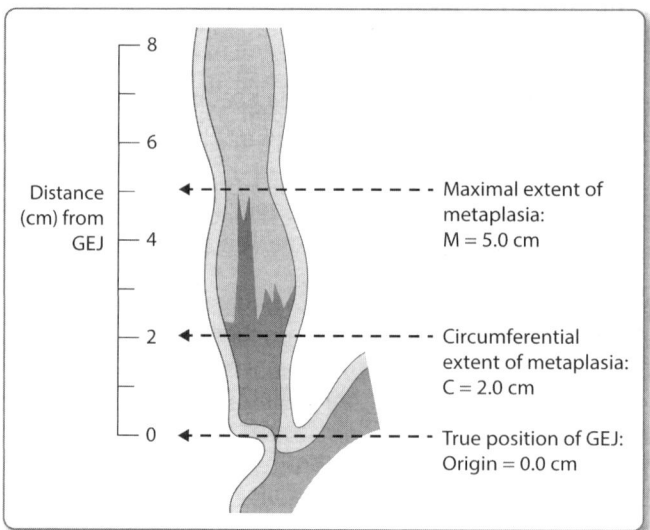

Prague classification criteria for extent of Barrett's oesophagus, image reference from Sharma P, et al.

Q. 6.5 This patient has an area of nodularity, which was biopsied. The report returns as low-grade dysplasia, what would you do?

The patient would need to be informed of the findings and counselled for the risks associated with progression of LGD to malignancy (40%), this is 80% for HGD.

Modifiable and life-style risk factors, such as smoking should be corrected. Double does PPI therapy should be instituted as best medical management. In this case, the nodule biopsied was taken as part of a 'targeted biopsy protocol' it does not confer the standard surveillance biopsy protocol advised for Barrett's oesophagus, which is discussed later. The initial management would be a repeat OGD and mapping biopsies as per the British Society of Gastroenterology Guidelines. Note, the Seattle biopsy protocol is utilised in North America.

The management for LGD varies between the UK and the US, the British Society of Gastroenterology revised guidelines suggest: Patients with LGD should have a repeat endoscopy in 6 months' time. If LGD is found in any of the follow-up OGD and is confirmed by an expert GI pathologist in at least two sets of biopsies (independent histopathologists), the patient should be offered endoscopic ablation therapy, preferably with radiofrequency ablation (RFA), after review by the specialist MDT. If ablation is not undertaken, 6-monthly surveillance is recommended.

Biopsy protocol

The advised protocol for Barrett's oesophagus biopsies varies between the UK and the US. For a featureless segment undergoing routine surveillance, mapping biopsies should be taken at 2-cm intervals from each quadrant as well as separate biopsies from the anatomic cardia.

For dysplastic segments biopsies should be taken at 1-cm intervals. This so-called Seattle protocol increases the yield of both low-grade and high-grade dysplasia by 17% and 3%, respectively, compared with random biopsies.

A minimum of eight biopsies are required in order to provide an acceptable degree of histological confirmation of BE. If only four biopsies are taken, BE is confirmed in only 34.7% of cases.

Q. 6.6 Explain how you would manage this patient?

Lifestyle and disease modifiable risk factors need to be corrected. Further management is directed according to the extent of disease and histological findings as per the biopsy protocol.

Medical management

All patients with a diagnosis of Barrett's oesophagus are on primary prevention of GORD with PPIs. In a randomised trial of twice-daily PPI use versus twice-daily H2-blocker use identify some regression in Barrett's noted in the twice-daily treatment group.

Fundoplication for Barrett's prevention

There are no randomised control trials for fundoplication showing the prevention or regression of Barrett's oesophagus. Parilla et al. compared the results of H2-receptor antagonists and PPIs versus open LNR with the outcome measure being preventing Barrett's oesophagus progressing to dysplasia and adenocarcinoma. The authors concluded that surgery cannot be advocated as the treatment of choice in patients with Barrett's oesophagus. In addition, PPI alone does not eliminate the risk of dysplasia or adenocarcinoma.

A schematic for the management of Barrett's metaplasia and associated histological variants.

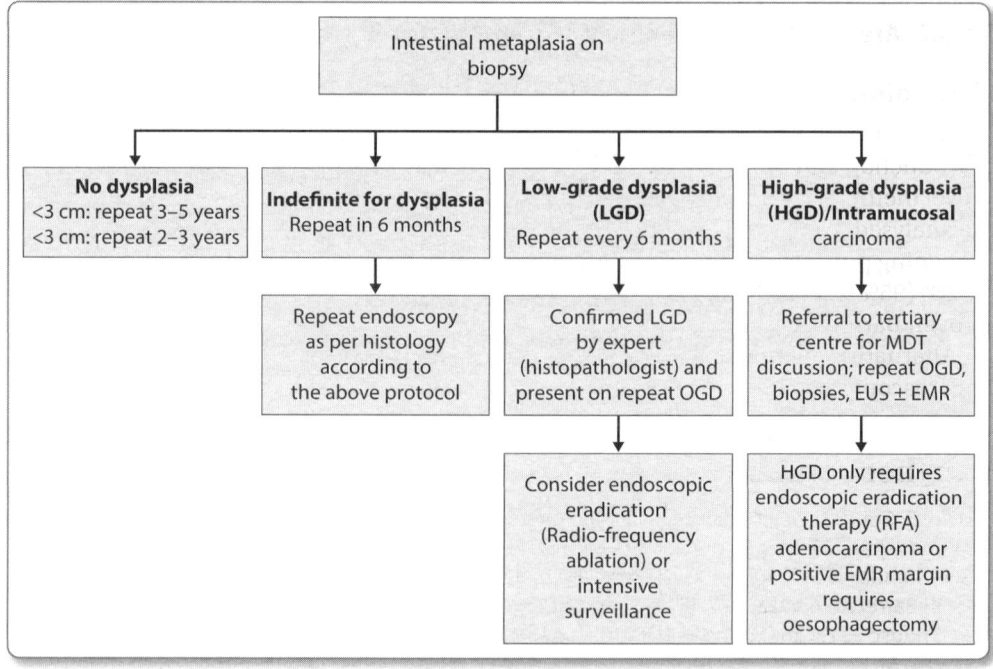

(EMR, endoscopic mucosal resection; EUS, endoscopic ultrasound; MDT, multidisciplinary team; OGD, oesophagogastro duodenoscopy)

Radiofrequency ablation

Radiofrequency ablation (RFA) utilises radiofrequency energy applied via a coiled electrode array to ablate the mucosal surface epithelium allowing replacement with neosquamous epithelium.

The RFA is performed along the entire segment of SIM with approximately 5 mm of overlap between ablated zones. After the initial ablation, the patient is treated with maximal acid suppression. Typical regimens should include a PPI at high dose twice daily or high-dose H2 blocker ± sucralfate suspension for a minimum of two or at least until eradication therapies are complete. The patient should avoid alcohol intake and cease smoking.

At 12 weeks, the patient should undergo a repeat OGD, and if nodular areas are identified within the previously ablated SIM segment, then these should be biopsied (targeted method) and endoscopically resected [endoscopic mucosal resection/endoscopic ultrasound (EMR/ESD)]. A further circumferential ablation is performed if there is >2 cm of circumferential featureless residual SIM or multiple islands of residual SIM.

The efficacy of RFA for Barrett's metaplasia was summarised in a meta-analysis by Orman et al. The analysis included 18 studies of 3,802 patients reporting efficacy and six studies of 540 patients reporting durability. The authors concluded that treatment of Barrett's oesophagus with RFA results in complete eradication of dysplasia and SIM in a high proportion of patients with few recurrences of SIM after treatment and a high safety profile.

Q. 6.7 Are there any screening programmes for Barrett's oesophagus?

Screening

There is currently no formal screening for Barrett's oesophagus in the UK, the introduction and utility of sampling devices such as 'Cytosponge™' provide future novel methods for non-invasive cellular sampling of the oesophagus which can then be analysed using cytology, immunohistochemistry or other genetic analysis for screening purposes. Cytosponge™ was evaluated in the BEST2 trial with a sensitivity of 79.9% (95% CI 76.4–83%) and specificity 92.4% (95% CI 89.5–94.7%) for endoscopically proven Barrett's oesophagus.

Alternative methods include capsule endoscopy; however, this is limited to macroscopic visualisation alone.

Further reading

Abela JE, Going JJ, Mackenzie JF, et al. Systematic four-quadrant biopsy detects Barrett's dysplasia in more patients than nonsystematic biopsy. Am J Gastroenterol 2008; 103:850–855.

ASGE Standards of Practice Committee; Buxbaum JL, Abbas Fehmi SM, et al. The role of endoscopy in Barrett's esophagus and other premalignant conditions of the esophagus. Gastrointest Endosc 2012; 76:1087–1094.

di Pietro M, Fitzgerald RC; BSG Barrett's guidelines working group. Revised British Society of Gastroenterology recommendation on the diagnosis and management of Barrett's oesophagus with low-grade dysplasia. Gut 2018; 67:392–393.

Fitzgerald RC, di Pietro M, Ragunath K, et al. British Society of Gastroenterology guidelines on the diagnosis and management of Barrett's oesophagus. Gut 2014; 63:7–42.

Harrison R, Perry I, Haddadin W, et al. Detection of intestinal metaplasia in Barrett's esophagus: an observational comparator study suggests the need for a minimum of eight biopsies. Am J Gastroenterol 2007; 102:1154–1161.

Orman ES, Li N, Shaheen NJ. Efficacy and durability of radiofrequency ablation for Barrett's Esophagus: systematic review and meta-analysis. Clin Gastroenterol Hepatol 2013; 11:1245–1255.

Peters FGS, Kuipers E, Sluiter W, et al. Endoscopic regression of Barrett's oesophagus during omeprazole treatment: a randomised double blind study. Gut 1999; 45:489–494.

Ross-Innes CS, Debiram-Beecham I, O'Donovan M, et al. Evaluation of a minimally invasive cell sampling device coupled with assessment of trefoil factor 3 expression for diagnosing Barrett's esophagus: a multi-center case-control study. PLoS Med 2015; 12:e1001780.

Sharma P, Dent J, Armstrong D, et al. The development and validation of an endoscopic grading system for Barrett's esophagus: the Prague C & M criteria. Gastroenterology 2006; 131:1392–1399.

Scenario 7

Oesophageal dysmotility

A 78-year-old female patient presents with progressive dysphagia and recurrent chest infections. She reports eating a normal volume but is losing weight and has noticed worsening halitosis over the past 2 months. She does not have a family history of UGI cancer but required several endoscopies in her childhood, for reasons she cannot recall.

Q. 7.1 What is your differential?

Complete a full history and examination primarily.

The differential diagnosis is an upper GI malignancy, which would need to be ruled out with an oesophagogastroduodenoscopy (OGD).

Further diagnoses include achalasia, peptic stricture, Barrett's oesophagus with stricturing, delayed caustic stricture (prior history of paediatric OGDs).

Q. 7.2 What is the epidemiology of achalasia; what are the clinical features and the natural history?

The pathophysiology is unclear, but it is postulated that it could be as a result of an autoimmune response to viral infections such as herpes simplex virus 1 (HSV-1). It is important not to confuse idiopathic achalasia with Chagas disease of the oesophagus, which is caused by the protozoan parasite *Trypanosoma cruzi,* which invades the myenteric nerve plexus of the oesophagus resulting in 'megaoesophagus'.

Clinical presentation

The incidence of achalasia increases with age, but does occur in any age group, including paediatric patients. It has no gender predilection. The classical symptoms are dysphagia, regurgitation, chest pain and weight loss.

Common complaints are the requirement to take a longer time than family members to finish a meal, as well as a need to wash most mouthfuls of food down with water. Regurgitation is the second most common symptom, occurring in approximately 80% of patients and is due to LOS obstruction as well as oesophageal dilatation and formation of a reservoir for food. Chest pain occurs in over half of achalasia patients and is found equally in all subtypes. Weight loss is secondary to poor nutritional input.

Achalasia leads to an increased risk of oesophageal cancer, both SCC and ACA histological subtypes. The risk of SCC is approximately 30–50-fold compared to the baseline population and is as a result of stasis and inflammation in the oesophagus. The increase in ACA risk is approximately 10-fold and associated with persistent gastro-oesophageal reflux, which is typical in all forms of achalasia.

Q. 7.3 How do you make a diagnosis of achalasia from your differential?

Investigations

The first diagnostic step is to rule out anatomical lesions, neoplasia, or pseudoachalasia using endoscopy or radiology. Pseudoachalasia should particularly be suspected in cases of rapidly progressing dysphagia, significant weight loss, and old age, and should be excluded by endoscopic ultrasound or CT scan. These investigations will reveal unusual thickening of the oesophageal wall, mass lesions, or even an infiltrating pancreatic carcinoma.

Radiology

In the early stage of achalasia, both endoscopy and radiology are less sensitive than manometry and only identify about half (or even less) of patients with early-stage of achalasia. In advanced cases, endoscopy might reveal a dilated oesophagus with retained food and increased resistance at the gastro-oesophageal junction. Radiological examination often shows a typical bird-beak image at the junction with a dilated oesophageal body, occasionally an air-fluid level and absence of an intragastric air bubble. In more advanced achalasia, severe dilatation with stasis of food and a sigmoid-like appearance can occur. To assess emptying of the oesophagus, a timed barium swallow can be done, in which the height of the barium column 5 minutes after ingestion of diluted barium is a measure of emptying.

Manometry studies

On conventional manometry, absence of peristalsis, sometimes with increased intra-oesophageal pressure owing to stasis of food and saliva, and incomplete relaxation of the LOS on deglutition (residual pressure > 10 mmHg) are the hallmarks of achalasia. Additionally, the resting tone of the LOS is often raised.

High-resolution manometry (HRM) is increasingly being used to provide more detailed information on oesophageal motility. This modality allows the placement of 36 or more pressure sensors spaced only 1 cm apart, HRM allows detailed pressure recording from the pharynx to the stomach and is regarded as the gold standard for diagnosis of achalasia.

The use of HRM has led to the sub-classification of achalasia into three clinically relevant groups on the basis of the pattern of contractility in the oesophageal body. **High-resolution manometry (HRM) dependent classification of achalasia.**

Achalasia classification	HRM features
Type 1	Classical achalasia; no evidence of pressurisation
Type 2	Achalasia with compression or compartmentalisation in the distal oesophagus > 30 mmHg
Type 3	Two or more spastic contractions

Q. 7.4 How would you manage this patient?

The management options should be presented in a stepwise process from medical, endoscopic to surgical intervention. Initial medical and endoscopic therapies may be used at temporising measures prior to definitive surgical management. The development of per-oral endoscopic myotomy (POEM) has introduced a further minimally invasive endoscopic option for the management of achalasia.

Medical therapy

The two most often used pharmacological drugs are nitrates and calcium-channel blockers. Nitrates inhibit normal LOS contraction by dephosphorylation of the myosin light chain. In a review by Wen Z, et al. only two randomised studies assessed the clinical success of nitrates with no significance in the intervention and control arm of the study. Nifedipine, in sublingual doses of 10–20 mg 15–60 minutes before meals, is the most widely used medical therapy for achalasia. It inhibits LOS muscle contraction by blocking cellular calcium uptake and lowers the LOS resting pressure by 30–60%.

Botulinum toxin

A more widely used pharmacological treatment is botulinum toxin A, a neurotoxin that blocks the release of acetylcholine from the nerve terminals. It is directly injected, at a dose of 80–100 units in four or eight quadrants, into the LOS through a sclerotherapy needle during upper-gastrointestinal endoscopy.

Botulinum toxin is a safe and effective treatment with few side effects. More than 80% of cases have a clinical response by 1 month, but response fades rapidly with <60% of patients in remission at 1 year. Leyden J et al. reviewed the randomised trials comparing botulinum toxin with pneumodilatation; Zaninotto G et al. compared botulinum toxin with laparoscopic myotomy, showing initially comparable relief from dysphagia, but a rapid deterioration in patients treated with botulinum toxin after 6–12 months. Therefore, it is used only as an interim option.

Pneumatic dilatation

Pneumatic dilatation, which tears the LOS by forceful stretching with air or fluid-filled balloons, has become standardised with the development of wire guided non-compliant endoscopic balloons (25–40 mm diameter).

The procedure is principally performed under fluoroscopic guidance with the balloon positioned across the LOS and gradually inflated until the waist is flattened. The most popular technique is a graded dilation protocol starting with a 25 or 30 mm balloon. Subsequent dilations are spaced over 2–4 week intervals on the basis of symptom relief or improvement in oesophageal emptying.

Pneumatic dilatation has been shown to have good to excellent symptom relief in 74%, 86%, and 90% of patients treated with 30, 35, and 40 mm balloons, respectively. Over 4–6 years, nearly a third of patients have symptom relapse. However, long-term remission can be achieved in nearly all these patients by repeat dilatation by an on-demand strategy on the basis of symptom recurrence.

Laparoscopic Heller's cardiomyotomy

Surgical management is by myotomy of the muscle layer of the distal oesophagus and LOS, with or without the addition of a fundoplication to reduce the risk of gastro-oesophageal reflux.

Procedure

The patient is set up for the standard approach to the hiatus as per the operating surgeon's preference. The phreno-oesophageal ligament is divided, and the lower oesophagus mobilised so that the myotomy can be performed from the gastric cardia to a point approximately 5 cm up the oesophagus while preserving the anterior vagus nerve. The posterior oesophagus does not require mobilisation unless the surgeon is planning a posterior 'Toupet' style fundoplication. Important steps during the procedure include:
- Full mobilisation of the oesophagus before the myotomy is begun, including mobilisation of the anterior fat pad
- Downward traction on the stomach by the surgical assistant to keep the muscular layers and mucosa on stretch thereby decreasing the risk of mucosal injury
- Careful dissection of oesophageal layers down to the mucosa in order to lift the muscle off the mucosa before division
- A myotomy extending up the oesophagus 5 cm and down 2 cm over the gastric cardia, starting with the oesophageal myotomy where the plane is easier to dissect

Laparoscopic Heller myotomy combined with partial fundoplication is a safe operation with Campos et al. reporting an operative mortality of 0.1% (three deaths in 3,086 patients). The most common complication of laparoscopic Heller myotomy is perforation of the oesophageal or gastric mucosa during the myotomy, which is usually recognised during the procedure and repaired immediately without any consequences.

Laparoscopic Heller's cardiomyotomy versus pneumatic dilatation

The best evidence comparing laparoscopic Heller myotomy + DOR fundoplication (LHM + DOR) with pneumatic dilatation (PD) comes from the European achalasia trial. This randomised clinical trial including 201 patients published 5-year results in 2015. The primary conclusions were:
- 5-year results after LHM + DOR and PD are equivalent (84% vs. 82% response rate)
- Pneumatic dilatation needs to be performed by a standardised technique to minimise the risk of perforation
- Patients who were treated with PD were considered to have equivalent results to LHM patients, 25% had required a median of three serial dilatations over the 5-year period to maintain clinical response
- The results of both treatments decline over time, confirming that achalasia is a chronic and progressive disease, even when treated aggressively

Per-oral endoscopic myotomy

Per-oral endoscopic myotomy is a recently developed endoscopic technique for treatment of achalasia. The technique involves the formation of a submucosal tunnel to reach the LOS and subsequent dissection of the circular muscle fibres over a 7-cm oesophageal and 2 cm gastric length.

Longer follow-up is needed and randomised studies to compare POEM with pneumatic dilatation or laparoscopic Heller myotomy.

Oesophagectomy

Despite the efficacy of pneumodilatation and laparoscopic Heller myotomy, 2–5% of patients will develop end-stage disease. This is defined as a massive dilatation of the oesophagus with retention of food, unresponsive reflux disease, or the presence of preneoplastic lesions. In these cases, oesophageal resection might be necessary to improve the patient's quality of life and avoid the risk of invasive carcinoma. Reconstruction options after oesophagectomy are similar to those utilised postcancer resectional surgery.

Q. 7.5 What is nutcracker, jackhammer and how does it compare to distal oesophageal spasm? How are these conditions classified?

Nutcracker or jackhammer oesophagus is diagnosed by high-amplitude contractions in the oesophagus. These motility disorders as well as achalasia are most commonly defined with the Chicago classification (version 3.0). This hierarchical analysis utilises HRM to determine an integrated relaxation pressure (IRP), distal contractile integer – a measure of the strength of peristaltic waves and distal latency – the identification of premature or spastic contractions.

Nutcracker oesophagus

Nutcracker oesophagus is a condition where, on HRM, there are waves of peristalsis in the distal oesophagus that display elevated mean amplitudes (more than two standard deviations above the mean of a normal group of individuals). The presenting complaint is usually one of chest pain.

Jackhammer oesophagus

Jackhammer oesophagus or hypercontractile oesophagus is defined in the Chicago classification as a condition which on high-resolution manometry displays at least one swallow with a distal contractile integer > 8,000 mmHg-s-cm with single-peaked or multi-peaked contractions. It is a rare condition and so there is little published.

Distal oesophageal spasm

Distal oesophageal spasm is defined on HRM as ≥20% premature contractions with maintenance of a normal integrated relaxation pressure. It is characterised by chest pain with or without dysphagia.

Q. 7.6 What are the surgical options?

The surgical management for nutcracker oesophagus incorporates the role of a 'long myotomy'. In very selected patients a myotomy extending the length of the smooth muscle in the distal oesophagus can be undertaken with the aim of interrupting the spastic activity. With the advent of HRM it seems logical to tailor the myotomy to the area of spasticity seen on the trace.

Further reading

Annese VBG, Coccia G, Dinelli M, et al. A multicentre randomised study of intrasphincteric botulinum toxin in patients with oesophageal achalasia. Gut 2000; 46:597–600.
Boeckxstaens GAV, des Varannes SB, Chaussade S, et al. Pneumatic dilation versus laparoscopic Heller's myotomy for idiopathic achalasia. N Engl J Med 2011; 364:1807–1816.
Boeckxstaens GE, Zaninotto G, Richter JE. Achalasia. The Lancet 2014; 383:83–93.
Campos GM, Vittinghoff E, Rabl C, et al. Endoscopic and surgical treatments for achalasia: a systematic review and meta-analysis. Ann Surg 2009; 249:45–57.
de Borst JM, Wagtmans MJ, Fockens P, et al. Pseudoachalasia caused by pancreatic carcinoma. Eur J Gastroenterol Hepatol 2003; 15:825–828.
Eckardt AJ, Eckardt VF. Current clinical approach to achalasia. World J Gastroenterol 2009; 15:3969–9975.
Fisichella PM, Raz D, Palazzo F, Niponmick I, Patti MG. Clinical, radiological, and manometric profile in 145 patients with untreated achalasia. World J Surg 2008; 32:1974–1979.
Herbella FA, Oliveira DRCF, Del Grande JC. Are Idiopathic and Chagasic Achalasia Two Different Diseases? Dig Dis Sci 2004; 49:353–360.
Howard PML, Pryde A, Cameron EW, Heading RC. Five year prospective study of the incidence, clinical features, and diagnosis of achalasia in Edinburgh. Gut 1992; 33:1011–1015.
Hulselmans M, Vanuytsel T, Degreef T, et al. Long-term outcome of pneumatic dilation in the treatment of achalasia. Clin Gastroenterol Hepatol 2010; 8:30–35.
Inoue H, Minami H, Kobayashi Y, et al. Peroral endoscopic myotomy (POEM) for esophageal achalasia. Endoscopy 2010; 42:265–271.
Kahrilas PJ, Bredenoord AJ, Fox M, et al. The Chicago Classification of esophageal motility disorders, v3.0. Neurogastroenterol Motil 2015; 27:160–174.
Kahrilas PJ. Esophageal motor disorders in terms of high-resolution esophageal pressure topography: what has changed? Am J Gastroenterol 2010; 105:981–987.
Leeuwenburgh ISP, Alderliesten J, Tilanus HW, et al. Long-term esophageal cancer risk in patients with primary achalasia: a prospective study. Am J Gastroenterol 2010; 105:2144–2149.
Leyden JE, Moss AC, MacMathuna P. Endoscopic pneumatic dilation versus botulinum toxin injection in the management of primary achalasia. Cochrane Database Syst Rev 2014; 12:CD005046.
Moonen A, Annese V, Belmans A, et al. Long-term results of the European achalasia trial: a multicentre randomised controlled trial comparing pneumatic dilation versus laparoscopic Heller myotomy. Gut 2016; 65:732–739.
Pandolfino JE, Kwiatek MA, Nealis T, et al. Achalasia: a new clinically relevant classification by high-resolution manometry. Gastroenterology 2008; 135:1526–1533.
Richter J. Update on the management of achalasia balloons surgery and drugs. Expert Rev Gastroenterol Hepatol 2008; 2:435–445.
Richter JE. Oesophageal motility disorders. The Lancet 2001; 358:823–828.
Roman S, Kahrilas PJ. Management of spastic disorders of the esophagus. Gastroenterol Clin North Am 2013; 42:27–43.
Triadafilopoulos G, Boeckxstaens GE, Gullo R, et al. The Kagoshima consensus on esophageal achalasia. Dis Esophagus 2012; 25:337–348.
Vaezi MB, Achkar E, Richter JE. Timed barium oesophagram- better predictor of long term success after pneumatic dilation in achalasia than symptom assessment. Gut 2002; 50:765–770.

Wen ZH, Gardener E, Wang YP. Nitrates for achalasia. Cochrane Database Syst Rev 2002;(4):CD002299.

Zaninotto G, Annese V, Costantini M, et al. Randomized controlled trial of botulinum toxin versus laparoscopic heller myotomy for esophageal achalasia. Ann Surg 2004; 239:364–370.

Zerbib FTV, Richy F, Benajah DA, Message L, Lamouliatte H. Repeated pneumatic dilations as long-term maintenance therapy for esophageal achalasia. Am J Gastroenterol 2006; 101:692–697.

Scenario 8

Paraoesophageal hernia

A 58-year-old male patient presents to your surgical clinic with intermittent retrosternal pain and postprandial fullness. He describes volume reflux with regurgitation of his evening meal when he lies down at night. He is known to have a hiatus hernia from an endoscopy performed many years ago. He takes a PPI regularly and is overweight.

Q. 8.1 How would you assess this patient?

Initial clinical assessment including history and examination, including review of regular medications.

Note: It is important to ensure that a broad differential diagnosis is adopted initially as the symptoms from a paraoesophageal hernia (PHH) may be similar to those of a myocardial infarction, peptic ulcer disease, pancreatitis or pneumonia.

A symptomatic hiatus hernia (HH) will present depending on the anatomy of the defect, type II hernias typically present without reflux symptoms, whereas type III hernias most typically present with postprandial chest pain with or without reflux symptoms (e.g. heartburn, dysphagia, and regurgitation).

Q. 8.2 This patient has a PHH, what is the epidemiology and how are these hernias classified?

Epidemiology

Hiatal hernias occur in approximately 10% of the population, 15% of these are PHH. Risk factors for HH include male gender, age above 50 years, body mass index > 25 kg/m^2.

Hiatal hernias are classified as type I–IV are given below.

Type I

Most HHs are of the sliding type (90%) hernias in which the gastric cardia herniates upwards with proximal migration of the lower oesophageal sphincter into the thorax. The phreno-oesophageal ligament is attenuated but remains intact. The term 'sliding hiatal hernia' is applied here because the gastric wall comprises a portion of the hernia sac, analogous to retroperitoneal structures in sliding inguinal hernias.

Type II
This is a true PHH hernia and constitutes approximately 3% of hiatal hernias. In type II HHs, the oesophagogastric junction remains anchored in its normal position, and the gastric fundus herniates through an enlarged hiatus. This defect is very rare because most PHHs evolve directly from type I (sliding hiatal hernia) to type III (mixed PHHs).

Type III
This is a combined HH and involves elements of both types I and II hernias and represents the majority of PHs presenting for surgical repair. The enlargement of a type I hernia defect allows cephalad migration of the stomach, there is a true hernia sac present with fundic herniation and proximal migration of the oesophagogastric junction into the thorax. This type of hernia can progress to complete gastric herniation. This increased gastric mobility predisposes patients to gastric volvulus.

Type IV
This HH refers to a large defect in the phreno-oesophageal membrane, allowing other organs, such as colon, spleen, pancreas and small intestine to enter the hernia sac.

Q. 8.3 How would you investigate this patient?

Oesophagogastroduodenoscopy (OGD)
This is the primary investigation of choice for anatomical definition of the hiatus and type; macroscopic assessment of oesophageal and gastric mucosal integrity; and to rule out an overt upper GI malignancy.

Imaging
In the acute setting of foregut obstructions, such as gastric volvulus, a chest radiograph may typically demonstrate a retrocardiac and infradiaphragmatic air-fluid level.

Barium studies will provide a functional roadmap, and in the acute setting will identify the level of obstruction in a volvulus.

CT imaging provides a higher resolution image and can be performed with oral contrast (gastrografin) in the context of suspected volvulus. This can guide further management and give a representative appearance of the visceral contents of the hernia sac.

Manometry studies
Manometry can be useful in identifying oesophageal motility disorders, therefore anti-reflux procedures such as a fundoplication must be considered carefully. The positioning of the catheter beyond the lower oesophageal sphincter can be challenging in the case of a type III and IV HH, thereby giving a false representation of oesophageal peristalsis and acid exposure.

Q. 8.4 What are the current recommendations for surgery?
The current consensus agreement (EAES and SAGES) for the surgical repair for HH outlines that all symptomatic type II–IV hernias should be repaired electively,

particularly patients with obstructive symptoms who have had an episode of volvulus.

Q. 8.5 What are the surgical options for repair?

Principles of repair

The repair of PHHs may be approached via a thoracotomy, laparotomy or laparoscopically. The primary principles of surgical repair remain the same with all approaches:
- Complete excision of the hernia sac
- Reduction of the herniated stomach with tension-free reconstruction of 3–4 cm of abdominal oesophageal length. The mobilisation and reduction of craniocaudal tension prevents wrap slippage
- Repair of the diaphragmatic hiatus (primary crural repair versus reinforcement with mesh, with the former reducing the radial tension on the hiatus.)

Transthoracic repair

This was historically advocated for most PHHs, approaching the oesophagus via a thoracotomy provides excellent visualisation of the hernial sac and access for dissection and mobilisation of the oesophagus or herniated stomach. It requires one-lung ventilation, which may add to the morbidity of the procedure in the acute setting on in an anaesthetically unfit patient. This approach is rarely used now and as is typical of open surgery, it is associated with increased pain and longer hospital length of stay.

Transabdominal repair

Paraoesophageal hernia may be approached by a laparotomy, which provides anatomical access to the hiatus – best achieved by a rooftop incision. This access allows the placement of the stomach in its correct orientation and does not require one-lung ventilation. The primary disadvantage is access to the thorax to dissect or mobilise the oesophagus. This approach makes it difficult to perform a Collis gastroplasty if required for short oesophagus.

Laparoscopic repair

Laparoscopic PHH hernia repair is now the gold-standard method for elective and emergency surgery. The major advantages are from access to the hiatus and the thoracic oesophagus from the abdomen. There is no need for one-lung ventilation and postoperatively the morbidity rate is significantly less. This approach is also better suited to patients with other significant co-morbidities and when performed in expert hands it carries a similar recurrence rate to open surgery.

Laparoscopic paraoesophageal hernia repair

Port placement

A pneumoperitoneum is secured by open cut down epigastrium 12 mm port, which is sited 8–10 cm below the Xiphoid process. Two ports are placed in the left sub-costal position (12 mm and 5 mm – lateral) and one port in the right sub-costal position (12 mm). A further 5-mm trochar is inserted 2 cm below the xiphoid process, 2 cm to the left of the midline in order to insert a Nathanson's retractor to elevate the liver and provides full exposure to the oesophageal hiatus.

Reduction of the hernia sac and gastric mobilisation

The stomach is reduced from the hernia sac to identify the left and right diaphragmatic pillars. The dissection continues along the left crus between the lung pleura and the hernial sac along the angle of Hiss. The anterior phreno-oesophageal membrane is divided and retracted to attain full exposure of the right crus. Pars flaccida is opened with special care to avoid injury to the anterior vagal branches and the right gastric artery and vein. The gastro-splenic omentum is divided, and the then short gastric vessels are ligated along the full length of the fundus. The posterior oesophageal fat pad is reduced, and a retro-oesophageal window is created to place a nylon tape to allow caudal retraction and left and right distraction of the oesophagus.

The dissection continues from right to left and into the thorax to reveal the plane between the peritoneal hernial sac and the mediastinal attachments (lung pleura or pericardium). The sac is reduced without tension and excised in entirety to reduce the risk of recurrence. When dissecting and excising the sac posteriorly, it is important to avoid injury to the left gastric origin.

Assessment of oesophageal length

Once the hernia sac has been excised, it is imperative to have at least 2.5 cm of tension-free intra-abdominal oesophageal length. If a shortened oesophagus is identified, an extensive circumferential mobilisation of the intrathoracic oesophagus is performed, which usually provides the desired oesophageal length.

Crural repair

After complete reduction of the hernia sac and identification of an adequate length of intra-abdominal oesophagus, attention is turned to the crural closure. This is performed using interrupted, braided non-absorbable suture such as 5-ethibond. It is important to place the majority of the stitches inferiorly in order to reconstruct the anterior oesophageal lie for LOS function. A perioperative OGD will assess for the adequacy of closure and risk of postoperative dysphagia caused by mechanical obstruction. This is a prerequisite prior to completion of the procedure.

In addition to suture repair, a biological mesh has been advocated routinely in order to reduce HH recurrence. This was typically by a porcine 'U-shaped' mesh covering the repair and was fixed by suture as opposed to laparoscopic 'tacking' devices. Recent studies no longer advocate the placement of a mesh to reinforce the crural repair, as there is no evidence to suggest that it decreases recurrence or other complications.

Fundoplication

After completion of the crural repair, an anti-reflux procedure is routinely performed ('floppy' Nissen fundoplication) because failure to do so has been associated with a 20–40% rate of postoperative reflux and preoperative testing cannot successfully predict postoperative reflux.

Further reading

Campos V, Palacio DS, Glina F, et al. Laparoscopic treatment of giant hiatal hernia with or without mesh reinforcement: A systematic review and meta-analysis. Int J Surg 2020; 77:97–104.

Fuchs KH, Babic B, Breithaupt W, et al. EAES recommendations for the management of gastroesophageal reflux disease. Surg Endosc 2014; 28:1753–1773.

Kahrilas PJ, Kim HC, Pandolfino JE. Approaches to the diagnosis and grading of hiatal hernia. Best Pract Res Clin Gastroenterol 2008; 22:601–616.

Kohn GP, Price RR, DeMeester SR, et al. Guidelines for the management of hiatal hernia. Surg Endosc 2013; 27:4409–4428.

Luketich JD, Raja S, Fernando HC, et al.Laparoscopic Repair of Giant Paraesophageal Hernia – 100 Consecutive Cases. Ann Surg 2000; 232:608–618.

Zehetner J, Demeester SR, Ayazi S, et al. Laparoscopic versus open repair of paraesophageal hernia: the second decade. J Am Coll Surg 2011; 212:813–20.

Scenario 9

Gastric volvulus

A 72-year-old female patient presents with severe retrosternal pain and absolute dysphagia. She has been unable to tolerate any oral intake for over 6 hours. She is tachycardic, tachypnoeic and febrile. She underwent an endoscopy many years ago which diagnosed a hiatus hernia.

Q. 9.1 What is your differential and how would you manage this patient?

The differential diagnosis remains broad for this patient and the acute presentation with sepsis may indicate pneumonia, duodenal or gastric ulcer perforation. Retrosternal pain may be cardiac with a myocardial infarction and an acute aortic dissection is also important to consider. The history of chronic HH suggests the dysphagia may be secondary to an acute HH ± gastric volvulus.

Completion of initial assessment

This includes an urgent review with history (including prior surgical procedures) and examination, the patient has signs if systemic inflammatory response and would require fluid resuscitation and early antibiotics as there are features of sepsis. After each intervention or episode of resuscitation, the patient should be re-assessed on the response to treatment.

An early naso-gastric (NG) tube should be inserted to decompress the stomach and may potentially correct the gastric volvulus in certain cases.

Q. 9.2 What is the background and mechanism for a gastric volvulus?

Epidemiology

The true incidence of gastric volvulus remains unknown, but it affects males and females equally. Approximately 20% of cases occur in infants and young children with the remainder occurring in adults older than 50 years of age.

Mechanism

The anatomical classification of gastric volvulus is based on the axis of rotation.

Organo-axial volvulus is the most common type (A), and it accounts for almost all cases of acute gastric volvulus. This involves rotation of the stomach around the anatomical (longitudinal) axis, represented as a line drawn from the cardia to the pylorus. This type of volvulus frequently results in gastric strangulation and mucosal compromise.

Mesenteroaxial volvulus (B) results in the antrum of the stomach rotates anteriorly and superiorly around a transverse axis that extends from the mid-lesser curvature to the mid-greater curvature. The rotation is typically incomplete and results in intermittent gastric obstruction, rather than acute strangulation.

Anatomical representation of gastric volvulus.

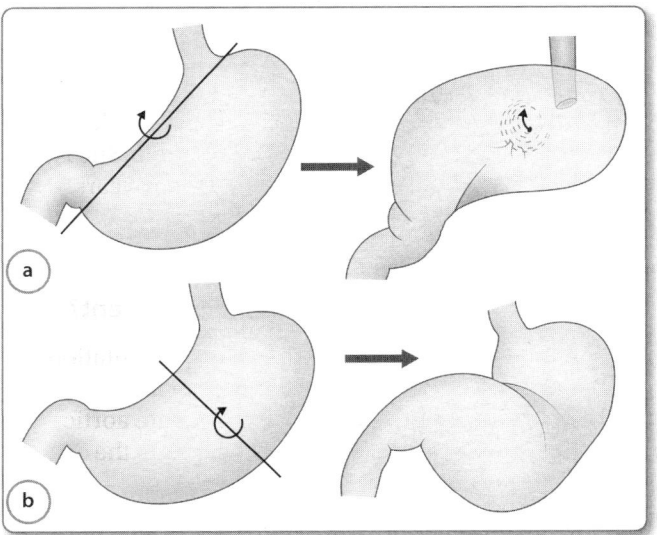

Presentation

Acute gastric volvulus is diagnosed with a combination of clinical history and a plain chest radiograph. The X-ray shows a retrocardiac air-fluid level, often with a second air-fluid level present below the diaphragm. If diagnostic uncertainty remains, a CT of the chest and abdomen + PO contrast will demonstrate the presence of the stomach within the chest and no oral contrast past the level of the diaphragm.

Q. 9.3 What is the management of acute gastric volvulus?

Once the diagnosis is confirmed, intravenous fluid resuscitation should be initiated. An attempt should be made to perform gastric decompression with a nasogastric tube. If successful, this results in rapid symptom improvement, and allows time for intravenous fluid resuscitation prior to surgical repair. It is important to carefully consider electrolyte replaccment as these patients typically experience metabolic shifts, presenting with hypochloraemic, hypokalaemic, metabolic alkalosis secondary to significant proton loss from vomiting.

If nasogastric decompression is unsuccessful, the patient must be taken to theatre immediately for emergency operative repair.

Surgical repair of gastric volvulus may be approached via thoracotomy, laparotomy or laparoscopy. The principles of repair include reduction of the hernia, release of the volvulus, debridement of all non-viable tissue, hiatal closure and anterior gastropexy or fundoplication to prevent recurrent volvulus. In cases where nasogastric decompression can be achieved preoperatively, and adequate intravenous fluid resuscitation accomplished, most can be managed laparoscopically. In the setting of acute peritonitis or gastric distension that cannot be relieved by decompression, laparotomy or thoracotomy may be required.

In high-risk patients deemed unfit for a laparoscopic or open approach, several authors have proposed the use of endoscopic reduction with gastropexy performed via either one or two percutaneous endoscopic gastrostomy tubes. When available, intraoperative endoscopy allows for assessment of viability of gastric mucosa and may facilitate gastrostomy placement for postoperative decompression and enteral access.

Further reading

Rashid F, Thangarajah T, Mulvey D, Larvin M, Iftikhar SY. A review article on gastric volvulus: a challenge to diagnosis and management. Int J Surg 2010; 8:18–24.

Scenario 10

Oesophageal perforation (Boerhaave's syndrome)

You review a 28-year-old male patient in A&E resus who has a history of an acute food bolus getting lodged yesterday while eating a piece of meat. He has attended with multiple episodes of vomiting.

His heart rate is 125 bpm, blood pressure 84/63 mmHg, and he is febrile. He is complaining of severe pain in his chest and abdomen. He has no past medical history. Fluid resuscitation is ongoing.

Q. 10.1 How would you manage this patient?

This patient is critically unwell and requires assessment and active resuscitation simultaneously.

Completion of initial assessment

This patient is unstable and requires active resuscitation, he has more than two markers of systemic inflammatory response syndrome (SIRS) and with a suspected perforation he has sepsis. His haemodynamic instability confirms septic shock, which has not been treated. He would require immediate management with fluid resuscitation with a 10 mL/kg STAT bolus of crystalloid. He will require broad-spectrum antimicrobial cover including cover for fungal pathogens. After each fluid bolus, the patient should be re-assessed on the response to treatment.

The primary differential is acute oesophageal perforation, a chest drain should be inserted into the left thorax for relief of any pneumothorax and sepsis control (5th IC space in the mid-axillary line).

A nasogastric (NG) tube should be inserted to allow aspiration of fluid contents in the oesophagus and stomach, this will also protect against aspiration during imaging especially CT.

The anaesthetist should be contacted urgently; and the patient consented for theatre, inclusive of laparotomy, thoracotomy, feeding jejunostomy and placement of T-tube. The theatre team need to be notified urgently so the patient can be prioritised as the next case in theatre.

Q. 10.2 What is the typical clinical presentation?

The clinical features depend upon the cause, site and time from injury. The classical Mackler's triad in spontaneous perforation of vomiting, chest pain and subcutaneous emphysema is actually an uncommon presentation.

Depending on the aetiology and amount of contamination, pain may be severe, constant, retrosternal or epigastric, distressing, exacerbated by movement and poorly relieved by analgesia. Dysphagia and odynophagia are common. Patients can be tachypnoeic and may sit up to splint their diaphragm. Subcutaneous emphysema takes time to develop; mediastinal emphysema precedes this and may be visible on a plain chest radiograph. With time the negative intrathoracic pressure draws air, food and fluid into the mediastinum and pleural cavities. A chemical and microbial pleuro-mediastinitis develops. This worsens as the SIRS response gives way to sepsis. Within 24–48 hours cardiopulmonary embarrassment and collapse develop as a consequence of overwhelming bacterial mediastinitis and septic shock. Survival is dependent on treating sepsis, providing organ support as required and evacuating contamination from the mediastinal and pleural cavities at the earliest possible opportunity.

Q. 10.3 What investigations should be arranged?

Radiograph
A plain erect chest radiograph may show subtle findings depending on the delay in onset and site of the perforation. It may be possible to identify mediastinal or subcutaneous emphysema, a pneumothorax or pleural effusion.

Computed tomography
Computed tomography (CT) is the first-choice imaging modality in patients stable enough to undergo imaging. It should not be delayed if an oesophageal perforation is suspected.

Contrast studies
Oral water-soluble contrast radiography ascertains the site, the degree of containment and the degree of drainage of the perforation. Aqueous agents are rapidly absorbed, do not exacerbate inflammation and have minimal tissue effects.

Endoscopy
Endoscopic assessment excludes the diagnosis if normal, influences or enables endoscopic management if underlying pathology is discovered and facilitates the placement of a naso-jejunal tube to allow enteral feeding.

It is often safest to perform endoscopy in suspected spontaneous perforation under a general anaesthetic with the patient intubated. This can allow for positive-pressure ventilation to reduce the risk of cardiorespiratory embarrassment by air insufflation into the mediastinum and pleural spaces.

Note: A chest tube may be required urgently if the patient is intubated and positive pressure ventilation results in respiratory or haemodynamic instability.

Q. 10.4 How would you manage this patient?
These patients are critically unwell with survival dependent on controlling mediastinal and pleural sepsis. Therefore, surgery remains mandatory when gross contamination is present. The patient will require postoperative critical care admission (CCU).

Patients require a multi-disciplinary approach with input from intensive care, radiology, physiotherapy, dieticians and rehabilitation services. Hospitals lacking these specialist facilities to deal with the oesophagus by abdominal or left or right thoracic operative approaches should transfer the patients to a specialist unit. This should occur at the earliest opportunity after stabilisation, as deterioration can be rapid and unpredictable. A summary of initial management is shown in **Box** below.

Initial management in spontaneous oesophageal perforation
Control airway and provide supplementary oxygen
Large-bore intravenous access and intravenous fluid resuscitation
Complete set of blood tests including arterial blood sampling and crossmatch
Intravenous broad-spectrum antibiotics and antifungals
Intravenous proton pump inhibitors
Strictly NBM
Urethral catheterisation and strict fluid balance
Early anaesthetic and critical care review
Insertion of chest drains, left primarily but likely bilaterally depending on contamination
Nasogastric tube insertion (placed under endoscopic or radiological guidance)
Enteral feeding adjunct, NJ if OGD performed
MDT approach with transfer to specialist centre and low threshold for surgical intervention in event of acute deterioration
(MDT, multi-disciplinary team; NBM, nil by mouth; NJ, naso-jejunal; OGD, oesophagogastroduodenoscopy)

Non-operative management

Non-operative management, endoscopic and minimally invasive operative management have all been shown to be safe and feasible in carefully selected patients who have either been diagnosed with minimal contamination and no mediastinitis or with a contained perforation.

Non-operative treatment is not 'conservative'. Patients require intensive observation and a low threshold for intervention, with 20% of patients requiring aggressive surgical salvage.

Endoscopic adjuncts for non-operative management

An endoluminal approach can be used to support patients undergoing non-operative management. Endoscopy in this setting is very challenging and should only be undertaken by an expert. The use of endoclips and stents across the perforation may be deployed with appropriate endoscopist experience.

Endoscopic drainage and lavage of contained mediastinal perforations may be an adjunctive strategy. This process may be performed by endoscopic placement of a vacuum sponge drainage system (Endo-SPONGE®) across small perforations to control small volume liquid contamination. This is a novel approach but labour-intensive and not suitable for gross contamination.

Operative management

Surgery is advocated if the patient has overt signs of sepsis, shock, gross contamination or failure of non-operative management.

Q. 10.5 What is the operative strategy?

For unstable patients, the safest surgical strategy is sepsis control. This surgical intervention involves the drainage of sepsis at the level of the perforation with washout pleural and abdominal drain placement. A venting gastrostomy is typically used to control reflux of gastric contents; however, a proximal oesophageal diversion or oesophagostomy is rarely required in the acute setting.

A feeding jejunostomy is universally sited for continuity of enteral feeding. Depending on the location of the perforation (mid to distal oesophagus), this procedure can be performed as a transhiatal approach via a rooftop incision or a right-sided thoracotomy.

Primary repair

In cases where a primary repair is being adopted, where there is minimal contamination, a posterolateral thoracotomy (left 7th of 8th IC space) is used to approach the oesophagus. Solid debris is removed, and the pleural cavity thoroughly cleaned. The mediastinal pleura is widely incised to expose the injury. Necrotic as well as devitalised tissue is debrided. A longitudinal myotomy is made as the mucosal injury is usually longer than the muscular one and the oesophagus repaired. A single- or two-layered, primary repair can be fashioned using 2/0 or 3/0 interrupted absorbable sutures with or without a small-diameter bougie in situ. However, primary repair is associated with a significant leak rate (20–50%) and should be reserved for those operated on rapidly with demonstrably healthy tissue and limited soiling.

T-tube repair

The concept of repair over a T-tube is to form a controlled oesophago-cutaneous fistula. A large-diameter (6–10-mm) T-tube is placed through the injury with the limbs lying beyond the boundaries of the perforation. The oesophageal wall is closed loosely around the tube with fine interrupted, absorbable sutures. The tube is externalised and secured. At least one further drain is placed around the repair. Apical and basal intercostal chest drains are sited. Healing is monitored by contrast radiology and CT scans. The T-tube is left until a defined tract is established with the majority removed endoscopically at around 6 weeks.

Resection

Oesophageal resection in the presence of a perforation is a major undertaking with an extremely high mortality. It is reserved for damage to a diseased oesophagus or in cases of extensive oesophageal trauma. This has even been performed in this setting as a minimally invasive approach.

Management algorithm

Diagnostic delay beyond 24 hours is classically associated with a poor outcome. Even when managed promptly and aggressively, perforation of the oesophagus, especially

Scenario 10 Oesophageal perforation (Boerhaave's syndrome)

spontaneous perforation such as Boerhaave's syndrome, carries a significant mortality rate. The management algorithm (see **Flowchart** below) is based on treatment following initial resuscitation and stabilisation as directed in **Box** mentioned above.

Management algorithm for spontaneous oesophageal perforation (Boerhaave's syndrome).

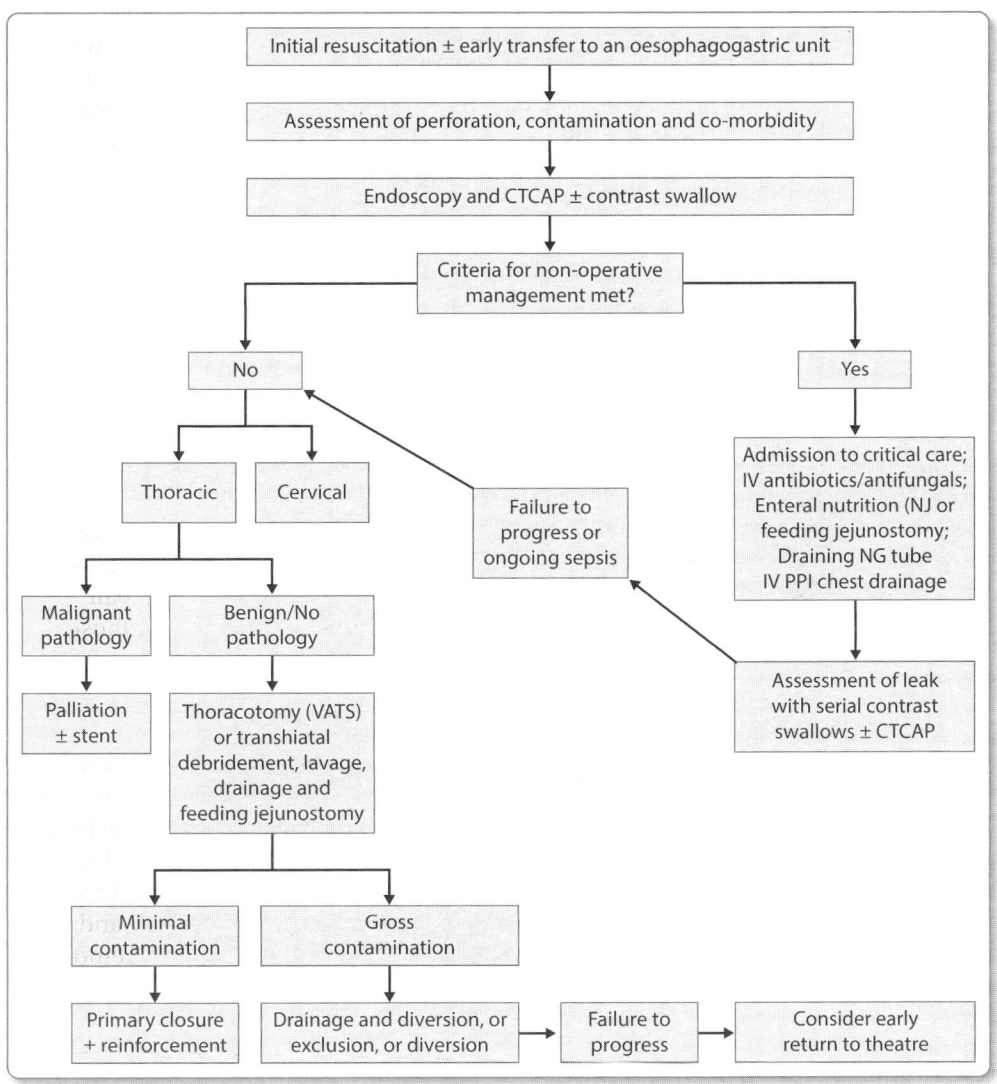

Further reading

de Schipper JP, Pull ter Gunne AF, Oostvogel HJ, van Laarhoven CJ. Spontaneous rupture of the oesophagus: Boerhaave's syndrome in 2008. Literature review and treatment algorithm. Dig Surg 2009; 26:1–6.

Jougon J, Mc Bride T, Delcambre F, Minniti A, Velly JF. Primary esophageal repair for Boerhaave's syndrome whatever the free interval between perforation and treatment. Eur J Cardiothorac Surg 2004; 25:475–479.

Kaman L, Iqbal J, Kundil B, Kochhar R. Management of Esophageal Perforation in Adults. Gastroenterology Res 2010; 3:235–244.

Kuppusamy MK, Felisky C, Kozarek RA, et al. Impact of endoscopic assessment and treatment on operative and non-operative management of acute oesophageal perforation. Br J Surg 2011; 98:818–824.

Moschler O, Nies C, Mueller MK. Endoscopic vacuum therapy for esophageal perforations and leakages. Endosc Int Open 2015; 3:E554–E558.

Sulpice L, Dileon S, Rayar M, et al. Conservative surgical management of Boerhaave's syndrome: experience of two tertiary referral centers. Int J Surg 2013; 11:64–67.

Chapter 11

Vascular surgery

Abdullah Jibawi, Mohamed Baguneid

Scenario 1

Deep vein thrombosis

A 32-year-old man is referred to your clinic by his general practitioner (GP) with a 3-day history of a painful swollen right lower leg. He had radiofrequency ablation of his right great saphenous vein 2 weeks earlier for large symptomatic varicose veins.

Q. 1.1 How would you assess this patient?

A comprehensive history would help to establish the onset, duration, and progression of the swelling and pain in the right lower leg. This would help to narrow down my differential diagnoses which include deep vein thrombosis (DVT), superficial thrombophlebitis, thigh haematoma or a soft-tissue infection. My main concern would be the DVT, and I would enquire if he was mobile after surgery, if he had a previous DVT or had a family history suggestive of thrombophilia. I would also check what form of thromboprophylaxis he may have had perioperative.

I would compare both legs for asymmetry, noting any redness, warmth, or prominent tender superficial veins. I would measure the circumference of both legs at fixed points, 10 cm below the tibial tuberosity and 10 cm above and assess for tenderness along the deep veins. I would use the Wells' score to stratify the clinical probability of DVT.

Q. 1.2 He was found to have an iliofemoral DVT on a venous duplex scan. How would you manage him now?

I would start anticoagulation therapy immediately to prevent thrombus propagation and reduce the risk of pulmonary embolism (PE). I would give a low-molecular weight heparin (LMWH) initially and then switch to either a direct oral anticoagulant (DOAC) such as rivaroxaban or apixaban or a vitamin K antagonist like warfarin targeting an international normalised ratio (INR) of 2–3. My management plan would also address his pain and swelling by giving analgesics and elevating his leg. He would need to be well hydrated. When the leg swelling has reduced and his pain is well controlled, I would measure him for Class 2 above knee graduated compression stockings.

If the patient's leg swelling was severe and particularly if he had features of phlegmasia cerulea dolens, then I would consider catheter-directed thrombolysis (CDT) or in combination with mechanical endovenous thrombectomy. This is because post-thrombotic limb syndrome can be debilitating and there is good evidence that decompressing the ilio-femoral DVT will reduce the risk of the post-thrombotic limb.

Q. 1.3 How would you reduce the risk of a preoperative DVT after surgery and what are the current guidelines?

I would start by doing a thorough preoperative risk assessment using validated tools such as the Caprini score to stratify patients based on their risk factors for venous thromboembolism (VTE). I would then determine the need for mechanical and pharmacological prophylaxis. Mechanical prophylaxis includes the use of graduated compression stockings and intermittent pneumatic compression devices. Pharmacological prophylaxis would depend on the patient's risk profile and surgical procedure. The American College of Chest Physicians (ACCP) guidelines recommend LMWH, unfractionated heparin (UFH), or direct oral anticoagulants (DOACs) based on the type of surgery and patient-specific factors. The risk of thrombosis would need to be balanced against the risk of bleeding.

I would encourage early mobilisation postoperatively and good hydration.

Further reading

Gloviczki P, Lawrence PF, Wasan SM, et al. The 2023 Society for Vascular Surgery, American Venous Forum, and American Vein and Lymphatic Society clinical practice guidelines for the management of varicose veins of the lower extremities. Part II: Endorsed by the Society of Interventional Radiology and the Society for Vascular Medicine. J Vasc Surg: Venous Lymph Disord 2024; 12:101670.

Kearon C, Akl EA, Ornelas J, et al. Antithrombotic Therapy for VTE Disease: CHEST Guideline and Expert Panel Report. Chest 2016; 149:315–352.

National Institute for Health and Care Excellence (NICE). (2020). Venous thromboembolism in over 16s: Reducing the risk of hospital-acquired deep vein thrombosis or pulmonary embolism. NICE Guideline [NG89]. [online] Available from NICE Website https://www.nice.org.uk/guidance/ng89 [Last accessed July, 2024].

Turner BR, Machin M, Jasionowska S, et al. Systematic review and meta-analysis of the additional benefit of pharmacological thromboprophylaxis for endovenous varicose vein interventions. Ann Surg 2023; 278:166–171.

Scenario 2

Abdominal aortic aneurysm

A 48-year-old man presents to your clinic having recently recovered from a chest infection and now has abdominal pains. He is known to have an abdominal aortic aneurysm (AAA) and is already on a surveillance programme with his last scan 6 months ago with his AAA measuring 4.5 cm in maximal diameter. His background includes hypertension, hypercholesterolemia, and coronary artery syndrome for which he required coronary angioplasty and stent insertion. He is an ex-smoker.

Q. 2.1 How would you assess him and what are the indications for treating patients with abdominal aortic aneurysm (AAA)?

I would begin by exploring the onset, duration and nature of his abdominal pains. I would enquire if his abdominal pains radiated to his back or if he had new onset back pains. I would try and establish if there were any associated nausea, vomiting, or changes in bowel habits. However, I would be concerned that his abdominal pains were related to his previously known AAA particularly as it was already 4.5 cm 6 months ago. I would establish his cardiovascular status, particularly establish his exercise tolerance and whether he had any symptoms relating to ischemic heart disease.

On examination, I would check his vital signs and examine his abdomen in general and in particular check for any tenderness over his AAA. He would require routine blood tests including amylase and I would arrange for imaging by means of a CT with contrast.

The indications for treating patients with AAA include size > 5.5 cm, rate of growth > 5 mm in 6 months or 10 mm in a year, presence of symptoms such as tenderness, ruptured AAA or embolisation from the AAA irrespective of size.

Q. 2.2 You find that his AAA is tender to palpation. What would you do?

Tenderness over an AAA is concerning and may indicate impending rupture. I would arrange an urgent CT angiography to assess the current state of the aneurysm, including its size, anatomical features, and any signs of rupture or leak. An ultrasound scan would not help to determine the morphology of the AAA or if it had ruptured.

I would contact the vascular surgery team to let them know that I had a patient with a tender AAA. The patient would need admission and urgent treatment. If the CT scan confirmed a contained ruptured, then treatment would be immediate. If there were no signs of rupture, then the patient should have treatment during the same admission.

Q. 2.3 What are the options for treating patients with symptomatic AAAs and how would you decide which option is best for any patient?

Treatment options include open surgical repair or endovascular aneurysm repair (EVAR). The choice between these options depends on various factors, including the patient's AAA anatomy, comorbidities, and overall fitness for surgery. There remains a lot of controversy as to which treatment option is best but in this case, the patient is young, and I would probably favour open surgical repair. However, this decision should be made at a multidisciplinary team meeting (MDT). Factors that are considered at MDT would include:

- *Anatomy:* The presence of adequate proximal and distal landing zones, the quality of the infra renal aortic neck and the iliac vessel diameter and tortuosity.
- *Comorbidities:* Such as severe cardio respiratory disease which may benefit more from a less invasive EVAR approach.
- *Age and life expectancy:* Younger patients with a longer life expectancy may be considered for open repair due to its durability.
- *Patient preference:* The risks and benefits of each approach should be discussed with the patient. Some patients prefer open surgical approach to avoid needing long-term surveillance. Some patients prefer EVAR because they can recover quicker and there are less immediate postoperative risks and less risk of erectile dysfunction and retrograde ejaculation.

Further reading

Patel R, Sweeting MJ, Powell JT, et al. Endovascular versus open repair of abdominal aortic aneurysm in 15-years' follow-up of the UK endovascular aneurysm repair trial 1 (EVAR trial 1): a randomised controlled trial. Lancet 2016; 388:2366–2374.

Powell JT, Wanhainen A. Analysis of the differences between the ESVS 2019 and NICE 2020 guidelines for abdominal aortic aneurysm. Eur J Vasc Endovasc Surg 2020; 60:7–15.

Schanzer A, Oderich GS. Management of abdominal aortic aneurysms. N Engl J Med 2021; 385:1690–1698.

UK Small Aneurysm Trial participants Powell JT. Final 12-year follow-up of surgery versus surveillance in the UK Small Aneurysm Trial. J Br Surg 2007; 94:702–708.

Scenario 3

Chronic limb-threatening ischaemia

A 65-year-old man presents to the emergency department with a 3-week history of rest pain in his right leg preceded by a 2-month history of short distance claudication. He has no symptoms in his left leg. He had a right axillo-bi femoral and a right femoral-popliteal bypass 4 years ago for an occluded aorta and occluded superficial femoral artery (SFA). His past medical history includes type 2 diabetes mellitus, stroke, hypertension and congestive cardiac failure.

Q. 3.1 What is the likely cause of his symptoms?

He currently presents with symptoms suggestive of chronic limb-threatening ischaemia (CLTI). It is likely that one or both of his bypass grafts are occluded. His left leg appears unaffected probably because the axillo-bi femoral graft has remained patent and it is the right femoro-popliteal bypass graft that has occluded. However, it is possible that the axillo-bi femoral bypass graft has also occluded but he is not experiencing symptoms in his left leg because the right leg is the most critical and limiting his walking abilities the most. Either way, his right leg is at risk from severe limb ischaemia.

Q. 3.2 How would you manage him?

He needs urgent management with the vascular surgical team to prevent ulceration or gangrene from developing. He would need to be admitted and after a detailed history and clinical examination, he should have routine bloods and vascular imaging. A bedside handheld Doppler assessment and 'ankle brachial pressure index' measurements would help to stratify the severity of his limb ischaemia. However, he needs urgent arterial duplex scan and a computed tomography angiography (CTA), or magnetic resonance angiography (MRA), to evaluate the patency of the bypass grafts and to identify the site of occlusion so that a plan for revascularisation can be made.

He needs pain relief and his legs should be kept warm and in a slightly dependent position to maximise blood flow. I would give him heparin to prevent thrombus propagation and plan for urgent revascularisation. In addition to revascularisation, we would need to manage his comorbidities aggressively. Antiplatelet therapy and statins should be continued. Smoking cessation is critical if he is still smoking.

Q. 3.3 You determine that his right axillo-bi femoral bypass graft is patent but his right femoral-popliteal bypass graft is occluded. He is suitable for a redo right femoral-popliteal bypass. What risks would you warn this patient in relation to this surgery?

I would first explain to him that redo femoral-popliteal bypass surgery is being proposed to save his limb but that it carries several risks such as:

- *Infection and seroma:* Surgical site infections are common in redo bypass surgery, especially in patients with diabetes. He is at risk from early or late prosthetic graft infection. These risks are greater if he develops a lymphatic leak or seroma which is higher in redo groin surgery.
- *Bleeding:* As with any major vascular surgery, there is a risk of bleeding intraoperatively and postoperatively. This is increased by the patient's need for anticoagulation and antiplatelet therapy.
- *Thrombosis and graft failure:* There is a risk of early or late graft thrombosis. This would lead to acute limb ischaemia.
- *Cardiovascular complications:* Given his history of congestive cardiac failure and previous stroke, he is at high risk for perioperative cardiovascular events.
- *Renal impairment:* The use of contrast and potential perioperative hypotension and reperfusion can worsen any underlying renal impairment.
- *Limb loss:* Despite a technically successful bypass surgery, there remains a risk of limb loss due to development of a complication, pressure sore and wound infection.

Further reading

Aboyans V, Ricco JB, Bartelink ML, et al. 2017 ESC guidelines on the diagnosis and treatment of peripheral arterial diseases, in collaboration with the European Society for Vascular Surgery (ESVS). Kardiologia Polska (Polish Heart J) 2017; 75:1065–1160.

Bradbury AW, Adam DJ, Bell J, et al. Bypass versus Angioplasty in Severe Ischaemia of the Leg (BASIL) trial: analysis of amputation free and overall survival by treatment received. J vasc surg 2010; 51:18S–31S.

Bradbury AW, Moakes CA, Popplewell M, et al. A vein bypass first versus a best endovascular treatment first revascularisation strategy for patients with chronic limb threatening ischaemia who required an infra-popliteal, with or without an additional more proximal infra-inguinal revascularisation procedure to restore limb perfusion (BASIL-2): an open-label, randomised, multicentre, phase 3 trial. Lancet 2023; 401:1798–1809.

Conte MS, Bradbury AW, Kolh P, et al. Global vascular guidelines on the management of chronic limb-threatening ischemia. Eur J Vasc Endovasc Surg 2019; 58:S1–S109.

Members WC, Gerhard-Herman MD, Gornik HL, et al. AHA/ACC Guideline on the Management of Patients With Lower Extremity Peripheral Artery Disease: Executive Summary: A Report of the American College of Cardiology/American Heart Association Task Force on Clinical Practice Guidelines. Circulation 2016; 135:e686.

Venermo MA, Farber A, Schanzer A, et al. Reduction of major amputations after surgery versus endovascular intervention: the BEST-CLI randomised trial. Eur J Vasc Endovasc Surg. 2024; S1078-5884(24)00492-1.

Scenario 4

Acute lower limb ischaemia

A 67-year-old male woke up at 2 AM with a painful, cold and numb left lower leg. He can move his left ankle and toes but weaker than the right. He attends the emergency department 8 hours later as his left calf is becoming more painful.

Q. 4.1 How will you assess him and what is the likely diagnosis?

I would take a focussed history and perform a comprehensive physical examination. I would confirm the onset, duration and progression of his symptoms. He is likely to have acute lower limb ischaemia and therefore the ischaemic time is important. He is now 8 hours following onset of pain and that raises concern that he may have developed irreversible ischaemia. However, it is reassuring that he can still move his ankle and foot albeit weak.

I would inquire whether he had any symptoms of claudication in the past and if he had a history of atrial fibrillation (AF) or other cardiac conditions. I would ask about his current medications, particularly if he is on any anticoagulants or antiplatelet agents. I would assess his left lower limb for signs of acute ischaemia, such as *p*allor, *p*ulselessness, *p*oikilothermia (coldness), *p*aralysis, *p*araesthesia and *p*ain—the 'six *P*s' of acute limb ischaemia. A comparison of these findings with his right leg would help to diagnose any underlying peripheral arterial disease.

Q. 4.2 You note that he is in AF and has no pulses in his left leg (absent left femoral, popliteal and foot pulses). He has normal palpable pulses in his right leg. How would you manage him?

It is likely that he has suffered acute lower limb ischaemia because of an embolus. This is because he is in AF and he has normal pulses on his right leg. He needs rapid revascularisation to salvage any viable muscle but I am conscious that he is likely to suffer significant reperfusion injury and be at risk of a compartment syndrome. I would immediately give him intravenous heparin to prevent further thrombus propagation. I would involve my vascular surgical colleagues and it is likely that they would obtain urgent imaging, most likely a computed tomography angiography (CTA), to confirm the location of the embolus which would guide the treatment approach. It is important that the imaging is immediate and does not delay treatment. If there are concerns on timing of the imaging, I would take him to theatre with the view to performing a femoral embolectomy and on-table angiogram. I would plan to perform a surgical revascularisation by femoral embolectomy and not catheter-directed thrombolysis or percutaneous mechanical thrombectomy because he needs rapid restoration of blood flow. Using a Fogarty catheter to remove the embolus, I would restore flow to his left leg and confirm with an on-table angiogram. I would go on to perform a prophylactic four compartment fasciotomy. He would be maintained on heparin infusion initially with the view to long-term anticoagulation. He would be transferred to a critical care bed postoperatively. He will also need cardiac investigations including an 'Echo'.

Q. 4.3 How does reperfusion injury manifest and what will you do to reduce its impact on the patient's outcome?

The effect of the reperfusion injury manifests locally by the development of compartment syndrome in the affected limb and systemically by causing acute lung injury, renal failure or myocardial suppression. It can also cause deranged electrolytes such as hyperkalaemia and acidosis.

Anticipating the reperfusion injury, particularly in patients with prolonged ischaemia and those who have weakness or tenderness in the affected muscles is important. I would perform a fasciotomy empirically in those who, I would suspect, will develop compartment syndrome such as this patient. I would hydrate patients well to reduce the risk of renal failure from myoglobinuria. Monitoring vital signs and electrolytes on an intensive care unit is essential. Avoiding hyperkalaemia and acidosis will reduce the risk of critical arrhythmias. I would avoid medications that are nephrotoxic.

Further reading

Björck M, Earnshaw JJ, Acosta S, et al. Editor's choice–European Society for Vascular Surgery (ESVS) 2020 clinical practice guidelines on the management of acute limb ischaemia. Eur J Vasc Endovasc Surg 2020; 59:173–218.

Juneja A, Garuthara M, Talathi S, et al. Predictors of poor outcomes after lower extremity revascularization for acute limb ischemia. Vascular 2024; 32:632–639.

Kithcart AP, Beckman JA. ACC/AHA versus ESC guidelines for diagnosis and management of peripheral artery disease: JACC guideline comparison. J Am Coll Cardiol 2018; 72:2789–2801.

Scenario 5

Popliteal aneurysm

An 83-year-old male referred by general practitioner (GP) due to prominent popliteal pulsatile lump. He has no history of intermittent claudication. He is not diabetic and ex-smoker. He has limited mobility.

Q. 5.1 What are key features in the history and examination and what are the differential diagnoses?

I would like to understand when the patient noticed this lump or was it an incidental finding on a routine clinical examination. I would like to know if there have been any changes in the size or nature of the popliteal lump. Does he have pain, swelling or numbness. I would try to establish if there was any history of trauma, recent infections, or systemic symptoms such as fever or weight loss. I understand that he does not suffer from claudication but at the same time it seems he has limited mobility. This could be due to many reasons, but I would enquire whether he had any arthritis in his knees or any previous knee surgery or injections.

On examination, I would inspect the lower limbs for asymmetry, discolouration and signs of ischaemia. I would look for evidence of arthritis in the knee. I would palpate the popliteal fossa to establish the size, pulsatility and compressibility of the lump. I would also examine distal pulses and perform a neurovascular examination of the foot and leg.

The differential diagnoses include popliteal artery aneurysm which would be the most likely diagnosis given the pulsatile nature of the lump. But, a Baker's cyst (popliteal cyst) could be possible because of his age and limited mobility which may relate to osteoarthritis of the knee. It could be a deep vein thrombosis (DVT) but this is less likely. A soft-tissue tumour could be possible, and it may feel pulsatile if it is close to the popliteal artery.

Q. 5.2 What are the risks of having a popliteal aneurysm?

Popliteal artery aneurysms are less likely to rupture than abdominal aortic aneurysms and more commonly present as an incidental finding or following thrombosis and embolisation with acute limb ischaemia. If the popliteal aneurysm is large, it can compress adjacent structures such as the nerves in the popliteal fossa causing pain or compressing the deep veins causing DVT. By far the greater risk is that of acute lower limb ischaemia. They usually embolise initially into the tibial vessels and then subsequently thrombose which is why the risk of major amputation from popliteal artery aneurysm thrombosis is high at around 15%.

Q. 5.3 What are the principles of management in this case?

Most popliteal artery aneurysms are asymptomatic and particularly those <2 cm in diameter. In asymptomatic cases, <2 cm in diameter, surveillance by means of arterial duplex scanning every 6–12 months is sufficient. I would also check the contralateral limb for a popliteal aneurysm which may be present in 30–50% of patients and check for abdominal aortic aneurysm (AAA) which may be present in 15–30%. As the underlying cause of popliteal aneurysms is atherosclerosis, cardiovascular medical therapy should be started including antiplatelet therapy, statins and managing smoking, BP and diabetes if present.

Surgical or endovascular intervention of popliteal aneurysms is indicated for symptomatic aneurysms, those larger than 2 cm, or if there is evidence of thrombus formation or distal embolisation. 'Open surgical repair' remains the gold standard with excision or ligation of the aneurysm and bypass grafting. Placement of a stent-graft within the aneurysm is a minimally invasive approach which is suitable for some patients particularly those considered high surgical risk, but long-term durability is a concern. In the case of emergency presentation of a thrombosed popliteal aneurysm, complex emergency surgical repair and thrombolysis or a hybrid approach are options depending on the situation.

Further reading

Beuschel B, Nayfeh T, Kunbaz A, et al. A systematic review and meta-analysis of treatment and natural history of popliteal artery aneurysms. J Vasc Surg 2022; 75:121S–125S.

Björck M, Earnshaw JJ, Acosta S, et al. Editor's choice–European Society for Vascular Surgery (ESVS) 2020 clinical practice guidelines on the management of acute limb ischaemia. Eur J Vasc Endovasc Surg 2020; 59:173–218.

Farber A, Angle N, Avgerinos E, et al. The Society for Vascular Surgery clinical practice guidelines on popliteal artery aneurysms. J Vasc Surg 2022; 75:109S–120S.

Jung G, Leinweber ME, Karl T, et al. Real-world data of popliteal artery aneurysm treatment: Analysis of the POPART registry. J Vasc Surg 2022; 75:1707–1717.

Scenario 6

Claudication

A 54-year-old postman complains of cramp in his right calf when he walks 50 m. He had an angioplasty of his right superficial femoral artery 2 years ago for similar symptoms and got a good clinical result. He is diabetic with glycated haemoglobin (HbA1c) of 8% and an ex-smoker of 2 years.

Q. 6.1 What are the risk factors for peripheral arterial disease (PAD), and how can you reduce the risk of future cardiovascular events in patients with PAD?

Modifiable risk factors include smoking, diabetes mellitus: dyslipidaemia, hypertension and obesity. Nonmodifiable factors include age, gender and family history. Patients with PAD should have a management strategy that includes risk factor modification and lifestyle adjustment. In addition, there is level 1A evidence to recommend the use of antiplatelet therapy and good level 1B evidence to recommend the use of clopidogrel over aspirin in patients with atherosclerosis and in particular PAD. The use of statins irrespective of the lipid panel is recommended for its plaque stabilisation affect. Supervised exercise programme not only help patients with claudication in terms of walking distance but also in terms of general cardiovascular health improvement.

Q. 6.2 You establish that he has lifestyle limiting claudication and at risk of losing his job. How would you manage this patient?

Risk factor optimisation and, in particular, his diabetes control need to be controlled. He would need to be seen and managed in a diabetes specialist clinic. Although supervised exercise programmes are beneficial in terms of improving his walking distance, it is likely that he will need to be considered for revascularisation as his lifestyle is limited and as a postman it could affect his ability to manage his work. I would arrange noninvasive investigations first including an arterial duplex scan with 'ankle brachial pressure index (ABPI)'. This will help to determine the site of the occlusive disease. It is possible that he would need computed tomography angiography (CTA) or magnetic resonance angiography (MRA) to understand the extent of the arterial disease better. We need to be cautious with contrast nephropathy if he has existing renal impairment as he is a poorly controlled diabetic. It is likely that his occlusive disease will be at the previous angioplasty site, but it may be multifocal. Depending on the extent and site of arterial occlusive disease based on the Trans-Atlantic Inter-Society Consensus (TASC) classification, he would be considered for further endovascular procedure or surgical bypass. The risks and benefits of intervening with his recurrent arterial disease would need to be discussed with the patient. This would also require a comprehensive general cardiovascular/respiratory and renal assessment.

Q. 6.3 What are the risks of performing femoral artery angioplasty?

When consenting for femoral angioplasty, it is important to consider risks at the puncture site including bleeding, groin haematoma and retroperitoneal haematoma. The risk of a pseudoaneurysm is around 0.2–8%. Uncommonly, an arteriovenous (AV) fistula can occur between the femoral artery and vein. If puncture occurs at a site of a calcified plaque, it could cause a dissection flap and occlude the artery or even cause micro-embolisation.

Risks at the angioplasty site include distal embolisation, dissection flaps, thrombosis, rupture and later can result in a re-stenosis.

There are also systemic complications related to the contrast agent used such as contrast nephropathy, contrast anaphylaxis and in patients with cardiac failure, it can cause exacerbation of the heart failure.

Further reading

Conte MS, Pomposelli FB, Clair DG, et al. Society for Vascular Surgery practice guidelines for atherosclerotic occlusive disease of the lower extremities: management of asymptomatic disease and claudication. J Vasc Surg 2015; 61:2S–41S.

Nordanstig J, Behrendt CA, Baumgartner I, et al. Editor's choice--European Society for Vascular Surgery (ESVS) 2024 clinical practice guidelines on the management of asymptomatic lower limb peripheral arterial disease and intermittent claudication. Eur J Vasc Endovasc Surg 2024; 67:9–96.

Tan LT, McDermott KM, Hicks CW. Overview and comparison of contemporary SVS, AHA, and ESVS guidelines for the management of patients with intermittent claudication. Semin Vasc Surg 2024.

Scenario 7

Carotid disease

A 62-year-old male heavy goods vehicle (HGV) driver attends your clinic for his long-standing right inguinal hernia. His hernia is reducible and not painful, but he wants it to be repaired. However, during the consultation he explains that he had two episodes of loss of vision in his left eye that lasted approximately 15 seconds each time 2 weeks ago.

Q. 7.1 How are you going to manage him?

The management of his inguinal hernia is not a priority as it is reducible and not painful. However, he has had two recent episodes suggestive of amaurosis fugax and so his risk of having a stroke is high without proper medical and may be surgical management. I would tell him that he needs urgent assessment of his transient mono-ocular blindness and refer him for immediate ophthalmology and transient ischaemic attack (TIA) clinic. He should be started on antiplatelet therapy, statin and have an urgent carotid duplex scan to evaluate for carotid disease. He needs a full cardiovascular risk assessment as atherosclerosis is likely to be the underlying aetiology. In terms of his hernia management, I would advise him to avoid activities that exacerbate the hernia, such as heavy lifting. I would ask him to monitor for symptoms of a strangulated or obstructed hernia which would necessitate emergency surgical intervention.

Q. 7.2 He had a carotid duplex scan which is reported as demonstrating an 80% right internal carotid artery stenosis and a 40% left internal carotid artery stenosis. How would you manage this now?

He has a high-grade stenosis on the right internal carotid artery but this is not the symptomatic side. He has a 40% symptomatic left internal carotid artery stenosis. This is not high grade and does not require carotid surgery and should be managed by medical treatment alone. He should have further investigations to look for other causes of amaurosis fugax including 'Echo' and thrombophilia.

I would still defer any plans to treat his hernia as it is not causing symptoms at present and he clearly has had a recent cerebrovascular event. His risk of a further cerebrovascular event remains high for at least the next 6 weeks even with medical management.

Q. 7.3 He attends your clinic 3 months later and his inguinal hernia is becoming more symptomatic. He is on clopidogrel and has had no new symptoms suggestive of TIA/stroke or any cardiovascular events. You agree that he should have his hernia repaired. How would you prepare him for his hernia surgery?

I would take a comprehensive history and establish whether he has had any new cerebrovascular or cardiovascular events. I would also try to establish whether he is truly having symptoms from his inguinal hernia. Assuming that he has a symptomatic hernia and had no further cerebrovascular or any new cardiovascular events, then I would arrange his preoperative evaluation with anaesthesia. I would consider open repair of his hernia under local anaesthetic. I would establish with the team who follows him for his carotid disease if he could temporarily stop his clopidogrel or switch to aspirin for his hernia surgery. He would need to stop his clopidogrel for at least 5 days before having his hernia surgery. I would be happy to operate on his hernia while he is on aspirin. I would examine him for peripheral arterial disease (PAD) and avoid compression stockings if there is evidence of significant PAD. When taking consent, I would inform him that he is at risk of perioperative cardiovascular and cerebrovascular events.

Further reading

AbuRahma AF, Avgerinos ED, Chang RW, et al. Society for Vascular Surgery clinical practice guidelines for management of extracranial cerebrovascular disease. J Vasc Surg 2022; 75:4S–22S.

Arasu R, Arasu A, Muller J. Carotid artery stenosis: An approach to its diagnosis and management. Aust J Gen Pract 2021; 50:821–825.

Bir SC, Kelley RE. Carotid atherosclerotic disease: A systematic review of pathogenesis and management. Brain Circ 2022; 8:127–136.

Bonati LH, Jansen O, de Borst GJ, et al. Management of atherosclerotic extracranial carotid artery stenosis. Lancet Neurol 2022; 21:273–283.

Scenario 8

Intravenous drug use and pseudoaneurysm

A 32-year-old woman presents to the 'emergency department' with a 10 cm painful red hot tender swelling in right groin. She admits that a swelling has been present for 2 months but it became red and painful for past 5 days. She is a known intravenous drug user (IVDU). She looks unwell with a pulse rate of 110 bpm, blood pressure (BP): 90/60 mmHg, respiratory rate (RR): 28 breaths/min and temperature of 38.5°C.

Q. 8.1 How would you manage her in the emergency department?

I would first prioritise stabilisation of her systemic symptoms which are indicative of infection or sepsis. I would establish intravenous access for fluid resuscitation and antibiotics. This would help to address her hypotension and sepsis. I would give empirical broad-spectrum antibiotics with microbiology advice and tailoring later based on culture results. I would send blood tests for complete blood count, blood cultures, urea and electrolytes and coagulation profile. She needs an immediate ultrasound scan to assess the nature of the groin swelling and may be a CT scan if further detail is needed. It is likely that she has an infected false aneurysm or a large groin abscess. The urgency of the surgical management of her infected groin swelling would depend on skin integrity, bleeding or discharge from the groin and systemic sepsis. She will also need pain relief, which may be complicated because of her previous opiate and substance use.

Q. 8.2 An arterial duplex is performed and confirms an 8 cm pseudoaneurysm at the origin of the right superficial femoral artery with an overlying abscess. What is a pseudoaneurysm and how would you treat it?

A pseudoaneurysm, or false aneurysm, occurs when an artery is injured, and blood is contained within a sac made by surrounding tissue. Unlike a true aneurysm, a pseudoaneurysm does not have all layers of the vessel wall as part of the sac wall.

This patient needs urgent treatment to repair the pseudoaneurysm and drainage of the abscess. Unlike pseudoaneurysms after cardiac catheterisation, this type of infected pseudoaneurysm cannot be treated by ultrasound-guided compression or thrombin injection. She will require ligation of the injured artery. I would get proximal and distal control first. This would involve a Rutherford–Morrison incision and extraperitoneal approach to the right external iliac artery to get proximal control. Then, I would make a longitudinal incision over the groin swelling and try and approach the superficial femoral and profunda femoral artery distal to the aneurysm to get control. The fibrosis and inflammation around the profunda femoral artery may make it difficult to get control and, in that situation, I would aim to pass a small Fogarty balloon from inside the artery to get control of it. After giving 5,000 units of heparin, I would then control proximal and distal arteries and open the pseudoaneurysm and excise the infected sac. I would send the infected sac and tissues to microbiology for culture and sensitivities. I would then ligate proximally and distally as close to the injured artery which in this case is the origin of the superficial femoral artery. I would try and spare as many collateral vessels as possible.

Closure of the groin may be difficult because of the induration and scarring and may necessitate a sartorius rotation flap. If it is not possible to safely close the groin over a drain, then I would leave the skin and subcutaneous tissues open to heal by granulation tissue. This may be managed by 'negative pressure wound therapy (NPWT)', if there is good coverage over the femoral vessels.

Postoperatively, the patient will need antibiotics, deep vein thrombosis (DVT) prophylaxis and wound care. She will likely have short distance claudication and there is a very small chance that she develops ischaemic ulceration and tissue loss in her right foot that may ultimately require an amputation.

There are occasions where it may be safe to revascularise the femoral artery but this is not very common in this type of presentation. If revascularisation is an option, saphenous vein would be used if possible and an extra-anatomical bypass by means of an obturator bypass could be considered.

Q. 8.3 What are concerns do you have with managing this patient and how would you manage those issues?

This type of patient has many other issues to consider in their management. It is often difficult to get IV access and may require an ultrasound-guided approach to a deeper peripheral vein or a central vein. Empirical antibiotics will need to cover resistant organisms which is often present in intravenous drug user (IVDU) patients.

There are frequently behavioural issues related to the addiction that will require specialist input during her hospital stay. Also, many IVDU patients will have hepatitis C or rarely human immunodeficiency virus (HIV) and therefore blood and tissue samples will need to be clearly marked as high risk and caution taken to avoid needle stick injuries in surgery and when taking blood samples.

Further reading

Quiroga E, Shalhub S, Tran NT, et al. Outcomes of femoral artery ligation for treatment of infected femoral pseudoaneurysms due to drug injection. J Vasc Surg 2021; 73:635–640.

Sarkar M, Fridling J, Nagarsheth K. Post-Operative Ischemia and Surgical Technique Affect Late Mortality of Femoral Artery Pseudoaneurysms Following Injection Drug Use. Ann Vasc Surg 2023; 92:231–239.

Singh AA, Ashcroft J, Stather PW. Ligation alone versus immediate revascularization for femoral artery pseudoaneurysms secondary to intravascular drug use: a systematic review and meta-analysis. Ann Vasc Surg 2021; 73:473–481.

Scenario 9

Varicose veins

A 34-year-old woman is referred to your clinic by her general practitioner (GP) for symptomatic varicose veins. She complains of aching and itching on the medial aspect of both legs, swelling that worsens over the course of the day. She has previously tried compression stockings and steroid creams but her symptoms have not improved and she is keen to discuss her options.

Q. 9.1 How would you assess this patient in clinic?

I would start by taking a detailed history focussing on her symptoms to establish if they relate to venous hypertension. Her description of aching, itching and swelling is typical of venous hypertension. I would establish how her symptoms affect her life and whether any other treatments apart from compression stockings have been tried. I would try to establish if she has suffered from any of the complications of varicose veins, e.g. bleeding, superficial thrombophlebitis or venous ulcers. Finally, I would enquire about her past medical history including any contributing conditions such as previous deep vein thromboses (DVTs), and her functional status to assess which interventions may be appropriate. I would then examine the patient taking note of any skin changes of venous hypertension such as venous eczema, ulcers, haemosiderin deposition and lipodermatosclerosis. I would assess the location of varicose veins in order to determine which system was affected (great or short saphenous vein). I would then establish if there are any sites of venous reflux using a hand-held Doppler and, in particular, assess for sapheno femoral or saphenopopliteal junction reflux.

Q. 9.2 If the patient is confirmed to have varicose veins with great saphenous vein reflux, what treatment options are available to her?

I would follow the guidance of the National Institute for Health and Care Excellence (NICE) and offer this patient endothermal ablation of the great saphenous vein and multiple phlebectomy of larger varicosities. However, if this was not possible to treat by endothermal ablation, for example, because of the degree of tortuosity I would offer ultrasound-guided foam sclerotherapy. Another option would be surgery in the form of saphenofemoral junction ligation, stripping of the great saphenous vein and multiple phlebectomy. If the patient was not suitable for these options, then I would recommend wearing graduated compression stockings as long as she did not have any contraindications such as peripheral arterial disease. I would suggest using class 2 graduated compression stockings as she has varicose veins and oedema. They would provide a pressure of 25–35 mmHg at the ankle.

Q. 9.3 The patient is suitable and keen to have endothermal ablation. What risks would you consent her for?

Endothermal ablation can be done under local anaesthetic as a day case procedure. I would consent her for a recurrence rate of 3–5% each year following treatment and an initial treatment failure rate around 5%. I would explain to her that she may suffer some discomfort temporarily from bruising and superficial thrombophlebitis. She may also notice some skin pigmentation at the sites of treatment and, particularly, if she develops some phlebitis. There is a small risk of neuralgia, paraesthesia or anaesthesia from damage to the saphenous nerve particularly if treating below the knee. I would explain to her that the risk of DVT is around 0.5–1% depending on her risk factors and she would be offered DVT prophylaxis as appropriate.

Further reading

Gloviczki P, Lawrence PF, Wasan SM, et al. The 2023 Society for Vascular Surgery, American Venous Forum, and American Vein and Lymphatic Society clinical practice guidelines for the management of varicose veins of the lower extremities. Part II: Endorsed by the Society of Interventional Radiology and the Society for Vascular Medicine. J Vasc Surg: Venous Lymphat Disord 2024; 12:101670.

Hitchman LH, Mohamed A, Smith GE, et al. Provision of NICE-recommended varicose vein treatment in the NHS. Br J Surg 2023; 110:225–232.

O'Flynn N, Vaughan M, Kelley K. Diagnosis and management of varicose veins in the legs: NICE guideline. Br J Gen Pract 2014; 64:314–315.

The National Institute for Health and Care Excellence (NICE). (2013). Varicose veins: diagnosis and management. Clinical Guideline 168. [online] Available from https://www.nice.org.uk/guidance/cg168 [Last accessed July, 2024].

Scenario 10

Peripheral arterial disease and colorectal cancer

A 74-year-old man with newly diagnosed rectal cancer attends your clinic to discuss having a curative anterior resection. He underwent a colonoscopy that revealed the presence of a stenosing mass of the rectosigmoid junction, 15 cm from the anal margin, which was biopsied and determined to be an adenocarcinoma. Staging CT scan did not demonstrate any evidence of metastatic disease. However, it demonstrates that he has severe atherosclerotic disease in his aorta and iliac arteries. He is on aspirin and a statin by his general practitioner (GP) for claudication. He is an ex-smoker and does not have hypertension or diabetes.

Q. 10.1 What further considerations are necessary for this patient, given his peripheral arterial disease (PAD)?

He has been found to have PAD but I am also concerned that he will most likely have ischaemic heart disease and cerebrovascular disease. An anaesthetic review is required and a more detailed cardiovascular assessment. This may require a cardiac stress test if it is not possible to assess his exercise tolerance because of claudication. I would take advice from cardiology if he could stop his antiplatelet therapy for 5 days before his surgery. However, I would be happy to proceed with surgery on aspirin, if needed. I would be cautious about the risk of him developing lower limb ischaemia, ischaemic foot ulceration and pressure ulceration in the perioperative period. He would need to be considered high risk for pressure sore development and appropriate measures put in place to reduce this risk including the use of a pressure relieving mattress. I would avoid the use of compression stockings and be very cautious of keeping his legs elevated for long periods during surgery to avoid the development of compartment syndrome. Finally, as an arteriopath, he is at increased risk of anastomotic leak because of poor mesenteric blood flow. This would be considered when planning his surgery and creation of a colorectal anastomosis. He would be warned about the risk of an anastomotic leak and need for a temporary ileostomy. He would also need to be aware that he is at risk of developing an ischaemic limb.

Q. 10.2 He gets seen by a vascular surgeon and was noted to have bilateral lower limb claudication limiting him to 50 m but he has no rest pain or ulceration to his feet. A review of his CT scan demonstrates distal aortic occlusion and bilateral common iliac stenoses. They decide that there is no indication to treat his aortoiliac occlusive disease as he has good collaterals and only experiences claudication. How does this information affect the plan for his anterior resection?

He has severe PAD and this is concerning. Aortoiliac occlusive disease means that his internal iliac arteries are not contributing well to his pelvic blood flow, and it would be very likely that his mesenteric collateral flow is compromised. This makes the risk of a colorectal anastomotic leak high. He also has a high risk of developing sacral pressure sores due to the poor internal iliac flow and developing an ischaemic limb.

I would discuss his case in a multidisciplinary team meeting (MDT) again and consider whether he should have a permanent stoma to avoid the risk of anastomotic leak or if he has an anterior resection to perform a protective ileostomy. I would discuss with vascular surgery whether revascularisation of his aortoiliac occlusive disease would benefit him by helping his pelvic circulation sufficiently to reduce his risk of anastomotic leak. However, it is unlikely that vascular surgery would plan to prophylactically treat his aortoiliac disease before his colorectal cancer surgery as it would involve either a complex CERAB (covered endovascular reconstruction of aortic bifurcation) or an open surgical approach that would involve aorto-bi-iliac or aorto-bi femoral bypass. Surgical bypass is not a realistic option with him needing a colorectal procedure shortly afterwards and CERAB usually requires combination of anticoagulation and antiplatelet therapy for 3–6 months before downgrading to a single antiplatelet agent. The best option for him is to have colorectal cancer surgery that does not require a precarious colorectal or coloanal anastomosis. It would benefit him to have a shorter duration procedure with his legs not elevated for long periods and with his abdominal wall incisions and stoma avoiding any collaterals which usually include the epigastric arteries.

Q. 10.3 He had a Hartmann's procedure but developed postoperative chest infection 4 days later and deteriorated with sepsis requiring inotropic support in intensive care unit. One week later, he has dusky toes in both feet with evidence of dry gangrene to the tips of his toes on both feet. What would you do now?

This pattern of digital ischaemia described is typical of that seen from inotropic vasoconstriction on background of severe PAD. There is no realistic option for revascularisation particularly as it would involve at best a complex endovascular procedure which is not appropriate while a patient is on inotropic support. Therefore, the best plan would be to protect his pressure areas and optimise his cardiovascular status which is only likely to happen if his source of sepsis is managed and controlled. As long as his gangrenous toes are dry and not a source of sepsis themselves, then they are best left alone and allowed to demarcate as his condition improves and inotropes weaned off. When he has stabilised and recovered from his colorectal surgery, then he can be considered for revascularisation, if necessary, or may be simply manage with digital auto-amputation.

Further reading

Deguelte S, Besson R, Job L, et al. Assessing abdominal aortic calcifications before performing colocolic or colorectal anastomoses: A case–control study. J Res Med Sci 2021; 26:110.

Shen Z, An Y, Shi Y, et al. The Aortic Calcification Index is a risk factor associated with anastomotic leakage after anterior resection of rectal cancer. Colorect Dis 2019; 21:1397–1404.

Yamamoto K, Miyata T, Nagawa H. The high prevalence of colorectal neoplasms in preoperative patients with abdominal aortic aneurysm or peripheral artery disease. Eur J Vasc Endovasc Surg 2007; 33:397–400.

Index

Note: Page numbers in **bold** or *italic* refer to tables or figures, respectively.

A

ABCDE assessment 95, 97
Abdomen 135, 158, 557, 595
    acute 104
Abdominal aortic aneurysm 661, 668
    indications for treating 661
    repairs 251
    rupture 54
    symptomatic 662
Abdominal approach 398
Abdominal cavity 134, 138, 259
    volumes 259
Abdominal compartment syndrome 109, 165
Abdominal examination 192, 551
Abdominal mass, suspicious 432
Abdominal operations 152
Abdominal organs 517
Abdominal pressure, increased 275
Abdominal transplantation, application for 517
Abdominal wall
    closure 131
    compliance 166
ABO incompatible transplant 521, 522
Abscess
    groin 228
    intravenous drug user groin 203
    lactational 328
    overlying 673
    scrotal 146
Accessory nerve 183
Acetylcholinesterase, reversed with 60
Achalasia 636
    classification of 637
    diagnosis of 637
    early stage of 637
    epidemiology of 636
    increases, incidence of 636
    leads 636
Acid clearance 622
Acidic urine 304
Acidity 87
Acidosis 97, 109, 275
Actinomycosis 226

Acute coronary syndrome 41, 95, 100
Acute gastric volvulus 649
    management of 649
Acute kidney injury 90, 114, 200
    complications of 114
    development of 90
    management in 114
    network 91
Acute lower limb ischaemia 155, 665
    diagnosis 665
Acute respiratory distress syndrome 26, 104, 105
    pathophysiology of 106
Adenocarcinoma 631
Adenoma 461, 469
    removal of 475
Adenosine triphosphate 518
Adequate hydration 269
Adhesion formation 403
Adjuvant chemotherapy, risks of 332
Administering conscious sedation 57
Administering palliative chemotherapy 405
Adrenal 459
Adrenal gland, hormones secreted by 459
Adrenal lesion
    biopsy of 462
    incidental 460
Adrenal masses, proportion of 460
Adrenal phaeochromocytoma, bilateral 465
Adrenal vein sampling, selective 470
Adrenaline 68, 361
    administer 362
    injection 170
    intravenous 362
Adrenocortical cancer 461
Adrenocorticotrophic hormone measurement 460
Advanced trauma life support 30, 140
    principles 210
Advancement flap 413
    surgery 427
Aerodigestive injury 184
Air-filled stomach *563*

Index

Airway 25, 42
    adjuncts 30
    breathing, and circulation 557
    compromise 184
    protection 58
Alanine
    aminotransferase 529
    transaminase 157
Alcohol
    excess 239
    intake
        excess 157
        increased chronic 81
Alcoholic liver disease 71, 571
Aldosterone 63, 460
Alemtuzumab 506, 522
Alkaline
    environment 87
    phosphatase 157
Alkalosis 48
Allen's test, perform modified 531
Allergic reaction 361
    and treatment 361
    risk of serious 361
    type of 362
Allergy 233
Allograft loss 480
Alopecia 331
Alpha-fetoprotein 373
Altruistic donation
    directed 539
    non-directed 539
Alveolar gas 49
Amaurosis fugax, causes of 671
Amethocaine 86
Amiodarone 118
Amitriptyline 35
Amnesia 173
Ampullary tumour 567
Amylase 554
Anabolic phase 65
Anaerobic threshold measurement 259
Anaesthesia 60, 189
    general 60
    principles of general 59
Anaesthetic factors 316
Anal canal 409
Anal cancer 408, 409
Anal fissure 426
    pathophysiology of 426
Anal fistula treatment, video-assisted 449
Anal margin 409

Anal mass, unexplained 432
Analgesia 35, 59, 60
    patient-controlled 73
    perioperative 34
Anaphylactic reaction 361
Anaphylaxis, cause of 362
Anastomotic leak 603, 611
    classification of 612
Anastomotic strictures, benign 613
Anastrozole 331, 374
Androgen 460
    synthesis 297
Aneurysm
    false 673
    screening 189
    size of 189
Angiomyolipoma 540
    bilateral 540
Angioplasty site 670
Angiosarcoma 360
Angiotensin 63
Angiotensin-converting enzyme 63
Ankle brachial pressure index 669
Ann Arbor staging classification 266
Anorectal physiology 442
Anti-acid therapy 624
Antibiotic 158, 223, 328
    broad-spectrum 167
    prophylaxis 259
Antibody, donor-specific 504
Anticoagulants 35, 289
Anticoagulation, indication for 289
Antiembolism stockings 269
Antihistamines 361
Antiplatelet
    agents 665
    medications 81
Anti-reflux
    mechanisms 620
    surgery 624, 625, 627, 629
        technique of 627
Anti-resorptive therapies 479
Antisepsis 312
Antiseptic
    skin preparation, guidelines for 312
    solutions 312, 313
    wash 321
Anxiolytics 35
Aortic arch 177
Aortic valve closes 53
Apnoea test 84
Aponeurotic layer 254

Index

Appendages 280
Appendiceal carcinoid tumours 424
Appendiceal mucinous neoplasm, low-grade 424, 425
Appendiceal neoplasm, high-grade 424
Appendiceal tumours 424
Appendicectomy, interval 392
Appendicitis 206, 207, 390
    acute 390
    uncomplicated 206
Appendix mass 226
Appetite 304
Architectural atypia 343
Argon plasma coagulation 170, 440
Arimidex 331
Aromasin 331
Aromatase inhibitors 331
Arrhythmia 464
Arterial blood 49
    gas 96, 97, 559
Arterial duplex 673
Arterial line waveform 53
Arteriovenous fistula 531, 532, 670
Arthralgia 331
Ascites 71
Aseptic technique, use 110
Aspartate aminotransferase 529
Aspirin 81, 435
Asthenia 331
Asthma 58, 250
Atelectasis
    bilateral 210
    pathophysiology of 73
Atlanta criteria 157
Atmospheric air 49
Atracurium 60
Atrial fibrillation 118, 156, 665
    management of 118
    new onset of 156
Atrioventricular fistula
    creation 533
        complications of 533
    failure, primary 533
    stenosis 533
Attorney for health and welfare, lasting power of 39
Autoimmune haemolytic anaemia 285
Autologous 353
    reconstruction 353
Autonomic neuropathy 500
Autosomal recessive polyposis syndrome 436

Axilla 376
    management of 363
    surgical assessment of 363
Axillary clearance 365
Axillary core biopsies 377
Axillary nodes, enlarged 339
Axillary radiotherapy 365
Azygos vein 609

B

B3 lesions 342
Baclofen 626
Baker grading system 339
Bariatric
    operations 591
    surgery 591
Barium studies 644
Barrett's oesophagus 631, 633, 635, 636
    biopsies 633
    diagnosis of 633
Barrett's prevention, fundoplication for 633
Basal atelectasis 73
    management of 73
    risk of 73
Basal cell carcinoma 260
Basal metabolic rate 64
Basal skull fracture, signs of 173
Basiliximab 503, 506
Battle's sign 173
Beck depression inventory 272
Bedside index 560
Belly crosses, inferior 183
Benzodiazepine 57, 89, 297
Bernoulli's principle 27
Berry's ligament, posterior leaflets of 488
Beta-blockers 118, 482
Bias, type of 4, **4**, 5
Bile duct
    congenital abnormalities of 585
    dilated 552
    injury 138, 302, 557
Bile leak 22, 557, 589
Biliary anatomy, intact 557
Biliary colic 22
Biliary fistulas 128
Biliary sepsis 216
Biliary stricture, diagnosis of 530
Biliopancreatic diversion 592
Bilirubin 157, 530
Biofilm 339

Biopsy 439
    protocol 633
Bisacodyl 149
Bismuth classification 138
Bisphosphonate 331, 349, 473, 479
    treatment 332
Bladder
    damage 249
    injury 274
Bleeding 80, 275, 288, 664
    disorder 80
    duodenal ulcer 170
    peptic ulcer 236
    per rectum 287
Blood
    glucose and ketones, checking 524
    loss 117
    pressure 25, 68, 238
        diastolic 117
        systolic 117
    products, resuscitate with 587
    reflects light 46
    salts and electrolytes, disturbance of 112
    tests 120, 265, 373, 390
        routine 349
    transfusion 286
Blue dye 361
Blue naevus 260
Blunt chest trauma 140, 210
Blunt neck trauma 185
Blunt trauma 587
    mortality 590
Body mass index 495, 591
Body temperature 61, 64, 84
    normal parameters for 61
Boerhaave's syndrome 160, 651, 653, 655
Bogota bag 111, 168, 242
Bologna guidelines 401
Bone marrow failure 81
Bony regions 280
Botulinum toxin 638
Bougie placement 627
Bovine cough 488
Bowel ischaemia 399
    and infarction 400
Bowel obstruction 113
Bowel screening 432, 433
Brachial plexus trunks 183
Brachiobasilic fistula 532
Bradycardia, persistent profound 101

Brain
    haemorrhage 278
    injuries 176
Brainstem
    death 519
    function 84
    testing 83, 85
        criteria for 83
BRCA1 mutation 345, 347
BRCA2 mutation 345, 346
Breast 340, 345, 376
    abscess 327
        treatment for 327
    area 296
    conservation surgery 359
    disease, symptoms of 296
    disorders 334
    lumps 334
    malignancies 367
    multidisciplinary team 330
    reconstruction, delayed 352
    screening programme 355
    size 380
    surgery 325, 378
        risks, general 383
    swollen 340
    triple assessment of 322
    tumours of 329
Breast cancer 265, 329, 335, 346, 373, 375
    advanced 348, 377
    development of 345
    develops 347
    invasive 377
    recurrent 322
    risk assessment 344
    risk of developing 346
    treatment of 336
Breast implant 338
    round 339
    structure of 338
Breast-conserving surgery 330
Breastfeeding 328
Breathing 25, 31, 42
Breslow's depth 264
Bridging therapy 290
Bronchial veins 102
Bronchospasm 362
Brunner grading 323
    system 323
Bulky rectal tumour 240

Bullet
    cause injury 169
    injuries, types of 168
Bupivacaine 34, 86, 87
    isomeric forms of 86
Burn 42
    body surface area of 43
    causes of 44
    injury 42, 43
        depth of 44
Bypass procedures 322, 323

C

Cadaveric liver transplant 573
Cadet face right 48
Caecal pole close 154
Caecum 242
Calcitonin 473
Calcium sensing receptor gene 473
Cancer
    interval 356
    personal history of 462
    risks of developing 346
    screening 272
    triple negative 335
    type of 344
Capillary refill 116, 155
Caprini score 660
Capsular contracture
    causes of 339
    degree of 339
    grades of 339
Capsule endoscopy 237, 288
Carbohydrate load 613
Carbon monoxide 42
Carbonic anhydrase reaction 305
Carboxyhaemoglobin 42, 46
Carcinoembryonic antigen 265, 575
Carcinoma, histological confirmation of 605
Cardiac arrhythmias 88, 275
Cardiac assessment tools 597
Cardiac cycle, phase of 52
Cardiac death, donor after 495
Cardiac function 275
    assess 55
Cardiac output 47, 64, 67
Cardiac rhythm 259
Cardiac risk index, revised 597
Cardiac tamponade 107
Cardiac technician 280
Cardio respiratory disease, severe 662

Cardiopulmonary exercise testing 55, 253, 257, 259, 598
Cardiothoracic surgeons 220
Cardiovascular complications 480, 664
Cardiovascular disease 474, 520
Cardiovascular drugs 297
Cardiovascular dysfunction 218
Cardiovascular fitness 501
Cardiovascular monitoring 51, 52
    types of 51
Cardiovascular risk factors 156
Care
    levels of 45
    plan of 551
Caroli's disease 585
Carotid artery stenosis, right internal 671
Carotid disease 671
Carpal-tunnel syndrome 331
Catabolic phase 64
Catastrophic haemorrhage 30
Catecholamines 460
Catheter, two-way 144
Catheter-directed thrombolysis 102, 659
Cause-dependent advice 328
Caustic injuries, classify 178
CDK4/6 inhibitors 350
Cell
    lymphoma, large 339
    salvage machine, intraoperative 286
Cellular calcium, blocking 638
Cellular fibroepithelial lesion 342
Cellular rejection, acute 530
Cellulitis 322
Celox 30
Central catheter, peripherally inserted 113
Central nervous system 278
Central venous
    catheter complications 276
    pressure 51
        complications of 52
        line 113
        measure 51
        monitoring 51
Cerebrospinal fluid leakage 173
Cerebrovascular accident 155, 500
Cerebrovascular event 671
Cervical
    intraepithelial neoplasia 410
    oesophagus 620
Chaperone 376
Charcot's triad of fever 217
Charles procedure 323

Chemodectoma 300
Chemoradiotherapy 410
Cheng system 323
Cherry haemangioma 261
Chest
  physiotherapy 73, 251
  wall, segment of 141
  X-ray 96, 97
Chest drain
  bottle 108
  position of 221
Chest infection 40, 95
  developed postoperative 678
Chest pain 118
  postprandial 643
  sudden onset 160
Child's Pugh scoring systems 543
Chlorhexidine 312, 362
Cholangiocarcinoma 544
Cholangiogram 567
Cholangitis
  acute 218
  ascending 67
  severity of 217
Cholecystectomy 139, 303
Cholecystitis 22, 223
  acute 554
  diagnosis of acute 555
Cholestasis 217
Choline citrate 149
Chronic kidney disease 90, 534
Chronic limb-threatening ischaemia 663
  cause of 663
Chronic obstructive pulmonary disease 25, 26, 200, 250
Chylothorax 612
Ciclosporin 321
Cinacalcet 473
Circulatory arrest 88, 89
Circulatory support 67
Cirrhosis 498
Cisplatin 462, 597
Clark level 264
Clark naevus 260
Clavien–Dindo classification 277
Clopidogrel 81
Clostridium difficile 162, 291
  colitis 163
    causes of 163
  infection 162, 163
Clotting 559
  cascade 80

Coagulation profile 554
Cocaine 86
Codeine phosphate 35
Cold
  ischaemic time 512
  phase 512
Coldness 665
Colitis 201
  ischaemic 200
Collapse 459
Collis procedure 628
Colloids 362
Colon cancer 434
  diagnosis 434
  right-sided 451
Colonic injury 274
Colonic lesions 442
Colonic pseudo-obstruction, pathophysiology of 199
Colonic transit studies 442
Colonoscopy 271, 442
Colorectal cancer 677
  advanced 404
Colorectal endoscopic stenting trial 388
Colorectal liver metastases 575
Colorectal surgery 55, 385
Colostomy, reversal of 396
Colovesical fistula 453-455
Columnar epithelium 631
Combat action tourniquets 30
Common bile duct 139, 216, 303
Common duct, diverticulum of 585
Compartment syndrome, development of 666
Complex diverticular disease 453
Complex endovascular procedure 678
Computed tomography angiography 663, 665
Conduit necrosis 612
Congenital adrenal hyperplasia 297
Congenital bleeding disorders 81
Congenital neck lumps 300
Congestive heart failure 119
Conn's syndrome 470
Conscious sedation 58
Consciousness, loss of 88, 173
Consent, principles of 282
Consort statement 16, 18
Constipation 318, 441
Continuous ambulatory peritoneal dialysis 523
Continuous mandatory ventilation 29
Continuous positive airway pressure 28, 210, 257
Continuous venovenous haemofiltration 92

Contusion 187
Core biopsy 372
    confirms 330
Corneal reflex 85
Coronavirus disease-2019 392, 496
Corticosteroids 35, 349
Cough reflex 85
Cranial nerves 85
C-reactive protein 148, 554
Creatine kinase 69
Creatinine 91, 504, 508
Cricopharyngeus 177
Cricothyroidotomy 78
Critical care 23
    admission, postoperative 652
    unit 40
Critically ill surgical patient, care of 135
Crohn's disease 226, 320, 423
    ileocaecal resection for 422
Crura, dissection of both 627
Crural repair 646
    completion of 646
Crush injury 587
Cryoprecipitate 81
Cryotherapy 440
Cryptoglandular theory 412
Crystalloid 233, 587
    solution 115
Cushing's adrenal nodules 468
Cushing's disease 467
Cushing's syndrome 467
    causes 467
    diagnosis 467
Cutaneous squamous cell carcinoma 261
Cyclooxygenase enzyme 35
Cyclosporine 90
Cyst
    branchial 300
    choledochal 584, 585
    popliteal 667
    thyroglossal 300
    wall of 563
Cystic duct stump 303
Cystic hygroma 300, 301
Cytomegalovirus 496
Cytoreductive surgery 425

D

Dabigatran 82
Daily sodium requirement 122
Damage control laparotomy 131, 168
    benefits of 132

Damage control surgery, disadvantages of 132
Data, graphical representation of 8
Day surgery 316
D-dimer 75
Deaths, perioperative 411
Debulking 323
    procedures 322
Deep vein thrombosis 75, 555, 570, 667,
    674, 675
    prophylaxis 208
Dehydration 504
    assess for 304
    symptoms of 304
Delayed graft function 536
    cause of 536
Delorme's procedure 398
Dementia 378
Deoxygenated haemoglobin reflecting 46
Depression 331
Dermatofibroma 261
Dexamethasone 35
    suppression test 467
        high-dose 468
        low-dose 468
Diabetes 241
    complications to 500
    controlled 239
    mellitus 149, 520, 669
        type 2 250
    treatment 500
Dialysate 523
Dialysis, types of 115
Diamorphine 34
Diaphragmatic herniation 613
Diaphragmatic rupture 196
    traumatic 195
Diaphragmatic sphincter 621
Diaphragmatic splinting 259
Diarrhoea 504
    frequency of 292
    persistent 504
    severe 112
Diathermy 280
    plate placement 280
Diazepam 35
Dietary modification 440
Digoxin 118, 297
Diodes, light-emitting 46
Disability 25
Disease
    benign 454
    malignant 454
    pathophysiology of 69, 71

Disseminated intravascular coagulation 81, 120
Distal bile duct
　carcinoma 567
　cholangiocarcinoma 584
Distal fistula creations 532
Distal gastrectomy 598
Distal ileum approximately, loop of 241
Distal oesophageal
　compression 621
　spasm 640
　tumour 605
Distal oesophagus 632, 639
Diverticular disease 417
Diverticulectomy 288
Diverticulitis 291, 417
Diverticulum 288
Dobutamine 68
Donor
　availability, geographical differences in 544
　extended criteria 515
　potential 495
Dopamine 68
Dopexamine 68
Double cannula tracheostomy tube 79
Double duct sign 567
Down splenic flexure 454
Down-staging chemotherapy 576
Doxazosin 465
Doxorubicin 462
Drainage setons 413
Drug, type of 68
Dubious viability, bowel of 242
Duct of Luschka leak 303
Ductal cancer 363
Ductal carcinoma in situ 352, 358
　high-grade 330, 360
　pathology of high-grade 359
　surgical treatment for 359
Duodenal carcinoma 567
Duodenal diverticulum, presence of 167
Duodenal stump leak 603
Duodenal switch 592
Duodenal ulcer 73
Duodenal-jejunal flexure 402, 526
Duodenum 132, 177, 601, 605
　mobilisation of 600
　perforated 208
Duplex ultrasound 531
Duty of Candour 295
Dynamic high-pressure zone 620

Dyslipidaemia 669
Dysphagia 182, 184, 643, 652
　greater degree of 629
　postoperative 629
Dysphonia 485
Dysplasia
　high-grade 583, 631
　low grade 631, 632
Dysplastic naevus 260
Dysuria 455

E

Early nasogastric tube 648
Early rectal cancers 407
　management of 407
Ebb phase 64
Ebrospinal fluid 31
Efficacy 2
Egger's test 10
Elbow fistula over wrist 532
Electrical conductional abnormalities, identify 597
Electrocardiogram 25
Electrolyte 127, 554, 666
　disturbances, correct 56
Electronic offering system 495
Elevated respiratory rate 387
Embolic disease 90
Embolisation 131
Emergency laparoscopic cholecystectomy 22
Emergency laparotomy 399
Emergency surgery 129, 259
　indications for 194, 420
Emphysema, developing 141
Encapsulating peritoneal sclerosis 525
Encephalopathy 92
End colostomy 395
End ileostomy 193, 292
End-arterial organs 280
Endoanal ultrasound 442
Endocrine
　resistance 350
　surgery 457
　therapy, role for 375
　treatment 331
　　side effects of 331
　　types of 331
Endogenous catecholamine 68
Endogenous hormone 68
Endopredict test 332

End-organ dysfunction 67
Endoscopic assessment 612
Endoscopic drainage and lavage 653
Endoscopic mucosal resection 610, 634
Endoscopic resection 595, 610
Endoscopic retrograde
 cholangiopancreatography 67, 138, 303, 552
Endoscopic submucosal dissection 611
Endoscopic ultrasonography 606
Endoscopic ultrasound 595, 606, 616, 634
Endoscopy 428, 621, 652
 widespread availability of 621
Endothelial
 dysfunction 268
 injury 268
Endothermal ablation 676
Endotracheal tube 29
Endovascular aneurysm repair 662
Enteral nutrition 113
Enteritis, infective 201
Enterocele 441
Enterocutaneous fistula 113, 422
 causes for 423
Enzyme activity 64
Epididymitis 146
Epididymo-orchitis 147
Epidural technique deposits drugs 34
Epigastrium 304
Epinephrine 87
Epirubicin 597
Epistaxis 81
Epithelial atypia 342
Epithelial proliferation 343
 atypical 343
Epstein–Barr virus 496
 infection 266
Erythema 240
Erythropoiesis stimulating agents 286
Ethanol alcohol 200
Etomidate 59
Excision biopsy 341
Excisional haemorrhoidectomy 415
Exemestane 331
Extra-abdominal injury 131
Extracardiac monitoring 281
Extracorporeal membrane oxygenation 42
Extradural haematoma 33, 175
 large left 32
Extramural vascular invasion, evidence of 424
Extra-thyroid extension, gross 491
Extremity, lower 532
Eyes 551

F

Faecal immunochemical test 432
Faecal incontinence 444
Familial hypocalciuric hypercalcaemia 472
Fasciotomies 156
Fat 64
 and protein stores, replenishing of 65
Fatty liver disease, non-alcoholic 591
Feeding gastrostomy 113
Feeding jejunostomy 113
Femoral angioplasty, consenting for 670
Femoral artery
 angioplasty 670
 common 156
 superficial 156, 674
Femoral canal
 anatomy 246
 boundaries of 246
Femoral hernia 245
 prevalence of bilateral 246
 strangulated 190
Femoral line 92, 113
Femoral vein 51, 246
Fentanyl 36, 57, 60
Fibreoptic nasoendoscopy 489
Fibrin-degradation products, levels of 75
Fibroadenoma 371
Fibroproliferative phase 106
Fictitious meta-analysis **8**
Finger thoracostomy 108
Fistula 286, 411
 maturation 532
 plugs 413
 presence of 222
 proximal 532
Fistula-in-ano
 classify 412
 formation of 412
 surgical management for 413
Fistulectomy 413
Fistulotomy 413
Flail chest 26, 210
Flaps, dissection 670
Floppy Nissen fundoplication 646
Fluid 62, 361, 362
 balance, monitor 236
 overload 92, 535
 resuscitation 168, 362
  aggressive 70
  rules for 587
Fluorodeoxyglucose 569, 579
Fluorouracil 597

Follicle stimulating hormone 374
Fondaparinux sodium 269
Foreign body 177
    ingested 177
Forest plots 8
Fournier's gangrene 146, 240
Fowler–Stephens procedure 310
Fragility fractures 479
Frank-Starling mechanism 67
Fraser guidelines 284
Friedman's test 13
Full blood count 137, 554, 566
Full breast examination 371
Functional residual capacity 28
Fundoplication 646
    anterior partial 628
    partial 628
    posterior 628
    procedure 629
    total 628
Funnel plots 10
Furosemide 176

G

Gabapentin 35
Gag reflex 85
Gail model 345
Gallbladder 158, 224, 556, *564*
    entering 224
    fossa 557
    thick-walled 554
Gallium nitrate 473
Gallstone 157, 158, 552
    diagnose 552
    ileus 230
    large 564
    multiple 158
    pancreatitis, severe acute *564*
Gamma-glutamyl transferase 530
Gastrectomy
    during 285
    extended total 609
    proximal 598
    total 598, 599, 601, 602
Gastric band 592
Gastric cancer 595, 597, 599, 601, 603
    classification of 598
Gastric conduit 613
    necrosis 611
Gastric contents, control reflux of 654

Gastric emptying, delayed 613
    incidence of 613
Gastric injury 274
Gastric lymphoma 615
Gastric mobilisation 646
Gastric protection 349
Gastric tip necrosis, potential increased risk of 610
Gastric vein, left 600
Gastric volvulus 648, 649
    anatomical
        classification of 648
        representation of 649
    surgical repair of 649
Gastritis 157
Gastrocolic
    omentum 613
    trunk vessels 600
Gastroduodenal artery 170, 564
Gastroepiploic vessels, left 600
Gastrografin 644
Gastrointestinal bleed, massive 236, 237
Gastrointestinal cancer, lower 432
Gastrointestinal stromal tumour 615-617
    malignant 615
    surgery, surgical principles of 617
Gastrointestinal tracts 134
Gastro-oesophageal
    reflux disease 607, 619, 621, 623
    regurgitation 625
General surgery 243
Genes tested 465
Genetic mutations, specific 375
Gillick competent 283
Gillick test 284
Gland disease, multiple 475
Glandular density 380
Glandular origin, epithelial tissue of 429
Glasgow coma scale 25
Glomerular disease 90
Glucocorticoids 460, 473
Glucose 64
    production 64
Glycerine suppositories 443
Glycerol 64
Glycolytic pathway, by-product of 49
Goligher's classification system 415
Goodsall's rule 413
Gord and Barrett's oesophagus 631
Graft
    dysfunction 508
    failure 664

kidney 537
pancreatitis 501
thrombosis 664
Graves' disease 481
Groin hernia 248
management of 246
repair 249
Groin lump, acute 228
Groshong catheter 113
Guillain–Barré syndrome 26
Gum, perioperative chewing of 149
Gunshot wounds 168
Gynaecomastia 296, 297, 374
bilateral 374
causes of 297

H

Haematemesis 170, 564
Haematological dysfunction 218
Haematology 289
Haematoma 187, 205, 233, 249
infected 204
Haemodialysis 92, 93, 115
Haemodynamic
changes 268, 275
instability 118, 237
status 172, 179
Haemofiltration 115
Haemoglobin
amount of 46
beta chain of 49
concentration 47
Haemolytic uraemic syndrome 90, 537
Haemophilia 80
A 81
B 81
Haemophilus 77
influenzae 583
B 235
vaccinations 285
Haemorrhage 149, 464, 603
evidence of 131
intracranial 175
major 212
protocol, major 236
Haemorrhagic brain injuries, types of 174
Haemorrhagic shock 116
Haemorrhoid 318, 319, 408, 415
artery ligation 415, 416
external 319
grade 3 415
internal 319

management of 318
risk factors for 318
surgery 416
surgical management of 415
Haemostatic dressings 30
Haemothorax 219
Haggitt classification 431
Hair, free of 280
Halo naevus 261
Halothane 60
Hamartoma 429
Hand 551
dominance 531
Hannover classification 138
Harmless acute pancreatitis score 560
Harmonic scalpel 281
Hartmann's pouch 224
Hartmann's procedure 394, 418, 678
Haustral markings, loss of 292
Head injury 173
evidence of 31
Headache 331, 459, 464
Heart
disease, ischaemic 155
failure 464
rate 117
Heartburn 643
Heat loss, mechanisms of 61
Heater probe 170
Heidelberg pouchitis activity score 438
Helicobacter pylori eradication therapy 171
Hemicolectomy
elective right 25
open right 34
Hemithyroidectomy 487
specimen 492
Heparin 81, 82, 270
in coagulation cascade, mechanism of action of 269
reversal 270
Hepatectomy 580
Hepatic ducts, injury to 303
Hepatic dysfunction 218
Hepatic failure 57
Hepatic function 275
Hepatic vein, right *576*
Hepaticojejunostomy 586
Hepatitis
acute alcoholic 71
C 498
virus, donor 498
E virus 496, 499
ischaemic 542

Hepatobiliary dysfunction 277
Hepatocellular carcinoma 573, 574
  sign of 497
Hepatocystic triangle 224, 303
Hepatoma 573
Hepato-pancreato-biliary 568
Hepatopancreatobiliary surgery 549
Hepatopulmonary syndrome 527
Hepatorenal syndrome 71
  types of 72
Hereditary
  colon cancer syndromes 435
  colorectal cancer 434
  nonpolyposis colorectal cancer 435
Hernia 395, 541, 643
  clinical examination of 245
  female groin 245
  incarcerated 228
  management 671
  paraoesophageal 643-645, 647
  parastomal 19, 395
  recurrence 253
  sac
    portion of 643
    reduction of 646
  symptoms 245
  type of 644
Hernial sac
  large 253
  radiological measurement of 259
Hiatal dissection 608
Hiatal hernias 643
  symptomatic 643
Hickman line 113
Hidradenitis suppurativa 320
Hierarchical system 7
High-dependency unit 45, 200
  care 259
High-resolution manometry 622, 637
Hilar cholangiocarcinoma, classification of 579
Hilar mass 578
Hinchey classification 417
Hinchey diverticulitis 417
Hodgkin's disease 285
Hodgkin's lymphoma 266
  staging of 266
Homan's procedure 323
Hormonal treatment 374
Hormone replacement therapy 329
Horner's sign 184
Hospital-acquired pneumonia 76

Human immunodeficiency virus 674
Human leukocyte antigens antibodies 521
Human Tissue Act 520
Human Tissue Authority Guidelines 513
Humidified tracheal gas 49
Hyaluronidase 87
Hydrocoele 308
  operative options for 309
  secondary 308
  types of 308
Hydrogen drives, loss of 305
Hydrophilic portion 86
Hyperacute rejection 536
Hypercalcaemia 546
  causes of 472
  management of 473
  severe 473
Hypercapnia 176, 275
  permissive 176
Hyperchloraemic acidosis, causes of 127
Hypercholesterolaemia 155
Hypercoagulability 268, 269
Hyperkalaemia 69, 92, 535
Hyperparathyroidism 472, 474, 478
  biochemical evidence of 478
  persistent 478
  primary 472, 474, 476
  recurrent 478
  secondary 479
Hyperphosphatemia 69, 479, 535
Hyperplasia 334
Hypertension 119, 155, 200, 520, 669
  leads, portal 71
  portal 71, 528
Hyperthermic intraperitoneal chemotherapy 425
Hyperthyroidism 297
Hypertrophic scar 261
Hypnosis 59
  maintain 59
Hypocalcaemia 479
Hypoglycaemic unawareness 501
Hypokalaemia 113, 149, 570
Hypomagnesaemia 113
Hyponatraemia 122, 570
  causes of 122
  management of 123
  metabolic alkalosis 304
  symptoms of 122
Hypophosphataemia 113
Hypotension, permissive 188

Hypothalamic pituitary adrenal axis 459
Hypothermia 48, 62, 84, 519
  in theatres, prevent 62
  physiological responses to 62
  prevent 62
Hypothesis 18
Hypothetical meta-analyses 10
Hypothyroidism 297
Hypovolaemia 100
Hypoxemia, acute onset with 105
Hypoxia 97
  primary 105

I

Iatrogenic bile leak 138
Ibuprofen 35
Idiopathic seroma, unilateral 340
Idiopathic thrombocytopenic purpura 81, 285
Ileocaecal junction 177
Ileocolic intussusception 151, 153
  diagnosis of 152
Ileostomy, defunctioning 404
Ileus
  causes of postoperative 149
  postoperative 148
  prolonged 112, 150
  radiological features of 149
  risk of postoperative 149
Iliac fossa mass, right 226
Imatinib 618
Immobilise C-spine 186
Immune-mediated contracture 339
Immunosuppression 112
  complications of 502
  long-term 545
Immunosuppressive agents
  common induction 506
  common maintenance 505
Implant 353
  based, pros and cons of 353
  donor liver 528
  types of 339
Implant-based reconstruction 338
Incidentaloma 459, 461
Incisional hernia 250, 251, 256-258
  management of 256
  massive 258
  risk of 250
Induction agents 503
Induction therapy 503

Infarcted descending 202
Infarction 334
Infected liquid, drainage of 315
Infection 52, 112, 149, 276, 308, 664
  primary source of 98
Inflammatory bowel disease 291, 392
Inflammatory breast cancer 352, 367, 376, 377, 379, 381
Inflammatory conditions 334
Infrahyoid muscle 183
Infra-pyloric lymphadenectomy 600
Inguinal approach 310
Inguinal hernia 245, 310
  repair, consent for 248
  strangulation for 248
Inguinal ligament 246
Inguinoscrotal hernia 308
Injury
  patterns of 185
  serious 181
Inotropes 52, 67, 68
Inspired oxygen, fraction of 27, 28
Insulin levels, suppressed 65
Integrated relaxation pressure 640
Intensive care unit 278
Intensive therapy units 423
Intention-to-treat analysis 19
Intercostal blood vessel 220
Intercostal chest drains
  apical 654
  basal 654
Intercostobrachial nerve 365
Intersphincteric fistula tract procedure 413
Intersphincteric tract, ligation of 449
Interstitial fibrosis 508
Interstitial oedematous pancreatitis, acute 563
Intestinal failure 526
Intestinal transplant 523, 526
Intestine, segment of 525
Intoxication 519
Intra-abdominal adhesion formation 275
Intra-abdominal hypertension 109, 165
Intra-abdominal lesions 149
Intra-abdominal malignancies 265
Intra-abdominal pressure 109, 110, 165
Intra-abdominal sepsis 201, 501
Intracellular toxins, subsequent release of 69
Intracranial pressure 32
Intractable bleeding 194
Intra-ductal epithelial proliferation, atypical 342

Intra-ductal papillary mucinous neoplasm 581-583
Intraoperative haemostasis, methods of 281
Intraperitoneal techniques, types of 394
Intravenous
    drug 673
        user 673, 674
    fluids 127
    hydrocortisone 361
Intussusception 151
    cause of 154
    types of 152
Invasive ductal carcinoma 378
Iron-deficiency anaemia 432
Ischaemia 242
Ischaemic bowel 230, 241
    concerning for 241
Isoflurane 60

J

Jackhammer oesophagus 640
Japanese severity score 560
Jaundice 566, 571, 578
    duration of 551
Jehovah's witness 286
Jejunal interposition after total gastrectomy 602
Jugular vein, internal 51
Juxta-hepatic venous injury 132

K

Kaffes stent 530
Kaplan–Meier curves 10
Kaplan–Meier survival curves *11*
Kehr T tube 139
Keloid 261
Ketamine 59
Kidney 534, 540
    biopsy 508, 509
    disease 479
    graft, marginal 515
    physiology in 305
    transplant 500
        service 534
        type of 539
    transplantation 514
        pre-emptive 535
Klebsiella 77
Kolmogorov–Smirnov test 21
Kudo pit pattern 429

L

Laceration 187
Lactate 97
    adenomas 334
    dehydrogenase 69
        normal 263
Lacunar ligament 191, 246
Laparoscopic access 274
Laparoscopic adhesiolysis, role for 402
Laparoscopic appendectomy 206
Laparoscopic approach 402
Laparoscopic cholecystectomy 137, 159, 289, 302, 552
    acute 555
Laparoscopic distal pancreatectomy 583
Laparoscopic donor nephrectomy 540
Laparoscopic Heller's cardiomyotomy 639
Laparoscopic Heller's myotomy 640
Laparoscopic injuries 134
Laparoscopic lavage 418
Laparoscopic Nissen fundoplication 626
Laparoscopic paraoesophageal hernia repair 645
Laparoscopic peritoneal lavage 418
Laparoscopic repair 249, 253, 255, 645
Laparoscopic right hemicolectomy 80
Laparoscopic rives 257
Laparoscopic splenectomy 286
Laparoscopic surgery 149, 250, 274
    complications of 134
    generic complications of 134
    hostile abdomen for 275
Laparoscopic techniques 629
Laparoscopic *vs.* open repair 253, 255
Laparoscopy 138, 274, 606
    staging 595
Laparotomy 166, 525
    difficult 165
    lower midline 258
    steps of 213
Laryngeal entry point 488
Laryngeal nerve, right recurrent 609
Lasofoxifene 350
Latissimus dorsi resurfacing 378
Laurén classification 596
L-bupivacaine 87
Lead time bias 356
Learning difficulties, severe 283
Left breast
    malodorous large lesion 378
    nodularity 373

Index

Left thoracoabdominal
  approach 609
  oesophagectomy 609
Leiomyoma 615
Leiomyosarcoma 615
Lesions, classification of 424
Lesser curve tumour 598
Letrozole 331, 350
Leucopenia 331
Lidocaine 86, 87
  infusions 149
Lifestyle factors 320
Lifestyle measures 622
Ligament of berry 488
Ligatures 281
Limb
  ischaemia, acute 155
  ischaemic 677, 678
  loss 664
Lipolysis 64
Liposuction 297
Live donor blood pressure 539
Liver
  abscess formation 589
  cirrhosis 297
  damage, wide spectrum of 591
  first surgery 575
  function suppression 62
  function tests 112, 373, 554
  metastases 575
Liver disease
  advanced chronic 71
  intestinal failure with 526
  score, model for end-stage 543
  severity of alcoholic 571
  stigmata of 373
Liver failure 82, 589
  causes of acute 542
  chronic 527, 541
  transplantation for 542
Liver transplant
  curative treatment 72
  indications for 527
  super urgent 528
Liver transplantation 514, 527, 528, 541-543
  contraindications for 543
  Milan criteria for 543
Liver trauma 212, 213, 587
  classification of 588
  complications of 589
  management of 213

Living donor
  kidney 536
  liver transplant 573
  renal transplantation assessment 538
  transplant 522
Living kidney donor 539
Living over deceased donation, advantage of 539
Lobar collapse 105
Local anaesthetic 86
  agent 86
  types of 86
  block action potential 87
  toxicity
    signs of 88
    symptoms of 88
Lockwood infrainguinal approach 229
Loco-regional disease 617
Loop of Henle 70
Lord's procedure 309
Lotheissen transinguinal approach 229
Low-molecular-weight heparin 40, 269
Lump, biopsy of 335
Lung
  collapse 105
  function tests 55
  function, assess 55
  tissue formation 106
Lung injury
  causes of direct 106
  diffuse 105
  direct 106
  transfusion-related acute 106
Luteinizing hormone 374
Lyapunov stability reducing tremor 452
Lymph node 263, 490
  appearing 335
  in axilla 367
  locoregional 371
  metastases 492
  multiple abnormal 377
  reactive 300, 301
Lymphadenectomy 598, 599, 608
  station dissection and excision 599
Lymphadenopathy 228, 265
Lymphatic vessels, subdermal plexus of 361
Lymphocyte
  depleted 267
  rich 266
Lymphoedema 322, 365
  rarely occurs 364
  systems for 323

Index

Lymphoscintigram 364
Lymphoscintigraphy 322
Lymphovenous anastomosis 323

M

Mackler's triad 160
Macrophage migration inhibitory factor 98
Magnesium oxide 149
Magnetic resonance
  cholangiopancreatography 552
Major trauma centre 42
Malaria 496
Male breast cancer 346, 375
  incidence of 375
  risk of 375
Malignancy 226, 230, 585
  high incidence of 153
Mammograms, bilateral 372
Mammography 352, 358
Manchester score 344
Mannitol 70, 176
Mann–Whitney U test 13, 22
Manometry 442
  studies 637, 644
Marshall's hypertonic citrate 516
Massive blood
  loss 125
  transfusion 126
Mastectomy 352
  indications for 352
  risk-reducing 352
Mastitis 327, 328
  lactational 328
McEvedy suprainguinal approach 228
Meckel's diverticulum 237, 287, 288
Medical management 613, 622, 633
Medical therapy 624, 638
  failure of 420
Medical treatment, evidence for 626
Medullary thyroid carcinoma 492
Megaoesophagus 636
Melanoma 260-262
  in situ 262
  malignant 260
  occur, types of 261
Membrane, layers of 33
Membranoproliferative glomerulonephritis 537
Meninges 33
Meningococcal 285
Meningococcus 235

Mental Capacity Act 38
Mental capacity, altered 37, 39
Mental health 294
Mepivacaine 87
Mesenteric artery, superior 241, 512, 564, 569
Mesenteric catheter angiogram 237
Mesenteric vein, superior 569
Mesenteroaxial volvulus 649
Mesh
  infection 249
  insertion, technique of 19
  repair 257
Metabolic abnormality 540
Metabolic acidosis 92
  respiratory compensation for 95
Metabolic complications 277
Metabolic picture 97
Metabolic rate 64
Metabolic risks 112
Metal implants 280
Metallic taste 88
Metaplastic replacement 631
Metastasectomy 404
Metastasis 461
  distant 263, 491
Metastatic colorectal cancer, advanced 576
Metastatic disease 617
  absence of 597
Metastatic lymph node 300, 301
Methotrexate 321, 336
Metoclopramide 149, 613
Microcirculatory changes 98
Micrometastasis 332
Micro-polyurethane 340
Microsatellite instability pathway 435
Midazolam 57
Mid-rectal cancer 405
Milan criteria 574
Milrinone 68
Minimal abdominal distension 152
Minimally invasive
  oesophagectomy 608
  parathyroidectomy 474
Mitochondria 49
Mitomycin 410
Mitotane 462
Mobilisation 73
Mobilise pedicle 383
Monoclonal antibodies 522
Monoclonal protein 546
Monopolar diathermy, use of 280
Monro–Kellie doctrine 176

Index

Montreal classification 448, 619
Morbidity, enumeration of 55
Morphine 36, 60
Mortality 249
    enumeration of 55
    estimate of operative 135
    scoring 38
mTOR inhibitors 350
Mucinous cystic neoplasm 581
Multi-channel intra-luminal impedance 622
Multidisciplinary team
    discussion 259
    meeting 662, 678
Multinodular goitre 486
Multiorgan failure 464
Mural thrombus 156
Muscle 183
    breakdown, direct consequence of 70
    layer, myotomy of 639
    relaxants 59, 60, 362
Mycophenolate mofetil 503
MYH polyposis 436
Myocardial
    depression 57
    infarction 31, 40, 241, 464
    suppression 666
Myoglobin 70
Myosin light chain, dephosphorylation of 638
Myotomy extending up oesophagus 639

N

Nagano classification 589
Nail varnish 46
Naproxen 35
Nasal cannulae oxygen 95
Nasogastric
    decompression 649
    feeding tube 488
    suctioning 128
    tube 113, 148, 152, 525, 651
Nasojejunal tube 113
National Audit of Breast Cancer in Older Patients 332
National Audit of Small Bowel Obstruction 231, 402
National Emergency Laparotomy Audit 37, 152, 231
National Health Service 294, 338
National Institute for Health and Care Excellence 312, 330, 675
    guidelines 377

National Institute of Clinical Excellence Guidelines 246, 621
Nausea 504
    persistent 504
Neck
    anterior triangle of 183, 300
    injury 181
    left side of 181, 610
    lumps 299
    midline of 299
    posterior triangle of 183, 301
    swelling 481
    trauma 181, 182
    triangles of 183
    veins, distended 107
Necrotic collection, acute 562, *564*
Necrotic gallbladder 223
Necrotic patches, multiple 224
Necrotic terminal ileum 242
Needle cricothyroidotomy 78
Negative nitrogen balance 65
Negative predictive value 3, 15
Negative pressure wound therapy 674
Neisseria meningitidis 583
Neoadjuvant chemotherapy 367, 569, 577
    indications for 367
Neonatal intensive care unit support 197
Neoplasia 637
Nephrotic syndrome 90
Nerves 183
Neural monitoring, intraoperative 487
Neuralgia 360
Neuroendocrine tumours 424
Neuroleptic drugs 149
Neurological criteria 83, 85
Neurological dysfunction 218
Neuromuscular blocking agents 519
Neuromuscular junction 60
Neurone
    cell membrane of 86
    nerve sheath of 87
Neuropathic pain 35
Neuropraxia 365
Neurotrauma 30
New organ failure, developing 109
Nicotine-stained fingers 46
Nifedipine 638
Nipple
    discharge 341
        pathological 341
    soreness 328

Index

Nissen fundoplication 627, 628
Nitrates inhibit 638
Nodal status 409
Nodular sclerosing 266
Non-accidental injury, sign of 180
Non-lactational mastitis 328
Non-local causes 286
Non-parametric statistical tests 13, **13**
Non-radical lymphadenectomy 611
Non-ST elevation myocardial infarction 41
Non-steroidal anti-inflammatory drugs 35, 81, 170, 328
Noradrenaline 68, 72
    endogenous precursor of 68
Noradrenergic tissue 464
Normothermic machine perfusion 517
Norovirus 291
Nosocomial pneumonia 76
Null hypothesis 3, 18
Numbness 249
Nutcracker oesophagus 640
    surgical management for 640
Nutrition 112, 276

O

Obesity 87, 318, 520, 533, 669
Obstructed defecation syndrome 442
    treatment of 443
Obstructing colon cancer 387
Obstructive defecation 441
Obstructive jaundice 551, 567
    cause of 567
    symptoms of 551
Obstructive uropathy 91
Odynophagia 182, 652
Oesophageal anatomy, normal 620
Oesophageal cancer 605, 607, 609, 611, 613
    risk factors for 607
    staging 606
Oesophageal diversion, proximal 654
Oesophageal dysmotility 636, 637, 639, 641
Oesophageal impedance monitoring 622
Oesophageal injury 182
Oesophageal length, assessment of 646
Oesophageal manometry 622
Oesophageal perforation 160, 651, 653, 655
    causes of 161
Oesophageal resection 654
Oesophageal sphincter, lower 620
Oesophagectomy 118, 611, 640
    complications of 611
    three-phase 610
    two-phase 611
Oesophago-cutaneous fistula, controlled 654
Oesophagogastric junction 160, 644
Oesophagogastric surgery 55, 593
Oesophagogastro duodenoscopy, diagnostic 605
Oesophagogastroduodenoscopy 621, 634, 636, 644
Oesophagus 177, 178, 620
    abdominal 620
    Barrett's disease of 631
    lower 160
    mobilisation of 639
Ogilvie syndrome 198
Omental injury 275
Omeprazole 626
Omohyoid 183
Omphalomesenteric duct 287
Oncoplastic
    breast reconstruction 352
    surgery 380
    techniques 380
Onlay mesh augmentation 257
Open surgical repair 668
    techniques of 249
Open technique 274
Operating theatre 61
Operation, relevant risks of 282
Operative strategy 654
Operative technique 259
Opiates 87
Opioids 362
    use of 149
Optical access technique 274
Optimal bone health, management of 332
Optimization, principle of 56
Oral anticoagulant, direct 82, 659, 660
Oral contraceptive
    pill 321, 329
    use of 371
Oral vancomycin, use of 163
Orchitis 308
Organ 517
    and tissue involvement 98
    donation 83, 540
        specialist nurse for 496
        types of 83
    dysfunction 97
    failure persists 111
    pancreas transplantation 501
    preservation 515

Index

retrieval 511
space 314
Osmotherapy 33
Osteoclast function 473
Osteoporosis 331
  presence of 479
Ovarian analysis 345
Ovarian cancer 346
Ovarian malignancy 367
Overwhelming postsplenectomy 285
  infection 286
Oxygen 57
  carried in blood 47
  cascade 49
  consumption 64
  delivery 47
    devices 27, 28
  dissociation curve 48
  flow 27, 28
  masks 27
  percentage saturation of 46
  saturation 47
    monitoring of 57
  therapy, long-term 38
Oxygenation 30

P

Pacemaker 280
Paediatric end-stage kidney disease, cause of 534
Paediatric kidney
  transplant, contraindications for 535
  transplantation 534
Paediatric pyloric stenosis, epidemiology of 305
Paediatric transplant recipient 536
Paediatric trauma 179
Paget–Schroetter disease 322
Pain 665
  abdominal 217, 432, 661
  absence of 551
  chronic 249
  pathways, descending 35
  via stimulation, modulation of 35
Palliative chemotherapy 405
Palliative mastectomy 378
Pallor 665
Palmer's point 274
Palpitations, cause of 481
Pancreas
  acute inflammatory process of 560
  carcinoma, head of 567
  classify cystic neoplasms of 581
  cystic neoplasm of 581
  head and tail of *563*
  implantation, preventing safe 501
  mass, head of 569
  mucinous cystic neoplasm of 582
  pseudocyst of 562
  thrombosis 501
  transplantation 502, 514
    indications for 500
    potential complications of 501
  tumour, head of 585
Pancreatic cancer 346
  infiltrating 637
Pancreatic duct, main 583
Pancreatic fistula 128, 603
Pancreatic leak 286
Pancreatic necrosis 562
Pancreatic oedema 131
Pancreatic parenchyma 131
Pancreatic pseudocyst *563*
Pancreaticoduodenal artery
  inferior 564
  superior 564
Pancreaticoduodenal complex injury 132
Pancreatitis 22
  acute 157, 158, 559
  causes of 559
  common causes of 157
  CT evidence of 157
  diagnosis of acute 157
  mild 560
    acute 560
  severe acute 560, 562, 564
Panproctocolectomy 435
Papillary thyroid carcinoma 490
Paracetamol 35, 328, 542
Paraesthesia 665
Paralysis 665
Paralytic ileus 198
Parametric data, used for 22
Parametric statistical tests 13, **13**
Parametric tests 12
Paraphimosis 143
Parathyroid 472
  glands, constant stimulation of 479
  surgery 489
  tissue 476
Parathyroidectomy 476
Parenchymal fractures 588
Paris classification 429
Parkland formula 43
Parotid lesion 300
Patent airway, maintenance of 30, 42

Pathogen stimulates host defence cells 98
Patient's fluid status 52
Pectineal ligament 246
Pelvic
　　dyssynergy 441
　　floor surgery 397
　　fracture 131
　　prolapse 441
Pelvis 595
Penetrate platysma 181
Penetrating injuries 181
Penetrating mortality 590
Penetrating platysma 181
　　significance of 181
Penicillin V 285
Peptic oesophageal strictures, treatment of 625
Peptic stricture 636
Percutaneous coronary intervention, primary 41
Percutaneous drain 302
Percutaneous endoscopy gastrostomy tube 488
Percutaneous ethanol injection 573
Percutaneous transhepatic
　　biliary drainage 567
　　cholangiography 530
Perianal Crohn's disease 448, 449
Perianal sepsis 239, 411
Perianal skin and scrotum 240
Perianal surgery 397
Pericarditis 92
Pericholecystic fluid 554
Perihilar cholangiocarcinoma 580
Perineal procedures 398
Perineum 240
Periorbital tingling 88
Peri-pancreatic collection 501
　　large 563
Peripheral arterial
　　catheter 53
　　disease 669, 672, 677
Peritoneal dialysis 523
　　catheter 523
　　types of 523
Peritonitis 100
　　complicated 104
Per-oral endoscopic myotomy 639
　　development of 638
Persistent hyperparathyroidism, biochemical diagnosis of 478
Petechiae 81
Pethidine 57

Peutz–Jeghers syndrome 436
Phaeo crisis 464
Phaeochromocytoma 464
　　classical presentation of 464
　　planning surgery for 465
　　unilateral 465
Pharyngeal pouch 301
Pharynx, inferior constrictor of 488
Phimosis 143
Phosphate 69
　　buffer system 516
Phreno-oesophageal ligament 627, 639
Phyllodes tumour 372
　　malignant 372
PIK3CA inhibitors 350
Pilonidal disease 446
　　management 446
　　procedures 447
　　risk factors for 446
Pilonidal sinus, chronic 446
Pituitary adenoma 467
Plain erect chest radiograph 652
Plasmapheresis 522
Platelet
　　activating factor 98
　　consumption, increased 81
　　dysfunction 81
　　longevity, decreased 81
　　production, decreased 81
Pleural effusion 652
Plicamycin 473
Pneumatic dilatation 638, 639
Pneumaturia 455
Pneumococcal 285
Pneumococcus 235
Pneumonia 26, 73
　　diagnosis of 74
Pneumoperitoneum 645
Pneumothorax 100, 107, 112, 221, 652
　　radiological assessment of 141
Poikilothermia 665
Polycystic liver disease 527
Polyp 430
　　cancers, classification systems for 430
　　screening 428
　　surveillance, guidelines for 430
Polypropylene mesh 18
Popliteal aneurysm 667
　　differential diagnoses 667
　　management of 668
Porcelain gallbladder 556
Port placement 645

Post-adrenal vein ligation 465
Post-endoscopic retrograde
    cholangiopancreatography perforation 167
Post-hemithyroidectomy 491
Post-liver transplantation 545
Postneoadjuvant stage groups 595
Post-pancreatitis 137
Post-splenectomy 235
    management 285
Post-thrombotic limb syndrome 659
Post-transplant lymphoproliferative disorder
    545, 546
    pathogenesis of 545
    signs of 546
    symptoms of 546
    treatment for 547
    types of 546
Potassium 69, 113
Pouch failure 437
Pouchitis 437, 438
    disease activity index 438
P-POSSUM score 55
Prague classification 631, 632
Prednisolone 506
Pre-emptive recipient hepatectomy 528
Pre-emptive transplants, contraindications of
    535
Pregnancy 206, 318
    safe in 206
Prehabilitation programmes 250
Prehn's sign 147
    positive 146
Pressure
    support ventilation 29
    transducer and tubing 110
Pre-transplant evaluation 536
Prilocaine 86, 87
Priori hypotheses 1
Prisma 16
Procaine 86
Proctogram, defecating 442
Profunda femoral artery distal 673
Proinflammatory mediators 98
Prophylactic mesh 250
Prophylactic reinforcing mesh, use of 18
Propofol 59, 89
Prostaglandin
    inhibition of 35
    synthesis, inhibition of 35
Prostate
    enlarged 144
    specific antigen 272
Prostatic hyperplasia 143

Prosthetic material 314
Protamine sulphate 270
Protein 65
    production of acute phase 64
Proteus mirabilis 328
Prothrombin concentrate complex 289
Prucalopride 149
Pseudo Cushing's 468
Pseudoaneurysm 673
    infected 228
    risk of 670
Pseudogynaecomastia 296
Pseudomembranous colitis 162
Pseudomonas 147
    aeruginosa 77
Pseudomyxoma
    peritonei 424
    tertiary 425
Pseudo-obstruction 198, 199
Psychiatric drugs 297
Ptosis, grade of 380
Pulmonary angiogram, CT 40
Pulmonary embolism 26, 74, 100, 570
    risk of 659
Pulmonary embolus 40
Pulmonary function 275
    testing 259
Pulmonary oedema 92
Pulse oximetry 46
Pulselessness 665
Pupillary reaction 85
Purified protein derivative test 272
P-value 4
Pyloric procedures 613
Pyloric stenosis 304
Pylorus 605
    preserving 598

R
Rabbit anti-thymocyte globulin 506
Racoon' eyes 173
Radial scar 343
Radiation 61
    exposure 375
    proctitis 439
Radical lymphadenectomy 611
Radiofrequency 573
    ablation 440, 634
Radiology 637
Radiotherapy 336, 410, 462
    side effects of 359
Ramstedt's pyloromyotomy 305

Re-bleeding on endoscopy, risk of 170
Receiver operating characteristic
    analysis 20
    curves 11
Recreational drugs 58
Rectal cancer 406
Rectal compliance 442
Rectal intussusception 441
Rectal mass 432
Rectal prolapse 397, 398
Rectal stump 420
Rectocele 441
Recurrent laryngeal nerves 488
    injury, incidence of 489
Recurrent umbilical hernia 252
Red flag signs 84
    presence of 99
Red flag symptoms 415
Reduction mammaplasty 297
Re-feeding syndrome 276
Reflex tachycardia 465
Reflux control, less effective for 629
Reflux with Barrett's disease 625
Reflux with respiratory complications 625
Reflux with stricture formation 625
Regional lymph nodes 261
Regional wall motion abnormality 41
Regression
    analysis 11
    multiple 11
    types of 11
Regurgitation 643
Remifentanil 60
Remnant radio iodine ablation therapy 491
Renal dysfunction 218
Renal failure 69, 297, 666
    complex 479
    development of 71
    end-stage 501
    history of 500
Renal function 69, 275
    indicates 515
    suppression 62
Renal hyperparathyroidism 479
Renal impairment 664
Renal perfusion, reduced 71
Renal replacement therapy 114
    acute 115
    methods of 92
    types of 115

Renal transplant biopsy, Banff classification of 509
Renal transplantation 495
Renal trauma 186
    classify 186
    complications of 187
    manage 187
Renal vasoconstriction 71
Renin converts angiotensinogen 63
Renin-angiotensin
    aldosterone system 63
    system, activation of 71
Reperfusion injury 666
Resistant ventricular arrhythmias 88
Respiratory assessment tools 597
Respiratory complications, postoperative 73
Respiratory compromise 181
Respiratory depression 57, 58
    potential for 57
Respiratory distress 181
Respiratory dysfunction 218
Respiratory failure 25, 28, 105
    causes of 26
    treatment of 26, 27
    types of 26
Respiratory illness, chronic 58
Respiratory pattern 25
Respiratory problems 249, 253
Respiratory support 28
    advanced 28
Retinopathy 500
Retro-areolar area 342
Retroperitoneal duodenal perforation 167
Retroperitoneal lesions 149
Retroperitoneal perforations 167
Retrosternal goitres 487
Rhabdomyolysis 69
    diagnosis of 69
Ribs, osteonecrosis of 360
RIFLE, limitations of 91
Rituximab 547
Rivaroxaban 289
Road traffic collision, low speed 31
Roberts clip 108
Robotic colorectal surgery 450
Robotic surgery, advantages of 452
Rocuronium 60
Rooftop incision 654
Ropivacaine 86, 87
Roux-en-Y reconstruction after subtotal
    gastrectomy 601

Rubber band ligation 415, 416
Rule of Nines 43
Rupture
　abdominal aortic aneurysm 188
　signs of 661
　spontaneous 285
　traumatic 285
Rutherford-Morrison incision 673

S

Sac, contents of 253
Saline 339
Salmonella 226, 291
Scalpel 108
Scandinavian quality register reports 489
Scapula, winging of 365
Scar tissue, areas of 280
Scarring around implant 339
Sclerosing peritonitis 525
Scrotum 240
　relieves pain 146
Sedation 57
　high risk for 58
Sedative drugs 519
Sedative medications, common 57
Seek urgent advice 118
Seizures, control 89
Selection bias 356
Selective oestrogen receptor modulators 331
Sensitivity 3, 14, 21
Sentinel lymph node biopsy 261
Sentinel node
　biopsy 330
　identification of 361
　localization, types of 363
Sepsis 81, 95, 97, 98, 240, 276, 542, 678
　circulatory support in 68
　pathophysiology of 98
　rapid diagnosis of 99
　risk of developing overwhelming 235
　signs of 209, 239, 327, 387, 654
　source of 99
　treatment of 99
Septic shock 68, 98
Serology 541
Seroma 249, 664
　formation 253
Serous cystic neoplasm 581
Serrated adenoma 429
Serrated polyp 429

Serrated polyposis syndrome 436
Serum 546
　amino acids 65
　calcium 483
　creatinine 91
　dehydroepiandrosterone 460
　investigations 551
　lactate dehydrogenase, elevated level of 546
　magnesium 84
　phosphate 84
　potassium 84
　sodium 84
Sessile
　polyps 431
　serrated 429
Sevoflurane 60
Shigella 291
Shock 67, 116, 654
　life-threatening causes of 117
　presence of 107
　stage of 116
　type of 116
Short bowel syndrome 112
Shotgun wound 169
Shoulder stiffness, risk of 365
Shunt, physiological 102
Siewert grading 605
Sigmoid colectomy 418
Sigmoid colon 202
Sigmoid volvulus 198
Sigmoidoscopy 434
　flexible 318, 319
Silicone 339
　gel, microscopic diffusion of 339
Silk sutures 108
Sirolimus 506
Sistrunk procedure 300
Skeletal muscle, breakdown of 69
Skin
　lesion 260
　prick testing 361
Sliding inguinal hernias 643
Small bites suture technique 251
Small bowel
　injury 274
　obstruction 230, 258, 387, 401
　rest of 242
Small gallstones 158
Small periampullary tumour 584
Society of Emergency Surgeons 400

Index

Sodium 63
   low 122
   plasma concentration of 122
Soft signs, presence of 185
Somatostatin analogues 72
Sphincters
   external 427
   internal 427
Spigelian fascia 254
Spigelian hernia 226, 254
Spinal anaesthesia 87
Spinal regional anaesthetic technique 34
Spinal space 34
Spirometry 55
Spironolactone 297
Splanchnic vasodilation 71
   effects of 71
Splanchnic vasopressors 72
Splenectomy 285
   indications for 285
Splenic artery 564
Splenic injury, grade of 234
Splenic trauma 233
Splenic vein 131
Split kidney functions 539
Spontaneous oesophageal perforation 655
Sputum 99
Squamous intraepithelial lesion, high-grade 408
Standard chemotherapy agents 405
Staphylococcus
   aureus 77, 328
   epidermidis 328
Starling's law of heart 67
Stasis 268
Statistical error, types of 15
Statistical hypothesis testing 272
Statistical power 18
Statistical tests 12
Steal syndrome 533
   risk factors of 533
Stenosis, high-grade 671
Stereotactic core biopsy 359
Sterilisation 312
   methods of 313
Sternoclavicular joint 107
Sternocleidomastoid 181
Sternotomy, unplanned 487
Steroids 84, 157
Stewart–Way classification 138
Stoma 394
   diversion 413
   formation 250
   relocation of 396
   site, closure of 396
Stomach 305, 605, 609
   abdominal mobilisation of 608
   distal 563
   inferior retraction of 600
Stone weight loss 258
Strasberg classification 138
Stratified squamous epithelium 631
Streptococcus pneumoniae 583
Stress
   echocardiogram 597
   response to surgery 63
Stridor 181
Stroke, ischaemic 278
Stromal atypia 343
Sub-arachnoidal bleeding 278
Subclavian vein 51
Subcutaneous
   emphysema 652
   injection 87
   mastectomy 297
Subdural haematoma 174
Sub-glandular implant placement 339
Sub-group analysis 15
Submandibular gland 300
Subtotal colectomy 165, 193, 292
Subtotal gastrectomy 599, 602
Subtotal parathyroidectomy 480
Succinyl chlorine 362
Sunken fontanell 304
Superheated air, inhalational injury of 42
Superior mesenteric artery embolectomy 242
Supplemental oxygen 241
Supraclavicular node, left 265
Suprahyoid muscle 183
Supraorbital pressure 85
Suprascapular artery 183
Surgery, complications of major 502
Surgical clip application 281
Surgical complications, classification of 278
Surgical management, urgency of 673
Surgical options 480, 640
Surgical procedures 599
Surgical pulmonary embolectomy 102
Surgical renal transplant assessment clinic 520
Surgical site infection 253, 314, 664
   types of 314
Surgical technique 627
Surgical treatment, evidence for 626
Suxamethonium 60
Swelling, reduce 308

Synchronised intermittent mandatory
   ventilation 29
Systemic chemotherapy, role of 617
Systemic inflammation 217
Systemic inflammatory response
      early signs of 208
      syndrome 651, 557
Systemic thrombolysis 102

T

Tacrolimus 529, 530
Tamm–Horsfall protein 70
Tamoxifen 331, 336, 374
T-cell immune response 339
Technetium-99m pertechnetate scintigraphy
   288
Tenderness 661
Tenecteplase 102
Tension pneumothorax 107, 108, 181, 221
Tertiary oesophagogastric centre 160
Testicular cancer 308
Testicular complication 249
Testicular pain 146
      acute 283
      severe left-sided 146
Testicular torsion 146
Testicular ultrasound scan 374
Testosterone 373, 374
Thebesian veins 102
Therapeutic mammoplasty 380, 381
      risks of 383
      technique, use of 383
Therapeutic modalities 1
Thermoregulation 61
Thiopentone 60
Thiopurine methyltransferase 505
Thoracic duct 609
      damage to 612
Thoracic nerve 365
Thoracic oesophagus 620
Thoracic phase 608
Thoracodorsal pedicle limiting, injury to 365
Thoracoscopic surgery, video-assisted 487
Thoracotomy 220
      indications of 220
Thrombocytopenia 81, 331
      heparin-induced 124
Thrombosed external haemorrhoid 319
Thrombosis 664, 670
Thyroid 481
      artery, inferior 488
      cancer 300, 490, 491

capsule, condensation of true 488
function tests 373
malignancy, risk of 485
nodule 300
peroxidase, autoantibodies to 481
receptor antibodies 481
status examination 486
surgery and complications 488
swelling 484, 490
Thyroidectomy
   completion 492
   staged total 487
Thyroid-stimulating hormone concentrations
   481
Thyrothymic ligament 476
Thyrotoxicosis 481
Tissue
   cause heating of 280
   debridement of infected 315
   expanders 339
   oxygen delivery to 47
   repair of 65
Tongue, protrusion of 300
Topical formalin therapy 440
Torsion 147
Total parenteral nutrition 52, 276, 525, 526
Total thyroidectomy 482, 487
Totally extraperitoneal technique 255
Toupet style fundoplication, posterior 639
Toupet vs. Nissen fundoplication 629
Tourniquet test 531
Toxic megacolon 162, 192-194, 420
Toxin producing 162
Tracheostomy 78, 79
   insertion, complications of 79
Tramadol 36
Tranexamic acid 286, 587
Transabdominal repair 645
Transabdominal ultrasound 551
Transarterial chemoembolisation 573
Transhiatal mobilisation 627
Transhiatal oesophagectomy 610
Transient ischaemic attack 155, 500, 671
Transillumination 308
Transjugular intrahepatic portosystemic shunt
   72
Transmural ulceration 178
Transplant surgery 493
   immunosuppression for 503, 505, 507
Transplantation
   Bench prepare kidney for 516
   contraindications to 527
Transthoracic echocardiography 597

Transvaginal ultrasound 391
Transversus abdominis release 256
Trastuzumab 336
Trauma
    history of 348
    massive 54
Triglycerides 64
Triple assessment, steps of 376
Trocar injuries 134
Troisier's sign 265
Truelove and Witts criteria 194, 419
Trypanosoma cruzi 496, 636
T-tube repair 654
Tubercle of Zuckerkandl 488
Tubular atrophy 508
Tubular necrosis, ischaemic acute 536
Tumour
    benign 429
    location 380
    profiling tools 331
    size of primary 568
Tyrer–Cuzick model 345

U

Ulcer and necrosis, circumferential 178
Ulceration 432
Ulcerative colitis 419, 423
Unconsciousness 59
Undergoing emergency cholecystectomy 22
Undescended testis 310
Unkempt gentleman 239
Unstable angina 41
    conditions of 41
Upper gastrointestinal bleeds 171
Uraemia, complications of 92
Uraemic symptoms 535
Urea 148, 554
Ureteric stenosis 504
Urethral catheterisation 143, 653
Urethral stricture 143
Urgent trauma laparotomy 197
Urinalysis 495
Urinary catheter 236
    blocked 91
Urinary incontinence, episodes of 348
Urinary infection 286
Urinary retention 143, 249
    acute 144
    causes of 143
    indicative of chronic 144

Urinary steroid analysis, role of 469
Urinary tract 534
    infections 455
Urine 546
    alkalinisation of 70
    output
        measure 99
        reduced 63
Urolithiasis 143
Urology team 144
Urosepsis 201

V

Vaccinations 285
Vacuum-assisted
    closure 111
    excision 341
Vagus nerve, hepatic branch of anterior 627
Vaizey score 442
van Nuy's score 359
Vancomycin 163
Vancomycin-resistant enterococci,
    development of 163
Variant syndromes 527
Varicose veins 675
Vas injury 249
Vascular complication 504
Vascular injury 134, 275
Vascular surgery 55, 657
Vascularised lymph node flap transfer 323
Vasopressin 68
Vasopressors 52, 67
Vein 183
    diameter 532
Vena cava
    inferior 517
    venting of 512
Venous blood 49
    venting of 512
Venous duplex scan 659
Venous stasis 275
Venous thromboembolism 249, 268
    prophylaxis 259
    risk factors for 660
Venous thrombosis 322
Ventilation
    invasive 29
    non-invasive 28
Ventilator-associated pneumonia 76
    pathophysiology of 76

Veress needle 274
Vessel 183
    thrombosis of 52
Vestibulo-ocular reflex 85
Virchow's node 265
Virchow's triad 268
Virgin abdomen 152
Virology 508
Virus 496
Visceral perforation 286
Viscus, perforation of 104
Visible gastric peristalsis 304
Vital signs, monitoring 666
Vitamin
    D deficiency 479
    E supplements 440
    K 82, 289
        deficiency 82
Vitelline 287
Vomiting 304
    severe 112
von Hippel-Lindau disease 465
von Willebrand disease 81
Vulvar intraepithelial neoplasia 410

W
Walled-off necrosis *563*
Warfarin 82

Warm ischaemia 518
Weight gain 65
Weight loss 64, 432
Weight reduction 256, 259
Well's criteria 74
Well's score 74
Wexner score 442
Wilcoxon's matched pairs test 13
Wilson's disease 542
Withdraw tacrolimus 509
Worsening pain, complains of 209
Worsening renal vasoconstriction 71
Wound
    infection 249, 286, 482
    manager 242
Wrist fistula 532

X
X-linked recessive disorder 81

Y
Y-drainage tube, internal 139
Yellow card scheme 362
Yersinia 226

Z
Zona glomerulosa secretes 459